THE ILLUSTRATED CHINESE MATERIA MEDICA

THE ILLUSTRATED CHINESE MATERIA MEDICA

Crude and prepared

by

Kun-Ying Yen, Ph. D.
Professor of Taipei Medical College

translated by

Nigel Wiseman

238 Color Photographs

SMC PUBLISHING INC.

Taipei

SMC PUBLISHING INC.
P.O. Box. 13-342, Taipei 107
Taiwan, Republic of China
Tel (886-2) 2362-0190
Fax (886-2) 2362-3834

© 1992 by SMC Publishing Inc.
Second printed, 1997.

ISBN 957-638-076-6
LCCN 91-67121

Printed in Taiwan, R.O.C.

Contents

VII. FRUCTUS (Fruits) 119–158　　　　　　　　　果實類

Preface

Over recent years, Chinese medicine has become a new focus of world attention not only because it has made new advances through the application of modern research methods but no less importantly because of growing concern about the increasing health risks attached to the synthetic drugs used by Western medicine. New interest in an ancient healing art among both providers and consumers of health care is evidenced by its insertion into health private and public health insurance schemes in both the East and the West.

Chinese medicine takes a different approach to treating disease from that of Western medicine. It treats illnesses by devising formulae that addresses disease patterns. Formula science is founded on the principle of "determining what treatment is necessary by the pattern identified." Proficiency in devising or selecting the right formula for a given disease pattern is dependent upon on sound knowledge of drugs, and their properties and effects.

The task of matching formula to disease pattern requires a knowledge of the origin, characters, quality, properties, and functions of each agent. Without such knowledge, there can be no hope of providing effective treatment. Crude agents often have to undergo processing before they can be used, so as to make them produce the desire effect. Agents that are cut to a suitable size for decoction, and processed to modify their properties are called 飲片 yin³ pian⁴, literally "drink pieces," a term rendered in this text as decocting pieces.

With a knowledge of the pharmaceutical properties and actions of decocting pieces, it is possible to understand why a formula is suitable for a given pattern, and makes it possible to vary the formula to suit the needs of the patient. If the practitioner is to maximize the positive effects of a formula, he must understand the properties of both the raw materials and the processed agents. Information on both these items is rarely provided in a single volume. This book has been written with the aim of meeting this need. The present volume is intended as a reference for people interested in Chinese medicine, pharmateutical students, pharmacists, and clinical doctors of Chinese medicine. It is written in pharmacognosological style to provide knowledge not only of raw materials but the effect of decocting pieces. Even for concentrated extracts, the individual constituents of the whole prescription have to be understood.

The plates, shot in the brief moments that the busy life of a teacher gives me, provide a useful visual complement to the text, and are invaluable to the beginning student acquainting himself or herself with the Chinese materia medica for the first time. They naturally form the central focus of the book.

I would like to express my thanks to my teacher Koichi Kimura for reading the present text and for his suggestions. I also thank Wei Te-wen of SMC Publishing Inc., and Nigel Wiseman for their active help in completing this book. Not least, thanks also go to Ch'ien Yuan and Sheng Yuan drugstores and to the Sheng-Chang Drug Factory for supplying the materials that appear in the plates.

Kun-Ying Yen
Taipei Medical College
Taipei, Republic of China
October 10, 1992

Introduction

1. This illustrated guide includes full-color plates of the 238 most commonly used drugs in the Chinese pharmacopoeia used in Mainland China, Taiwan, Japan, Korea today.
2. The book is divided into thirteen sections according to part of the plant or animal used: a) Cortices; b) Caules et Ligna; c) Radices d) Rhizomata; e) Folia; f) Flores; g) Fructus; h) Semina; i) Herbae; j) Resinae et Balsami, etc; k) Materia medica animalis; l) Materia medica mineralis; m) Cryptogamae.
3. For each drug the following information is given: its names, origin, characters, production areas, quality, properties and action, indications, and formulas in which it is used.

   Names: The official Latin name (usually composed of a botanical, zoological, or mineralogical name, and the part used); the Chinese name, followed by its pinyin transcription; the vernacular English name; the Japanese phonetic transcription; and commonly used alternate Chinese names.

   Origin: The botanical, zoological, or mineralogical entity or entities from which the drug is derived are preceded by the family to which they belong. An asterisk following a botanical or zoological name indicates that this entity or relevant part thereof, is locally, occasionally, or wrongly used as the drug.

   Characters: Under this heading is a description of the macroscopic characteristics of the drugs, and their decocting pieces (yin^3 $pian^4$).

   Quality: Hints are given under this heading to judge the quality of raw materials.

   Production areas: The country of origin is given, and in the case of Chinese the province or region is specified.

   Properties and actions: Under this heading are listed: the nature (hot, cold, warm, cool, or balanced), the flavor, and toxicity of the agent, the channels which it enters (i.e., acts upon), and the functions of raw and processed drugs.

   Indications: The indications, i.e., the symptoms or diseases that the drug treats, are followed by the daily dosage, contradindications and one or more formulas in which the agent is used, referenced by number to a list of formulae at the back of the book.

   Remarks: Under this heading are allied drug (i.e., interchangeable), similar drugs, similar plants, chemical constituents, and remarks concerning clinical usage.

4. A list of 356 formula commonly used in China, Korea, and Japan, arranged in pinyin order. For each formula, there are ingredients, notes on preparation, functions, indications, and dosages. These are referenced to the items in the drugs section in which they are mentioned.
5. Tables comparing drugs of similar function.
6. Two indexes are provided for the reader's convenience at the end of the book — one in Roman characters, and the other in Chinese.

   Index I is a full list of Latin names, pinyin and Japanese transcription of drugs (and their variants and substitutes), names of botanical, zoological, and mineralogical entities, and English names of formulae. Numbers referring to the drugs section are preceded by the letter D, while those referring to the formulae section are preceded by the letter F.

   Index II is a Chinese listing of drug and formulae names, referenced to the drugs and formulae sections by the letters D and F respectively.

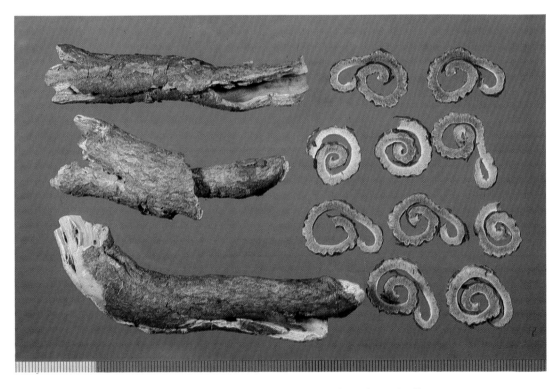

Acanthopanacis Radicis Cortex: crude and cut. (×1)

1   ACANTHOPANACIS RADICIS CORTEX

五加皮 *wu³ jia¹ pi²*. English: acanthopanax root bark. Japanese: *gokahi*.

Alternate name: 南五加皮 *nan² wu³ jia¹ pi²*.

Origin: Araliaceae family. *Acanthopanax gracilistylus* W.W. Smith, *A. sessiliflorus* (Rupr. et Maxim.) Seem., *A. senticosus* (Rupr. et Maxim.) Harms., *A. henryi* (Oliv.) Harms., *A. verticillatus* Hoo., *A. giraldii* Harms,* *A. trifoliatus* (L.) Merr.,* *A. evodiaefolius* Franch. var. *ferrugineus* W.W. Smith,* *A. setchuenensis* Harms,* *A. leucorrhizus* (Oliv.) Harms.*

Characters: This bark comes in strips of varying lengths, coiled in tubular form. Its exterior surface is finely wrinkled, but generally smooth in texture and pierced with long lenticels, and is grayish brown in color; the interior surface is grayish white. This bark, which gives off a faint smell, is brittle, and leaves a jagged edge when snapped. The decocting pieces are slices 1 mm thick.

Quality: Long, thick, neat strips without any trace of wood.

Production areas: China (Jiangsu, Anhui, Zhejiang, Hubei, Hunan, Guangxi, Sichuan, Yunnan, Shaanxi, Henan, Shandong).

Properties and actions: Warm; acrid. Enters the liver and kidney channels. Dispels wind-damp; strengthens sinew and bone; quickens the blood and eliminates stasis.

Indications: Wind-cold-damp bi, leg qi, wind-damp in the skin, impotence, and scrotal damp. Daily dosage: 5–10 g. Contraindicated in effulgent yin vacuity fire. Used in *wu³-jia¹-pi² wan²* (Acanthopanax Pills, 278).

Remarks: Constituents: Phenylpropanoids: 4-methoxysalicylaldehyde. Acids: palmitic acid, linolenic acid. Tannoids.

* Similar plants.

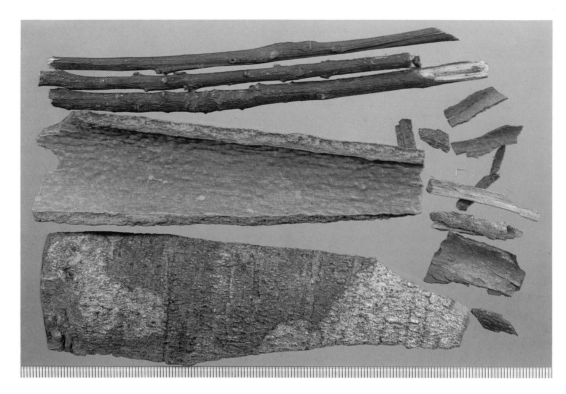

Top: Cinnamomi Ramulus. Bottom: Cinnamomi Cortex. (×7/8)

---

2 CINNAMOMI CORTEX

肉桂 *rou⁴ gui⁴*. (Including Cinnamomi Ramulus 桂枝 *gui⁴ zhi¹*.) English: cinnamon bark. Japanese: *nikkei (keishi)*.

Alternate name: 玉桂 *yu⁴ gui⁴*

Origin: Lauraceae family. *Cinnamomum cassia* Blume.

Characters: This bark comes in strips 6–40 cm long and 1–3 mm thick, and curled into trough or tube shapes. The outside is relatively smooth with inconspicuous lenticels. If the cork has not been stripped off, it is brown in color; if it has been stripped off, it is a dark, reddish brown. It is hard, and breaks into pieces when snapped. A pale line (the stone cell layer) can be observed on the fracture. The twigs (Cinnamomi Ramulus) are about 1 mm thick, straight, with a purplish cortex and pale brown interior wood. They are usually cut obliquely.

Quality: A strong, sweet, pungent taste and powerful aroma are signs of good quality.

Production areas: China (Guangdong, Guangxi, and Yunnan), Vietnam, India, and Cambodia.

Properties and actions: Bark: Hot; acrid and sweet; nontoxic. Enters the kidney, spleen, and bladder channels. Supplements original yang; warms the spleen and stomach; eliminates accumulated frigidity; frees the blood vessels. Twigs: warm and pungent. They promote sweating, and warm and free the channels.

Indications: The bark treats inversion cold in the limbs, upper body heat with lower body cold, lumbar and knee pain, vacuity cold with aversion to food, clear-food diarrhea, menstrual block, abdominal pain, shan-jia, and inhibited urination. The twigs treat wind-cold exterior patterns, with cold in the joints, as well as thoracic bi with phlegm and rheum, and menstrual block with concretions and conglomerations. Daily dosage: Bark 1–5 g; twigs 1.5–5 g. The bark is contraindicated in effulgent yin vacuity fire and pregnancy; the twigs are contraindicated in pregnancy, effulgent yin vacuity fire, and blood patterns. Used in *shi² quan² da⁴ bu³ tang¹* (Perfect Major Supplementation Decoction, 243), *ba¹ wei⁴ di⁴-huang² wan²* (Eight-Ingredient Rehmannia Pills, 6), *gui⁴-zhi¹ tang¹* (Cinnamon Twig Decoction, 114), *gui⁴-zhi¹ fu²-ling² wan²* (Cinnamon Twig and Poria Pills, 109).

Remarks: Constituents: Phenylpropanoids: (Volatile oil, 1–3.5%) *trans*-cinnamic aldehyde (cinnamaldehyde, 80–90%), cinnamic acid.

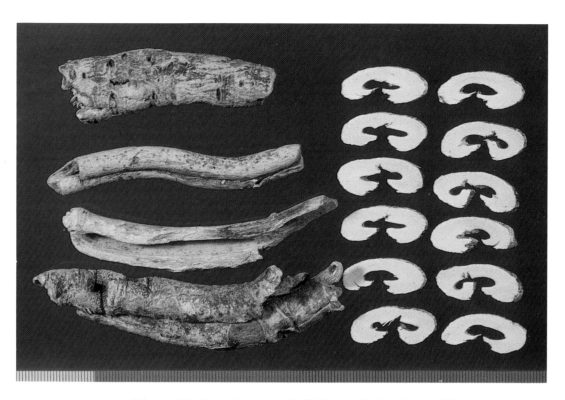

Dictamni Radicis Cortex: crude (left) and sliced (right) (×7/8)

3   DICTAMNI RADICIS CORTEX

白鮮皮 *bai² xian¹ pi²*. English: Chinese dictamnus root bark. Japanese: *hakusenpi*.
Alternate names: 白羶 *bai² shan¹*, 白薛皮 *bai² xian³ pi²*.
Origin: Rutaceae family. *Dictamnus dasycarpus* Turcz.
Characters: This root bark comes in quills 5–10 mm in diameter. The outer layer is peeled off, leaving a smooth, pale yellow surface with fine longitudinal wrinkles, and scars from small branch roots. Indented white speckles may be observed on gray black cork that has not been properly stripped away. The inner surface is smooth, earth-colored, and slightly fibrous. Though hard, it snaps easily, giving off white powder and leaving a whitish yellow fracture. The decocting pieces are transverse slices 1–2 mm thick.
Quality: Best if large, dry, and pale, without any wood.
Production areas: China (Manchuria, Hebei, Henan, Anhui, Jiangsu, and Hubei), and Korea.
Properties and actions: Cold; bitter and salty. Enters the spleen and stomach channels. Dispels wind; dries damp; clears heat; and resolves toxin.
Indications: Wind bi, damp sores, jaundice, jie and xian. Daily dosage: 6–10 g. Contraindicated in lower burner vacuity cold. Used in *bai²-xian¹-pi² san³* (Dictamnus Powder, 18).
Remarks: Constituents: Alkaloids: dictamnine, skimmianine. Triterpenoids: dictamnolactone, obakunone.
Allied drug: *D. angustifolius* G. Don. Triterpenoid: dictamnolactone, obakunone.

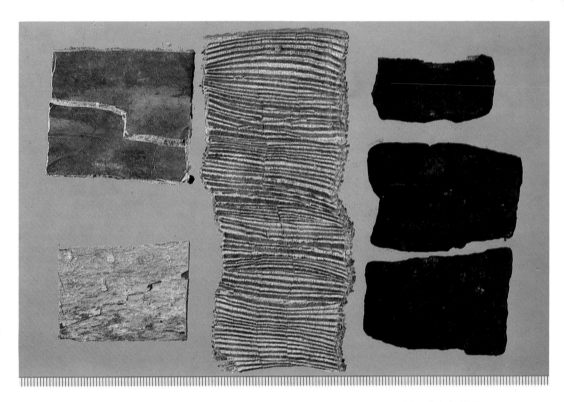

Eucommiae Cortex: crude (left); cut (middle); and carbonized (right) (×7/8)

4   EUCOMMIAE CORTEX

杜仲du⁴ zhong⁴. English: eucommia (or hardy rubber) bark. Japanese: tochū.

Alternate names: 思仙 si¹ xian¹, 思仲 si¹ zhong⁴, 絲棉皮 si¹ mian² pi².

Origin: Eucommiaceae family. *Eucommia ulmoides* Oliv.

Characters: This bark comes in flat strips with a slight curl, 1–6 mm thick, with pale gray-brown cork bearing longitudinal wrinkles and furrows, and transverse lenticels. Thicker areas of cork are often partly removed, leaving a flat, brown surface. The inner surface has a smooth texture, and is dark, purplish, or blackish brown in color. This bark is brittle, but when broken the parts are held together by silvery, extensible filaments. The decocting pieces are sections with multiple cuts allowing the filaments to be stretched. Carbonized pieces, made by stir-frying in brine, are brownish black in color.

Quality: Best when hard and dry, with rubbery threads that do not easily break.

Production areas: China (Sichuan, Shaanxi, Guizhou, Hunan, Henan, Hubei, and Yunnan).

Properties and actions: Warm; bitter and slightly acrid; nontoxic. Enters the liver and kidney channels. Supplements the liver and kidney; strengthens sinew and bone; quiets the fetus.

Indications: Lumbar and knee pain. Daily dosage: 6–10 g. Use with care in the presence of yin vacuity fire. Used in *du⁴-zhong⁴ san³* (Eucommia Powder, 74), *da⁴ zao⁴ wan²* (Greatly Supplementing Pills, 55), *du²-huo² ji⁴-sheng¹ tang¹* (Duhuo and Mistletoe Decoction, 73).

Remarks: Constituents: Lignoid: (+) pinoresinol. Polyterpenoid: gutta-percha (6–10%). Saccharide: glycans (0.26%). Iridoids: eucommioside I, eucommiol, geniposide. Triterpenoid: ulmoprenol.

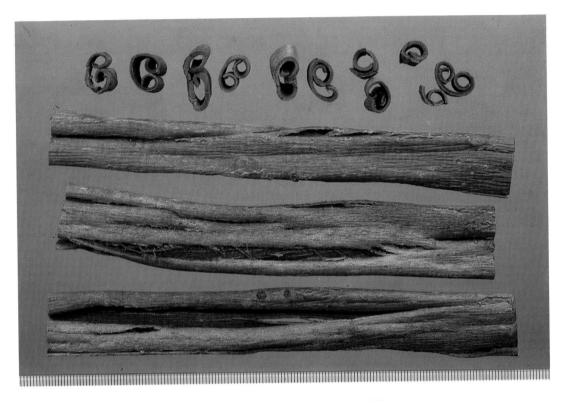

Fraxini Cortex: crude and cut. (× 7/8)

5 FRAXINI CORTEX

秦皮 *qin² pi²*. English: ash (or fraxinus bark). Japanese: *shinpi.*

Alternate name: 秦白皮 *qin² bai² pi².*

Origin: Oleaceae family. *Fraxinus rhynchophylla* Hance.

Characters: The dried bark of the branches comes in channeled sections, or in single or double quills, about 10–20 cm long, 1.5–3 cm in diameter, and roughly 3 mm thick. The exterior surface is rough in texture, and brown or gray in color with lighter speckles. The interior surface is yellowish white. Sometimes the exterior layer peels away to reveal the reddish brown color of the interior layer. This bark is hard, and snaps easily, leaving a fibrous fracture. It has a blue fluorescent appearance when soaked in water. The decocting pieces are 1 cm long sections.

Quality: Bark that comes in long, neat tubes is the best.

Production areas: *F. bungeana:* China (Liaoning, Jilin, Hebei, Henan, Shaanxi, Shanxi, Sichuan, and Inner Mongolia). *F. rhynchophylla:* China (Manchuria and the North).

Properties and actions: Cold; bitter; nontoxic. Enters the liver and gallbladder channels. Clears heat and dries damp; calms dyspnea and suppresses cough; brightens the eyes.

Indications: Bacterial dysentery; enteritis; vaginal discharge; chronic bronchitis; sore, red, swollen eyes and tearing on exposure to wind; oxhide xian. Daily dosage: 5–10 g. Contraindicated in stomach vacuity with low food intake. Used in *bai²-tou²-weng¹ tang¹* (Pulsatilla Decoction, 16).

Remarks: Constituents: Coumarins: aeseulin, aesculetin, fraxin, fraxetin.

Allied drug: Dried bark of *Fraxinus bungeana* DC.

Similar drug: *Juglans mandshurica* Maxim. (Juglandaceae).

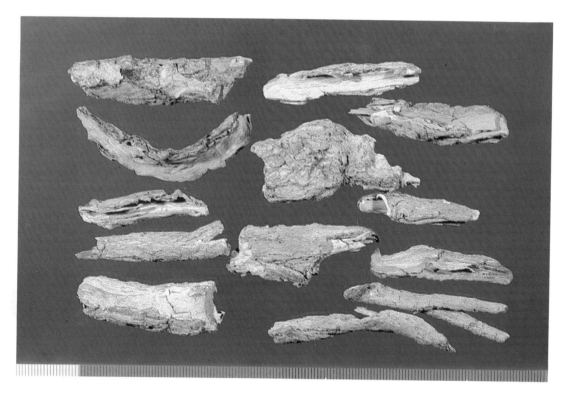

Lycii Radicis Cortex. (×7/8)

6 LYCII RADICIS CORTEX

地骨皮 *di⁴ gu³ pi²*. English: lycium (or matrimony vine) root bark. Japanese: *jikoppi*.
Alternate name: 枸杞根皮 *gou³ qi³ gen¹ pi²*.
Origin: Solanaceae family. *Lycium chinense* Mill.
Characters: This root bark comes in channeled sections or single quills of up to 12 cm in length,
2 cm wide, and 1–3 mm thick. The exterior is orange brown, with the cork layer peeling off or
having irregular fissures. The inside has a textured grain and is yellowish white, sometimes with
brown speckles. This root bark is light, and breaks easily, leaving a jagged fracture. The decocting
pieces are fine slices.
Quality: Dry, hard, thick pieces without wood or impurities are the best.
Production areas: China (Anhui, Jiangsu, Shandong, Shanxi, Gansu, and Inner Mongolia), and
Korea.
Properties and actions: Cold; sweet. Enters the lung, liver, and kidney channels. Clears heat;
cools the blood.
Indications: Cough, blood ejection; heat vexation; wasting thirst; taxation fever with perspira-
tion; steaming bone tidal fever; swollen yong and malign sores. Daily dosage: 6–10 g. Contrain-
dicated if construction heat is not present, and for spleen-stomach vacuity cold. Used in *xie⁴ bai²
san³* (White-Draining Powder, 303).
Remarks: Constituents: Alkaloid: kukoamine-A. Amino acid. Lyciumamide. Amine: betaine. Acid:
cinnamic acid.
Allied drug: Dried root bark of *Lycium barbarum* L., from China, is frequently utilized.
Lyciumamide. Amine: betaine. Acid: cinnamic acid.

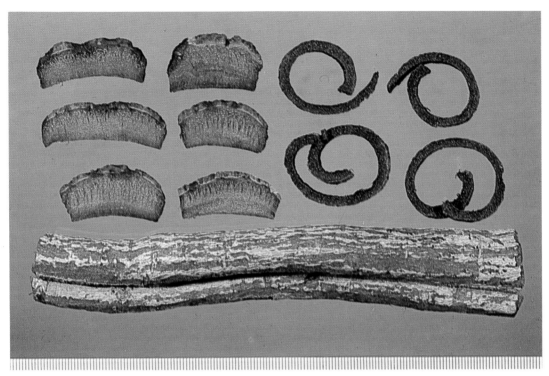

Magnoliae Cortex: crude (bottom); prepared in ginger juice (top left); and root bark prepared in ginger juice (top right). (× 5/6)

7 MAGNOLIAE CORTEX

厚朴 *hou⁴ po⁴*. English: magnolia bark. Japanese: *kōboku*.

Alternate names: 赤朴 *chi⁴ po⁴*, 厚樸 *hou⁴ po⁴*.

Origin: Magnoliaceae family. *Magnolia biloba* (Rehd. et Wils.) Cheng, *M. officinalis* Rehd. et Wils.

Characters: This product comes in the form of single or double quills, roughly 35 cm long, and 2–5 mm wide. The outer surface is a dull, grayish brown in color, and is rough and scaly in texture, with an irregular grain. The inner surface is a purplish brown with a straight grain. This bark is hard, and breaks to leave a jagged fibrous edge.

Quality: Good quality barks have an outer layer thicker than the inner layer, and have a clear reddish purple hue on the cross section. They have a high oil content, a strong smell, and a sweet, acrid taste.

Production areas: China (Anhui, Jiangsu, Shandong, Shanxi, Gansu, and Inner Mongolia), and Korea.

Properties and actions: Warm; bitter and acrid; non-toxic. Enters the spleen, stomach, and large intestine channels. Warms the center, precipitates qi, and dissipates fullness; dries damp; disperses stasis and breaks accumulations.

Indications: Painful distention and fullness in the chest, vomiting and diarrhea, and dyspnea and cough. Daily dosage: 3–8 g. Use with care in pregnancy. Used in *ban⁴-xia⁴ hou⁴-po⁴ tang¹* (Pinellia and Magnolia Bark Decoction, 25), *ping² wei⁴ san³* (Stomach-Calming Powder, 196), *xiao³ cheng² qi⁴ tang¹* (Minor Qi-Infusing Decoction, 299), *hou⁴-po⁴ san¹ wu⁴ tang¹* (Magnolia Bark Three Agents Decoction, 120).

Remarks: Constituents: Sesquiterpenoids and monoterpenoids (volatile oil, 0.24–0.36%): eudesmol (94–98%). Phenols: magnolol (1.8–2.6%), honokiol (0.34–1.2%). Alkaloids (0.07%). Tannoids. Allied drug: Dried bark of *Magnolia obovata* Thunb. (Japan).

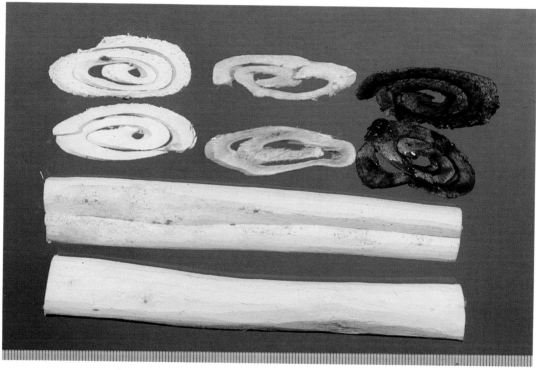

Mori Radicis Cortex: crude (bottom); slices (top left); stir-fried (top center); and honey mix-fried (top right). (× 6/7)

8 MORI RADICIS CORTEX

桑白皮 *sang¹ bai² pi²*. English: (white) mulberry root bark. Japanese: *sōhakuhi.*

Alternate name: 桑根白皮 *sang¹ gen¹ bai² pi².*

Origin: Moraceae family. *Morus alba* L.

Characters: This product is the dry root bark with the cork removed. It comes in double quills 20–50 cm long and 1.5–3 mm thick. It has a whitish, fibrous outer surface, and a yellow-brown fibrous inner surface. It is tough and stringy, and tends to rip lengthwise rather than snap. It has an unpleasant odor similar to that of soybean flour. The decocting pieces are fine slices that are either untreated or mix-fried with honey.

Quality: Dry, thick and white barks without impurities are the best.

Production areas: China (Anhui, Jiangsu, Zhejiang being the main areas, and Hubei, Guangdong, and Guangxi being secondary areas), Japan, and Korea.

Properties and actions: Cold; sweet; nontoxic. Enters the lung and spleen channels. Drains the lung and calms dyspnea; moves water and disperses swelling.

Indications: Lung heat cough, and blood ejection, water swelling, and abdominal distention. Mix-frying with honey adds a lung-moistening action suited to patients suffering from lung vacuity cough. Daily dosage: 5–10 g. Contraindicated for lung vacuity without fire, and cold cough. Used in *xie⁴ bai² san³* (White-Draining Powder, 303), *wu³ pi² san³* (Five Cortices Powder, 281), *huang²-qi² bie¹-jia³ san³* (Astragalus and Turtle Shell Powder, 132), *wu³ hu³ tang¹* (Five Tigers Decoction, 276).

Remarks: Constituents: Flavonoids: morusin, morusinol, cyclomorusin, kuwanons A-Z. Benzofurans: mulberrofuran A, B., G, I, M, P, and Q. Coumarins: umbellifierone, scopoletin. Allied drug: Dried root bark of *Morus bombycis* Koidz. (Japan).

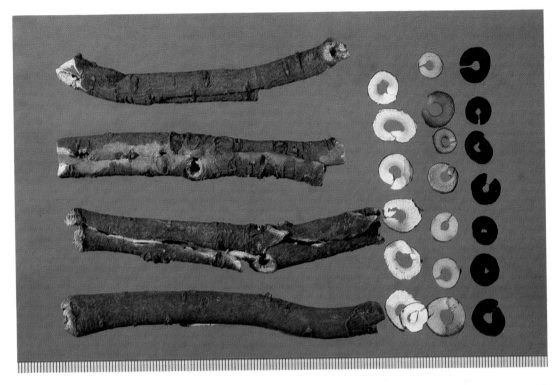

Moutan Radicis Cortex (left to right) crude, cut, stir-fried, and carbonized. (× 6/7)

9   MOUTAN RADICIS CORTEX

牡丹皮 *mu³ dan¹ pi²*. English: moutan (or tree peony) root bark. Japanese: *botanpi*.

Alternate names: 丹皮 *dan¹ pi²*, 牡丹根皮 *mu³ dan¹ gen¹ pi²*.

Origin: Paeoniaceae family. *Paeonia moutan* Sims. [= *P. suffruticosa* Andr.], *P. papaveracea* Andr.,* *P. lutea* Franch.,* *P. delavayi* Franch.,* *P. potanini* Kom., *P. szechuanica* Fang,* *P. thalictrumifolia* C. Ho et S.Y. Chen,* *P. yunnanensis* Fang,* *P. suffruticosa* Andr. var. *spontanea* Rehd.*

Characters: This bark resumes its original shape after being removed from the root by a single longitudinal cut. It is 2–4 mm thick, 0.6–1.4 cm in diameter, and comes in lengths of 10–20 cm. It is a grayish brown on the outside with a slight purple hue. The outer surface has conspicuous, long lenticels, and scars left where branch roots were removed. Sometimes the cork is stripped away, exposing a brighter red coloring. The flesh and inner surface is gray. This bark breaks cleanly, revealing a pale red fracture surface. The decocting pieces are slices 1–2 mm thick, appearing pinkish on the cut edge. Stir-frying and carbonizing darken the color.

Quality: Better barks are thick, evenly sized, round and straight, have a thin skin and thick flesh, do not become redder with time, and have no wood or fine roots attached.

Production areas: China (Shandong, Anhui, Shanxi, Hunan, Hubei, Sichuan, Gansu), Japan, and Korea.

Properties and actions: Slightly cold; bitter and acrid; non-toxic. Enters the heart, liver, and kidney channels. Clears heat, cools the blood, harmonizes the blood, and disperses stasis. Stir-frying enhances the stasis-dissipating action, and carbonizing adds a blood-staunching effect.

Indications: Heat entering construction, fright epilepsy, ejection of blood, nosebleed, and hemafecia, steaming bone tidal fever, menstrual block, shan-jian, yong, and impact injury; intestinal yong, and sores. Daily dosage: 6–10 g. Contraindicated in spleen-stomach vacuity cold and diarrhea. Used in *da⁴-huang² mu³-dan¹-pi² tang¹* (Rhubarb and Moutan Decoction 50), *gui⁴-zhi¹ fu²-ling² wan²* (Cinnamon Twig and Poria Pills, 109), *jia¹ wei⁴ xiao¹ yao² san³* (Supplemented Free Wanderer Powder, 143), *xi¹-jiao³ di⁴-huang² tang¹* (Rhinoceros Horn and Rehmannia Decoction, 284), *wen¹ jing¹ tang¹* (Channel-Warming Decoction, 269).

Remarks: Constituents: Phenylpropanoids: paeonol (1.3–2.5%), paeonoside, paeonolide. Monoterpenoids: paeoniflorin, oxypaeoniflorin, benozoylpaeoniflorin, benzoyloxypaeoniflorin. Steroid. Tannoid. Acid.

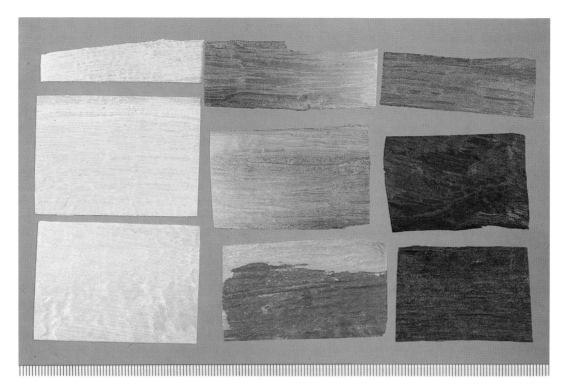

Phellodendri Cortex: (left to right) cut, stir-fried in brine, and carbonized. (×6/7)

10 PHELLODENDRI CORTEX

黃柏 *huang² bo²*. English: phellodndron bark. Japanese: *ōbaku*.

Alternate names: 檗皮 *bo⁴ pi²*, 黃檗 *huang² bo⁴*.

Origin: Rutaceae family. *Phellodendron amurense* Rupr., *P. chinense* Schneid., *P. chinense* Schneid. var. *glabriusculum* Schneid.,* *P. chinense* Schneid. var. *omeiense* Huang,* *P. chinense* Schneid. var. *yunnanense* Huang,* *P. chinense* Schneid. var. *falcatum* Huang.*

Characters: This product comes in flat pieces 1.5–4 mm thick, with the cork layer already removed. It is yellow with a green or brown tint. The outer surface is smooth and conspicuously fibrous; the inner surface is a dirty or grayish brown yellow. It is light, and is easily broken, leaving a fibrous fracture. The decocting pieces are thin strips or squares that are yellow if crude, and darker if stir-fried or carbonized.

Quality: Superior barks are dry, thick, solid, and finely grained, with the rough outer layer removed.

Production areas: *Phellodendron amurense:* China (Jilin, Liaoning, and Hebei). *P. chinense:* China (Sichuan, Guizhou, and Hubei).

Properties and actions: Cold; bitter; nontoxic. Enters the kidney and bladder channels. Clears heat, dries damp, drains the fire and resolves toxin. Use crude to clear heat and drain fire. Use stir-fried with brine to clear vacuity heat, especially in kidney vacuity. Use stir-fried with wine to treat the upper burner or for better blood-quickening action. Use mix-fried with honey for middle burner patterns, and carbonized to staunch bleeding.

Indications: Heat dysentery and diarrhea, jaundice, steaming bones, hemorrhoids, hemafecia, turbid strangury, vaginal discharge, and sores. Daily dosage: 5–10 g. Used only for repletion fire, and contraindicated for patients suffering from spleen vacuity diarrhea or a weak stomach. Used in *zhi¹ bo² di⁴-huang² wan²* (Anemarrhena, Phellodendron, and Rehmannia Pills, 337), *bai²-tou²-weng¹ tang¹* (Pulsatilla Decoction, 16), *huang²-lian² jie³ du² tang¹* (Coptis Toxin-Resolving Decoction, 130), *da⁴ bu³ yin¹ wan²* (Major Yin Supplementation Pills, 44), *wen¹ qing¹ yin³* (Warm Clearing Beverage, 271).

Remarks: Constituents: Alkaloids (1.5–4.5%): berberine (0.6–3.5%), palmatine, jateorrhizine, phellodendrine, candicine, menispermine, magnoflorine. Limonoids: obakunone, limonin (obakulactone), dictamnolide. Steroids (7–8%).

Allied drug: Dried bark of *Phellodendron wilsonii* Hayata et Kanehira (Taiwan).

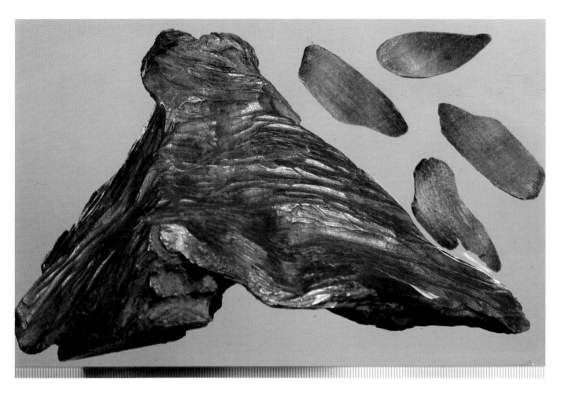

Aquilariae Lignum: crude and cut. (× 3/4)

11 AQUILARIAE LIGNUM

沉香 *chen² xiang¹*. English: aquilaria wood, aloeswood. Japanese: *jinkō*.

Alternate names: 沉水香 *chen² shui³ xiang¹*, 沉香木 *chen² xiang¹ mu⁴*.

Origin: Thymelaeaceae family. *Aquilaria agallocha* Roxb. [= *Aloexylon agallochum* Lour.], *A. sinensis* (Lour.) Gilg.

Characters: This product comes in irregular pieces roughly 10 cm long and 2–4 cm wide with knife marks at each end and sometimes signs of rotting. The surface is brown with darker lines in the grain marking the resinous medullary rays, which appear as black speckles on the transverse section. The wood is hard and heavy; it gives off a strong aroma, particularly when burning. The decocting pieces are fine shavings.

Quality: The best quality is hard, old wood that is the color of bull's horn, has a high oil content, sinks in water, ignites easily, and exudes oil and a powerful aroma when burning.

Production areas: *Aquilaria agallocha:* India, Indonesia, Vietnam, and Malaysia. *A. sinensis:* China (Hainan, Guangxi, and Guangdong).

Properties and actions: Warm; bitter and acrid; nontoxic. Enters the kidney, spleen, and stomach channels. Downbears qi and warms the center; warms the kidney and absorbs qi.

Indications: Vomiting, hiccough, pain in the abdomen and region of the heart, toxin dysentery with inability to eat, large intestinal vacuity constipation, vacuity cold of the lumbus and knees, counterflow qi dyspnea. Daily dosage: 1.5–3 g. Contraindicated in effulgent yin vacuity fire, and qi vacuity fall. Used in *chen²-xiang¹ jiang⁴ qi⁴ tang¹* (Aquilaria Qi-Downbearing Decoction, 39), *chen²-xiang¹ tian¹-ma² tang¹* (Aquilaria and Gastrodia Decoction, 40).

Remarks: Constituents: Sesquiterpenoids: α-, β-agarofurans, agarospirol, agarol. Polyketides: benzylacetone, *p*-methoxybenzylacetone. Coumarinolignoids: aquillochin.

Similar plants: *Aquilaria baillonii* Pierre (Cambodia), *A. bancana* Miq. (Malaysia), *A. crasna* Pierre (Vietnam), *A. microcarpa* Baill. (Borneo), *A. moszkowskii* (Sumatra), *A. pentandura* Blanco (Philippines).

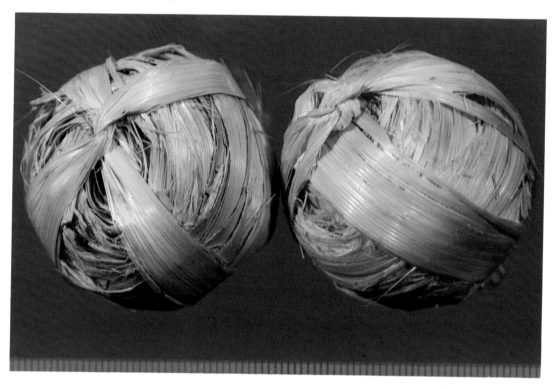

Bambusae Caulis in Taeniam: crude (left) and stir-fried in ginger juice (right). (×2)

12 BAMBUSAE CAULIS IN TAENIAM

竹茹 *zhu² ru²*. English: bamboo shavings. Japanese: *chikujo*.

Alternate names: 青竹茹 *qing¹ zhu² ru²*, 竹二青 *zhu² er⁴ qing¹*.

Origin: Bambusaceae family. *Phyllostachys nigra* (Lodd.) Munro var. *henonis* (Mitf.) Stapf ex Rendle.

Characters: This product comes in stringy strips bound in balls. The strips are about 5–7 mm wide, and are light brown with a greenish hue. They are fibrous and rough to the touch, but smooth when felt along the grain. They are stringy and tough, and do not break easily. The decocting pieces are fine shavings bound in balls.

Quality: The best quality is dry, light in color, finely shaved, supple and strong.

Production areas: China (Henan, Guangdong, Sichuan, Jiangsu, Zhejiang, Hebei, Anhui, Hubei).

Properties and actions: Slightly cold; sweet. Enters the stomach and gallbladder channels. Clears heat; cools the blood; transforms phlegm; checks vomiting. Used crude to clear heat and transform phlegm. Used stir-fried to moderate the cold nature. Used treated with ginger to reduce the cold nature and enhance the power to check vomiting.

Indications: Stomach heat with counterflow retching, heat vexation in the upper burner, blood ejection, nosebleed, profuse uterine bleeding, and stirring fetus. Daily dosage: 5–10 g. Contraindicated in spleen-stomach vacuity cold. Used in *wen¹ dan³ tang¹* (Gallbladder-Warming Decoction, 268), *ju²-pi² zhu²-ru² tang¹* (Tangerine Peel and Bamboo Shavings Decoction, 155), *ling²-jiao³ gou¹-teng² tang¹* (Antelope Horn and Uncaria Decoction, 164), *hao¹ qin² qing¹ dan³ tang¹* (Sweet Wormwood and Scutellaria Glallbladder-Clearing Decoction, 115).

Remarks: Constituents: Pentosan. Triterpene.

Similar plants: *Phyllostachys reticulata* K. Koch., *P. edulis* Houz. de Lehaie.

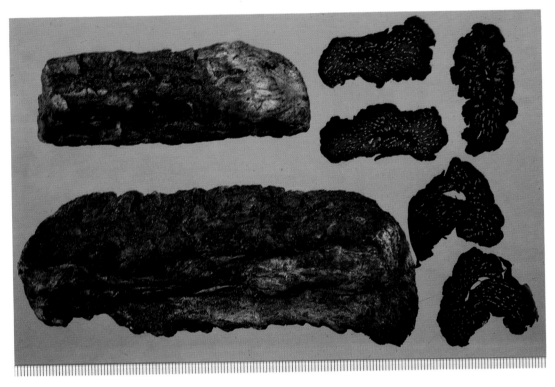

Cistanches Caulis: macerated in water (left) and treated with black beans (right). (× 7/8)

13 CISTANCHES CAULIS

肉苁蓉 *rou⁴ cong¹ rong²*. English: cistanche stem. Japanese: *nikujūyō*.

Alternate names: 大芸 *da⁴ yun²*, 苁蓉 *cong¹ rong²*.

Origin: Orobanchaceae family. *Cistanche salsa* (C.A. Mey.) G. Beck, *C. deserticola* Y.C. Ma, *C. ambigua* (Bge.) G. Beck.

Characters: This stalk takes the form of dark brown, slightly crooked lumps about 15–30 cm long, (10 cm long if broken), and 3–6 cm in diameter. The outer surface is densely covered with the remains of imbricate scaly leaf bases. The lumps are soft and fleshy, and break easily to reveal an uneven fracture. The decocting pieces are oblique slices 2 mm thick. On the cut edge, the skin and the medulla are blackish brown, while the vessels appear brown-white in radial formation.

Quality: 1) Cistanches Caulis Insulsa (non-salty): The best quality is soft, fat, oleaceous, and a rich dark brown in color on the outside. 2) Cistanches Caulis Salsa (salty): the best quality is of large diameter, soft, and black, with fine scales.

Production areas: China (Gansu, Xinjiang, and Inner Mongolia).

Properties and actions: Warm; sweet, sour, and salty. Enters the kidney and large intestine channels. Supplements the kidney and boosts essence; moistens dryness and lubricates the intestines. Treated with black beans, it has a greater supplementing and moistening action.

Indications: Impotence, cold pain in the lumbus and knees, dribble after urinary voiding, infertility, uterine bleeding, vaginal discharge, and constipation due to blood dryness. Daily dosage: 7–10 g. Contraindicated in constipation, heat in the kidney, impotence, and seminal emission. Used in *huan² shao⁴ dan¹* (Rejuvenation Elixir, 128).

Remarks: Constituents: Alkaloids.

Similar drug: Dried stalk of *Boschniakia rossica* B. Fedtsch.

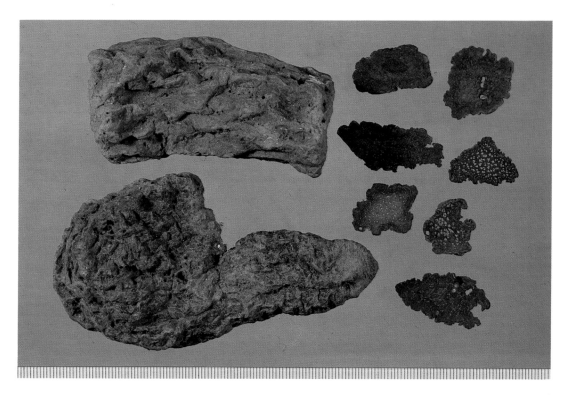

Cynomorii Caulis: crude (left) and prepared in wine (right). (× 6/7)

14 CYNOMORII CAULIS

鎖陽 *suo³ yang²*. English: cynomorium stem. Japanese: *sayō*.

Alternate name: 瑣陽 *suo³ yang²*.

Origin: Cynomoriaceae family. *Cynomorium songaricum* Rupr., *C. coccineum* L.

Characters: The body of this dried herb is roughly cylindrical in shape, with one end slightly thinner than the other. It is 8–21 cm long, and 2–5 cm in diameter. The exterior surface is red brown or dark brown, shrunken and wrinkled. Sometimes triangular scales are observable. It is hard, and not easily broken. The fracture is granular in texture, soft and brown. The decocting pieces are thin transverse slices, which are often threaded on a string.

Quality: Long, dry, hard, fat pieces that are a purplish or reddish brown in color, without any visible stringy sinews are best. When sliced, the cut face should be moist and slightly oily.

Production areas: China (Gansu, Xinjiang, Qinghai, and Inner Mongolia).

Properties and actions: Warm; sweet; nontoxic. Enters the liver and kidney channels. Supplements the kidney; invigorates yang and boosts essence; moistens the intestines.

Indications: Impotence, and weak lumbus and knees; seminal emission. Daily dosage: 5–10 g. Contraindicated in effulgent yin vacuity fire and in diarrhea. Used in *hu³ qian² wan²* (Hidden Tiger Pills, 123).

Remarks: Constituents: Anthocyanin. Triterpene. Tannoid.

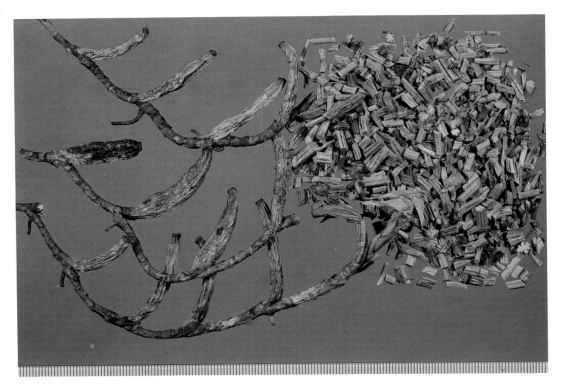

Dendrobii Caulis: crude (left) and cut (right). (× 6/7)

15 DENDROBII CAULIS

石斛 *shi² hu²*. English: dendrobium stem. Japanese: *sekkoku*.

Alternate names: 金釵花 *jin¹ chai¹ hua¹*, 吊蘭花 *diao⁴ lan² hua¹*.

Origin: Orchidaceae family. *Dendrobium nobile* Lindl., *D. linawianum* Reichb. f., *D. officinale* K. Kimura et Migo, *D. moniliforme* (L.) Sw., *D. hercoglossum* Reichb. f., *D. aduncum* Wall. et Lindl., *D. wilsonii* Rolfe, *D. hancockii* Rolfe, *D. lohohense* Tang et Wang, *D. loddigesii* Rolfe, *D. bellatulum* Rolfe.

Characters: These are fine, curved stems that are often split. Sometimes there are many stalks branching from one rhizome, with the stubble of fine roots. Stems vary from 20 to 45 cm in length, and from 5mm in diameter. The external surface is a golden yellow with conspicuous, brown nodes at 1–2.5 cm intervals. The stems are supple, and when snapped reveal a loose, fibrous interior. The decocting pieces are usually 1–2 cm lengths.

Quality: The best quality is a bright golden color, and highly supple.

Production areas: China (Hubei, Sichuan, and Taiwan).

Properties and actions: Cold; sweet, bland and slightly salty. Enters the stomach, lung, and kidney channels. Engenders liquid and boosts the stomach; clears heat and nourishes yin. Stir-frying with brine enhances the power to supplement the kidney, and clear kidney and stomach fire.

Indications: Damage to liquid in heat diseases, dry mouth, thirst, vexation, and vacuity heat after illness. Daily dosage: 5–10 g. Contraindicated in damp warmth and warm heat before transformation into dryness. Used in *gan¹ lu⁴ yin³* (Sweet Dew Beverage, 96), *shi²-hu² san³* (Dendrobium Powder. 241).

Remarks: Constituents: Alkaloid: dendrobine (0.3–0.5%), nobilonine, dendrine, dendramine, dendroxine, 6-hydroxydendroxine, 4-hydroxydendroxine.

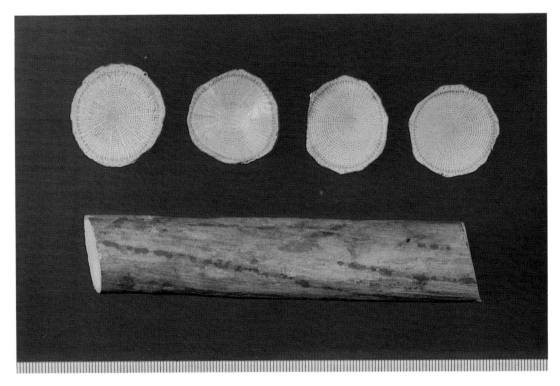

Hocquartiae Caulis: crude (bottom) and cut (above) (×6/7)

16 HOCQUARTIAE CAULIS (MUTONG CAULIS)

木通 *mu⁴ tong¹*. English: hocquartia (or mutong) stem. Japanese: *mokutsū.*

Alternate names: 萬年藤 *wan⁴ nian² teng².*

Origin: Aristolochiaceae family. *Hocquartia manshuriensis* (Kom.) Nakai [= *Aristolochia manshuriensis* Komarov], *Akebia trifoliata* (Thunb.) Koidz.,* *A. quinata* (Thunb.) Decne.,* *A. trifoliata* (Thunb.) Koidz. var. *australis* (Diels) Rehd.,* *Clematis armandi* Franch.,* *C. montana* Buch.-Ham.,* *Aristolochia kaempferi* Willd.,* *Aristolochia moupinensis* Franch.*

Characters: *Hocquartia manshuriensis*, traditionally called *guan¹ mu⁴ tong¹*, is now the most commonly used form of Mutong Caulis. Its straight or flexuose wood stem is about 1–2.5 cm in diameter, swelling to up to 3.5 cm at the nodes or branching points. The exterior surface is a grayish or yellowish brown, sometimes with horizontal fissures. The thicker cork is removed to reveal a lustrous, pale brown endodermis with longitudinal ridges (the stele sheath fiber bundles). The stems are hard, although the finer ones break easily and smoothly. The decocting pieces are slices 2–4 mm thick. They reveal Mutong's most distinctive quality: the light, airy structure of the woody part of the stem.

Quality: A fresh yellow color of the cut surface is a sign of superior quality.

Production areas: China (Heilongjiang, Jilin, Liaoning, Shanxi, Gansu, and Shaanxi).

Properties and actions: Cold; bitter. Enters the heart, small intestine, and bladder channels. Drains fire and moves water; frees the blood vessels.

Indications: Damp-heat strangury, inhibited urination, water swelling, menstrual block, and absence of breast milk. Daily dosage: 3–5 g. Contraindicated in the absence of damp-heat. Used in *ba¹ zheng⁴ san³* (Eight Corrections Powder, 7), *dao³ chi⁴ san³* (Red-Abducting Powder, 64), *long²-dan³ xie⁴ gan¹ tang¹* (Gentian Liver-Draining Decoction, 172), *dang¹-gui¹ si⁴ ni⁴ tang¹* (Tangkuei Counterflow Frigidity Decoction, 62).

Remarks: Constituents: aristolochic acid, oleanolic acid, hederagenin.

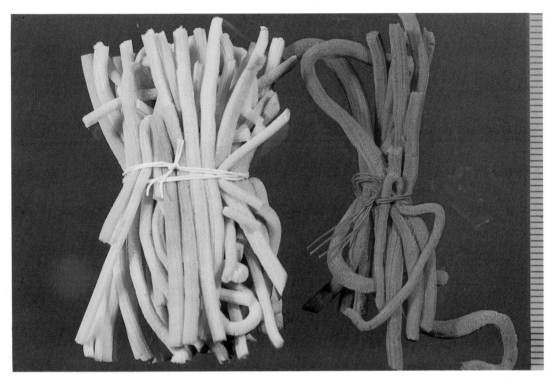

Junci Medulla: crude (left) and prepared with cinnabar (right). (×5/3)

17 JUNCI MEDULLA

燈心草 *deng¹ xin¹ cao³*. English: juncus (or bog rush) pith. Japanese: *tōshinsō*.

Alternate names: 燈草 *deng¹ cao³*, 燈芯草 *deng¹ xin¹ cao³*.

Origin: Juncaceae family. *Juncus effusus* L. var. *decipiens* Buchen. [= *J. decipiens* (Buchen.) Nakai].

Characters: This product has the form of cylindrical stalks of varying length, 2–3 mm in diameter. The outer surface is yellowish white, with a fine longitudinal grain and diffuse lenticels. The stems, which have no smell, are light in structure, and snap easily, revealing a spongy fracture. The decocting pieces are 3 cm lengths, usually bound in bundles.

Quality: Stems of the best quality are long and thick, light in structure, and whitish in color.

Production areas: China (Jiangsu produces the greatest quantity and the best quality; other production areas include Sichuan, Fujian, Guizhou, Shensi), and Japan.

Properties and actions: Cold; sweet, bland; nontoxic. Enters the heart, lung, and small intestine channels. Clears the heart and downbears fire; disinhibits urine and frees strangury. Coated in cinnabar, it quiets the spirit. Charred, it cools the blood and staunches bleeding, clears heat and resolves toxin.

Indications: Strangury; water swelling; inhibited urination; damp-heat jaundice; vexation and insomnia; night crying in infants; throat bi; and wounds. Daily dosage: 1.5–3 g. Contraindicated in vacuity cold. Used in *ba¹ zheng⁴ san³* (Eight Corrections Powder, 7), *jia¹ wei⁴ jie³ du² tang¹* (Supplemented Toxin-Resolving Decoction, 141), *dao³ shui³ fu² ling² tang¹* (Water-Abducting Poria Decoction, 66).

Remarks: Constituents: Flavone: luteolin. Fixed oil. Proteins.

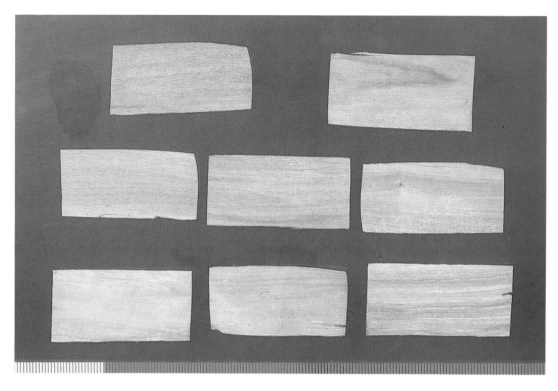

Santali Albi Lignum in slices. (× 6/7)

18 SANTALI ALBI LIGNUM

檀香 *tan² xiang¹*. English: sandal wood. Japanese: *danko*.

Alternate name: 眞檀 *zhen¹ tan²*.

Origin: Santalaceae family. *Santalum album* L.

Characters: Sandalwood comes in chunks of varying lengths, often prepared commercially in lumps 4cm long, 1 cm wide, and 2–5 mm thick. The color is a pale yellow brown. The wood is solid and heavy, but is easy to chop. It has a distinctive, long-lasting smell. The decocting pieces are planed off slices.

Quality: The best quality is heavy and hard, with a strong aroma.

Production areas: India, Indonesia, Malaysia, and China (cultivated in Guangdong, Yunnan, and Taiwan).

Properties and actions: Warm; acrid; nontoxic. Enters the spleen, stomach, and lung channels. Rectifies qi and harmonizes the stomach.

Indications: Pain in the venter and abdomen, esophageal constriction, and retching and vomiting. Daily dosage: 1.5–3 g. Contraindicated in exuberant yin vacuity heat. Used in *dan¹-shen¹ yin³* (Salvia Beverage, 56).

Remarks: Constituents: Volatile oil (1.6–6.0%): α-, β-santalol (ca. 90%), santene, santenone, α-, β-santalene. Pigment: santalin-A, -B.

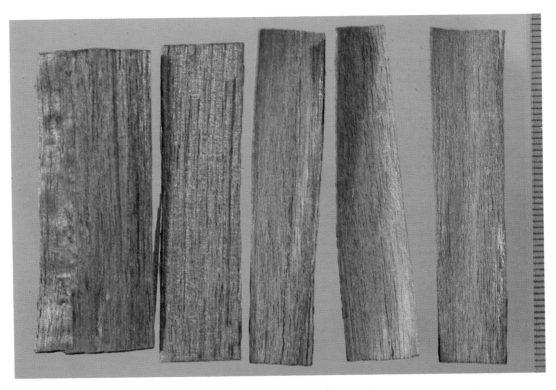

Sappan Lignum in slices. (× 8/5)

19 SAPPAN LIGNUM

蘇木 *su¹ mu⁴*. English: sappan wood. Japanese: *soboku.*
Alternate names: 蘇仿 *su¹ fang³*, 蘇仿木 *su¹ fang³ mu⁴.*
Origin: Leguminosae family. *Caesalpinia sappan* L.
Characters: Sappan wood comes ready-cut for decoction in irregular rectangles of wood about 0.5 mm thick, and usually about 1 cm wide, and dark or light tan in color, some being yellowish white at the edges. The pieces break easily.
Quality: The best quality comes from firm, large branches. It is hard and bears a reddish hue.
Production areas: India, Malaysia, and China (cultivated in Guangxi, Yunnan, Guangdong, and Taiwan).
Properties and actions: Balanced; sweet, salty; nontoxic. Enters the heart and liver channels. Moves the blood, breaks stasis, disperses swelling, and relieves pain.
Indications: Postpartum stasis obstruction, menstrual block with qi congestion, swollen yong, and stasis and stagnation due to injury. Daily dosage: 3–5 g. Contraindicated in blood vacuity. Used in *shu¹ jin¹ yao⁴ shui³* (Sinew-Soothing Medicinal Water, 249), *ba¹ li² san³* (Eight Pinches Powder, 4).
Remarks: Constituents: Volatile oil: α-, β-phelandrene. Pigment: brasilin (2.0%).
Similar plant: *Caesalpinia echinata* Lamarck (Brasil wood).

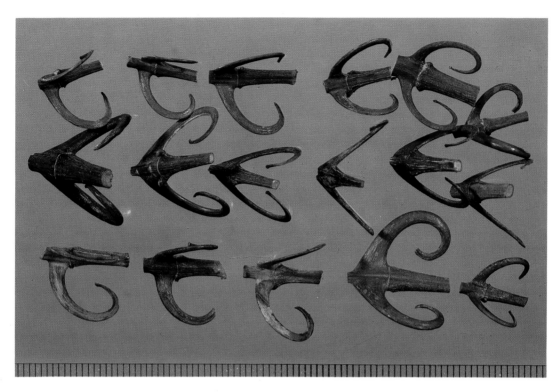

Uncariae Ramulus et Uncus in slices. (× 8/5)

20 UNCARIAE RAMULUS ET UNCUS

鉤藤 *gou¹ teng²*. English: uncaria stem and thorn. Japanese: *kōtō*.

Alternate names: 釣鉤藤 *diao⁴ gou¹ teng²*, 釣藤 *diao⁴ teng²*, 釣藤鉤 *diao⁴ teng² gou¹*.

Origin: Rubiaceae family. *Uncaria rhynchophylla* (Miq.) Jacks, *U. sinensis* (Oliv.) Havil., *U. lancifolia* Hutch.,* *U. rhynchophylloides* How,* *U. macrophylla* Wall,* *U. hirsuta* Havil.,* *U. sessifructus* Roxb.,* *U. scandens* (Smith) Hutch.*

Characters: This product is a stalk bearing thorns shaped like fish hooks. The thorns spring from the stalk in twos, at 90 degrees to each other, and are 1.2-2 cm long, and 2 mm wide at the base. The stems bear slight longitudinal ridges, and share with the thorns a smooth, lustrous reddish brown surface. Below the thorns are marks where stipules were once attached. The transverse section of the stem is a whitish brown. The decocting pieces are short sections of the stem, each with two hooks.

Quality: Unbroken hooks and a reddish luster are marks of good quality.

Production areas: *Uncaria rhynchophylla:* China (Guangxi, Jiangxi, Hunan, Zhejiang, and Guangdong, and Japan. *U. sinensis:* China (Sichuan, Guizhou, Yunnan, Hubei).

Properties and actions: Cold; sweet. Enters the liver and heart channels. Clears heat and calms the liver; extinguishes wind and settles fright.

Indications: Dizziness and infantile fright epilepsy. Daily dosage: 5-10g. Contraindicated in the absence of wind-heat or repletion heat. Used in *yi⁴ gan¹ san³* (Liver-Repressing Powder, 315), *gou¹-teng² tang¹* (Uncaria Decoction, 103), *qi¹ wu⁴ jiang⁴ xia⁴ tang¹* (Seven Agents Downbearing Decoction, 197).

Remarks: Constituents: Alkaloids: rhynchophylline, corynoxeine, isorhynchophylline, isocorynoxeine, hirsutine, hirsuteine, dihydrocorynantheine, corynantheine.

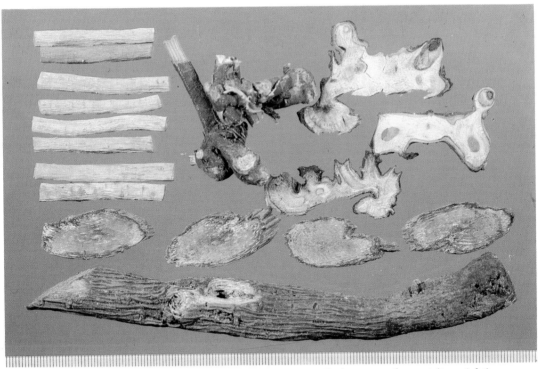

Achyranthis Bidentatae Radix (top left); Cyathulae Radix cut and uncut (top right);
Achyranthis Radix cut and uncut (bottom). (×6/7)

21   ACHYRANTHIS BIDENTATAE RADIX

牛膝 *niu² xi¹*. (Including Cyathulae Radix 川牛膝 *chuan¹ niu² xi¹*, Achyranthis Radix 土牛膝 *tu³ niu² xi¹*) English: achyranthes root. Japanese: *goshitsu*.

Alternate names: 牛七 *niu² qi¹*, 淮牛膝 *huai² niu² xi¹*, 懷牛膝 *huai² niu² xi¹*.

Origin: Amaranthaceae family. *Achyranthes bidentata* Blume.

Characters: This root comes in sections 30–50 cm long, and 4–8 mm in diameter. The outer surface is flesh or earth-colored with a meandering grain and long, horizontal lenticels, and conspicuous scars where fine branch roots have been removed. The root is soft, and breaks easily, leaving a smooth fracture and revealing the yellow-brown inside of the flesh with whitish vascular bundles appearing as speckles. The decocting pieces are short sections or thick slices.

Quality: Long, thick, pale-colored roots with a fine cortex, firm flesh and no speckles or dirt are the best quality.

Production areas: China (Henan, Shanxi, Shandong, Jiangsu, Anhui, Zhejiang, Hunan, Hubei, Sichuan, Yunnan, and Guizhou).

Properties and actions: Balanced; sweet and sour. Used crude, it dissipates stasis and disperses yong swelling. With wine, its channel-freeing and blood-quickening action is enhanced. Roasted or stir-fried, it supplements the liver and kidney, and strengthens the sinews and bones. Treated with brine, its bone and sinew strengthening action is enhanced.

Similar products: Achyranthis Radix (*tu³ niu² xi¹*) has the same function as Achyranthis Bidentatae Radix, while Cyathulae Radix (*chuan¹ niu² xi¹*) has a stronger stasis-dispelling effect.

Indications: Used crude it treats menstrual block, strangury, hematuria, swollen yong, difficult delivery. When roasted, stir-fried, or treated with brine, it treats pain and weakness in the knee and lumbus. Daily dosage: 5–10 g. Contraindicated in spleen vacuity diarrhea, and in pregnancy. Used in *niu²-xi¹ san³* (Achyranthes Powder, 194), *niu² che¹ shen⁴ qi⁴ wan²* (Achyranthes and Plantago Kidney Qi Pills, 192), *da⁴ zao⁴ wan²* (Greatly Supplementing Pills, 55).

Remarks: Constituents: Triterpenoids: saponin. Steroids (arthropod molting hormone) ecdysterone, inokosterone. Amino acids: α-aminobutyric acid; betaine.

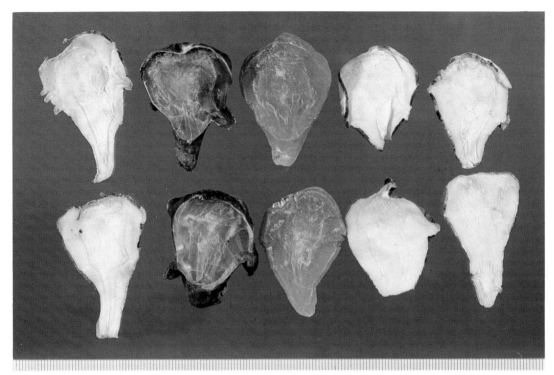

Aconiti Tuber Laterale (left to right): Taiwan stone-baked;
black; blast-fried; white; treated with ginger. (×6/7)

22 ACONITI TUBER LATERALE

附子 *fu⁴ zi³*. English: aconite accessory tuber. Japanese: *bushi*.

Alternate name: 附片 *fu⁴ pian⁴*.

Origin: Ranunculaceae family. *Aconitum carmichaeli Debx.*

Characters: The dried root is roughly spindle-shaped, about 1.5–3 cm long, and 1.5 cm in diameter. It has shoot scars at the top and a pointed tip at the bottom, and is covered with numerous tumorous protuberances. It comes ready-prepared in several forms. Taiwanese stone-baked: 1 mm thick longitudinal slices, farinaceous in texture. Black: skinned, cut in 2-5 mm longitudinal slices, black on the outside and blackish yellow on the cut edge. Blast-fried: skinned, cut in 3–4 mm thick slices, yellow and slightly translucent. White: skinned, cut in 5 mm transverse slices, treated with sulfur and sundried.

Quality: Fat hard tubers are the best.

Production areas: China (Sichuan, Shaanxi).

Properties and actions: Hot; acrid, sweet; toxic. Enters the heart, spleen, and kidney channels. Returns yang and supplements the fire; dissipates cold and eliminates damp.

Indications: Exuberant yin repelling yang; profuse sweating in yang collapse; blood conglomerations; cold-damp atony; hypertonicity; pain in the knees with difficulty in walking. Daily dosage: 2–5 g. Contraindicated in yang exuberance due to yin vacuity, in true heat and false cold, and in pregnancy. Used in *gan¹-cao³ fu⁴-zi³ tang¹* (Licorice and Aconite Decoction, 92), *si⁴ ni⁴ tang¹* (Counterflow Frigidity Decoction, 253) *zhen¹ wu³ tang¹* (True Warrior Decoction, 335), *bai¹ wei⁴ di⁴-huang² wan²* (Eight-Ingredient Rehammia Pills, 6)

Remarks: Constituents: Aconite alkaloids: aconitine, mesaconitine, hypaconitine, deoxyaconitine, benzoylaconine.

Allied drug: Tuber of *Aconitum japonicum* Thunb. (Japan).

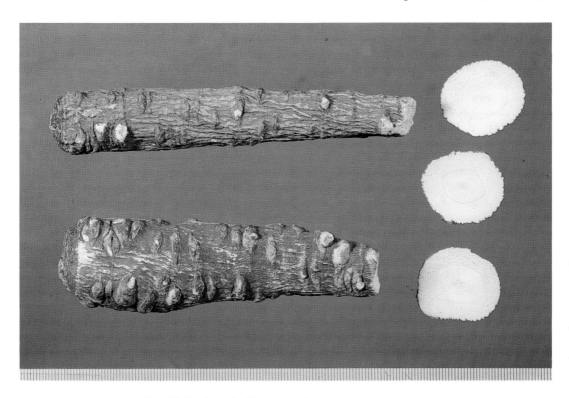

Angelicae Dahuricae Radix: crude (left) and sliced (right). (× 5/6)

23 ANGELICAE DAHURICAE RADIX

白芷 *bai² zhi³*. English: angelica root. Japanese: *byakushi*.

Alternate name: 香白芷 *xiang¹ bai² zhi³*.

Origin: Umbelliferae family. *Angelica dahurica* Benth. et Hook. var. *paichi* Kimura, Hata et Yen, *A. anomala* Lallem.,* *Heracleum scabridum* Franch.*

Characters: Roots shaped like a mallet head with four corners at the head, about 10–20 cm long, and about 1.5–2 cm in diameter at the head and tapering to the tip. There is an indentation on the head where the stalk was removed. The outer surface is a yellowish or pale brown, with a longitudinal grain, and scars on prominences where the fine roots were removed. The root is hard and heavy. The fracture is white and mealy with annular markings. The decocting pieces are 1 mm transverse slices, which reveal the annular markings even more clearly.

Quality: Dry, hard, fat roots with good farinaceous texture and full aroma are the best.

Production areas: China (Sichuan, Zhejiang, and Hebei).

Properties and actions: Warm; acrid. Enters the lung, spleen, and stomach channels. Dispels wind; dries damp; disperses swelling; relieves pain. Char-fry for vaginal discharge.

Indications: All diseases of the head and face including headache and toothache; red and white vaginal discharge; dry itchy skin. Daily dosage: 3–7 g. Contraindicated in yin vacuity and depressed fire. Used in *qiang¹-huo² bai²-zhi³ san³* (Notopterygium and Angelica Powder, 202), *wu³ ji¹ san³* (Five Accumulations Powder, 277), *cang¹-er³ san³* (Xanthium Powder, 34), *tuo¹ li³ xiao¹ du² yin³* (Internal Expulsion Toxin-Dispersing Beverage, 265).

Remarks: Constituents: Furocoumarins: byakangelicin, byakangelicol, oxypeucedanin, imperatorin, phellopterin, isoimperatorin.

Allied drug: Dried root of *Angelica dahurica* Benth. et Hook. var. *formosana* Yen (Taiwan).

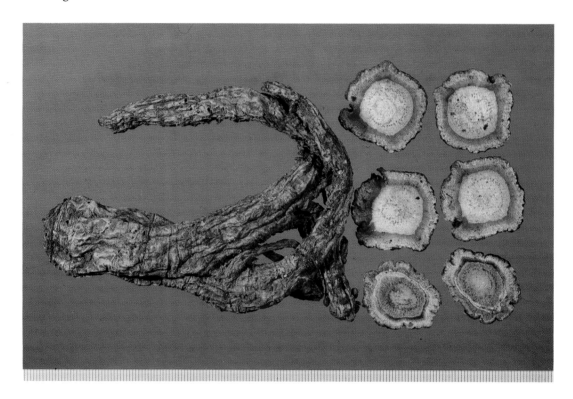

Angelicae Laxiflorae Radix: crude (left) and sliced (right). (× 5/6)

24   ANGELICAE LAXIFLORAE RADIX (ANGELICAE TUHUO RADIX)

川獨活 *chuan¹ du² huo²*. English: angelica laxiflora (or tuhuo angelica root.) Japanese: *sendokkatsu*.

Origin: Umbelliferae family. *Angelica laxiflora* Diels, *A. pubescens* Maxim.,* *A. porphyrocaulis* Nakai et Kitag.,* *Heracleum hemsleyanum* Diels.,* *H. lanatum* Michx.,* *Aralia cordata* Thunb.*

Characters: *Angelica laxiflora* is the most common type of *du² huo²* used. Its dried root is spindle-shaped, 5–10 cm long, and 1.5–3 cm thick. There is a scar left by the stem at the head. The exterior surface is a yellow brown, with irregular wrinkles, and sparse lenticels located on tumorous protuberances. It easily snaps to reveal a pale yellow-brown interior. The decocting pieces are transverse slices 1.5 mm thick. On their cut edge are clear annular markings.

Quality: Hard, solid, farinaceous roots with a strong aroma are best.

Production areas: China (Hubei and Sichuan).

Properties and actions: Warm; bitter, acrid; nontoxic. Enters the kidney and bladder channels. Dispels wind, percolates damp, dissipates cold and relieves pain.

Indications: Wind-cold-damp bi, especially damp bi of the lower limbs; painful, swollen knees; hypertonicity of the limbs. Daily dosage: 3–5 g. Contraindicated in effulgent yin vacuity fire and in high fever without aversion to cold. Used in *du²-huo² ji⁴-sheng¹ tang¹* (Duhuo and Mistletoe Decoction, 73).

Remarks: Constituents: Coumarins: bergapten, umbelliferone, angelol, columbianetin, columbianentin acetate, columbianadin.

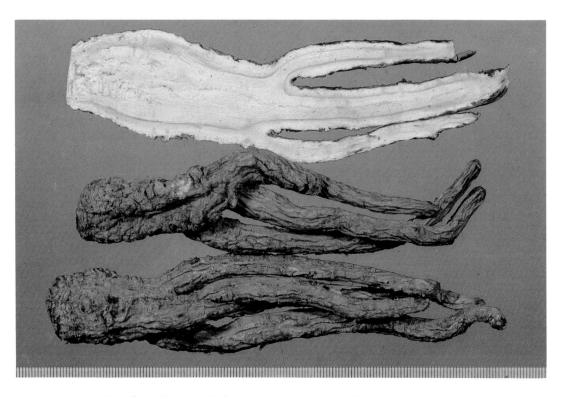

Angelicae Sinensis Radix: crude (bottom) and sliced (above). (× 5/6)

25 ANGELICAE SINENSIS RADIX

當歸 *dang¹ gui¹*. English: tangkuei (or Chinese angelica) root. Japanese: *tōki*.

Alternate name: 乾歸 *gan¹ gui¹*.

Origin: Umbellliferae family. *Angelica sinensis* (Oliv.) Diels.

Characters: The main root is short, with ten or more finer roots branching from its extremity, each of which is more or less the same length. The entire root is about 15–25 cm long, and about 2–3.5 cm thick at the head. The outer surface is middle brown, with irregular wrinkles. The flesh is yellow or pale brown. The decocting pieces are transverse, oblique, or longitudinal slices about 0.5–1 mm thick. They are pale yellow on the cross section. The branch roots are cut in transverse or oblique slices that have irregular margins. Annular markings are clear on the transverse slices.

Quality: A large, fat main root, pale flesh, and strong smell are the signs of superior quality.

Production areas: China (Gansu, Yunnan, Shaanxi, Guizhou, Sichuan, and Hubei).

Properties and actions: Warm; sweet, acrid; nontoxic. Enters the heart, liver, and spleen channels. Supplements and harmonizes the blood, regulates menstruation, relieves pain, moistens dryness, and lubricates the intestines. The head staunches bleeding; the body nourishes the blood, and the ''tails'' (branch roots) move the blood. The whole root is used to harmonize the blood. Angelica Sinensis supplements the blood and moistens the intestines when used crude, frees the channels and quickens the blood when treated with wine, and has a greater intestine-moistening power when mix-fried with honey.

Indications: Menstrual irregularities, menstrual pain, uterine bleeding, bi, impact injury, yong and ju, and blood vacuity constipation. Daily dosage: 5–10 g. Contraindicated in spleen damp. Used in *si⁴ wu⁴ tang¹* (Four Agents Decoction, 256), *dang¹-gui¹ shao¹-yao⁴ san³* (Tangkuei and Peony Powder, 60), *dang¹-gui¹ jian⁴ zhong¹ tang¹* (Tangkuei Center-Fortifying Decoction, 57).

Remarks: Constituents: Voltaile oil(0.1–0.3%): ligustilide, *n*-butylidenephthalide, *n*-butylphthalide, *n*-valero-phenone-O-carboxylic acid.

Allied drugs: Dried root of *Angelica acutiloba* Kitagawa (Japan); *A. gigas* Nakai (Korea).

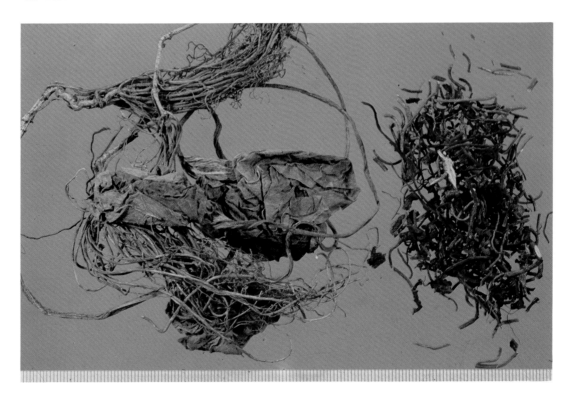

Asiasari Radix: crude (left) and sliced (right). (× 1)

26 ASIASARI RADIX (ASARI RADIX)

細辛 *xi⁴ xin¹*. English: asiasarum (or asarum) root. Japanese: *saishin*.
Alternate names: 小辛 *xiao³ xin¹*, 少辛 *shao⁴ xin¹*.
Origin: Aristolochiaceae family. *Asiasarum heterotropoides* F. Schm. var. *mandshuricum* (Maxim.) Kitag. [= *Asarum heteropoides* F. Schm. var. *mandshuricum* Kitag.], *Asarum sieboldii* Miq., *A. forbesii* Maxim.,* *A. maximum* Hemsl.,* *A. geophilum* Hemsl.,* *A. caudigerum* Hance,* *A. himalacicum* Hook. f. et Thoms.,* *A. longiflorum* C.Y. Cheng et C.S. Yang,* *A. insigne* Diels.*
Characters: The dried plant consists of up to three gray-green shrivelled cordate leaves mounted on long petioles. The rhizome is an irregular cylindrical shape, 1–4 cm long, 2–3 mm thick, sometimes with branches. Numerous yellow-brown cylindrical roots, 5–10 cm long, and 1 mm thick, with short branches spring from the lower side of the rhizome. The plant is cut into 1–3 cm lengths. The decocting pieces are sections 1–3 cm in length, appearing white on the cut edge.
Quality: Large leaves and absence of earth are signs of good quality.
Production areas: China (Liaoning, Jilin, and less importantly Shaanxi and Gansu).
Properties and actions: Warm; acrid; nontoxic. Enters the lung and kidney channels. Dispels wind, dissipates cold, moves water, and opens the portals.
Indications: Wind-cold headache; deep-source nasal congestion; toothache; phlegm-rheum; counterflow cough; wind-damp bi pain. Daily dosage: 1–3 g. Contraindicated in qi vacuity sweating, blood vacuity headache, and yin vacuity cough. Used in *xiao³ qing¹ long² tang¹* (Minor Green-Blue Dragon Decoction, 302), *ma²-huang² fu⁴-zi³ xi⁴-xin¹ tang¹* (Ephedra, Aconite, and Asarum Decoction, 174), *dang¹-gui¹ si⁴ ni⁴ tang¹* (Tangkuei Counterflow Frigidity Decoction, 62).
Remarks: Constituents: Phenylpropanoids and monoterpenoids (volatile oil 2.5–5.5%); methyleugenol, safrole, elemicin; α-, β-pinenes, eucarvone.

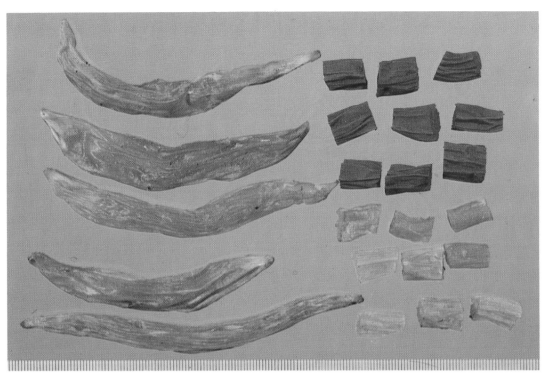

Asparagi Tuber: crude (left); treated with cinnabar (top right); cut (bottom right). (×5/6)

27 ASPARAGI TUBER

天門冬 *tian¹ men² dong¹*. English: (Chinese) asparagus tuber. Japanese: *tenmondo*.
Alternate name:天冬 *tian¹ dong¹*.
Origin: Liliaceae family. *Asparagus cochinchinensis* (Lour). Merr. [= *A. lucidus* Lindley].
Characters: The tuber is cylindrical or spindle-shaped, sometimes slightly contorted. It is 4–10 cm long, and 0.5–1.5 cm in diameter. Its surface is pale yellow, glossy, and semitranslucent, bearing irregular wrinkles of varying depth. Its flesh is whiter than the surface, and is sticky. The decocting pieces are short sections about 1.5–2 cm long.
Quality: Large, full, shiny, light-colored tubers with sticky flesh are the best quality.
Production areas: China (Guizhou, Yunnan, and Sichuan, and less importantly Jiangsu, Anhui, and Guangxi).
Properties and actions: Cold; sweet and bitter; nontoxic. Enters the lung and kidney channels. Enriches yin and moistens dryness; clears the lung and downbears fire. Mix-frying with honey enhances the lung-moistening and cough-suppressing action. Coating in cinnabar adds a spirit-quieting action.
Indications: Yin vacuity fever; cough; blood ejection; pulmonary atony; pulmonary yong; sore, swollen throat; wasting thirst; constipation. Daily dosage: 1.5–10 g. Contraindicated in spleen-stomach vacuity cold with diarrhea. Used in *zi¹ yin¹ jiang⁴ huo³ tang¹* (Yin-Enriching Fire-Downbearing Decoction, 351), *da⁴ zao⁴ wan²* (Greatly Supplementing Pills, 55), *gan¹ lu⁴ yin³* (Sweet Dew Beverage, 96), *di⁴-huang² yin³ zi³* (Rehmannia Drink, 68) *huang²-qi² bie¹-jia³ san³* (Astragalus and Turtle Shell Powder, 132), *zhen⁴ gan¹ xi² feng¹ tang¹* (Liver-Settling Wind-Extinguishing Decoction, 336).
Remarks: Constituents: mucilage, aspargine, β-sitosterol.
Similar plants: *Asparagus meioclados* Lévl.; *A. racemosus* Willd.

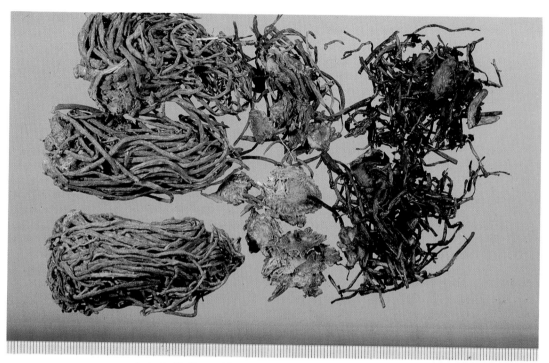

**Asteris Radix et Rhizoma: crude (left); cut (middle);
stir-fried with honey (right). (× 5/6)**

28 ASTERIS RADIX ET RHIZOMA

紫菀 *zi³ wan³*. English: aster root. Japanese: *shion*.

Alternate names: 紫蒨 *zi³ qian⁴*, 青菀 *qing¹ wan³*.

Origin: Compositae family. *Aster tataricus* L. f., *A. souliei* Franch.,* *A. diplostephioides* (DC.) C.B. Clarke,* *Ligularia fischeri* (Ledeb.) Turcz.,* *L. sibirica* (L.) Cass,* *L. intermedia* Nakai,* *L. hodgsoni* Hook var. *sutchuenensis* (Franch.) Henry,* *L. macrophylla* (Ledeb.) DC.,* *L. przewalskii* (Maxim.) Diels.

Characters: This product comprises numerous supple, wrinkled, brown roots, 6–15 cm long and 1.5–2 mm thick, with flesh slightly darker than the surface, springing from a gray-brown rhizome that is smoother than the roots, varies from 1 to 7 cm in length and from 1 to 5 mm in thickness, and bears leaf bases on its upper extremity. The decocting pieces are 1.5 cm lengths that are brown on the cut edge.

Quality: Dry, thick, long, tidy roots that are clean of earth are the best.

Production areas: China (cultivated in Northeast, Hebei, and Anhui).

Properties and actions: Warm; bitter; nontoxic. Enters the lung channel. Warms the lung, precipitates qi, disperses phlegm, and suppresses cough. Use crude to diffuse the lung and disperse phlegm. Stir-fry for stronger lung-warming action. Mix-fry with honey for greater lung-moistening action.

Indications: Wind-cold cough and dyspnea; coughing of blood and pus in vacuity taxation; throat bi; inhibited urination. Daily dosage: 5–10 g. Contraindicated in yin vacuity lung heat. Used in *zi³-wan³ san³* (Aster Powder, 353), *zhi³ sou⁴ san³*, (Cough Powder, 343).

Remarks: Constituents: astersaponin, shionone, quercetin.

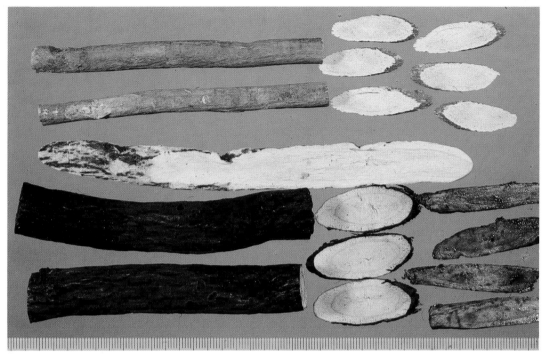

Jin qi *(Hedysarum mongholicum)* crude and sliced (top);
black-skinned Astragali Radix crude and honey-fried slices (bottom). (×3/4)

29 ASTRAGALI RADIX (1)

黄耆 *huang² qi²*   English: astragalus root. Japanese: *ogi.*

Alternate names: 晉耆 *jin⁴ qi²*, 黃芪 *huang² qi²*, 綿黃耆 *mian² huang² qi².*

Origin: Leguminosae family. *Astragalus membranaceus* (Fisch.) Bge., *A. mongholicus* Bge., *Hedysarum mongholicum* Turcz. [= *H. polybotrys* Hand.-Mazz.], *Astragalus tongolensis* Ulbr.,* *A. tibetanus* Benth. ex Bge.,* *A. yunnanensis* Franch.,* *A. camptodontus* Franch.,* *A. aksuensis* Bge.,* *A. chrysopterus* Bg.*

Characters: The roots are cylindrical in shape, 20 to 40 or sometimes 60 cm in length and from 0.6 to 2.5, and sometimes even 4 cm in thickness. Their outer surface is gray-brown, and they bulge slightly at the head. They may bear wrinkles, horizontal lenticels, and the marks of removed finer roots. The skin of thicker roots is easily removed revealing a reticular fiber structure. The flesh is hard and crisp, and snaps easily. It is a yellowish white, and lighter in the woodier parts. The decocting pieces are transverse or oblique slices 1 mm thick, showing annular markings on the cut edge.

Quality: The best roots are long, dry, and unwrinkled, and have no black or hollow core. They are supple and resist snapping, and have a floury texture.

Production areas: *Astragalus membranaceus*: China (Heilongjiang, Shanxi, Hebei, Shandong, Shaanxi, Gansu, and Inner Mongolia). *A. mongholicus*: China (Jilin, Hebei, Xinjiang, Shanxi, Inner Mongolia *H. mongholicum:* China (Mancharia, Inner Mongolia, Shaanxi, southern Gansu).

Remarks: Constituents: *A. membranaceus:* Triterpenoids; (saponins) astragalosides I, II, III, IV, V, VI, VII, VII, VIII, acetylastragaloside I, isoastragalosides I. II. Steroids: β-sitosterol. Flavonoids: kumatakenin, formononetin, calycosin. Amines: choline. Amino acids: α-aminobutyric acid (0.024–0.036%); betaine. Saccharides: sucrose.

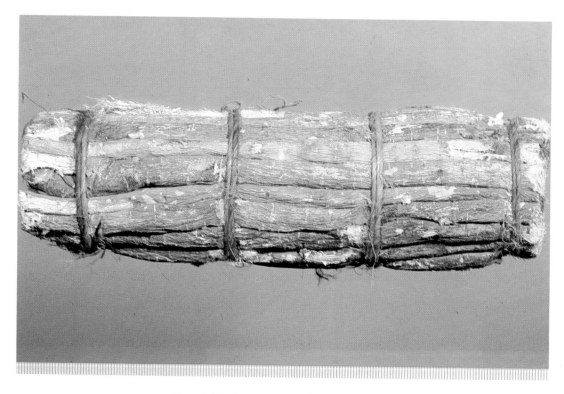

Jin qi (*Hedysarum mongholicum*). (×5/6)

30 ASTRAGALI RADIX(2)

黄耆(Cont.) *huang² qi²*. English: astragalus root. Japanese: *ogi*.

Characters: Black-skinned astragalus is *A. mongholicus* dyed with the decocted fluid of *Koelreuteria paniculata* (*wu¹ la¹ ye⁴*). The outer skin is gray-black in color, and is loose. The firmer interior wood is deep yellow, with pronounced medullary rays. White-skinned astragalus has a pale yellow-brown skin tightly attached to the wood. The cross section shows a pale outer layer surrounding a deep yellow central core. Jin qi, the root of *Hedysarum mongholicum*, is mostly produced in southern Gansu province and has a reddish skin and a white, farinaceous core.

Properties and actions: Slightly warm; sweet; nontoxic. Enters the lung and spleen channels. Boosts defense qi and secures the exterior; disinhibits water and disperses swelling; expels sore toxin and engenders flesh; supplements the center and boosts qi. Use crude both to promote and check sweating according to need. Use mix-fried with honey to supplement the center, boost original qi, warm the triple burner, and strengthen the stomach and spleen.

Indications: Spontaneous external bleeding; night sweating; blood bi; water swelling; persistent yong and ju. Daily dosage: 5–10 g. Contraindicated in repletion patterns and yang exuberance due to yin vacuity. used in *fang²-ji³ huang²-qi² tang¹* (Fangji and Astragalus Decoction, 85), *huang²-qi² gui⁴-zhi¹ wu³ wu⁴ tang¹* (Astragalus and Cinnamon Twig Five Agents Decoction, 133), *huang²-qi² jian⁴ zhong¹ tang¹* (Astragalus Center-Fortifying Decoction, 134), *yu⁴ ping² feng¹ san³* (Jade Wind-Barrier Powder, 327), *gui⁴-zhi¹ jia¹ huang²-qi² tang¹* (Cinnamon Twig Decoction Plus Astragalus, 111).

Remarks: Constituents: *A. mongholicus*: Steroids: β-sitosterol. Flavonoids: isorhamnetin, rhamnocitrin, formononetin, calycosin, 3′-hydroxy-formononetin, 7,3′-dihydroxy-4′,5′-dimethoxy-isoflavane, 7-hydroxy-3′4′-dimethoxy-pterocarpan-7-0-glucoside, 3-hydoxy-9,10-dimethoxy-pterocarpan, isoliquiritigenin.

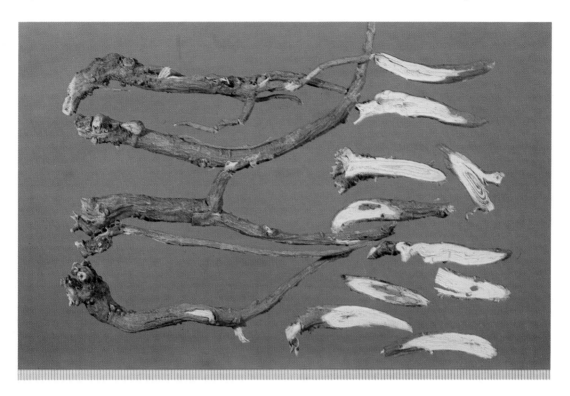

Bupleuri Radix: crude (left) and sliced (right). (× 5/6)

31 BUPLEURI RADIX

柴胡chai² hu². English: bupleurum (or hare's ear) root. Japanese: *saiko*.

Alternate name:茈胡*chai² hu²*.

Origin: Umbelliferae family. *Bupleurum chinense* DC., *B. scorzoneraefolium* Willd.

Characters: The roots are long and contorted, 5–10 cm long and 0.6–1.5 cm, sometimes with branch roots. The head of the root has the remains of leafstalks. The skin is brown with marked transverse creases near the head. The lower half of the root has irregular lengthwise wrinkles. Any branch roots are usually removed. Bupleurum root is light and brittle, and snaps to reveal a pale brown and white wood. It is cut into fine slices, which clearly reveal the medullary rays and the layered quality of the wood.

Quality: Good quality roots are long and thick, without any fine roots. They should be pale in color, slightly aromatic, and have a slightly bitter flavor.

Production areas: *Bupleurum chinense:* China (Liaoning, Gansu, Hebei, and Henan); *B. scorzoneraefolium:* China (Hubei, Jiangsi, and Sichuan).

Properties and actions: Cold; bitter; nontoxic. Enters the liver and gallbladder channels. Harmonizes exterior and interior, courses the liver, and upbears yang. Use crude for strong exterior-resolving action. Stir-fry to moderate the effusing and dissipating action. Mix-fry with honey for greater center-supplementing, lung-moistening, and cough-suppressing action. Prepare with wine to move the blood and free the channels. Prepare with vinegar to soothe the liver, quicken the blood, and relieve pain. Stir-fry in turtle's blood for greater yin-supplementing action.

Indications: Alternating fever and chills; thoracic fullness; pain in the lateral costal region; bitter taste in the mouth; deafness; headache and dizziness; malarial and dysenteric disease; menstrual irregularities; prolapse of the uterus. Daily dosage: 3–5 g. Contraindicated in intense yin vacuity fire. Used in *xiao³ chai²-hu² tang¹* (Minor Bupleurum Decoction, 298), *xiao¹ yao² san³* (Free Wanderer Powder, 296), *da⁴ chai²-hu² tang¹* (Major Bupleurum Decoction, 45), *chai²-hu² gui⁴-zhi¹ tang¹* (Bupleurum and Cinnamon Twig Decoction, 37).

Remarks: Constituents: Triterpenoids: (saponins, ca. 3%), saikosaponins a, c, d, e, acetylsaikosaponins 1, 2, 3. Steroids (ca. 0.07%): α-spinasterol, stigmasterol, stigmast-7-enol, stigmast-22-enol. Allied drugs: Dried root of *Bupleurum falcatum* L. (Japan).

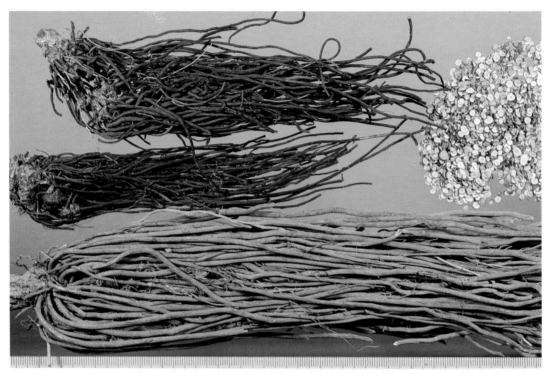

Clematidis Radix: crude (top left) and cut (top right); type grown
in Taiwan (bottom). (× 3/5)

32 CLEMATIDIS RADIX

威靈仙 *wei¹ ling² xian¹*. English: (Chinese) clematis root. Japanese: *ireisen*.

Alternate names: 鐵靈仙 *tie³ ling² xian¹*, 靈仙藤 *ling² xian¹ teng²*.

Origin: Ranunculaceae family. *Clematis chinensis* Osbeck, *C. hexapetala* Pall.,* *C. armandi*
Franch.,* *C. uncinata* Champ. ex Benth.,* *C. meyeniana* Walp.,* *C. henryi* Oliv.,* *C. finetiana*
Levl. et Vant.,* *C. manshurica* Rupr.,* *C. paniculata* Thunb.,*

Characters: This product is composed of numerous roots springing from a transversely growing
root tuber. The roots are slightly contorted and cylindrical, 10–20 cm long and 1–2 mm thick.
They are dark brown in color and bear fine longitudinal wrinkles. They are dark brown in color,
and snap easily to reveal the yellow wood. They have a slightly fetid smell. The tuber is cylindrical, 1.5–3.5 cm in length, and 2.5 cm thick, its skin often peeling away to reveal a fibrous interior. At the top end are the remains of a woody stem. The decocting pieces are fine transverse
slices.

Quality: Superior quality roots are clean, long, firm, and dark in color. They should be attached
to a tuber, but the tuber is best if there is no remains of the stem.

Production areas: China (all provinces of the Northeast, Anhui, Zhejiang, and Jiangsu).

Properties and actions: Warm; acrid, salty; toxic. Enters the bladder channels. Dispels wind-
damp, frees the channels, disperses phlegm, and dissipates elusive masses. Prepare with wine
to dispel wind and free the channels.

Indications: Cold pain in the lumbus and knees; leg qi; stubborn xian; gout; malarial disease;
concretions and gatherings; tetanus; tonsillitis; bones stuck in the throat. Daily dosage: 3–10 g.
Contraindicated in hypertonicity of the sinews due to blood vacuity, and pathogen repletion patterns without wind-damp. Used in *shu¹ jin¹ li⁴ an¹ san³*. (Sinew-Soothing Peace-Bringing Powder,
248).

Remarks: Constituents: saponin, anemonin.

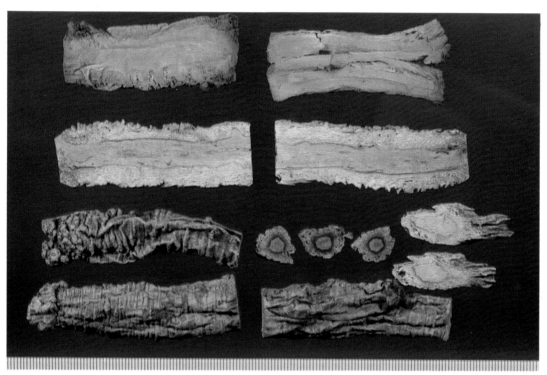

Codonopsitis Radix: longitudinal slices stir-fried in earth (top);
crude, longitudinal slices (middle); crude uncut lengths, transverse
and oblique slices (bottom). (×6/7)

33 CODONOPSITIS RADIX

黨參 *dang³ shen¹*. English: codonopsis root. Japanese: *tojin*.

Alternate names: 川黨 *chuan¹ dang³*, 潞黨 *lu⁴ dang³*.

Origin: Campanulaceae family. *Codonopsis pilosula* (Franch.) Nannf., *C. tubulosa* Kom.,* *C. viridiflora* Maxim,* *C. tsinlingensis* Pax. et Kin. Hoffm.,* *C. clematidea* (Schrenk.) Clarke,* *C. nervosa* (Chipp.) Nannf.*

Characters: The roots are cylindrical, though have sometimes been flattened. They are roughly 1.5 cm thick, and may be up to 30 cm long. The outer surface is an earth brown or dark brown, and bears irregular, deep furrows. The head of the root bears the dense scars left by the stalk and shoots, and close to the head are dense transverse creases that grow scarcer further down. The roots often have breaks in the skin. They are light and supple, and snap with difficulty to reveal a rough fracture that is whitish in color. They are cut into fine transverse or oblique slices, or into sections that are then sliced lengthwise. The skin accounts for the greater part of the cross section. Slices that are stir-fried in earth are golden brown.

Quality: The best roots are clean, long, and of even thickness, and are sweet to the taste. The heads should be small and the skin should be a light, fresh color.

Production areas: China (cultivated with Shanxi, Ṣhaanxi, Gansu, Manchuria).

Properties and actions: Balanced; sweet; nontoxic. Enters the lung and spleen channels. Supplements the center, boosts qi and engenders liquid.

Indications: Spleen-stomach vacuity; dual depletion of qi and blood; fatigue and lack of strength; low food intake; thirst; enduring diarrhea; prolapse of the rectum. Daily dosage: 5–10 g. Contraindicated in pathogen repletion patterns. Used in *da⁴ jian⁴ zhong¹ tang¹* (Major Center-Fortifying Decoction, 51), *si⁴ jun¹ zi³ tang¹* (Four Gentlemen Decoction, 251), *sheng¹ mai⁴ san³* (Pulse-Engendering Powder, 239), *qiong² yu⁴ gao¹* (Fine Jade Paste, 212), *shi² quan² da⁴ bu³ tang¹* (Perfect Major Supplementation Decoction, 243).

Remarks: Constituents: atractylenolids II, III; tangshenoside I, II; (Z)-3-hexenyl-β-D-glucopyranoside, (E)-2-hexenyl-β-D-glucopyranoside.

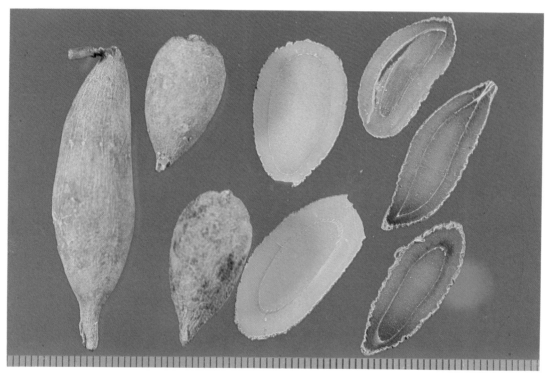

Curcumae Tuber (left to right): *Curcuma aromatica; Curcuma longa;*
crude slices; slices treated with vinegar. (× 5/3)

34 CURCUMAE TUBER

鬱金 *yu⁴ jin¹*. English: curcuma tuber. Japanese: *ukon*.

Alternate names: 郁金 *yu⁴ jin¹*.

Origin: Zingiberaceae family. *Curcuma aromatica* Salisb., *C. longa* L. [= *C. domestica* Valeton],
C. zedoaria (Berg.) Rosc.*

Characters: The main tubers are roughly 6 cm long and roughly 3 cm wide, while branches or
"fingers" are smaller. Both are grayish brown in color and ovate in shape. They are hard, and
break with difficulty to reveal a smooth, yellow or reddish fracture. The decocting pieces are fine
transverse, oblique, or longitudinal slices that are slightly translucent. A clear line separates the
skin from the central core.

Quality: The best tubers are hard, and yellowish on the inside.

Production areas: *Curcuma longa*: China (Sichuan); *C. aromatica*: China (Zhejiang).

Properties and actions: Cold; acrid, bitter; nontoxic. Enters the heart, lung, and liver channels. Moves qi and resolves depression; cools the blood and breaks stasis. Use crude to move qi
and resolve depression, to cool the blood and break stasis. Stir-fry to reduce the cold, bitter properties. Stir-fry with vinegar to treat upward surge of qi and blood. Stir-fry with wine to enhance
the qi-moving action.

Indications: Pain in the chest, abdomen, and lateral costal region; mania and withdrawal; clouding
of the spirit in febrile disease; blood ejection; spontaneous external bleeding; blood in the urine;
blood strangury; vicarious menstruation; jaundice. Daily dosage: 5–10 g. contraindicated in yin
vacuity without stasis and stagnation, and in pregnancy. Used in *yu⁴-jin¹ san³* (Curcuma Powder,
325), *an¹ gong¹ niu²-huang² wan²* (Peaceful Palace Bovine Bezoar Pills, 1), *bai² jin¹ wan²* (Alum
and Curcuma Pills, 15), *yu⁴-jin¹ yin³ zi³* (Curcuma Drink, 326).

Remarks: Constituents: Curcuminoids (0.3–48%): curcumin (0.8–5.4%), dihydrocurcumin, di-*p*-
coumaroylmethane, *p*-coumaroylferuloylmethane. Sesquiterpenoids and monoterpenoids (volatile
oil, curcuma oil, 1–6%): turmerone (58%), dehydroturmerone, zingiberene (25%).

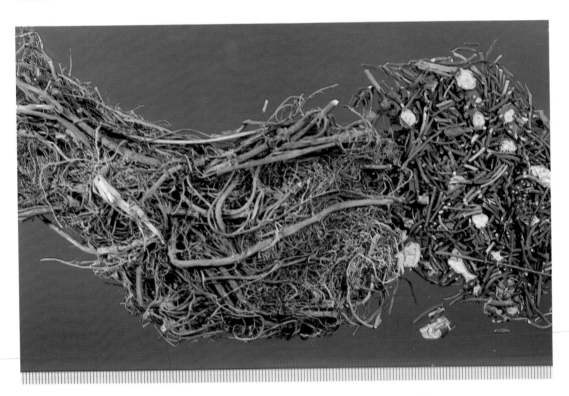

Cynanchi Radix: crude (left) and sliced (right). (×6/7)

35 CYNANCHI RADIX

白薇 *bai² wei²*. English: (cynanchum) bai wei root, swallow wort. Japanese: *byakubi.*
Alternate names: 白微 *bai² wei²*, 香白薇 *xiang¹ bai² wei²*.
Origin: Asclepiadaceae family. *Cynanchum atratum Bge., C. versicolor* Bge.
Characters: This product takes the form of multiple roots attached to the extremity of a small rhizome. The rhizome is noded, with a rounded head bearing the scar of the removed stem. The roots are fine and cylindrical, and often contorted. They are earth brown in color, and 10–16 cm long, and roughly 1.5 mm in diameter. They break easily, revealing a whitish yellow interior, with a darker woody core. The crude materials are roughly cut into 2–3 mm lengths. The best quality is yellow in color, with unbroken roots.
Production areas: China (Shandong, Liaoning, Anhui).
Properties and actions: Cold; bitter and salty; nontoxic. Enters the lung, stomach, and kidney channels. Use crude to clear heat and cool the blood. Use mix-fried with honey for external contraction with fever, cough, and dyspnea.
Indications: Yin vacuity heat; wind warmth with high fever and tendency to sleep; lung heat and coughing of blood; warm malaria; postpartum vacuity vexation and blood inversion; heat and blood strangury; rheumatic pain; scrofulous lumps. Daily dosage: 5–10 g. Contraindicated in the absence of heat in the blood aspect and center cold with diarrhea. Used in *bai²-wei² tang¹* (Baiwei Decoction, 17).
Remarks: Constituents: Cardiotonic glycosides.

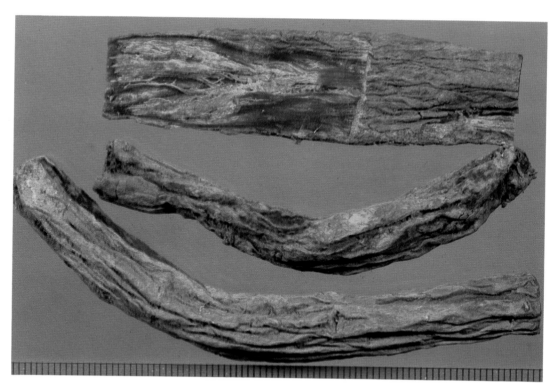

Dipsaci Radix: crude (bottom) and in fine slices (above). (× 5/3)

36 DIPSACI RADIX

續斷 *xu⁴ duan⁴*. English: dipsacus (or Japanese teasel) root. Japanese: *zokudan*.
Alternate names: 川續斷 *chuan¹ xu⁴ duan⁴*, 六汗 *liu⁴ han⁴*.
Origin: Dipsacaceae family. *Dipsacus asper* Wall., *D. japonicus* Miq. *
Characters: The roots are cylindrical, of varying length, and 0.4–1 cm in diameter. Their surface is earth brown in color, and bears longitudinal wrinkles or furrows and transversely configured lenticels 2–4 mm in length. They are soft and supple, and break with difficulty to reveal an uneven fracture. The decocting pieces are oblique slices or longitudinal slices of short sections.
Quality: Dry, fat roots with sticky, but not stringy flesh that has a slightly green tinge are the best.
Production areas: China (Hubei, Sichuan, Hunan, Guizhou, Shaanxi, Yunnan).
Properties and actions: Slightly warm; bitter, acrid; nontoxic. Enters the liver and kidney channels. Supplements the liver and kidney, joins sinew and bones, and regulates the blood vessels.
Indications: Aching pain in the lumbus and back; lack of strength in the knees and foot; uterine bleeding in pregnancy; profuse uterine bleeding and vaginal discharge; seminal emission; impact injuries; incised wounds; hemorrhoids and fistulae; yong, ju, and sores. Stir-fry to treat uterine bleeding. Mix-fry with brine for lower burner patterns (stirring fetus, and precipitation of blood). Daily dosage: 5–10 g. Contraindicated in intense yin vacuity fire. Used in *xu⁴-duan⁴ wan²* (Dipsacus Pills, 309).
Remarks: Constituents: Alkaloids. Volatile oil.
Allied drug: Root of *Dipsacus chinensis* Bat.

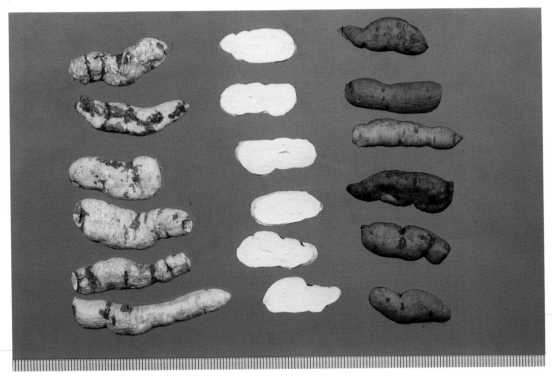

Euphorbiae Kansui Radix: crude (left); treated with vinegar (middle); roasted (right). (× 5/6)

37 EUPHORBIAE KANSUI RADIX

甘遂 *gan¹ sui⁴*. English: kansui root. Japanese: *kansui.*

Alternate names: 甘澤 *gan¹ ze²*, 重澤 *chong² ze²*.

Origin: Euphorbiaceae family. *Euphorbia kansui* Liou.

Characters: The root is composed of a series of globular, spindle-shaped, or oval sections 3–9 cm long and 0.6–1.5 cm in diameter. It has fibrous roots that have usually been removed. The skin is pale brown. Cut into transverse or oblique slices, the white, farinaceous flesh is revealed.

Quality: Dry, fat, farinaceous roots are the best.

Production areas: China (Shaanxi, Shandong, Gansu, Henan).

Properties and actions: Cold; bitter and sweet; toxic. Enters the spleen, lung, and kidney channels. Drains water-yin, breaks accumulations and gatherings, frees the urine and stool. Stir-frying with vinegar, roasting, and boiling with beancurd (tofu) reduces toxicity. Boiling with Glycyrrhizae Radix (*gan¹ cao³*) and Platycodonis Radix (*jie² geng³*) reduces the side-effect of vomiting.

Indications: Water swelling; phlegm-rheum; chest bind; mania and withdrawal; esophageal constriction; concretions, conglomerations, accumulations, and gatherings; urinary and fecal stoppage. Daily dosage: 1.5–3 g. Contraindicated for pregnant women and weak patients. Used in *shi² zao³ tang¹* (Ten Jujubes Decoction, 245), *da⁴-huang² gan¹-sui⁴ tang¹* (Rhubarb and Kansui Decoction, 49), *kong⁴ xian² dan¹* (Drool-Controlling Elixir, 159), *da⁴ xian⁴ xiong¹ tang¹* (Major Chest Bind Decoction, 54).

Remarks: Constituents: tirucallol (= kanzuiol), α-euphol, α-euphorbol, 20-*epi*-euphol.

Similar plants: *Euphorbia pekinensis* Ruprecht, *E. formosana* Hayata (Taiwan).

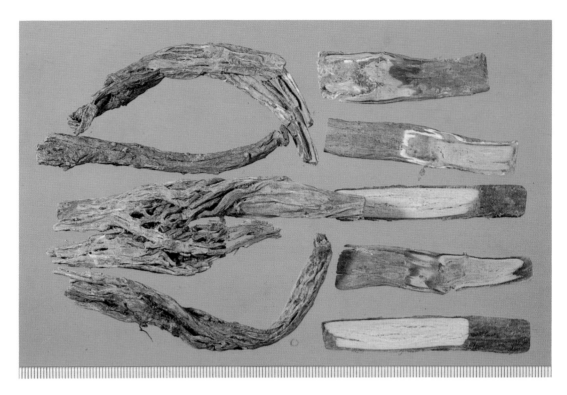

Gentianae Macrophyllae Radix: crude and sliced. (× 5/6)

38 GENTIANAE MACROPHYLLAE RADIX

秦艽 *qin² jiao¹*. English: macrophylla root. Japanese: *jingyō.*

Alternate names: 大艽 *da⁴ jiao¹*, 秦艽王 *qin² jiao¹ wang².*

Origin: Gentianaceae family. *Gentiana macrophylla* Pall., *G. crassicaulis* Duthie ex Burkill,* *G. tibetica* King,* *G. straminea* Maxim.*

Characters: The root is cylindrical and slightly contorted, 6–20 cm long, and roughly 0.5–1 cm thick at the top. The exterior surface is a yellowish brown, with pronounced furrows. At the head are the remains of the leafstalk bases. There are many branch roots that branch again into fine roots, but these have often been removed, Macrophylla root is supple, and breaks with difficulty to leave an uneven fracture. The decocting pieces are oblique slices about 1 mm thick, on whose cut edge the skin is seen to be darker than the wood.

Quality: Large, fat, dry, oleaceous roots with short heads stem base are the best.

Production areas: China (Gansu, Shaanxi, Shanxi, Inner Mongolia).

Properties and actions: Balanced; acrid, bitter; nontoxic. Enters the liver, stomach, and gallbladder channels. Dispels wind and eliminates damp; harmonizes the blood and soothes the sinews; clears heat and disinhibits urine.

Indications: Wind-damp bi pain; hypertonicity of the sinews and bones; jaundice; blood in the stool; steaming bone tidal fever; child gan heat; inhibited urination. Daily dosage: 5–10 g. Contraindicated in persistent pain in the limbs due to inability of qi and blood to provide adequate nourishment. Used in *qin²-jiao¹ bie¹-jia³ san³* (Macrophylla and Turtle Shell Powder, 205), *da⁴ qin²-jiao¹ tang¹* (Macrophylla Decoction, 52).

Remarks: Constituents: Alkaloids: gentianine A, B, C. Volatile oils. Saccharides.

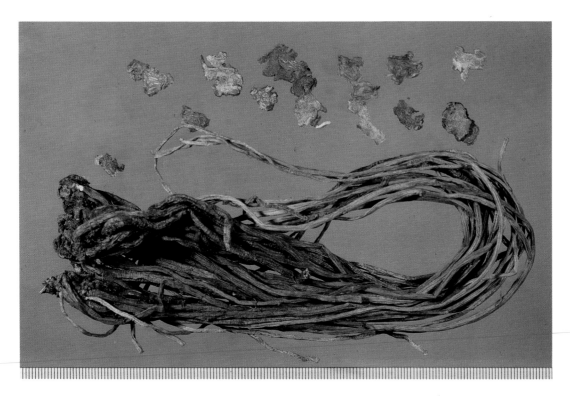

Gentianae Scabrae Radix: crude (bottom) and sliced (above). (× 5/6)

39 GENTIANAE SCABRAE RADIX (GENTIANAE RADIX)

龍膽 *long² dan³*. English: (Chinese) gentian root. Japanese: *ryūtan.*

Alternate names: 草龍膽 *cao³ long² dan³*, 龍膽草 *long² dan³ cao³*.

Origin: Gentianaceae family. *Gentiana scabra* Bge., *G. triflora* Pall.,* *G. manshurica* Kitag.,* *G. rigescens* Franch.,* *G. rigescens* Franch. var. *stictantha* Marquand,* *Gentianopsis paludosa* (Munro) Ma.*

Characters: This product is composed of multiple roots attached to both sides and extremity of a rhizome. The rhizome is 1-2 cm long and 4-7 mm thick, and is pale brown with regular annular creases. At the end are the remains of the stalk or the scar left after its removal. The roots are 10-20 cm long and about 2 mm thick. They are pale brown or grayish brown on the outside, bearing fine longitudinal creases and scant transverse creases. They are supple and not easily broken. The decocting pieces, 1 mm thick transverse slices, show clearly the spongy appearance of the woody core.

Quality: Fat, dry, supple roots that bear a deep yellow hue are best.

Production areas: China (Heilongjiang, Jilin, Liaoning, Inner Mongolia, Hebei, Shandong, Jiangsu, Anhui, Zhejiang, Fujian, Jiangxi, Hunan, Hubei, Guizhou, Sichuan, Guangdong, Guangxi).

Properties and actions: Cold; bitter; nontoxic. Enters the liver and gallbladder channels. Drains liver-stomach repletion fire; eliminates lower burner damp-heat. Use crude to make it act on the lower body, and stir-fry with wine to make it act on the upper body. Stir-fry with honey to make it act on the middle burner. Stir-fry with pig's bile to enhance the fire-downbearing action.

Indications: Exuberant heat in the liver channel; fright epilepsy; manic agitation; encephalitis B; headache; reddening of the eyes; sore throat; jaundice; heat dysentery; swollen yong and sores; painful swelling of the scrotum; genital damp itch. Daily dosage: 3-5 g. Contraindicated in spleen-stomach vacuity diarrhea, and in repletion fire patterns without cold-damp. Used in *long²-dan³ xie⁴ gan¹ tang¹* (Gentian Liver-Draining Decoction, 172), *dang¹-gui¹ long² hui⁴ wan²* (Tangkuei, Gentian, and Aloe Pills, 58).

Remarks: Constituents: Iridoids: gentiopicrin (gentiopicroside, 0.35-4%; 7-10% in fresh root), swertiamarin. Xanthones: gentisin. Alkaloids: gentianine (0.05%). Saccharides: gentianose, sucrose.

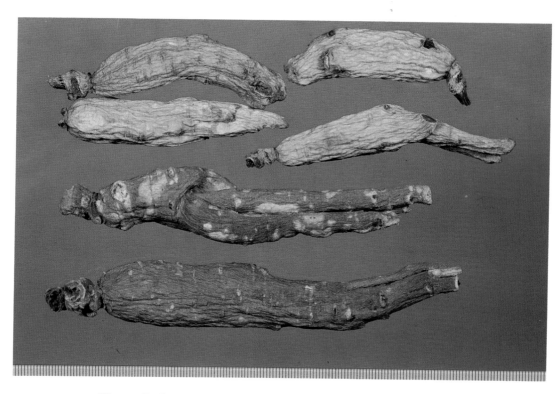

Ginseng Radix: Korean white (bottom); Japanese white (top). (× 5/6)

40 GINSENG RADIX

人参 *ren² shen¹*. English: ginseng root, white ginseng. Japanese: *ninjin*.

Alternate name: 神草 *shen² cao³*.

Origin: Araliaceae family. *Panax ginseng* C.A. Mey.

Characters: This product is the 4–5 year old root of the ginseng plant, washed, stripped of fine roots, and sun or oven dried. It is cylindrical or spindle-shaped, often dividing into two branch roots. The overall length is 5–20 cm. The surface is a pale or whitish yellow-brown, and bears longitudinal creases. It is hard and breaks with difficulty to reveal a granular fracture with the resin ducts appearing as brown speckles. For decoction, it is cut into fine oblique slices, on which an annular marking clearly delineates the woody core.

Quality: Undamaged roots with large branches, a long stem base, fine yellowish skin, and fine, but pronounced wrinkles are the best.

Production areas: China, North and South Korea, and Japan.

Properties and actions: Warm; sweet and slightly bitter; nontoxic. Enters the spleen and lung channels. Greatly supplements original qi, stems desertion and engenders liquid, and quiets the spirit.

Indications: Taxation damage with low food intake and lassitude; stomach reflux; efflux diarrhea; vacuity cough with rapid, distressed, dyspneic breathing; spontaneous sweating; fulminant desertion; fright palpitation; dizziness; impotence; frequent urination; uterine bleeding; chronic fright wind; enduring vacuity; insufficiency of qi, blood, and fluids. Daily dosage: 1.5–10 g. Contraindicated in pathogen repletion patterns. Used in *si⁴ jun¹ zi³ tang¹* (Four Gentlemen Decoction, 251), *sheng¹ mai⁴ san³* (Pulse-Engendering Powder, 239), *ren²-shen¹ tang¹* (Ginseng Decoction, 216), *liu⁴ jun¹ zi³ tang¹* (Six Gentlemen Decoction, 166), *ren²-shen¹ yang³ rong² tang¹* (Ginseng Construction-Nourishing Decoction, 217), *bai² hu³ jia¹ ren²-shen¹ tang¹* (White Tiger Decoction Plus Ginseng, 10)

Remarks: Constituents: Triterpenoids: (saponins, 4–5.2%) ginsenosides $Ra_{1, a2, a3}$, $Rb_{1, b2, b3}$, Rc, Rd, Re, Rf, $Rg_{1, g2}$, Rh_1, malonyl-ginsenosides Rb_1, Rb_2, Rc, Rd, quinquenoside R_1, notoginensosides $R_{1, 4}$, 20-glucoginsenoside Rf, ginsenoside Ro. Sesquiterpenoids (volatile oil, 0.005%).

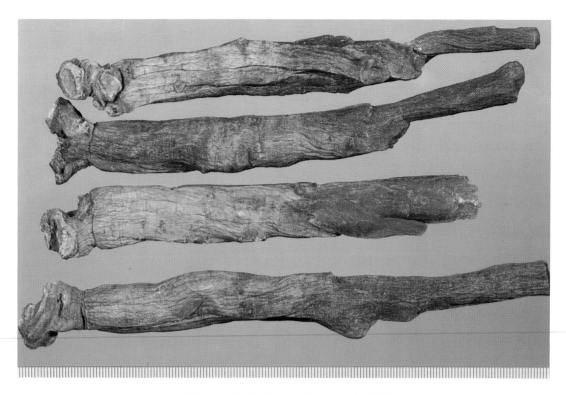

Ginseng Radix Rubra (Korean). (× 5/6)

41 GINGSENG RADIX RUBRA

紅參 *hong² shen¹*. English: red ginseng root. Japanese: *kojin*.

Alternate name: 紅人參 *hong² ren² shen¹*.

Origin: Araliaceae family. *Panax ginseng* C.A. Mey.

Characters: This product is the steamed root of the ginseng plant. It is a deep reddish brown, bears longitudinal wrinkles, and at the head a number of transverse wrinkles. Sometimes the branch roots have broken off. The root is very hard, but softens in damp weather. Like the white ginseng, it is cut into fine transverse slices for decoction. However, the steaming process makes the slices smooth and translucent. It is usually heated in an oven or over a flame to make cutting easier.

Quality: The best quality is a rich red in color, and has few but large branches, and a tough skin.

Production areas: China (Heilongjiang, Jilin, Liaoning), Korea, Japan.

Properties, actions, and indications: Red ginseng has the same nature and flavor as white ginseng, but has a stronger supplementing action. It is especially suitable for yang vacuity patterns with inversion cold in the limbs. Daily dosage: 1.5–10 g. Contraindicated in pathogen repletion patterns.

Remarks: Constituents: Same as Ginseng Radix (No. 40) except for the following: Triterpenoids: (saponins) ginsenosides Ra$_1$, a$_2$, b$_1$, b$_2$, b$_3$, c, d, e, f, g$_1$, g$_2$, g$_3$, h$_1$, h$_2$, s$_1$, s$_2$, 20 (S) ginsenosides Rg$_3$, 20(R)-ginsenosides g$_2$, h$_1$, h$_2$, quinquenosides R$_1$, notoginsenosides R$_{1, 4}$, 20-glucoginsenoside Rf, ginsenoside Ro. Glycerides: 2,3-dilinoleoyl, dilinolenoyl, dioleoyl, dipalmito-glycerol, 1-β-D-galactopyranosides. Saccharides: 2, 4-dihydroxy-2-methyl-6H-3-pyrone-4-O-α-D-glucoside, maltol; acetal-α-D-glucoside.

Similar drug: Codonopsitis Radix. (No. 33)

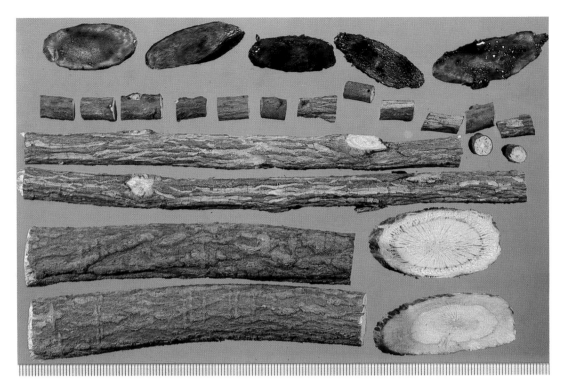

Glycyrrhizae Radix: mix-fried with honey (top); cut and uncut (bottom). (×5/6)

42 GLYCYRRHIZAE RADIX

甘草 *gan¹ cao³*. English: licorice root. Japanese: *kanzō*.

Alternate names: 國老 *guo² lao³*, 甜草 *tian² cao³*.

Origin: Leguminosae family. *Glycyrrhiza uralensis* Fisch. et DC., *G. glabra* L. var. *glandulifera* Regel et Herder, *G. echinata* L.,* *G. inflata* Batal.,* *G. glabra* L.*

Characters: The roots are long and cylindrical, and usually have no branches. They are are 1–2.5 cm in diameter. The exterior surface is a reddish or earth brown, with pronounced wrinkles or furrows, and transverse lenticels. The decocting pieces are transverse or oblique slices about 2 mm thick. Slices stir-fried in honey are a reddish brown in color, and are sticky to the touch.

Quality: Sweet, farinaceous roots are the best.

Production areas: *Glycyrrhiza uralensis:* China (all provinces of Manchuria, Hebei, Shanxi, Shaanxi, and Inner Mongolia). *G. glabra:* China (Gansu, Xinjiang).

Properties and actions: Balanced; sweet; nontoxic. Enters the spleen, stomach, and liver channels. Harmonizes the center and moderates tension; moistens the lung; resolves toxin. Harmonizes all drugs. Use crude to drain fire and resolve toxin, relieve pain and tension, stir-fried to fortify the stomach and spleen, and boost original qi, and mix-fried with honey to supplement the center and boost qi, as well as to eliminate unpleasant odors or flavors of decoctions.

Indications: Used crude for sore throat, yong, ju, digestive tract ulcers and food poisoning. Used mix-fried for spleen-stomach vacuity, low food intake, abdominal pain and thin stool, fatigue and fever, pulmonary atony with cough, and for palpitations and epilepsy. Daily dosage: 1.5–10 g. Contraindicated in spleen-stomach damp and center fullness with nausea and retching. Used in *si⁴ jun¹ zi³ tang¹* (Four Gentlemen Decoction, 251), *gan¹-cao³ gan¹-jiang¹ tang¹* (Licorice and Dried Ginger Decoction, 93), *gan¹ mai⁴ da⁴-zao³ tang¹* (Licorice, Wheat, and Jujube Decoction, 97), *zhi⁴-gan¹-cao³ tang¹* (Honey-Fried Licorice Decoction, 345), *gan¹-cao³ xie⁴ xin¹ tang¹* (Licorice Heart-Draining Decoction, 94), *tiao² wei⁴ cheng² qi⁴ tang¹* (Stomach-Regulating Qi-Infusing Decoction, 263).

Remarks: Constituents: Triterpenoids: (saponins) glycyrrhizin (glycyrrhizic acid 0–14%). Flavonoids (4–13%):liquiritin, neoliquiritin, isoliquiritin, neoisoliquiritin. Coumestans: glycyrol. Coumarins: liqcoumarin.

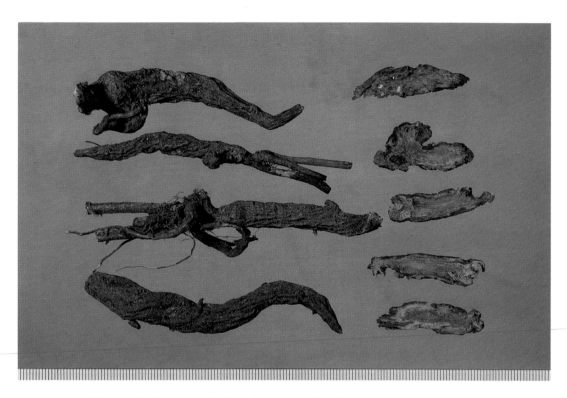

Knoxiae Radix: crude (left) and cut treated with vinegar (right). (×5/6)

43 KNOXIAE RADIX

紅大戟 *hong² da⁴ ji³*. English: knoxia root. Japanese: *kōdaigeki, kōgadaigeki*.

Origin: Rubiaceae family. *Knoxia valerianoides* Thorel.

Characters: The root is 6–8 cm long and 1 cm thick. It often bears a scar where the stem was removed. It is supple and usually slightly contorted, and at its lower end are 2–3 branch roots with numerous fine roots growing from them. The exterior surface has longitudinal wrinkles and is reddish brown, sometimes with a faint purple hue. The decocting pieces are transverse or oblique slices about 1–3 mm thick. On their cut surface, the skin is dark brown while the wood is a yellowish brown.

Quality: Large, firm, fat, reddish brown roots without fine roots are the best.

Production areas: China (Guangxi, Guangdong, Yunnan, Guizhou).

Properties and actions: Cold; bitter, acrid and sweet. Expels water and phlegm-drool; disperses swelling and fullness. Use roasted to reduce toxicity and enhance water-moving effects.

Indications: Pain in the chest, back, lumbus and the lateral costal region; dry retching. Daily dosage: 1.5–3 g. Contraindicated in yin water due to vacuity cold. Used in *shi² zao³ tang¹* (Ten Jujubes Decoction, 245), *kong⁴ xian² dan¹* (Drool-Controlling Elixir, 159).

Remarks: Constituents: Anthraquinones.

Similar drug: Root of *Euphorbia pekinensis* Ruprecht.

Similar plants: *E. soongarica* Boiss.; *E. pontica* Prokh.; *E. pekinensis* Rupr. var. *japonensis* Makino.; *E. sieboldiana* Morr. et Decne.

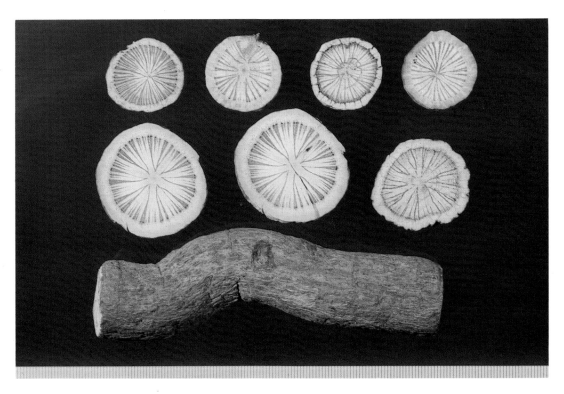

Kwangfangchi Radix: crude (bottom) and sliced (above). (× 5/6)

44 KWANG-FANG-CHI RADIX (FANGJI RADIX)

廣防己 *guang³ fang² ji³*. English: kwang-fang-chi (or southern fangji) root. Japanese: *kōboi*.

Origin: Aristolochiaceae family. *Aristolochia fangchi* Wu.

Characters: This product is a hard, contorted, cylindrical root, 8–15 cm long and 1.5–4.5 cm thick. The exterior surface is gray-brown, with thick cork and coarse longitudinal furrows. It is cut into thin transverse slices. On the transverse section, the woody part accounts for the larger part of the area, and is grayish white in color and slightly farinaceous in texture. The ducts appear gray-brown forming a radial configuration.

Production areas: China (Guangdong, Guangxi).

Properties and actions: Cold; bitter; slightly toxic. Resolves heat; disinhibits urine; relieves pain. Use crude for damp-heat and roasted or stir-fried for wind-damp.

Indications: Water swelling, leg qi, bi pain in the flesh, rheumatic arthritis, and inhibited urination. Daily dosage: 5–10 g. Contraindicated in the absence of damp-heat. Used in *fang²-ji³ fu²-ling² tang¹* (Fangji and Poria Decoction, 84), *fang²-ji³ huang²-qi² tang¹* (Fangji and Astragalus Decoction, 85).

Remarks: Allied drugs: Root of *Stephania tetranda* S. Moore; rhizome of *Sinomenium acutum* Rehder et Wilson; rhizome of *Cocculus trilobus* DC., all three plants of the Menispermaceae. These items as well as *Aristolochia fangchi* Wu are all collectively referred to as Fangji Radix. Constituents: Phenanthrenes: aristolochic acid and aristolactam. Alkaloids.

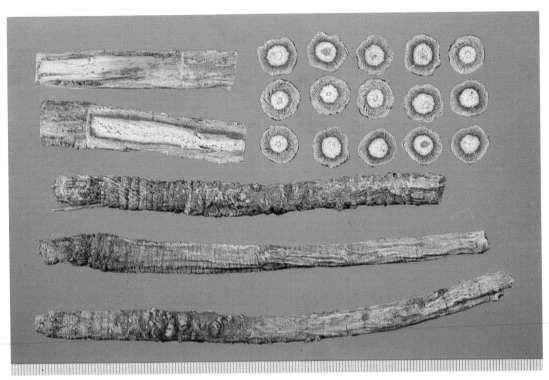

Ledebouriellae Radix: oblique and transverse slices (top); uncut (bottom). (×5/6)

45 LEDEBOURIELLAE RADIX (SAPOSHNIKOVIAE DIVARICATAE RADIX)

防風 *fang² feng¹*. English: ledebouriella root. Japanese: *bofu*.

Alternate names: 唐防風 *tang² fang² feng¹*, 關防風 *guan¹ fang² feng¹*.

Origin: Umbelliferae family. *Ledebouriella seseloides* Wolff. [= *Siler divaricatum* Benth. et Hook.; *Saposhnikovia divaricata* Schischkin], *Ligusticum brachylobum* Franch.,* *Seseli mairei* Wolff.,* *S. yunnanense* Franch.*

Characters: This product is a cylindrical root about 20 cm long and 1 cm thick, with dense annular nodes bearing scaly hairs. The exterior surface is brown or grayish brown with wrinkles. There are many protuberant lenticels and scars left by the fine roots. This root is soft and spongy, and when broken, the cork easily peels away. The decocting pieces are thin transverse slices. On the cut surface of these, the skin is dark brown, while the wood is pale yellow. Numerous fissures give the cross section a lace-like appearance.

Quality: The best roots have a yellow core on the cross section. The decocting pieces are longitudinal or transverse slices.

Production areas: China (grows wild in Heilongjiang, Jilin, Inner Mongolia, Shanxi, Hebei, Shandong).

Properties and actions: Warm; sweet, acrid; nontoxic. Enters the bladder, lung, and spleen channels. Effuses the exterior, dispels wind, percolates damp, relieves pain. Use crude to resolve the exterior, dispel wind-damp, and relieve tetany. Use stir-fried to check diarrhea and dispel wind. Stir-fry with wine to check perspiration, and char to staunch bleeding.

Indications: Headache, dizziness, and stiffness of the neck in external wind-cold patterns; wind, cold, and damp bi; aching pain in the joints; hypertonicity of the limbs; lockjaw. Daily dosage: 5–10 g. Contraindicated in effulgent yin vacuity fire, and pathogen patterns without wind. Used in *fang²-feng¹ tong¹ sheng⁴ san³* (Ledebouriella Sage-Inspired Powder, 83), *yu⁴ ping² feng¹ san³* (Jade Wind-Barrier Powder, 327).

Remarks: Constituents: Coumarins: bergapten, imperatorin, psoralen, phellopterin, deltoin, scopoletin, anomalin, xanthotoxin. Chromones: hamaudol, cimifugin. Volatile oil (0.3–0.6%). Saccharides: mannitol.

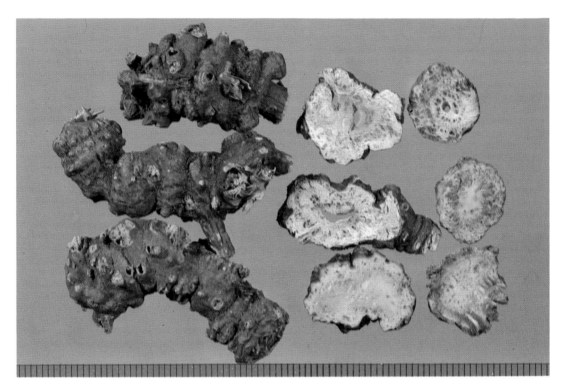

Ligustici Sinensis Radix et Rhizoma crude (left) and sliced (right). (×5/3)

46 LIGUSTICI SINENSIS RADIX ET RHIZOMA

藁本 *gao³ ben³*. English: Chinese lovage (or Chinese ligusticum) root. Japanese: *kōhon.*
Alternate name: 唐藁本 *tang² gao³ ben³.*
Origin: Umbelliferae family. *Ligusticum sinensis* Oliv., *L. jeholense* Nakai et Kitag.,* *L. tenuissimum* (Nakai) Kitag.*
Characters: This product has an irregular cylindrical rhizome, 5–9 cm in length and 0.5–2 cm in diameter. Its exterior surface is blackish brown, with longitudinal wrinkles. It bulges at the head, and at the top are the remains of the stem base. It often has branch roots that can be large enough to be confused with it. It is supple and does not break easily. The decocting pieces are thin oblique slices 1–2 mm thick. They are irregular in shape, and on the cut edge the skin appears a reddish brown, while the wood appears yellow, or even white. The heart is often empty.
Quality: The best quality is yellow in color, with a hollow core, and has a clean shiny appearance.
Production areas: China (Liaoning, Shanxi, Shaanxi, Hubei, Sichuan).
Properties and actions: Warm; acrid. Enters the bladder channel. Dissipates wind, cold and damp pathogens.
Indications: Wind-cold headache; vertex headache; cold-damp abdominal pain; diarrhea; concretions and conglomerations; jie and xian. Daily dosage: 3–3 g. Contraindicated in internal yin vacuity heat. Used in *qiang¹-huo² fang²-feng¹ tang¹* (Notopterygium and Ledebouriella Decoction, 203), *qiang¹-huo² sheng⁴ shi¹ tang¹* (Notopterygium Dampness-Overcoming Decoction, 204).
Remarks: Constituents: Volatile oil (0.5%): butylidenephthalide, cnidilide.

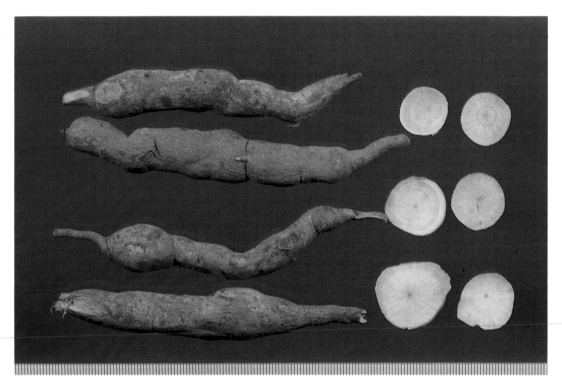

Linderae Radix: crude (left) and sliced (right). (×5/6)

47 LINDERAE RADIX

烏藥 *wu¹ yao⁴*. English: lindera root. Japanese: *uyaku*.

Alternate names: 天台烏藥 *tian¹ tai² wu¹ yao⁴*, 台烏藥 *tai¹ wu¹ yao⁴*.

Origin: Lauraceae family. *Lindera strychnifolia* (Sieb. et Zucc.) F. Villars.

Characters: This root is cylindrical or spindle-shaped and slightly contorted, with scant bulging nodes. It is 6–15 cm long and 0.5–2.5 cm thick. Its exterior surface is a yellowish, reddish or blackish brown, with fine wrinkles and the scars of removed roots. It bears annular fissures, and the skin often peels away to reveal a fibrous woody interior. This root is hard, and does not break easily. It is cut into oblique slices, the cut edge of which is pale yellow in color, with clearly observable medullary rays and annual rings.

Quality: The best quality is pale yellow in color.

Production areas: China (Zhejiang, Hunan, Anhui, Guangdong, Guangxi; if from Tiantai in Zhejiang, it is called Linderae Radix Tiantai).

Properties and actions: Warm; acrid; nontoxic. Enters the lung, spleen, kidney, and bladder channels. Normalizes qi, opens depression, dissipates cold, and relieves pain. Stir-fry with brine to warm the kidney and contain urine, or with bran to disinhibit qi.

Indications: Wind stroke; pain in the abdomen and region of the heart; thoracic glomus; perduring food; stomach reflux; vomiting; frequent urination; cold shan; qi counterflow. Daily dosage: 5–10 g. Contraindicated in qi vacuity with internal heat. Used in *wu¹-yao⁴ shun⁴ qi⁴ san³* (Lindera Qi-Normalizing Powder, 273).

Remarks: Constituents: Monoterpenoids: (–) borneol. Sesquiterpenoids: lindenene, linderene, lindenenone, lindestrene, linderane. Alkaloids: coclaurine, laurolitsine. Acids: linderic acid. Similar drug: Dried root of *Cocculus laurifolius* DC. (Menispermaceae).

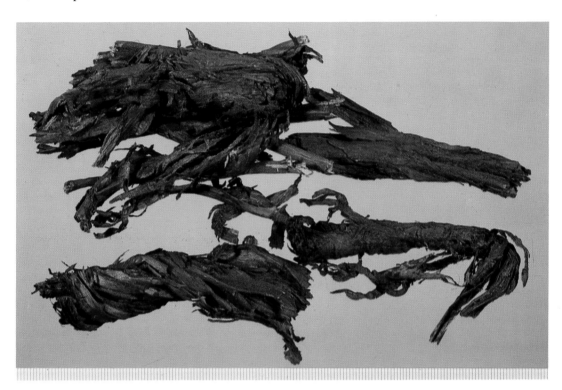

Lithospermi Radix, (*Lithospermum euchroma*) crude (left) and cut (right). (×5/6)

48 LITHOSPERMI RADIX

紫草zi³ cao³. English: lithospermum root, puccoon. Japanese: *shiso, shikon*.

Alternate names: 紫草根 *zi³ cao³ gen¹*, 紫根 *zi³ gen¹*.

Origin: Borraginaceae family. *Lithospermum euchroma* Royle [= *Macrotomia euchroma* Pauls], *L. erythrorhizon* Sieb. et Zucc., *Onosma paniculatum* Bur. et Franch.,* *Lithospermum tschimganicum* B. Fedtsch.,* *L. arvense* L.,* *Arnebia guttata* Bge,* *Onosma hookeri* Clarke var. *longiflorum* Duthie.*

Characters: The root of *Lithospermum euchroma* is contontored, spindle-shaped, 8–15 cm long and 1.5–2 cm in diameter. It has a blackish maroon or purple coloring. It has a loose skin, and the interior is composed of 10 or more flaky layers. It is light, and easily breaks, and has a slightly sour smell. The decocting pieces are 1.5 cm sections.

Production areas: Japan, and China (Xinjiang, Tibet, Gansu).

Properties and actions: Cold; bitter; nontoxic. Enters the liver and pericardium channels. Cools the blood, quickens the blood, clears heat, and resolves toxin.

Indications: Maculopapular eruptions in warm heat disease; damp-heat jaundice; purple patches; blood ejection; spontaneous external bleeding; blood in the urine; turbid strangury; blood dysentery; heat bind constipation; burns; eczema; cinnabar toxin; yong. Daily dosage: 5–10 g. Contraindicated in gastrointestinal vacuity with diarrhea. Used in *zi³ yun² gao¹* (Purple Clouds Paste, 355), *zi³-gen¹ mu³-li⁴ tang¹* (Puccoon [Lithospermum] and Oyster Shell Decoction, 352).

Remarks: Constituents: Naphthoquinones (up to 1.1%): acetylshikonin, shikonin, deoxyshikonin, isobutylshikonin, β,β-dimethylacrylshikonin, lithospermidins A and B. Phenols: shikononfurans A, B, C, D, E. Saccharides: lithospermans A, B, C.

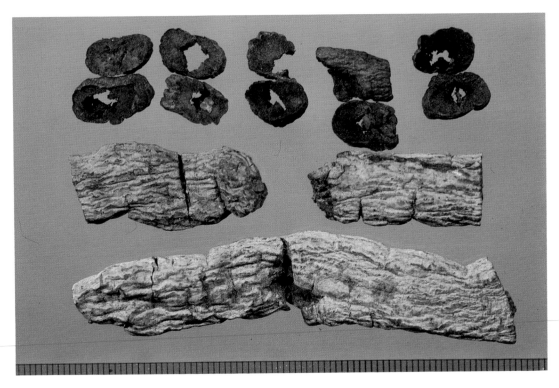

Morindae Radix: treated with wine (top); crude (bottom)., (×5/6)

49 MORINDAE RADIX

巴戟天 ba¹ ji³ tian¹. English: morinda root. Japanese: *hagekiten.*

Alternate names: 巴戟 *ba¹ ji³*, 巴戟肉 *ba¹ ji³ rou⁴*.

Origin: Rubiaceae family. *Morinda officinalis* How.

Characters: This root is cylindrical and contorted in shape. It varies from 1–2.5 cm in length, and has transverse fissures and longitudinal creases. The woody interior is tough and supple. The decocting pieces are short sections, which are dark brown on the cut edge with a well developed cortex.

Quality: The best quality roots are fat, clean and with a thin core. The should be moist and sweet.

Production areas: China (cultivated in Guangdong and Guangxi).

Properties and actions: Warm; acrid and sweet; nontoxic. Enters the spleen and kidney channels. Supplements kidney yang; strengthens the sinews and bone; dispels wind-damp.

Indications: Impotence; wind-damp leg qi; weak, aching sinews and bones; pain in the lumbus and knees. Stir-fry with brine to supplement the kidney. Boil in licorice water to reduce toxicity. Stir-fry with wine to dissipate wind-damp. Daily dosage: 5–10 g. Contraindicated in exuberant yin vacuity fire patterns with dry, bound stool. Used in *huan² shao⁴ dan¹*, (Rejuvenation Elixir, 128), *er⁴ xian¹ tang¹* (Two Immortals Decoction, 82).

Remarks: Similar plants: *Morinda citrifolia; M. tinctoria; M. lucida; M. umbellata* (Rubiaceae). Constituents: Vitamin C. Saccharides.

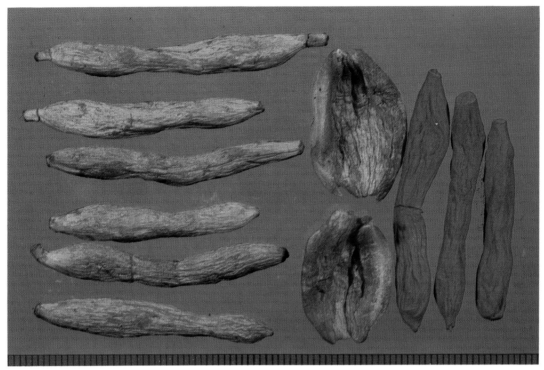

Ophiopogonis Tuber: crude (left); with hearts removed (middle);
coated with cinnabar (righ). (×5/3)

50 OPHIOPOGONIS TUBER

麥門冬*mai⁴ men² dong¹*. English: ophiopogon (or lilyturf) tuber. Japanese: *bakumondo*.
Alternate names: 寸冬 *cun⁴ dong¹*, 麥冬 *mai⁴ dong¹*.
Origin: Liliaceae family. *Ophiopogon japonicus* Ker-Gawl.
Characters: This is a spindle-shaped tuber 1.0–2.5 cm long, and 3–5 mm thick. It is a pale yellowish brown, and slightly translucent. It bears irregular longitudinal wrinkles. It is soft, and can be broken open to reveal a whitish, sticky flesh. Ophiopogonis Tuber is small enough to be decocted whole.
Quality: The best quality tubers are fat, light in color, and semi-translucent. They are soft and supple, have a sticky texture in the mouth, and give off a pleasant scent.
Production areas: China (Zhejiang, Sichuan, and less importantly Jiangsu, Guizhou, Yunnan, Guangxi, Anhui, Hubei, Hunan).
Properties and actions: Cold; sweet and slightly bitter; nontoxic. Enters the lung, stomach, and heart channels. Nourishes yin and moistens lung, clears the heart and eliminates vexation, boosts stomach and engenders liquid. Remove the heart to treat vexation. Stir-fry with rice to moderate the cool nature. Cover with cinnabar to quiet the heart-spirit.
Indications: Pulmonary dryness; dry cough; blood ejection; expectoration of blood; pulmonary yong and atony; vacuity taxation; heat vexation; wasting thirst; damage to liquid in febrile disease; dry mouth and throat; constipation. Daily dosage: 5–10 g. Contraindicated in spleen-stomach vacuity cold with diarrhea. Used in *mai⁴-men²-dong¹ tang¹* (Ophiopogon Decoction, 180), *mai⁴-men²-dong¹ yin³ zi³* (Ophiopogon Drink 181), *sheng¹ mai⁴ san³* (Pulse-Engendering Powder, 239), *zeng¹ ye⁴ tang¹* (Humor-Increasing Decoction, 334), *zhi⁴-gan¹-cao³ tang¹* (Honey-Fried Licorice Decoction, 345).
Remarks: Constituents: Steroids: (saponins) ophiopogonins A (0.05%), B (0.01%), C, D, B', C', D'; β-sitosterol, stigmasterol. Flavonoids: ophiopogonones A, B, methylophiopogonones A, B. Saccharides: β-$(2\rightarrow1)$-fructan; sucrose.
Similar drug: Dried tuber of *O. chekiangensis* K. Kimura (Zhejiang).

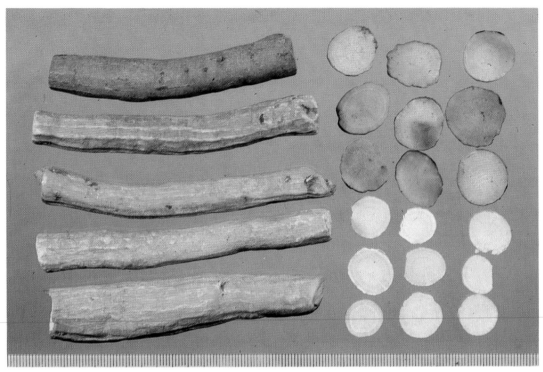

Paeoniae Radix Alba: crude (left); transverse slices stir-fried (top right); transverse slices crude (bottom right). (× 5/6)

---

51 PAEONIAE RADIX ALBA

白芍藥 *bai² shao² yao⁴*. English: white peony root. Japanese: *byakushakuyaku*.

Alternate names: 金芍藥 *jin¹ shao² yao⁴*, 白芍 *bai² shao²*.

Origin: Paeoniaceae family. *Paeonia lactiflora* Pall. [= *P. albiflora* Pallas var. *trichocarpa* Bunge].

Characters: This cylindrical root 1–2 cm thick comes in the form of 10–15 cm sections with the bark removed. The exterior surface is smooth and white, with transverse lenticels faintly visible. It is hard and solid, and does not break very cleanly. It is cut into transverse, oblique, or longitudinal slices about 1 mm thick. The cut surface is whitish, sometimes with a pink hue, and is smooth to the touch. The annular markings are clearly visible, and the medullary rays are broad and white, and have a farinaceous texture. Stir-fried slices a golden brown in color.

Quality: Long, thick, hard, straight roots with a farinaceous texture are the best.

Production areas: China (Zhejiang, Anhui, Sichuan, and less importantly in Shandong, Guizhou, Hunan, Hubei, Gansu, Shaanxi, and Yunnan), and Japan.

Properties and actions: Slightly cold; bitter and sour; nontoxic. Enters the liver and spleen channels. Nourishes the blood and emolliates the liver; moderates the center and relieves pain; constrains yin and sweat. Use crude to calm the liver. Use stir-fried to nourish the blood and harmonize the liver, free the blood vessels and relieve pain. Use roasted to moderate the cold nature, direct the effect toward the upper body, and enhance the blood-quickening action. Use stir-fried in earth to enhance pain-relieving and spleen-fortifying qualities.

Indications: Thoracic, lateral costal, and abdominal pain; diarrhea with abdominal pain; spontaneous or night sweating; yin vacuity fever; menstrual irregularities; vaginal discharge. Daily dosage: 5–10 g. Contraindicated for patients suffering from thoracic fullness. Used in *dang¹-gui¹ shao²-yao⁴ san³* (Tangkuei and Peony Powder, 60), *si⁴ wu⁴ tang¹* (Four Agents Decoction, 256) *si⁴ ni⁴ san³* (Counterflow Cold Powder, 252), *shao²-yao⁴ gan¹-cao³ tang¹* (Peony and Licorice Decoction, 229), *gui⁴-zhi¹ jia¹ shao²-yao⁴ tang¹* (Cinnamon Twig Decoction Plus Peony, 113).

Remarks: Constituents: Monoterpenoids: paeoniflorin (1.5–10.9%), albiflorin (0–1.7%), oxypaeoniflorin, benzoylpaeoniflorin, paeoniflorigenone. Volatile oil: benzoic acid (main), paeonol. Tannoids.

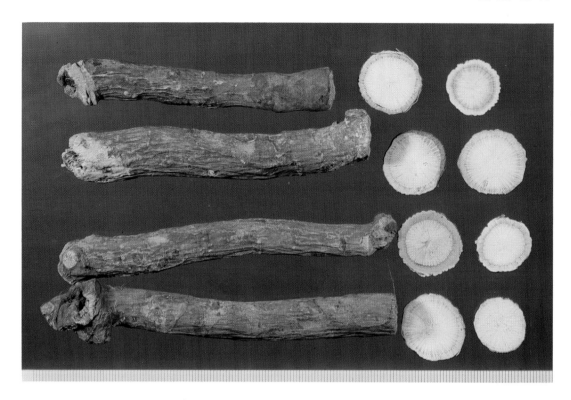

Paeoniae Radix Rubra: crude (left); transverse slices (right). (×5/6)

52 PAEONIAE RADIX RUBRA

赤芍藥chi⁴ shao² yao⁴. English: red peony root. Japanese: *sekishakuyaku*.

Alternate names: 木芍藥 *mu⁴ shao² yao⁴*, 赤芍 *chi⁴ shao²*.

Origin: Paeoniaceae family. *Paeonia lactiflora* Pall. [= *P. albiflora* Pallas var. *trichocarpa* Bunge.], *P. obovata* Maxim., *P. veitchii* Lynch, *P. anomala* L.*

Characters: This root is cylindrical and hard, and has a pinkish bark that bears longitudinal wrinkles. The decocting pieces are oblique or transverse slices. The cut edge is smooth and has a yellowish or pinkish hue and clearly visible annular markings. Stir-fried slices are brown in color.

Production areas: *Paeonia lactiflora:* China (Inner Mongolia, Zhejiang, Anhui, Hebei, Sichuan). *P. obovata:* China (Heilongjiang, Jilin, Liaoning, Inner Mongolia, Xinjiang, Hebei, Gansu). *P. veitchii:* China (Sichuan, Yunnan, Guizhou, Shanxi).

Properties and actions: Cool; sour, bitter; nontoxic. Enters the liver and spleen channels. Moves stasis, relieves pain, cools the blood, and disperses swelling. Use crude to clear heat and cool the blood. Stir-fry without additives to moderate the cool nature, or stir-fry with wine to enhance the blood-quickening and stasis-dispelling action.

Indications: Menstrual block due to blood stagnation; concretions and gatherings; pain in the abdomen and lateral costal region; spontaneous external bleeding; blood dysentery; intestinal wind bleeding; reddening of the eyes; yong swelling. Daily dosage: 5–10 g. Contraindicated in blood vacuity. Used in *du²-huo² ji⁴-sheng¹ tang¹* (Duhuo and Mistletoe Decoction, 73), *bai²-ji²-li² san³* (Tribulus Powder, 12).

Remarks: Constituents: paeoniflorin, mucilage, volatile oil, saccharides.

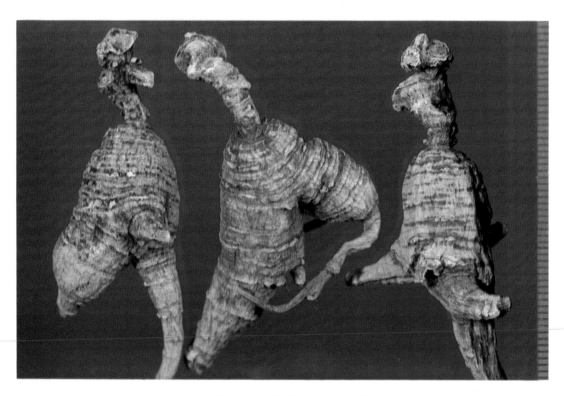

Panacis Quinquefolii Radix: crude. (×5/3)

53 PANACIS QUINQUEFOLII RADIX

西洋參 xi^1 $yang^2$ $shen^1$. English: American ginseng root. Japanese: *seiyojin*.

Alternate names: 花旗參 hua^1 qi^2 $shen^1$, 廣東人參 $guang^3$ $dong^1$ ren^2 $shen^1$,

Origin: Araliaceae family. *Panax quinquefolium* L.

Characters: This root is cylindrical or spindle-shaped, 2–6 cm long and 0.5–1 cm in diameter. The exterior surface is earth brown and has transverse wrinkles that have an annular appearance at the head of the root where they are densest. If the bark has been removed, the white flesh is revealed. This root breaks smoothly to reveal a pale yellowish white fracture with darker annular markings and reddish brown resin ducts. It is light and hard, and sticky in texture.

Quality: Evenly sized roots that are hard, light, but moist on the inside are the best.

Production areas: North America; China (cultivated in Jiangxi).

Properties and actions: Cool; sweet and slightly bitter; nontoxic. Enters the heart, lung, and kidney channels. Boosts lung yin and clears vacuity fire; engenders liquid and allays thirst.

Indications: Enduring cough; pulmonary atony; vacuity vexation; thirst with scant liquid; toothache due to stomach fire. Daily dosage: 3–5 g. Contraindicated in spleen-stomach cold-damp. Used in $qing^1$ shu^3 yi^4 qi^4 $tang^1$ (Summerheat-Clearing Qi-Boosting Decoction, 210).

Remarks: Constituents: Triterpenoids: (saponins, 6.4–7.3%) ginsenosides Rb_1 (1.6%), Re (0.9%), Rd (0.8%), Rc (0.2%), Rg, (0.0–0.2%), Ro (0.1%), Rb_2 (0.02%), Rg_2, Rb_3, F_2., pseudo-ginsenoside F_{11}, quinquenoside R_1. Saccharides: quinquefolans A, B, C.

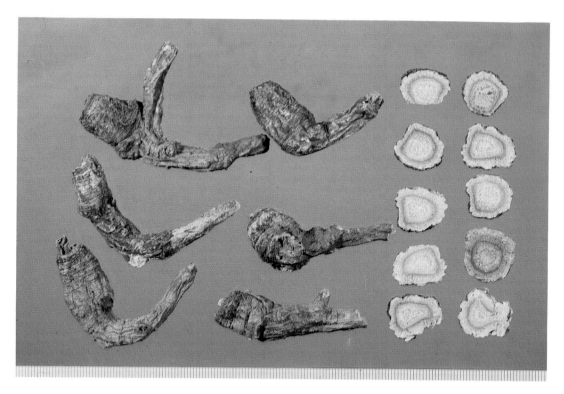

Peucedani Radix: crude (left); transverse slices (right). (×5/6)

54 PEUCEDANI RADIX

前胡 *qian² hu²*. English: peucedanum root, Japanese: *zengo*.

Origin: Umbelliferae family. *Peucedanum praeruptorum* Dunn.

Characters: This is a spindle-shaped root, about 2–5 cm long, and 1–2 cm in diameter. The exterior surface is a blackish brown. At the top, it bears scars where the stem and leaf bases were removed, and on the head are dense annular wrinkles. There are longitudinal furrows, and the cork easily peels off. Lateral roots are more cylindrical in shape, springing from the main root at a wide angle. The decocting pieces are transverse or oblique slices about 1–2 mm thick. The cut surface is yellowish white to brown, and shows cracks in the bark and annular markings in the wood. The medullary rays are more contorted in the bast.

Quality: Dry roots with dark skin and pale flesh, and without fine roots are the best.

Production areas: China (Zhejiang, Anhui, Hunan, Yunnan, Sichuan).

Properties and actions: Slightly cold; bitter, acrid; nontoxic. Enters the lung and spleen channels. Diffuses wind-heat, precipitates qi, and disperses phlegm. Use crude to diffuse wind-heat, or mix-fried with honey to moisten the lung, downbear qi, and transform phlegm.

Indications: Wind-heat cough and headache; phlegm dyspnea and fullness; counterflow retching; fullness and oppression in the chest and diaphragm. Daily dosage: 5–10 g. Contraindicated in the absence of repletion heat. Used in *shen¹ su¹ yin³*, (Ginseng and Perilla Beverage, 232), *ren²-shen¹ bai⁴ du² san³* (Ginseng Toxin-Vanquishing Powder, 214), *jing¹ fang² bai⁴ du² san³* (Schizonepeta and Ledebouriella Toxin-Vanquishing Powder, 150).

Remarks: Allied drug: Root of *Peucedanum decursivum* Maxim. (Japan).

Constituents: Coumarins: anomarin, peupraerin I, II, (+)-praeruptorins A, (±)-praeruptorins C, D, marmesin, rutarin, isorutarin, skimmin, praerosides I, II, III, IV, V, scopolin.

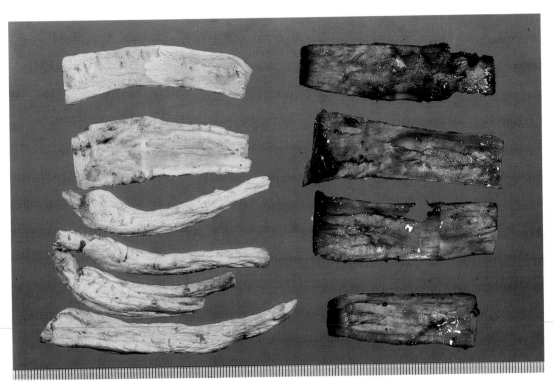

Platycodonis Radix: crude (left); slices and mix-fried with honey (right). (×5/6)

55 PLATYCODONIS RADIX

桔梗 jie[2] geng[3]. English: platycodon (or balloonflower, bellflower) root. Japanese: *kikyo*.
Alternate names: 白藥 *bai[2] yao[4]*, 苦桔梗 *ku[3] jie[2] geng[3]*.
Origin: Campanulaceae family. *Platycodon grandiflorum* (Jacq.) A. DC.
Characters: This spindle-shaped root has an overall length of 6–15 cm, and is 1–2 cm in diameter. The upper portion has the saucer-shaped stem base and bud traces. The exterior surface is a pale whitish yellow, and has deep, contorted longitudinal creases, as well as fine transverse wrinkles. It is hard and breaks easily producing a coarse fracture, and revealing the pale yellow wood of the interior. The decocting pieces are fine longitudinal slices.
Quality: Dry, firm, white, evenly sized roots are the best.
Production areas: China (Anhui, Jiangsu, Shandong, Hebei, Henan, Guizhou), Korea, and Japan.
Properties and actions: Slightly warm; acrid, bitter. Enters the lung and stomach channels. Opens and diffuses lung qi, eliminates phlegm, and expels pus. Use crude to diffuse the lung and dispel phlegm, to expel pus and disperse swelling, and to disinhibit the throat and relieve pain. Mix-fry with honey to moisten the lung.
Indications: External contraction cough; throat bi; sore throat; pulmonary yong; blood ejection; coughing of blood and pus; fullness in the chest; pain in the lateral costal region; dysenteric disease; abdominal pain. Daily dosage: 3–5 g. Contraindicated in yin vacuity cough. Used in *shi[2] wei[4] bai[4] du[2] tang[1]* (Ten-Ingredient Toxin-Vanquishing Decoction, 244), *ren[2]-shen[1] bai[4] du[2] san[3]* (Ginseng Toxin-Vanquishing Powder, 214).
Remarks: Constituents: Triterpenoids: (saponins, ca 2%) platycoside C, platycodins A, C, D, D2, polygalacins D, D2; betulin. Steroids (ca. 0.03%): α-spinasterol, α-spinasterol-β-D-glucoside, 7-dehydrostigmasterol. Saccharides: inulin, platycodin. Fixed oil (0.93%).

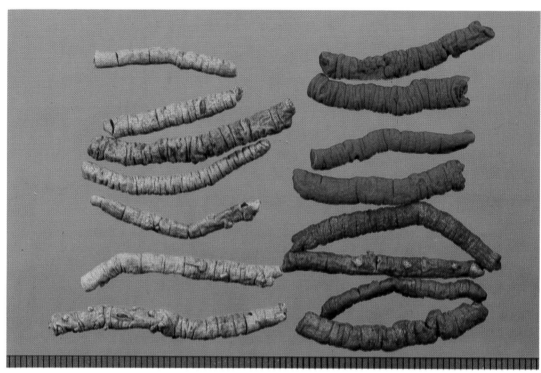

**Polygalae Radix: crude (left); coated in cinnabar (top right);
stir-fried with bran (bottom right). (×5/3)**

56 POLYGALAE RADIX

遠志 *yuan³ zhi⁴*. English: polygala (or Chinese senega) root. Japanese: *onji*.
Alternate names: 遠志肉 *yuan³ zhi⁴ rou⁴*, 遠志筒 *yuan³ zhi⁴ tong³*.
Origin: Polygalaceae family. *Polygala tenuifolia* Willd.
Characters: This product is a cylindrical root, up to 10 cm in length, and 3–6 mm in thickness.
The exterior surface is light brown, and rough in texture, bearing the scars of removed branch
roots. It has deep transverse creases. The skin is thick, and easily removed from the wood. This
root is hard. The decocting pieces are 2.5 cm lengths, which are processed to become soft and sticky.
Quality: The best quality roots are thick and soft, and have a thin, pale skin.
Production areas: China (Shanxi, Shaanxi, Hebei, Henan, and less importantly Shandong, Inner
Mongolia, Anhui, Hubei, Jilin).
Properties and actions: Warm; bitter, acrid; nontoxic. Enters the heart and kidney channels.
Quiets the spirit and sharpens the wits; dispels wind and resolves depression.
Indications: Fright palpitations; poor memory; wet dreams; insomnia; coughing with copious
phlegm; swollen yong, ju and sores. Stir-fry with honey to increase the moistening and spirit-quieting
effect. Coat in cinnabar for a powerful spirit-quieting effect. Daily dosage: 3–5g. Contraindicated
in repletion fire. Used in *ding⁴ zhi⁴ wan²* (Orientation-Stabilizing Pills, 72), *tian¹ wang² bu³ xin¹*
dan¹ (Celestial Emperor Heart-Supplementing Elixir, 262), *gui¹ pi² tang¹* (Spleen-Returning Decoction, 108).
Remarks: Constituents: Triterpenoids: (saponins, ca. 7–4%) onjisaponins A, B, C, D, E, F, G
(A=senegin IV, B=senegin III); β-amyrin.
Similar drugs: Dried root of *Polygala senega* L., *P. sibirica* L.

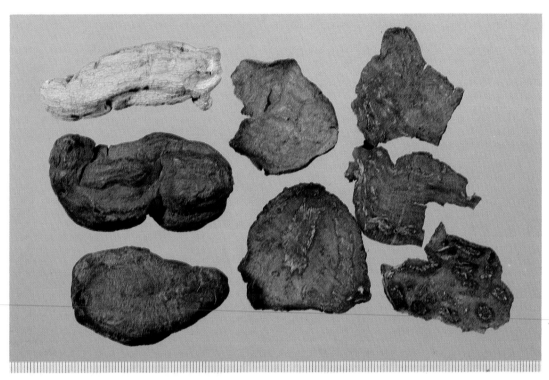

Cynanchi Bungei seu Auriculati Radix (top left). Polygoni Multiflori
Radix: crude (bottom left); steamed with black beans (right). (× 5/6)

57 POLYGONI MULTIFLORI RADIX

何首烏 *he² shou³ wu¹*. (Including Cynanchi Bungei seu Auriculati Radix 白首烏 *bai² shou³ wu¹*.) English: flowery knotweed, (or polygonum) root. Japanese: *kashuu*.

Alternate names: 夜合 *ye⁴ he²*, 首烏 *shou³ wu¹*.

Origin: Polygonaceae family. *Polygonum multiflorum* Thunb., *Cynanchum bungei* Decne,* *C. auriculatum* Royl. ex Wight.*

Characters: Polygoni Multiflori Radix is a fat spindle-shaped root tuber that is dark reddish brown with irregular wrinkles and the remains of the rhizome at one end. It is hard and difficult to break. It usually comes in the form of ready cut decocting pieces, both crude and processed slices being available. Crude slices are about 2 mm thick, and the cut surface is reddish brown in color. Processed slices are usually a little thicker, and are darker in color. Cynanchi Bungei seu Auriculati Radix is similar but a yellowish white in color, and is sometimes used as a substitute for Polygoni Multiflori Radix.

Quality: Solid roots that are black on the outside and reddish on the inside are best.

Production areas: China (Henan, Hubei, Guizhou, Sichuan, Guangxi, Jiangsu), and Korea.

Properties and actions: Slightly warm; bitter, sweet and astringent; slightly toxic. Enters the liver and kidney channels. Supplements the liver and boosts the kidney; nourishes the blood and dispels wind. It is used crude to moisten the intestines and free the stool, steamed in wine to increase humor, and treated with black beans to enhance the channel-freeing action.

Indications: Liver-kidney yin depletion with signs such as premature graying of the hair, weak lumbus and knees, and seminal emission; blood vacuity dizziness; uterine bleeding; vaginal discharge; enduring malaria; swollen yong; intestinal wind; hemorrhoids. Daily dosage: 10–15 g. Contraindicated in damp-phlegm and watery diarrhea. Used in *he² ren² yin³* (Flowery Knotweed and Ginseng Beverage, 117), *dang¹-gui¹ yin³ zi³* (Tangkuei Drink, 63)

Remarks: Constituents: Anthraquinones: chrysophanol, emodin. Tannoids.
Similar drugs: Cynanchi Bungei seu Auriculati Radix (*bai² shou³ wu¹*), the dried root of *Cynanchum bungei* Decne., or *C. auriculatum* Royl. ex Wight.

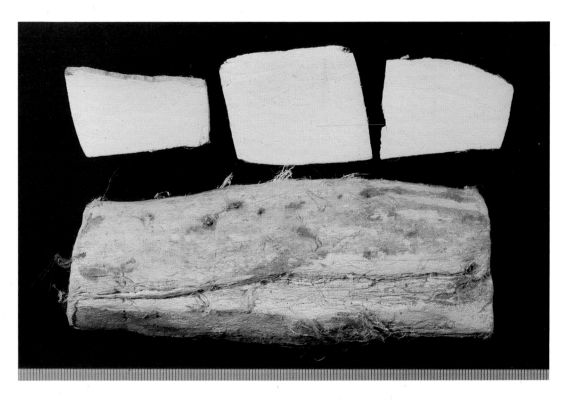

Puerariae Radix: sliced (top); crude (bottom). (×5/6)

58   PUERARIAE RADIX

葛根 *ge² gen¹*. English: pueraria (or kudzu) root, Japanese arrowroot. Japanese: *kakkon*.
Alternate names: 刈根 *yi⁴ gen¹*, 甘葛 *gan¹ ge²*, 粉葛 *fen³ ge²*.
Origin: Leguminosae family. *Pueraria lobata* (Willd.) Ohwi [= *P. pseudo-hirsuta* Tang et Wang],
P. omeiensis Wang et Tang,* *P. edulis* Pamp.,* *P. thomsonii* Benth.,* *P. phaseoloides* (Roxb.) Benth.*
Characters: This root is always sold ready cut into decocting pieces, which take the form large
longitudinal slices of the root 10-20 cm long, 5–10 cm wide, and 1–2 mm thick. The wood is white,
and highly fibrous, and turns pale yellow when roasted.
Quality: The best quality is white, adequately farinaceous, and not stringy.
Production areas: China (Jiangsu, Zhejiang, Anhui, Guangdong), Japan, and Korea.
Properties and actions: Balanced; sweet, acrid; nontoxic. Enters the spleen and stomach channels. Raises yang and resolves the muscles; outthusts papules and checks diarrhea; eliminates vexation and allays thirst. Use crude to resolve the exterior, outthrust macules, and engender liquid.
Roast to moderate the diaphoretic action and help supplement stomach qi.
Indications: Headache and stiffness of the neck in cold damage or warm heat; heat vexation;
wasting thirst; diarrhea; dysenteric disease; non-eruption of measles; hypertension; angina pec-
toris; deafness. Daily dosage: 3–7 g. Use with care in flaming yin vacuity fire and in upper body
exuberance with lower body vacuity. Used in *ge²-gen¹ tang¹* (Pueraria Decoction, 101), *ge²-gen¹
huang²-qin² huang²-lian² tang¹* (Pueraria, Scutellaria, and Coptis Decoction, 100), *sheng¹-ma²
ge²-gen¹ tang¹* (Cimicifuga and Pueraria Decoction, 238).
Remarks: Constituents: Flavonoids (1.8–12%): daizein, puerarin, 4′, 6″-di-O-acetylpuerarin, genistein, formononetin, miroestrol, daizin, daizein 7,4′-diglucosde. Triterpenoids: sophoradiol,
soyasapogenols A, B. Saccharides: starch (10–14%); D-mannitol, D-(±)-pinitol.

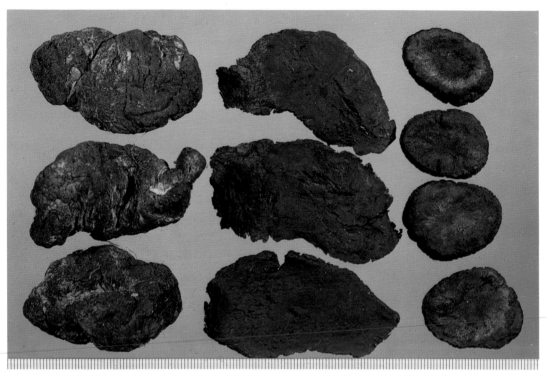

**Rehmanniae Radix Exsiccata (left), Conquita (middle),
Carbonisata (right). (×5/6)**

59 REHMANNIAE RADIX

地黃*di⁴ huang²*. (Including Rehmanniae Radix Exsiccata 乾地黃*gan¹ di⁴ huang²*, and Rehmanniae Radix Conquita熟地黃*shou² di⁴ huang².*) English: rehmannia root. Japanese: *jiō*.

Origin: Scrophulariaceae family. *Rehmannia glutinosa* (Gaertn.) Libosch., *R. glutinosa* (Gaertn.) Libosch. var. *hueichingensis* (Chao et Schih) Hsiao.

Characters: This root is an irregular spherical or cylindrical mass, about 6–12 cm long, and 3–6 cm thick. The outer surface is dark brown or gray, and is wrinkled, with irregular transverse creases. It is soft and heavy, becoming denser and harder as it dries. It is not easy to break, and does not break smoothly. Inside it is shiny, moist, and sticky, and is black or purple black in color. The cooked form is darker in color, stickier in substance, and sweeter to the taste. The decocting pieces are irregularly shaped slices 2–5 mm thick.

Quality: Fat, heavy roots that are dark in color and moist and oily in texture are the best.

Production areas: China (Henan, Zhejiang, Jiangsu, Anhui, Shandong, Hebei, Liaoning, Shanxi, Shaanxi, Inner Mongolia, Hunan, Hubei, and Sichuan). *Rehmannia glutinosa* Libosch. var. *hueichingensis* (Chao et Schih) Hsiao is cultivated in Huaiqing in Henan.

Properties and actions: Dry form: Cold; sweet, bitter; nontoxic. Enters the heart, liver, and kidney channels. Cooked form: Slightly warm, and sweet. Both forms enrich yin and nourish the blood. Carbonize to supplement the spleen and stomach. Stir-fry with wine to move the blood and check bleeding.

Indications: The dry form treats blood vacuity with fever, menstrual irregularities, stirring fetus, frenetic blood heat, blood ejection, spontaneous upper portal bleeding, precipitation of blood, uterine bleeding. The cooked form treats uterine bleeding, wasting thirst, yin vacuity cough, dyspnea, and blood vacuity. Daily dosage: 5–10 g. Contraindicated in spleen-stomach vacuity cold. Used in *xi¹-jiao³ di⁴-huang² tang¹* (Rhinoceros Horn and Rehmannia Decoction, 284), *si⁴ wu⁴ tang¹* (Four Agents Decoction, 256), *liu⁴ wei⁴ di⁴-huang² wan²* (Six-Ingredient Rehmannia Pills, 168).

Remarks: Constituents: Iridoids: catalpol, 6'-O-acetylcatalpol, aucubin, melittoside, rehmanniosides A, B, C, D, rehmaglutins A, B, C, D, glutinoside, Saccharides: rehmannans A, B, C; stachyose, D-mannitol.

Allied drug: Dried root of *Rehmannia glutinosa* (Gaertn.) Libosch. var. *purpurea* Makino (Japan).

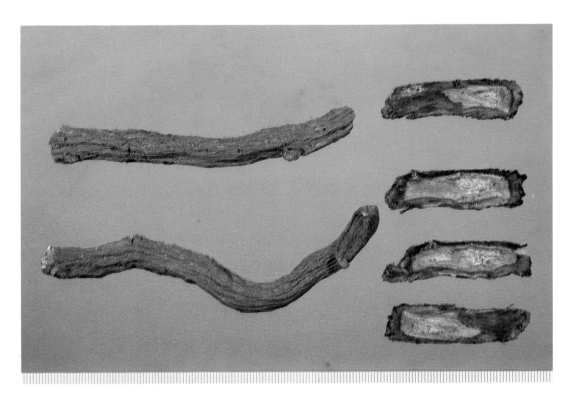

Salviae Radix: crude (left); sliced and washed in wine (right). (×5/6)

60 SALVIAE RADIX

丹参 *dan¹ shen¹*. English: salvia root, red-rooted sage. Japanese: *tanjin*.

Alternate names: 赤参 *ch⁴ shen¹*, 紫丹参 *zi³ dan¹ shen¹*.

Origin: Labiatae family. *Salvia miltiorrhiza* Bge.

Characters: This product is a cylindrical root is up to 25 cm long, and is 4–10 mm thick. The exterior is red-brick or rust red, and bears irregular longitudinal wrinkles. Sometimes fine roots are still attached. Older roots have a coarse, scaly skin that has peeled off in places. Saviae Radix is quite brittle, and the fracture reveals the fibrosity of the wood. The decocting pieces are 1–2 mm thick slices with wavy edges. On the cut edge, the bark appears red, while the vascular bundles in the wood, forming a radial configuration, appear yellow or white.

Quality: Dry, large, solid roots with a red bark are the best.

Production areas: China (Anhui, Hebei, Shanxi, Sichuan).

Properties and actions: Slightly cold; bitter. Enters the heart and liver channels. Quickens the blood and dispels stasis; quiets the heart and spirit; expels pus and relieves pain. Use crude to quicken and cool the blood, and dispel stasis. Char-fry to staunch bleeding. Stir-fry with rice to harmonize the stomach. Stir-fry with wine to enhance the effects. Mix-with turtle's blood to enter the liver. Stir-fry with pig's blood to enter the heart and calm the spirit.

Indications: Menstrual irregularities; concretions and gatherings; swollen yong; cinnabar toxin (erysipelas); malign sores; heat vexation; wind bi. Daily dosage: 5–10 g. Use with care in the absence of blood stasis. Used in *dan¹-shen¹ yin³* (Salvia Beverage, 56), *yi⁴-mu³ sheng⁴ jin¹ dan¹* (Leonurus Metal-Overcoming Elixir, 316).

Remarks: Constituents: Diterpenoids (ca. 2%): tanshinones I, IIA (0.85%) IIB, methylenetanshiquinone, dihydrotanshinone I, cryptotanshinone (0.71%), neocryptotanshinone.

Similar plants: *Salvia przewalskii* Maxim.; *S. przewalskii* Maxim. var. *mandarinorum* Sieb.; *S. yunnanensis* C.H. Wight.

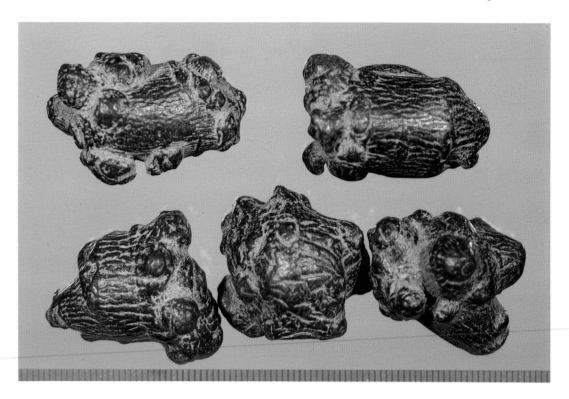

San-chi Ginseng Radix: crude. (×5/3)

61 SAN-CHI GINSENG RADIX (NOTOGINSENG RADIX)

三七 *san¹ qi¹*. English: notoginseng (or sanchi) root. Japanese: *sanshichi*.

Alternate names: 人參三七 *ren² shen¹ san¹ qi¹*, 田三七 *tian² san¹ qi¹*.

Origin: Araliaceae family. *Panax notoginseng* F.H. Chen [= *P. pseudo-gineseng* Wall. var. *notoginseng* (Burkill) Hoo et Tseng, and *P. sanchi* Hoo].

Characters: This is a spindle-shaped or tapered root, 2–4 cm long, and 1.2–2 cm thick. Knobby branch roots spring mostly from the upper part of the root. At the top are the remains of the base of the rhizome. The outer surface is a gray yellow, which, particularly on the protuberances, becomes blackish brown and shiny as a result of friction. When cracked open, the bark easily separates from the wood. The decocting pieces are transverse slices on whose cut surface, the skin appears whitish, while the wood appears gray with annular markings, and speckles indicating the resin ducts.

Production areas: China (East Yunnan, Southwest Guangxi).

Properties and actions: Warm; sweet and slightly bitter; nontoxic. Enters the liver, stomach, and large intestine channels. Staunches bleeding, dissipates stasis, disperses swellings, and relieves pain.

Indications: Blood ejection; coughing of blood; spontaneous external bleeding; blood in the stool; blood dysentery; uterine bleeding; concretions and conglomerations; postpartum blood dizziness; retention of the lochia; impact injury and stasis; bleeding due to trauma. Daily dosage: 5–10 g. Contraindicated in blood vacuity without blood stasis. Used in *yun² nan² bai² yao⁴* (Yunnan White, 331).

Remarks: Constituents: Triterpenoids (saponins, 3–12%); ginsenosides Rg_1, b_1, e, d, b_2, c, h_1, g_2, 20-glucoginsenoside Rf, notoginsenosides $R_{1,2,3,4,5,6}$, gypenoside XVII. Amino acids: dencichine. Polyenyes: panaxynol. Saccharides: sanchinan-A; starch.

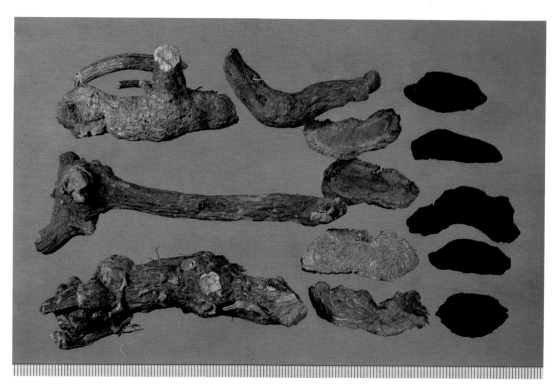

Sanguisorbae Radix: crude (left); sliced (middle); carbonized (right). (×5/6)

62 SANGUISORBAE RADIX

地楡 *di⁴ yu²*. English: sanguisorba root. Japanese: *chiyu*.

Alternate names: 紫地楡 *zi³ di⁴ yu²*, 酸赭 *suan¹ zhe³*.

Origin: Rosaceae family. *Sanguisorba officinalis* L.

Characters: This is a cylindrical root of varying length and thickness. The exterior surface is brown with longitudinal wrinkles. Sometimes a rhizome is attached. It is hard, and does not break easily. The decocting pieces are slices 2–4 mm thick, which are dark brown with irregular yellow or white markings on the cut edge.

Quality: The best roots are dry, thick, and solid with a blackish skin, and without rhizome or fine roots.

Production areas: China (Hebei, Jiangsu, Anhui, Zhejiang, Henan, Hunan, Guizhou), and Korea.

Properties and actions: Slightly cold; bitter and sour; nontoxic. Enters the liver and large intestine channels. Cools the blood and staunches bleeding; clears heat and resolves toxin.

Indications: Blood ejection; spontaneous external bleeding; blood dysentery; uterine bleeding; intestinal wind; hemorrhoids and fistulae; incised wounds; burns. Use crude for all blood patterns and burns. Char-fry to cool the blood and staunch bleeding. Stir-fry with vinegar to treat uterine bleeding and blood dysentery. Daily dosage: 5–10 g. Contraindicated in profuse uterine bleeding due to qi vacuity fall, and in dysentery with dark colored pus and blood in the stool. Used in *di⁴-yu² wan²* (Sanguisorba Pills, 69).

Remarks: Constituents: Saponins: sangisorbin (genin–sanguisorbigenin), ziyuglycoside I, II (genin–pomolic acid). Tannoid (17%). Vitamin-A (0.04%).

Similar plants: *Sanguisorba parviflora* Takeda (Mongolia); *S. grandiflora* Mak. (Mongolia).

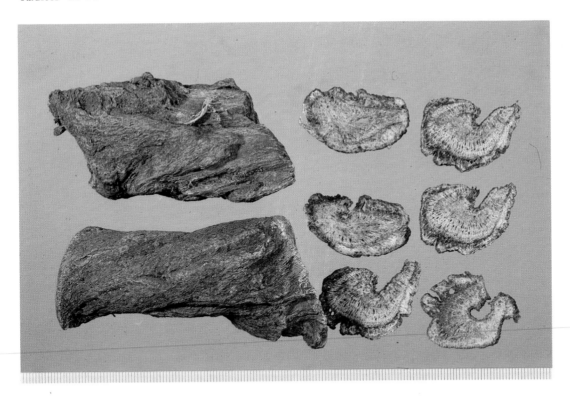

Saussureae Radix: crude (left); sliced (right). (×5/6)

63 SAUSSUREAE RADIX

木香 *mu⁴ xiang¹*. English: saussurea (costus) root, Japanese: *mokko*.
Alternate name: 老木香 *lao³ mu⁴ xiang¹*.
Origin: Compositae family. *Saussurea lappa* Clarke [= *Aucklandia lappa* Decne.], *Vladimiria denticulata* Ling,* *V. souliei* (Franch.) Ling.*
Characters: This is a spindle-shaped or cylindrical root, with irregular contours, usually 6–20 cm long, and 1.5–6 cm thick. The exterior surface is brown, and if split longitudinally as is often the case, the whitish yellow to dark brown wood can be seen. This root is heavy and hard, and does not break easily. On the transverse section, the skin is thin, and the larger woody area appears yellow or white, with dark brown annular markings and radial medullary rays. The decocting pieces are transverse slices 1–2 mm thick.
Quality: The best quality is dry and hard, and gives off a strong odor.
Production areas: China (Yunnan), Burma, and India.
Properties and actions: Warm; acrid and bitter; nontoxic. Enters the lung, liver, and spleen channels. Moves qi and relieves pain; warms the center and harmonizes the stomach. Use crude to rectify qi and relieve pain. Stir-fry with Coptidis Rhizoma (*huang² lian²*) to check dysentery. Roast to check diarrhea and allay thirst.
Indications: Fullness pain in the chest and abdomen; dysenteric disease with tenesmus; cold shan. Daily dosage: 1.5–5 g. Contraindicated in blood vacuity and damage to liquid. Used in *mu⁴-xiang¹ bin¹-lang² wan²* (Saussurea and Areca Pills, 190), *xiang¹ sha¹ er⁴ chen² tang¹* (Saussurea and Amomum Double Vintage Decoction, 289), *xiang¹ lian² wan²* (Saussurea and Coptis Pills, 286).
Remarks: Constituents: Monoterpenoids (volatile oil, 0.3–3%): α-, β-costenes, α-, β-ionones. Sesquiterpenoids: dehydrocostus lactone, mokkolactone (costus lactone), isodehydrocostus lactone. Triterpenoids: betulin, taraxasterol. Steroids: stigmasterol. Alkaloids: saussurine (0.05%). Saccharides: inulin (18%).

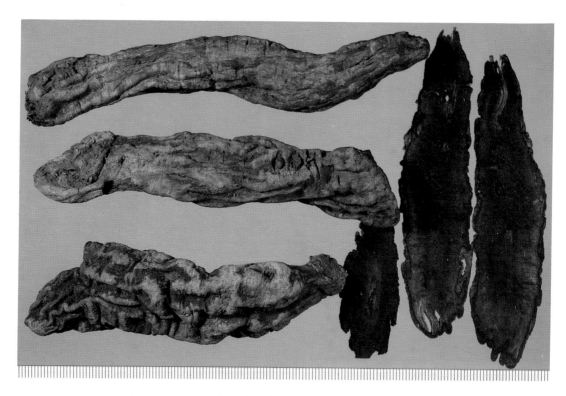

Scrophulariae Radix: crude (left); sliced and treated in brine (right). (×5/6)

64 SCROPHULARIAE RADIX

玄參 *xuan² shen¹*. English: scrophularia (or Ningpo figwort) root. Japanese: *genjin*.

Alternate names: 元參 *yuan² shen¹*, 黑參 *hei¹ shen¹*.

Origin: Scrophulariaceae family. *Scrophularia ningpoensis* Hemsl.

Characters: This root is spindle-shaped and slightly fatter in the middle. It is about 10–14 cm long, and 2–2.5 cm thick. The exterior surface is brown, and bears large wrinkles or folds, and lenticels in transverse configuration. The top bears the remains of the stem base, and is sometimes densely noded. This root is hard, and does not break easily. It is processed by soaking in brine and steaming. It then is cut into slices, which are black, with light flecks.

Quality: Soft, fat roots with fine skin and sweet flavor are the best.

Production areas: China (Zhejiang, Anhui, Shandong, Hebei, Hubei, Jiangxi, Shaanxi, Guizhou, Jilin, Sichuan), and Korea.

Properties and actions: Slightly cold; bitter and salty; nontoxic. Enters the lung and kidney channels. Enriches yin; downbears fire; eliminates vexation; resolves toxin. Use crude to drain fire, resolve toxin, and disinhibit the throat. Stir-fry with brine to enhance the yin-enriching action.

Indications: Vexation and thirst in febrile disease; swelling of yong; macular eruption; sore, swollen throat; scrofulous lumps; constipation. Daily dosage: 5–10 g. Contraindicated in spleen vacuity diarrhea. Used in *xuan²-shen¹ sheng¹-ma² tang¹* (Scrophularia and Cimicifuga Decoction, 313), *zeng¹ ye⁴ tang¹* (Humor-Increasing Decoction, 334), *xuan²-shen¹ san³* (Scrophularia Powder, 312).

Remarks: Constituents: Glycosides: harpagoside. Fatty acids; oleic acid, linoleic acid, stearic acid. Saccharides.

Similar drug: Dried root of *Scrophularia buergeriana* Miq. (Japan, Korea).

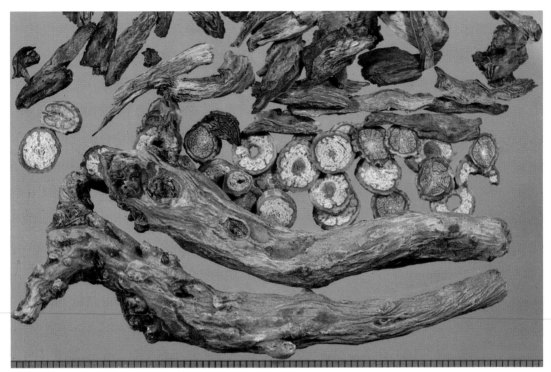

Scutellariae Radix: sliced and stir-fried in wine (top); crude slices (middle);
crude (bottom). (×5/3)

65 SCUTELLARIAE RADIX

黃芩 *huang² qin²*. English: scutellaria (or Baikal skullcap) root. Japanese: *ogon*.
Alternate names:腐腸 *fu³ chang²*,元芩 *yuan² qin²*.
Origin: Labiatae family. *Scutellaria baicalensis* Georgi, *S. viscidula* Bge.,* *S. amoena* C.H. Wright,*
S. hypericifolia Level.*
Characters: This is a cylindrical or spindle-shaped root up to 5–20 cm long and 1–4 cm thick. The
head has usually suffered damage. Older roots often have rotted wood exposed. The outer surface
is yellow, with contorted longitudinal wrinkles. It has numerous wart-like scars from removed branch
roots. The decocting pieces are 1 mm thick transverse or oblique slices, whose cut face is yellowish
green, with clearly visible brown annular markings, yellowish green bark, yellow wood, distinct ducts
configured in broken circles, and a brownish core.
Quality: Hard, long, yellow roots with few stem bases and with hard cores are the best.
Production areas: China (Hebei, Inner Mongolia, Shanxi, Shandong, Shaanxi), and Korea.
Properties and actions: Cold; bitter; nontoxic. Enters the heart, lung, gallbladder, and large in-
testine channels. Drains the fire, eliminates damp-heat, staunches bleeding and quiets the fetus.
Use crude to clear heat and drain fire. Stir-fry to moderate its cold nature and quiet the fetus.
Stir-fry with wine to clear upper-burner damp-heat and lung heat, with ginger juice to clear
heat and dispel phlegm, or with bran to reduce the agent's cold nature and minimize damage
to the stomach. Carbonize to clear heat and staunch bleeding.
Indications: Vigorous fever, vexation, and thirst; lung heat cough; damp-heat diarrhea; jaundice;
heat strangury; blood ejection; uterine and spontaneous external bleeding; red, sore, swollen eyes;
yong and ju; stirring fetus; swollen yong and clove sores. Daily dosage: 3–6 g. Contraindicated
in spleen-stomach vacuity cold, and in repletion fire patterns without damp-heat. Used in
huang²-qin² tang¹ (Scutellaria Decoction, 135), *xie⁴ xin¹ tang¹* (Heart-Draining Decoction, 304),
huang²-lian² jie³ du² tang¹ (Coptis Toxin-Resolving Decoction, 130), *xiao³ chai²-hu² tang¹* (Minor
Bupleurum Decoction, 298), *ge²-gen¹ huang²-qin² huang²-lian² tang¹* (Pueraria, Scutellaria, and
Coptis Decoction, 100).
Remarks: Constituents: Flavonoids: baicalein, 7-methylbaicalein, baicalin, wogonin, wogonoside,
oroxylin-A, skullcapflavones I, II.

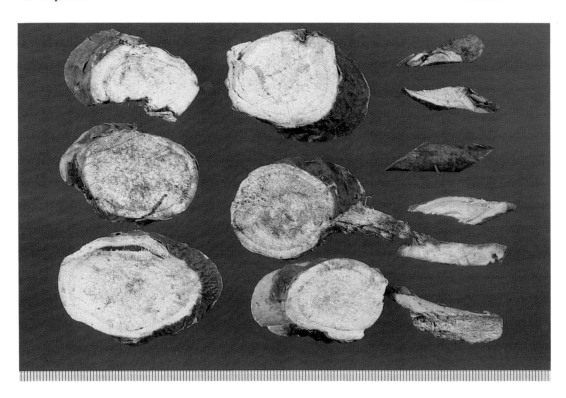

Sophorae Radix: sliced. (×5/3)

66 SOPHORAE RADIX (SOPHORAE FLAVESCENTIS RADIX)

苦参 *ku³ shen¹*. English: bitter ginseng root, sophora (flavescens) root. Japanese: *kujin*.
Alternate names: 苦骨 *ku³ gu³*, 苦参根 *ku³ shen¹ gen¹*.
Origin: Leguminosae family. *Sophora flavescens* Aiton [= *S. angustifolia* Sieb. et Zucc.].
Characters: This product is a irregular cylindrical root that bulges at the top, and often forking at the bottom. The exterior surface is brown, with unpronounced wrinkles, and a scar where the stem was removed. This root is hard and does not break easily. The decocting pieces are thin, oblique slices, whose cut face is pale yellow in color with annular rings, and a radial configuration in the woody part. Sometimes annual rings are clearly visible.
Quality: Pale-colored roots without mold and with a bitter flavor are the best.
Production areas: China (Shanxi, Hubei, Henan, Hebei), Japan, Korea.
Properties and actions: Cold; bitter; nontoxic. Enters the liver, kidney, large intestine, and small intestine channels. Clears heat, dries damp, and kills worms.
Indications: Heat toxin and blood strangury; intestinal wind bleeding; jaundice; red and white vaginal discharge; itchy skin; jie and xian; malign sores; scrofulous lumps; scalds. Soak in wine to treat malign sores. Stir-fry without additives to treat intestinal wind. Stir-fry with wine to treat heat bind, or with vinegar to treat lower abdominal heat pain. Char-fry to staunch bleeding. Daily dosage: 5–10 g. Contraindicated in stomach cold. Used in *ku³-shen¹ tang¹* (Bitter Ginseng Decoction, 160), *san¹ wu⁴ huang²-qin² tang¹* (Three Agents Scutellaria Decoction, 224).
Remarks: Constituents: Alkaloids: (+)-matrine, (+)-oxymatrine, (+)-allomatrine, (+)-isomatrine, (−)-sophoramine, (−)-anagyrine. Flavonoids: kushenols A, B, C, D, E, F, G, H, I, J, K, L, M, N, O, kurarinol, formononetin, (−)-maackiain. Triterpenoids: (saponins) soyasaponin I. Steroids.

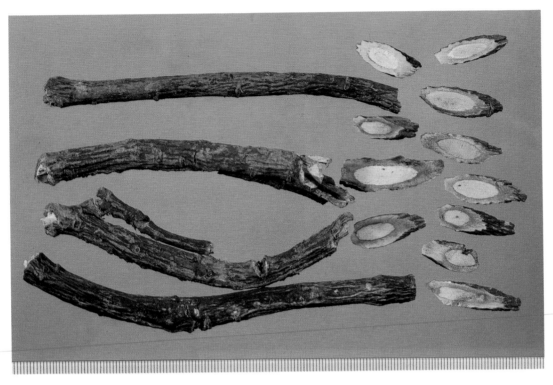

Sophorae Subprostratae Radix: crude (left); sliced (right). (×5/6)

67 SOPHORAE SUBPROSTRATAE RADIX

山豆根*shan¹ dou⁴ gen¹*. English: bushy sophora (or sophora subprostrata) root. Japanese: *sanzukon.*

Alternate name:廣豆根 *guang³ dou⁴ gen¹.*

Origin: Leguminosae family. *Sophora subprostrata* Chun et T. Chen.

Characters: This root is cylindrical, 10–15 cm long and about 7 mm in diameter, and often has branch roots. It is blackish brown in color, with coarse longitudinal wrinkles and long transverse lenticels that protrude slightly. It breaks to leave a granular fracture. The decocting pieces are thin oblique slices, whose cut face is smooth and light brown with annular markings.

Quality: Fat, farinaceous roots are the best.

Production areas: China (Guangxi).

Properties and actions: Cold; bitter; nontoxic. Enters the heart, lung, and large intestine channels. Clears fire, resolves toxin, disperses swelling, and relieves pain.

Indications: Throat yong; throat wind; throat bi; sore, swollen gums; heat cough with dyspnea and fullness; jaundice; dyspnea; hemorrhoids; heat swelling; bald scalp sores; jie and xian; snake, insect and dog bites. Daily dosage: 3–10 g. Contraindicated in spleen-stomach vacuity cold with thin stool. Use in *shan¹-dou⁴-gen¹ tang¹* (Bushy Sophora Root Decoction, 228).

Remarks: Constituents: Alkaloids; matrine, oxymatrine, anagyrine, methylcytisine. Flavonoids: sophoranone, sophoradochromene.
Allied drugs: Roots of *Menispermum dauricum* DC., *Indigofera fortunei* Craib., and *Dunbaria circinalis* Bak.

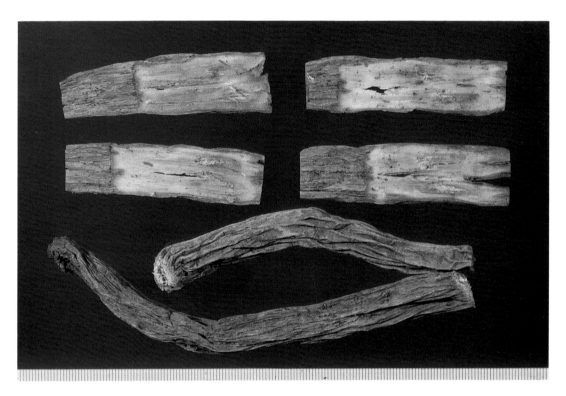

Stemonae Radix: oblique slices (top); crude (bottom). (× 5/6)

68 STEMONAE RADIX

百部 bai³ bu⁴. English: stemona root. Japanese: byakubu.

Alternate name: 百步 bai³ bu⁴.

Origin: Stemonaceae family. *Stemona tuberosa* Lour., *S. japonica* (Bl.) Miq.,* *S. sessilifolia* (Miq.) Franch. et Sav.*

Characters: This product is a long spindle-shaped, snake-like root. Its exterior surface is brown and bears deep creases. It is supple and difficult to break. The decocting pieces are sliced longitudinal sections of the root. Their cut face is yellowish white to brown.

Quality: Large, fat, white roots without stem bases are the best.

Production areas: China (Taiwan, Hubei, Guangdong, Yunnan, Sichuan, Guangxi, Anhui, Guizhou, Fujian).

Properties and actions: Slightly warm; sweet and bitter; nontoxic. Enters the lung channels. Warms and moistens lung qi; suppresses cough; kills worms. Use crude for roundworm and pinworm. Mix-fry with honey to moisten the lung and suppress cough.

Indications: Cold cough; hookworm or pinworm infestation; jie and xian; pulmonary consumption; fulminant cough. Daily dosage: 3–10 g. Contraindicated in spleen-stomach vacuity with diarrhea. used in *bai³-bu⁴ san³* (Stemona Powder, 19), *zhi³ sou⁴ san³* Cough Powder, 343).

Remarks: Constituents: Alkaloids: hypotuberostemonine, oxotuberostemonine, tuberostemonine, isotuberostemonine.

Similar plants: *Stemona parviflora* Wright, *S. vagula* W. Smith.

Similar drugs: Tuber of *S. japonica* (Bl.) Miq. and *S. vagula* W.W. Smith.

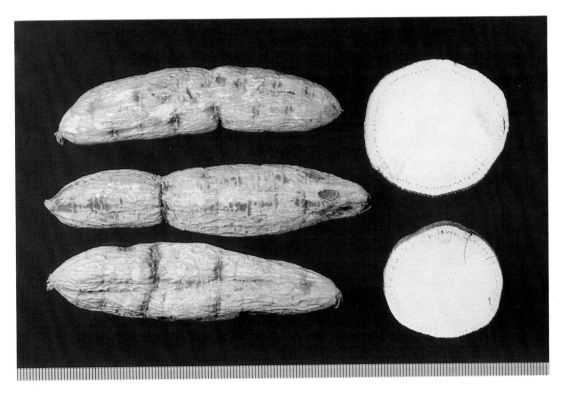

Trichosanthis Radix: crude (left); sliced (right). (× 5/6)

69 TRICHOSANTHIS RADIX

天花粉 *tian¹ hua¹ fen³*. English: trichosanthes root. Japanese: tenkafun, *karokon*.
Alternate names: 花粉 *hua¹ fen³*, 栝樓根 *gua¹ lou² gen¹*.
Origin: Cucurbitaceae family. *Trichosanthes kirilowii Maximowicz*.
Characters: Trichosanthes roots are cylindrical or irregularly shaped, 5–13 cm long and 1–6 cm in diameter. Most have the cork removed and have a whitish yellow surface with fine wrinkles. They are firm and farinaceous in substance and do not easily break. The decocting pieces are fine transverse slices, which reveal a whitish, fibrous interior with numerous small holes.
Quality: Large, fat roots that are fibrous in substance are the best.
Production areas: China (Henan, Guangxi, Shandong, Jiangsu, Guizhou, Anhui), and Korea.
Properties and actions: Cold; sweet, bitter and sour. Enters the lung and stomach channels. Engenders liquid and allays thirst; downbears fire; moistens dryness; expels pus; disperses swelling.
Indications: Thirst in febrile disease; wasting thirst; jaundice; lung dryness; coughing of blood; swollen yong; hemorrhoids. Daily dosage: 10–12 g. Contraindicated in spleen-stomach vacuity cold with diarrhea, and in patterns without repletion heat. Use in *gua¹-lou² gui⁴-zhi¹ tang¹* (Trichosanthes and Cinnamon Twig Decoction, 104), *mai⁴-men²-dong¹ yin³ zi³* (Ophiopogon Drink, 181).
Remarks: Constituents: Triterpenoids: 11-oxo-cucurbita-5-ene-3β, 24, 25 -triol. Steroids: $\triangle^7$ stigmasterol, α-spinasterol. Saccharides: trichosans A, B, C, D, E; starch. Amino acids: β-aminobutyric acid, citrulline. Protein: trichosanthin. Amines: choline.

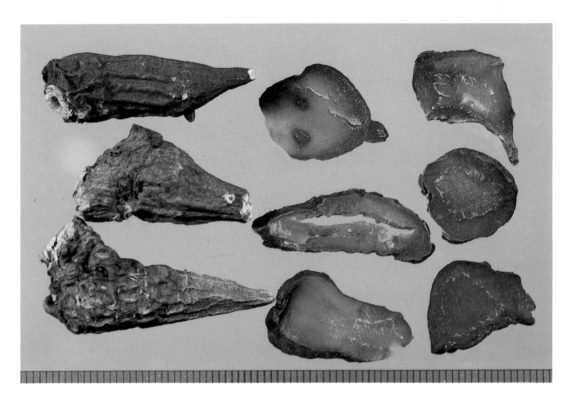

Tsao-Wu-Tou Tuber: crude (left); treated in ginger juice (right). (× 5/3)

70 TSAO-WU-TOU TUBER (ACONITI TSAO-WU-TOU TUBER)

草烏頭 *cao³ wu¹ tou²*. English: wild aconite tuber. Japanese: *souzu.*

Alternate names: 烏頭 *wu¹ tou²*, 草烏 *cao³ wu¹*.

Origin: Ranunculaceae family. *Aconitum kusnezoffi* Rehb., *A. carmichaeli* Debx., *A. hensleyanum* Pritz.

Characters: The mother root is spindle-shaped, about 4–6 cm long, and swelling to about 2 cm thick. Its surface is dark brown. The base of the rhizome is usually to be seen, and in some cases one or two secondary roots, 1–3 cm long and 1–1.5 cm thick, are still attached. The decocting pieces are slices 1 mm thick, that have been soaked, boiled with ginger, and then dried. The slices reveal an interior flesh that is paler than the skin, and semitranslucent.

Quality: Large, firm, farinaceous roots are the best.

Production areas: China (Heilongjiang, Jilin, Liaoning, Inner Mongolia, Hebei, Shanxi, Henan, Shandong, Shaanxi, Gansu, Jiangsu, Anhui, Zhejiang, Jiangxi, Fujian, Hunan, Hubei, Sichuan, Guizhou, Yunnan, Guangxi).

Properties and actions: Hot; acrid; toxic. Enters the liver, spleen, and lung channels. Tracks down wind and percolates damp; dissipates cold and relieves pain; sweeps phlegm, and disperses swelling.

Indications: Wind, cold, and damp bi; wind stroke paralysis; lockjaw; head wind; frigid pain in the venter and abdomen; phlegm pi; qi lumps; cold dysentery; throat bi; yong and ju; clove sores; scrofulous lumps. Daily dosage: 1–3 g. Contraindicated in severe vacuity, pregnancy, effulgent yin vacuity fire, and in heat patterns with pain. The crude form should be administered with care owing to its toxicity. Used in *cao³-wu¹-tou² san³* (Wild Aconite Powder, 35).

Remarks: Constituents: Alkaloids (aconite alkaloids, 0.82-1.6%): aconitine, mesaconitine, hypaconitine, deoxyaconitine, benzoylaconine, benzoylmesaconine, benzoylhypaconine, lipoaconitines. Saccharides: aconitans A, B, C.

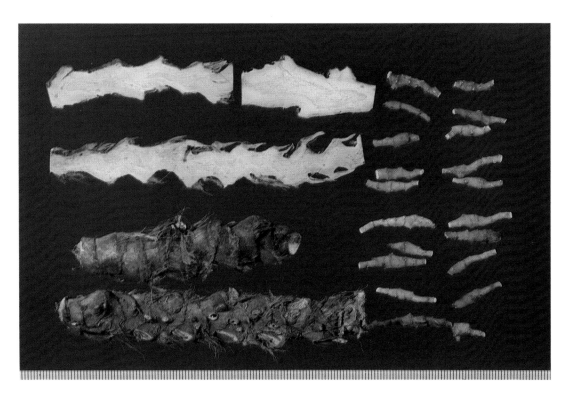

Acori Graminei Rhizoma: sliced (top left); crude (bottom left); Anemones Altaicae Rhizoma (right). (× 5/6)

71 ACORI GRAMINEI RHIZOMA

石菖蒲 *shi² chang¹ pu²*. (Including Anemones Altaicae Rhizoma 九節菖蒲 *jiu³ jie² chang¹ pu²*)
English: acorus rhizome, Japanese: *sekishobu.*
Alternate names: 菖蒲 *chang¹ pu²*, 劍菖 *jian⁴ pu²*.
Origin: Araceae family. *Acorus gramineus* Soland., *Anemone altaica* Fisch.* (Ranunculaceae)
Characters: This is a cylindrical, slightly crooked rhizome, 10-20 cm long and 0.3–1 cm in diameter.
It often has branch roots. The exterior surface is brown with distinct nodes and triangular scars
left by the leafstalk bases that form a crisscross pattern. Sometimes there are scaly hairs, and at
the lower extremity, fine roots, or the scars left by them. This rhizome is hard and does not break
easily. The decocting pieces are thin longitudinal slices that reveal the yellowish or grayish white
color and fibrous nature of the wood. Note: Anemones Altaicae Rhizoma *(jiu³ jie² chang¹ pu²)*
of the Ranunculaceae family is a common substitute.
Quality: The crude root should be dry, fat, and clean of roots.
Production areas: China (Sichuan, Zhejiang, Jiangsu).
Properties and actions: Slightly warm; acrid; nontoxic. Enters the heart, liver, and spleen channels. Opens the portals; sweeps phlegm; rectifies qi; quickens the blood; dissipates wind; eliminates
damp. Stir-fry with ginger juice to open the chest and relieve pain, warm the stomach and open
the portals. Mix-fry with bran and honey to open the portals and fortify the spleen. Coat in cinnabar for a stronger spirit-quieting action.
Indications: Mania and withdrawal; phlegm inversion; clouding inversion in febrile disease; poor
memory; qi block deafness; vexation and oppression in the chest; stomach pain; abdominal pain;
wind, cold, and damp bi; swelling and toxin of yong and ju; impact injury. Daily dosage: 3–6
g. Contraindicated in yang exuberance due to yin vacuity with cough and expectoration of blood.
Used in *ding⁴ zhi⁴ wan²* (Orientation-Stabilizing Pills, 72), *tian¹ wang² bu³ xin¹ dan²* (Celestial
Emperor Heart-Supplementing Elixir, 262).
Remarks: Constituents: Volatile oil 0.5–0.8% (asarone 86%).

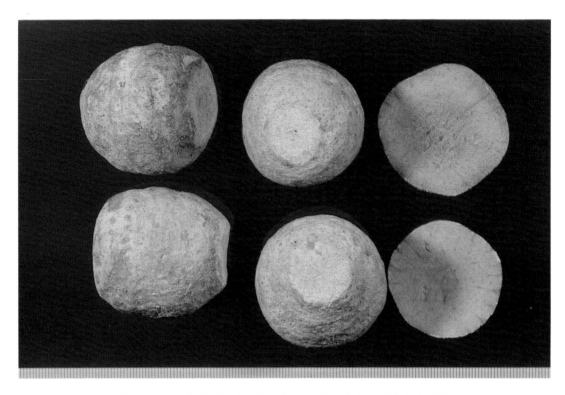

Alismatis crude (left); sliced and treated in brine (right). (×5/6)

72 ALISMATIS RHIZOMA

澤瀉 *ze² xie⁴*. English: alisma (or water plantain) rhizome. Japanese: *takusha*.
Alternate names: 澤芝 *ze² zhi¹*, 水瀉 shui³ *xie⁴*.

Origin: Alismataceae family. *Alisma plantago-aquatica* L. var. *orientale* Samuels.

Characters: This rhizome is spheroid or oval in shape, about 4–7 cm long. The exterior surface is pale brown, with irregular, annular, transverse furrows or indentations, and prominences bearing the scars left by fine roots (especially apparent at the lower end). This rhizome is hard, and breaks with difficulty to reveal a white, granular fracture. The decocting pieces are transverse slices, which reveal irregular vascular bundles. Slices that have been treated with brine are darker in color.

Quality: Large, hard, farinaceous rhizomes that are yellow-white in color are the best.

Production areas: Fujian Alisma: Fujian, Jiangxi. Sichuan Alisma: Sichuan, Yunnan, Guizhou.

Properties and actions: Cold; sweet; nontoxic. Enters the kidney and bladder channels. Disinhibits water, percolates damp, and drains heat.Use crude to fortify the spleen and disinhibit water. Stir-fry with brine to make it act on the kidney and have an even stronger water-disinhibiting effect. Stir-fry with wine and brine for use in supplementing formulae.

Indications: Inhibited urination; water swelling; distention and fullness; diarrhea; phlegm-rheum; leg qi; strangury; blood in the urine. Daily dosage: 6–12 g. Contraindicated in liver or kidney vacuity in the absence of damp-heat. Used in *ze²-xie⁴ tang¹* (Alisma Decoction, 333), *wu³ ling² san³* (Poria Five Powder, 280), *fu²-ling² ze²-xie⁴ tang¹* (Poria and Alisma Decoction, 90), *zhu¹-ling² tang¹* (Polyporus Decoction, 346).

Remarks: Constituents: Triterpenoids: alisols A, B, C, alisol-A monoacetate, alisol B monoacetate, alisol C monoacetate. Sesquiterpenoids: alismol, alismoxide. Saccharides: starch (ca. 25%). Acids: palmitic acid. Amines: choline, lecithin.

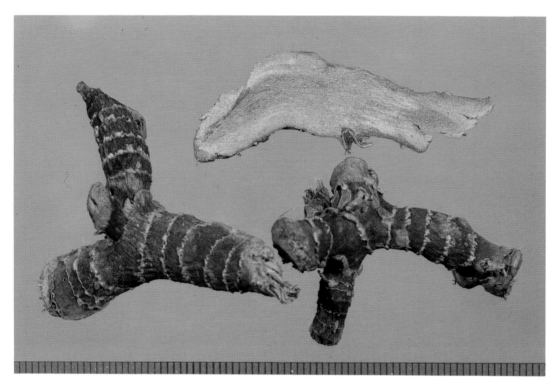

Alpiniae Officinarum Rhizoma: sliced (top); crude (bottom). (× 5/3)

73 ALPINIAE OFFICINARUM RHIZOMA

高良薑 *gao¹ liang² jiang¹*. English: lesser galangal rhizome. Japanese: *koryokyo.*

Alternate name: 良薑 *liang² jiang¹.*

Origin: Zingiberaceae family. *Alpinia officinarum* Hance.

Characters: This rhizome is cylindrical and branching. It is 5–12 cm in length and 1–2 cm in diameter. The exterior surface is a reddish brown, with longitudinal wrinkles, and leaf scars forming pale wavy markings about 5 mm apart, encircling the rhizome. At the lower end are scars left by the fine roots. This rhizome is hard, and breaks with difficulty to reveal an uneven, fibrous, orange-brown fracture. The decocting pieces are oblique or longitudinal slices 1–2 mm thick, and irregular in shape. The cut edge reveals diffuse vascular bundles. The inner layers of skin and the central core of the wood are slightly darker in color.

Quality: Hard, solid rhizomes that have a bright, fresh color, and a strong smell are the best.

Production areas: China (Guangdong, Guangxi, Taiwan).

Properties and actions: Warm; acrid. enters the spleen and stomach channels. Warms the stomach; dispels wind; dissipates cold; moves qi; relieves pain.

Indications: Spleen-stomach cold; frigid pain in the venter and abdomen; vomiting and diarrhea; esophageal constriction; food stagnation; miasmic malaria; cold pi. Daily dosage: 3–5 g. Contraindicated in vomiting due to stomach heat, summerheat damage or choleraic disease, diarrhea due to heat or fire, and in heart vacuity. Used in *gao¹-liang²-jiang¹ tang¹* (Lesser Galangal Decoction, 98), *an¹ zhong¹ san³* (Center-Quieting Powder, 3).

Remarks: Constituents: Volatile oil (0.5–1.0%): 1.8-cineole, methylcinnamate, α-cadinene. Acrids: galangol. Flavonoids: alpinin, galangin, kaempferid.

Similar drug: Rhizome of *Alpinia galanga* (L.) Swartz.

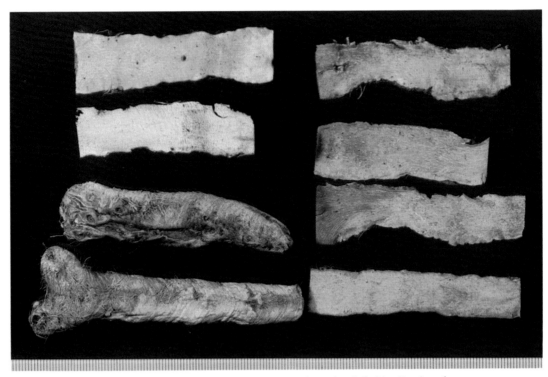

Anemarrhenae Rhizoma: crude sliced and unsliced (left); sliced and
stir-fried in brine (right). (× 5/6)

74 ANEMARRHENAE RHIZOMA

知母 zhi¹ mu³. English: anemarrhena rhizome. Japanese: *chimo*.

Alternate name: 知母肉 zhi¹ mu³ rou⁴.

Origin: Liliaceae family. *Anemarrhena asphodeloides* Bunge.

Characters: This is a flat, contorted, ribbon-like rhizome, with roots branching from it. It is 0.8–1.5 cm in diameter. The exterior surface is brown. The upper side is rounded and bears scars left by the bases of the leafstalks, while the under surface bears scars where the fibrous roots have been removed. This rhizome is soft, and breaks easily to reveal a pale yellowish brown, slightly spongy interior, and the dotted formation of the vascular bundles. The decocting pieces are longitudinal slices 1–2 mm thick.

Quality: Large, fat, smooth rhizomes that are pale yellow on the inside and that have little hair are the best.

Production areas: China (Hebei, Shanxi, Inner Mongolia, Gansu, Shaanxi, Manchuria).

Properties and actions: Cold; bitter; nontoxic. Enters the lung, stomach, and kidney channels. Enriches yin and downbears fire; moistens dryness and lubricates the intestines. Use crude to drain heat. Stir-fry to moderate the cold effect, with wine to make it act on the upper body and with brine to make it enter the kidney, moisten dryness, and enrich yin.

Indications: Vexation and thirst; steaming bone and taxation heat; lung heat cough; dry, bound stool; inhibited urination. Daily dosage: 5–10 g. Contraindicated in spleen-stomach vacuity with indigestion and thin-stool diarrhea. Used in *da⁴ bu³ yin¹ wan²* (Major Yin Supplementation Pills, 44), *bai² hu³ jia¹ ren²-shen¹ tang¹* (White Tiger Decoction Plus Ginseng, 10), *bai² hu³ tang¹* (White Tiger Decoction, 11).

Remarks: Constituents: Steroids: (saponins, ca. 6%): timosaponins A-I, A-II, A-III, A-IV, B-I, B-II, markogenin-3-O-β-glucopyranosyl (1–2)-β-galactopyranoside; sarsasapogenin, markogenin, neotigogenin. Saccharides: anemarans A, B, C, D.

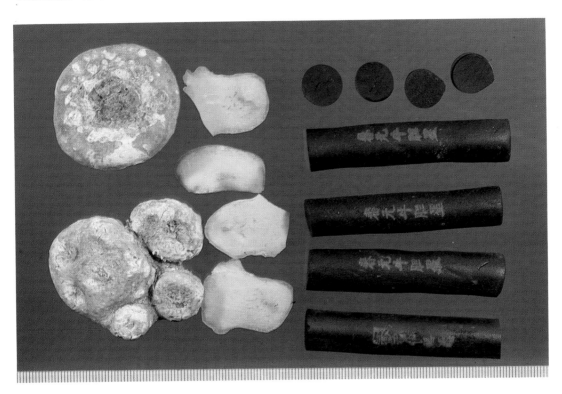

Arisaematis Rhizoma: crude and slices treated with ginger (left); with bovine bile (right). (× 5/6)

75 ARISAEMATIS RHIZOMA

天南星 *tian¹ nan² xing¹*. English: arisaema rhizome. Japanese: *tennansho*.
Alternate names: 虎掌南星 *hu³ zhang³ nan² xing¹*, 南星 *nan² xing¹*.
Origin: Araceae family. *Arisaema consanguineum* Schott, *A. amurense* Maxim., *A. heterophyllum* Bl., *A. ambiguum* Engl.,* *A. peninsulae* Nakai,* *A. japonicum* Bl. *
Characters: This is spheroid in shape, 1.5–6.5 cm in diameter. The exterior surface is brownish white, with a depression at the top that is surrounded by indented scars left by the fibrous roots. It is hard, heavy, and the fracture is white. It is commercially available treated with ginger or bovine bile. The type treated with ginger comes in slices that are pale in color, and slightly darker and translucent at the edges. Bile-processed arisaema (*dan³ xing¹*) takes the form of hard, dark brown, cylindrical sticks.
Quality: Evenly sized, dry, solid, farinaceous rhizomes are the best.
Production areas: China (Sichuan, Henan, Guizhou, Yunnan, Guangxi).
Properties and actions: Warm; bitter and acrid; toxic. Enters the lung, liver, and spleen channels. Dries damp and transforms phlegm; dispels wind and calms fright; disperses swelling and binds. Use the processed forms for reduced toxicity. Use stir-fried with ginger, for a warming and dissipating action to dispel phlegm, or processed in bile to reduce its dryness and harshness.
Indications: Wind stroke hemiplegia and deviation of the eyes and mouth; epilepsy; child fright wind; lockjaw; wind-phlegm dizziness; throat bi; scrofulous lumps; swollen yong; impact injury and bone fractures; snake and insect bites. Bile processed arisaema is the best type to treat fright, epilepsy, and dizziness. Daily dosage: 3–5 g. Contraindicated in yin vacuity and dryness phlegm. Used in *yu⁴ zhen¹ san³* (True Jade Powder, 329), *san¹ sheng¹ yin³* (Three Raw Agents Beverage, 222), *qing¹ shi¹ hua⁴ tan² tang¹* (Dampness-Clearing Phlegm-Transforming Decoction, 209).
Remarks: Constituents: Saponins. Starch.

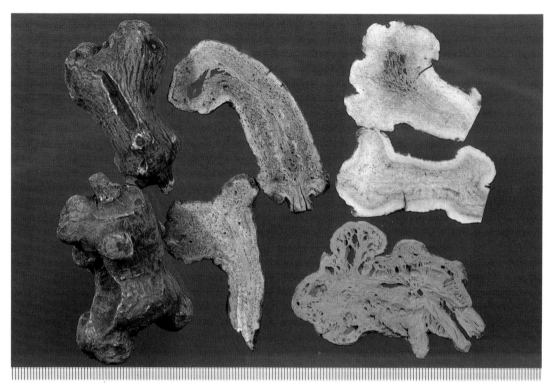

Atractylodis Ovatae Rhizoma: crude (left); stir-fried (middle); crude slices
(top right); stir-fried with earth (bottom right). (× 5/6)

76 ATRACTYLODIS OVATAE RHIZOMA

白朮 bai^2 zhu^2. English: atractylodes ovata rhizome. Japanese: $byakujutsu$.
Alternate name:於朮 yu^2 zhu^2.
Origin: Compositae family. *Atractylodes ovata* De Candolle [= *A. macrocephala* Koidz.].
Characters: This rhizome has the remains of one or two stalks at the top, and has knobbly protuberances toward the lower extremity. The surface is a grayish or yellowish brown. It is 4–8 cm
long and 2–5 cm thick. It is hard, and breaks with difficulty. On the fracture the skin is granular
in texture, while the wood is fibrous, hollow in places, and whitish in color. It is cut into oblique
or longitudinal slices 2–4 mm thick. These are used crude, or stir-fried to a golden brown. Also
available commercially are slices stir-fried in earth, which have a homogeneous rusty brown
coloration.
Quality: Large, dry rhizomes with fine light brown skin and white interiors are the best. They
should break cleanly, unimpeded by any stringy fibers.
Production areas: China (Zhejiang, Anhui, Hunan, Hubei, Jiangxi, Fujian).
Properties and actions: Warm; bitter and sweet; nontoxic. Enters the heart, spleen, stomach,
and triple burner channels. Supplements the spleen and boosts the stomach; dries damp; harmonizes
the center. Use crude to dry damp and disinhibit water. Use stir-fried for greater spleen-fortifying
action. Use stir-fried with earth to fortify the spleen and check diarrhea. Use stir-fried with bran
to disperse fullness and distention and to supplement the spleen.
Indications: Spleen vacuity with fullness and distention; vexation and oppression in the chest
and diaphragm; diarrhea; water swelling; phlegm-rheum; spontaneous sweating. Daily dosage:
5–10 g. Contraindicated in yin vacuity with thirst. Used in $dang^1$-gui^1 san^3 (Tangkuei Powder, 59),
si^4 jun^1 zi^3 $tang^1$ (Four Gentlemen Decoction, 251), wu^3 $ling^2$ san^3 (Poria Five Powder, 280),
shi^2 $quan^2$ da^4 bu^3 $tang^1$ (Perfect Major Supplementation Decoction, 243), bu^3 $zhong^1$ yi^4 qi^4 $tang^1$
(Center-Supplementing Qi-Boosting Decoction, 33).
Remarks: Constituents: Sesquiterpenoids (volatile oil, 0.9–3%): atractylon, 3-β-hydroxyatractylon,
3-β-acetylatractylon, atractylenolides I, II, III.
Allied drug: Dried rhizome of *Atractylodes japonica* Koidz. (Japan).

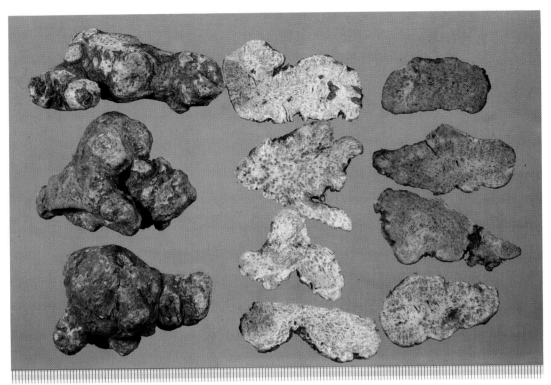

Atractylodis Rhizoma: crude (left); crude slices (middle); stir-fried
slices (right). (×.5/6)

77 ATRACTYLODIS RHIZOMA

蒼朮 *cang¹ zhu².* English: atractylodes rhizome. Japanese: *sojutsu.*
Alternate names: 赤朮 *chi⁴ zhu²,* 仙朮 *xian¹ zhu².*
Origin: Compositae family. *Atractylodes lancea* (Thunb.) DC., *A. .chinensis* Koidz*., *A. japonica*
Koidz. (Japan).,* *A. koreana* Nakai (Korea).*
Characters: This is a knobbly rhizome about 4–10 cm long and 1–2 cm thick. The exterior surface
is dark brown, dry and brittle. At the top are the remains of the stem base and scars where shoots
have been removed. At the lower end are the remains of the short, hard fine roots. This rhizome
is hard and solid, and breaks unevenly to reveal a pale interior and supple fibers. It is cut into
thin oblique or longitudinal 1–3 mm thick slices, which are irregular in shape. The cut edge has
orange brown spots, which are less apparent when the general coloration is darkened by stir-frying.
Quality: Large, firm rhizomes with dark skin, numerous oil sacs, and a sweet aroma are best.
Growing of fine white hairs in storage is also a sign of good quality.
Production areas: China (Jiangsu, Hubei, Henan, Zhejiang, Anhui, Jiangxi).
Properties and actions: Warm; acrid, bitter; nontoxic. Enters the spleen and stomach channels. Fortifies the spleen, dries damp, resolves depression, and repels foulness. Stir-frying with
rice water, earth, or bran removes oil and reduces the dry quality. Scorch-frying warms the spleen,
dispels damp, and checks diarrhea.
Indications: Exuberant damp encumbering spleen; lassitude; somnolence; glomus in the venter;
abdominal distention; loss of appetite; vomiting; diarrhea; dysenteric and malarial disease; phlegm-
rheum; water swelling; seasonal qi colds and flu; atony; night blindness. Daily dosage: 3–10 g.
Contraindicated in yin vacuity heat and conditions of dry bound stool and copious perspiration.
Used in *ping² wei⁴ san³* (Stomach-Calming Powder, 196), *bai² hu³ jia¹ cang¹-zhu² tang¹* (White
Tiger Decoction Plus Atractylodes, 8).
Remarks: Constituents: Sesquiterpenoids: (volatile oil, 3.5%): hinesol, β-eudesmol, elemol.
Polyenynes: atractylodin, atractylodinol, acetylatractylodinol.

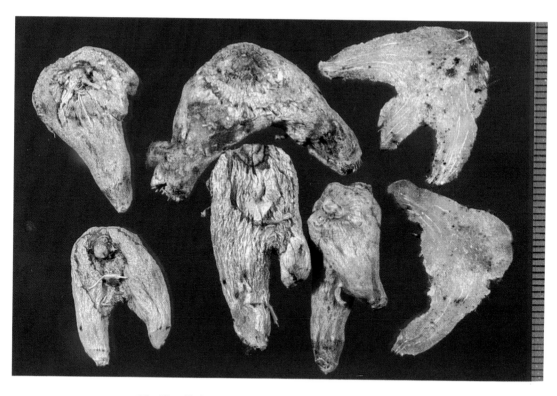

Bletillae Tuber: crude (left) and sliced (right). (×5/3)

78 BLETILLAE TUBER

白及 *bai² ji²*. English: bletilla tuber. Japanese *byakkyu*.

Alternate name: 白芨 *bai² ji²*.

Origin: Orchidaceae family. *Bletilla striata* (Thunb.) Reichb. f.

Characters: This is a fat, brown tuber with one or two branches and an overall length of 1.5–4 cm. At the top is a scar left by the stalk, and at bottom is the scar left where another tuber was attached. It is hard and horny, and does not break easily. It is cut into thin oblique or transverse slices, which are irregular in shape. The cut edge is white or pale yellow, horny, semitranslucent, with visible vascular bundles.

Quality: Tubers that are pale in color and semitranslucent when sliced are the best.

Production areas: China (Guizhou, Sichuan, Hunan, Henan, Zhejiang, and Shaanxi).

Properties and actions: Balanced; bitter and sweet; nontoxic. Enters the lung channels. Supplements the lung; staunches bleeding; disperses swellings; engenders muscle; closes sores.

Indications: Blood ejection; spontaneous external bleeding. Topically applied for incised wounds and swollen yong. Daily dosage: 3–5 g. Contraindicated in lung or stomach repletion heat. Used in *bai²-ji² pi²-pa² wan²* (Bletilla and Loquat Pills, 13).

Remarks: Allied drug: Tuber of *Bletilla ochraceae* Schltr.

Constituents: Mucilage: bletilla-glucomannan. Starch.

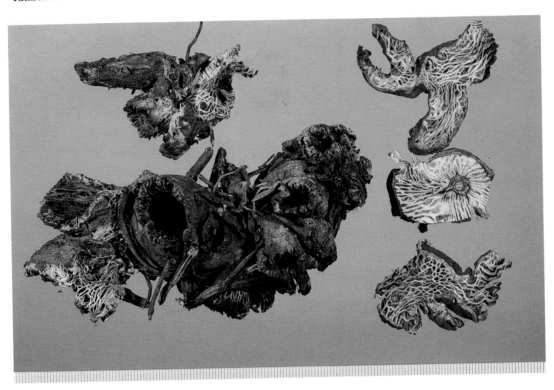

Cimicifugae Rhizoma: crude (left) and sliced (right). (× 5/6)

79 CIMICIFUGAE RHIZOMA

升麻 *sheng¹ ma²*. English: cimicifuga (or bugbane) rhizome. Japanese: *shoma*.

Alternate names: 綠升麻 *lü⁴ sheng¹ ma²*, 雞骨升麻 *ji¹ gu³ sheng¹ ma²*.

Origin: Ranunculaceae family. *Cimicifuga foetida* L., *C. dahurica* (Turcz.) Maxim., *C. heracleifolia* Kom.

Characters: This rhizome is roughly cylindrical, but very irregular in shape. The surface is blackish brown, sometimes with fine roots still attached. On the upper side are protuberances scars marking the place where stems were removed. The scars often take the form of holes, which reveal the reticular structure of the inner wood. This rhizome is light and vacuous, but hard and not easily broken. The decocting pieces are oblique or transverse slices 1–3 mm thick, which show the reticular structure of the yellowish white wood very clearly.

Quality: The best rhizomes are large, black, with stalks and hair removed. They should be light and loose in substance, and pale on the cross section.

Production areas: *Cimicifuga dahurica*: China (Liaoning, Helongjiang, Hebei, Shanxi). *C. foetida*: China (Shaanxi, Sichuan, Qinghai, Yunnan). *C. heracleifolia*: China (Liaoning, Jilin, Heilongjiang).

Properties and actions: Cold; sweet, acrid, slightly bitter. Enters the lung, spleen, and stomach channels. Upbears yang, promotes exterior effusion, outthrusts papules and resolves toxin. Use crude to outthrust papules, clear heat, resolve toxin, and effuse wind-heat. Use mix-fried with honey for stronger lung-moistening and cough-suppressing action.

Indications: Seasonal and epidemic pestilential qi; yang ming headache; sore throat; maculopapular eruption; wind heat sores; center qi fall; enduring diarrhea; prolapse of the rectum; uterine bleeding and vaginal discharge. Daily dosage: 3–5 g. Contraindicated upper body exuberance and lower body vacuity and effulgent yin vacuity fire. Used in *sheng¹-ma² ge²-gen¹ tang¹* (Cimicifuga and Pueraria Decoction, 238), *bu³ zhong¹ yi⁴ qi⁴ tang¹* (Center-Supplementing Qi-Boosting Decoction, 33).

Remarks: Constituents: Triterpenoids: cimigenol (cimicifugol), cimigol, dahurinol, isodahurinol, cimicifugenol, 25-O-methylcimigenol.

Allied drug: Dried rhizome of *Cimicifuga simplex* Worms. (Japan).

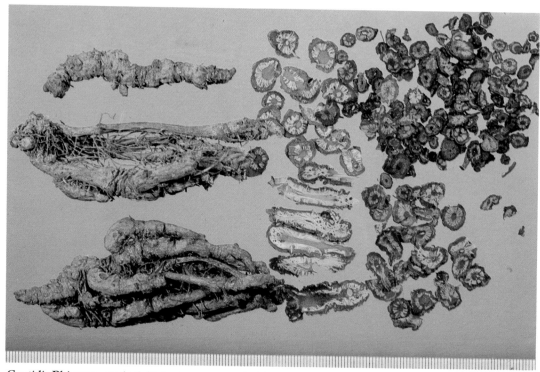

Coptidis Rhizoma: crude (left), in transverse and oblique slices (middle), stir-fried with evodia (top right), and stir-fried with ginger juice (bottom right). (× 5/6)

80 COPTIDIS RHIZOMA

黃連 *huang² lian²*. English: coptis (or goldthread) rhizome. Japanese: *oren*.

Alternate names: 味連 *wei⁴ lian²*, 雞連 *ji¹ lian²*.

Origin: Ranunculaceae family. *Coptis chinensis* Franch., *C. deltoides* C.Y. Cheng et Hsiao, *C. omeiensis* (Chen) C.Y. Cheng, *C. teetoides* C.Y. Cheng, *C. quinquesecta* W.T. Wang.*

Characters: This rhizome, with 3–6 firm, yellowish brown, cylindrical branches bearing irregular knobbles, often has the appearance of a closed chicken's foot. The decocting pieces are thin oblique slices, on whose cut edge the skin appears dark brown, and the wood, perforated with holes, appears golden yellow, sometimes with a slightly darker core.

Quality: Long, densely noded rhizomes without hair, having the appearance of the heart of a chrysanthemum flower on the cross section are best.

Production areas: China (Sichuan, Hubei, Shaanxi).

Properties and actions: Cold; bitter; nontoxic. Enters the heart, liver, stomach, and large intestine channels. Drains fire, dries damp, resolves toxin and kills worms. Use crude to break blood and qi. Stir-fry without additives to regulate the blood. Stir-fry with wine to move the blood and dispel stasis. Stir-fry in vinegar to calm the liver, staunch bleeding, and relieve pain. Boil with vinegar to nourish the liver. Stir-fry with wine and vinegar to relieve pain.

Indications: Seasonal heat toxin; cold damage; exuberant heat vexation; glomus and fullness; counterflow retching; bacillary dysentery; abdominal pain due to heat diarrhea; pulmonary tuberculosis; blood ejection; spontaneous external bleeding; precipitation of blood. Daily dosage: 1–3 g. Contraindicated in spleen vacuity diarrhea, and in vexation and fever due to either yin vacuity or postpartum blood vacuity. Used in *huang²-lian² e¹-jiao¹ tang¹* (Coptis and Ass Hide Glue Decoction, 129), *xie⁴ xin¹ tang¹* (Heart-Draining Decoction, 304), *huang²-lian² jie³ du² tang¹* (Coptis Toxin-Resolving Decoction, 130), *zuo³ jin¹ wan²* (Metal-Assisting Pills, 356), *huang²-lian² tang¹* (Coptis Decoction, 131), *xiang¹ lian² wan²* (Saussurea and Coptis Pills, 286).

Remarks: Constituents: Alkaloids: berberine (3–8%), palmatine, coptisine, jateorrhizine, worenine, columbamine, magnoflorine.

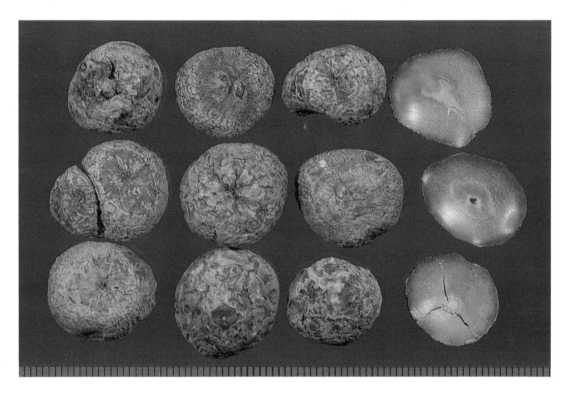

Corydalis Tuber: crude (left) and treated with vinegar (right). (×5/3)

81 CORYDALIS TUBER

延胡索 *yan² hu² suo³*. English: corydalis (or yanhusuo) tuber. Japanese: *engosaku.*

Alternate names: 元胡索 *yuan² hu² suo³*, 玄胡索 *xuan² hu² suo³*.

Origin: Papaveraceae family. *Corydalis yanhusuo* W.T. Wang.

Characters: This tuber is spheroid or ovate, sometimes single, and sometimes attached to another. It is about 1.5–2.5 cm in diameter, and a yellowish brown in color. On one side it has a depression where the base of the stalk was removed, and on the other, numerous tuberous protuberances. It is hard, and breaks to reveal a smooth, granular fracture that is a greenish yellow in color. It is cut into thin transverse slices, which are then stir-fried until they turn dark brown, or mix-fried with vinegar or wine until light brown.

Quality: Firm, large, plump tubers that have finely wrinkled wax-yellow skin, and golden yellow interiors are the best.

Production areas: China (cultivated in Dongyang and Panan in Zhejiang).

Properties and actions: Warm; bitter; nontoxic. Enters the liver and stomach channels. Quickens the blood and dissipates stasis; rectifies qi and relieves pain.

Indications: Pain in the chest and abdomen; menstrual irregularities; concretions and conglomerations; profuse uterine bleeding; postpartum blood dizziness; lochiorrhea; impact injury. Daily dosage: 5–10 g. Contraindicated in heat stasis and blood vacuity. Used in *san¹ shen² wan²* (Three Spirits Pills, 221), *an¹ zhong¹ san³* (Center-Quieting Powder, 3).

Remarks: Constituents: Alkaloids (0.59–0.74%): (–)-tetrahydrocolumbamine, (–)-tetrahydroberberine, (–)-tetrahydrocoptisine, (±)-tetraydropalmatine, (+)-corybulbine, (+)-corydaline, columbamine, coptisine, palmatine, dehydrocorybulbine, dehydrocorydaline.

Allied drugs: Tuber of *Corydalis turschaninovii* Besser, *C. ternata* Nakai, and *C. ambigua* Chamisso et Schlechter.

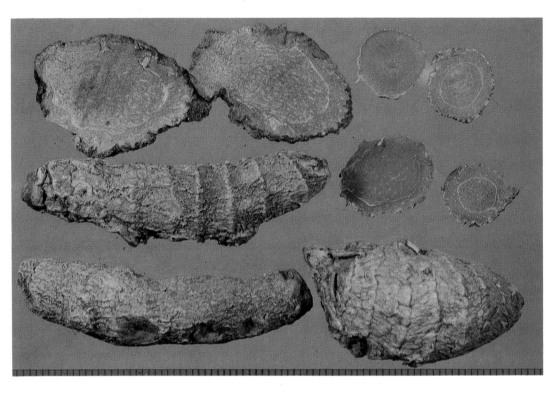

Curcumae Longae Rhizoma: long type (left) and round type (right). (×5/3)

82 CURCUMAE LONGAE RHIZOMA

薑黃 *jiang¹ huang²*. English: turmeric. Japanese: *kyoo.*

Alternate names: 川薑黃 *chuan¹ jiang¹ huang²*, 黃薑 *huang² jiang¹.*

Origin: Zingiberaceae family. *Curcuma longa* L., *C. aromatica* Salisb.

Characters: There is both a long and a round type. The long type is a straight or contorted cylindrical rhizome, tapering slightly at each end. Its exterior surface is a deep yellow-brown, with longitudinal wrinkles and transverse annular nodes that mark the places where the leaf stalks were attached. Sometimes there are tumorous branch roots, or the scars that they leave when they break off. This rhizome is hard and heavy. It is cut into thin transverse slices, 1–4 mm thick. The cut surface is a deep yellow brown, with a clearly defined skin layer and vascular bundles appearing as speckles. The round type is similar to the long type, but is shorter and fatter. It is about 4 cm long and 3 cm thick.

Quality: Dry, hard, yellow rhizomes with annular nodes are the best.

Production areas: China (southern mainland and Taiwan), Japan, Burma, Indonesia, and Mexico.

Properties and actions: Warm; bitter, acrid; nontoxic. Enters the spleen and liver channels. Breaks blood, moves qi, promotes menstruation and relieves pain.

Indications: Painful glomus and fullness in the abdomen and region of the heart; pain in the kidney; concretions and conglomerations; menstrual block due to stasis; postpartum abdominal stasis pain; impact injuries swollen yong. Daily dosage: 3–5 g. Contraindicated in the absence of stasis and stagnation. Used in *jiang¹-huang² san³* (Turmeric Powder, 144).

Remarks: Constituents: Volatile oil (1–5%): turmerone, dihydroturmerone, zingiberene, cineole. Yellow pigment: curcumin.

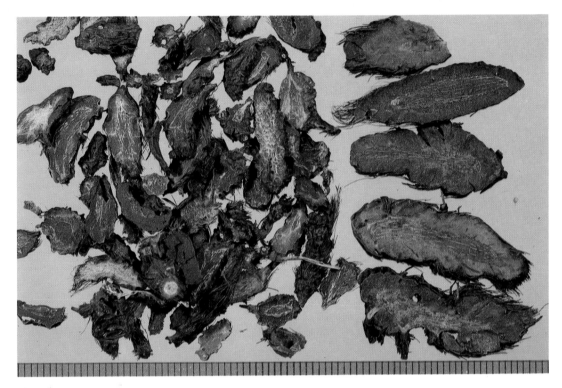

Cyperi Rhizoma: cut and treated. (×5/3)

83 CYPERI RHIZOMA

香附子 *xiang¹ fu⁴ zi³*. English: cyperus (or nut-grass) rhizome. Japanese: *kōbushi.*

Alternate names: 香附 *xiang¹ fu⁴*, 莎草根 *sha¹ cao³ gen¹.*

Origin: Cyperaceae family. *Cyperus rotundus* L.

Characters: This is a spindle-shaped or cylindrical rhizome, 2–3.5 cm long, and 8–10 mm thick. The exterior surface is purplish black, and sometimes has a blackened appearance. It usually has 6–10 protuberant annular nodes 2–4 mm apart, from which flat-lying hairs spring. There are invariably remains of fine roots, or the scars they leave behind after breaking off. This rhizome is hard, and breaks with difficulty to reveal a granular fracture. The decocting pieces are transverse, oblique, or longitudinal slices about 1–3 mm thick. The cut edge is a blackish brown at the edges and paler at the center. On it, the cortex is clearly defined, and the vascular bundles of both the cortex and core appear as speckles.

Quality: Large, firm, red rhizomes with a strong aroma are the best.

Production areas: China (Shandong, Zhejiang, Hunan, Henan), Korea, Japan.

Properties and actions: Balanced; acrid, slightly bitter, sweet; nontoxic. Enters the liver and triple burner channels. Rectifies qi and resolves depression; relieves pain and regulates menstruation. Use crude to resolve depression. Stir-fry with vinegar to enter the liver, rectify qi and blood, and relieve pain. Treat with wine to move channel and vessel flow. Stir-fry with brine to enter the blood aspect and moisten dryness. Stir-fry with ginger juice to transform phlegm and rheum. Char-fry to staunch bleeding.

Indications: Menstrual irregularities; qi depression; distention and pain in the chest and abdomen; liver-stomach disharmony; phlegm-rheum; glomus and fullness; uterine bleeding and vaginal discharge; yong and ju. Daily dosage: 5–10 g. Contraindicated in yin vacuity blood heat. Used in *xiang¹ su¹ san³* (Cyperus and Perilla Powder, 294), *xiang¹ sha¹ yang³ wei⁴ tang¹* (Saussurea and Amomum Stomach-Nourishing Decoction, 292), *xiang¹ sha¹ ping² wei⁴ san³* (Saussurea and Amomum Stomach-Calming Powder, 291), *xing² qi⁴ xiang¹ su¹ san³* Qi-Moving Cyperus and Perilla Powder, 305), *xiang¹ xiong¹ tang¹* (Cyperus and Ligusticum Decoction, 295).

Remarks: Constituents: Sesquiterpenoids and monoterpenoids (volatile oil, 0.5%): α-cyperone (main), β-cyperone, cyperol, α-, β-rotunols, cyperene, kobusone, isokobusone.

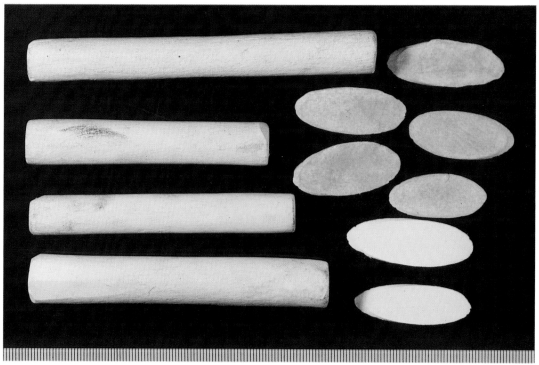

Dioscoreae Rhizoma: crude (left), sliced and stir-fried in earth (top right),
and crude slices (bottom right). (× 5/6)

84 DIOSCOREAE RHIZOMA

山藥 *shan¹ yao⁴*. English: dioscorea (or Chinese yam) rhizome. Japanese: *sanyaku*.
Alternate names: 淮山藥 *huai² shan¹ yao⁴*, 薯蕷 *shu³ yu⁴*, 懷山藥 *huai² shan¹ yao⁴*.
Origin: Dioscoreaceae family. *Dioscorea batatas* Decaisne [= *D. opposita* Thunb.].
Characters: This is a cylindrical rhizome about 20 cm long and 1.3–4 cm in diameter, with flat
ends. The exterior surface is smooth, chalky, and white, with vascular bundles appearing as faint,
fine markings. It is hard and heavy, and breaks to reveal a white granular, chalky fracture. The
decocting pieces are oblique slices 1–3 mm thick. Their cut edge is smooth, white and chalky,
occasionally with visible brown vascular bundles. When stir-fried in earth, the slices turn a slightly mottled yellow-brown.
Quality: Firm, straight, pure white, highly farinaceous rhizomes are the best.
Production areas: China (Henan, Hunan, Hubei, Shanxi, Guizhou, Yunnan, Shaanxi, Jiangsu,
Zhejiang, Jiangxi, Sichuan).
Properties and actions: Balanced; sweet; nontoxic. Enters the lung, spleen, and kidney channels. Fortifies the spleen, supplements the lung, secures the kidney and boosts essence. Use crude
to enrich yin. Stir-fry (with or without bran or earth) to harmonize the stomach and spleen.
Indications: Spleen vacuity diarrhea; enduring dysentery; cough due to vacuity taxation; wasting
thirst; seminal emission; frequent urination. Daily dosage: 10–15 g. Contraindicated in damp-heat
repletion patterns. Used in *ba¹ wei⁴ di⁴-huang² wan²* (Eight-Ingredient Rehmannia Pills, 6), *zhi¹
bo² di⁴-huang² wan²* (Anemarrhena, Phellodendron, and Rehmannia Pills, 337).
Remarks: Constituents: Saccharides: starch (16%), dioscorea-mucilage-B, mannan, phytic acid. Sesquiterpenoids: (+)-abscisin II. Stilbenes: batatasins I, II, III, IV, V. Steroids. Amines. Enzymes:
amylase.
Allied drugs: Rhizome of *D. japonica* Thunb. (Japan), *D. alata* L. (Taiwan), and *D. doryophora*
Hance (Taiwan).

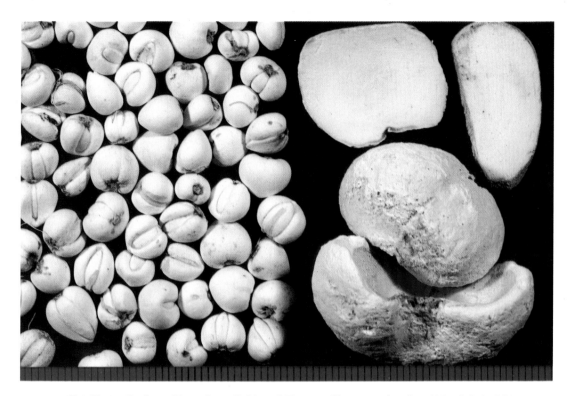

Fritillariae Bulbus: *F. cirrhosa* (left) and *F. verticillata* var. *thunbergii* (right). (×5/3)

85 FRITILLARIAE BULBUS

貝母 *bei⁴ mu³*. English: fritillaria bulb. Japanese: *baimo*.

Origin: Liliaceae family. *Fritillaria cirrhosa* D. Don, *F. verticillata* Willd. var. *thunbergii* Bak.

Characters: Sichuan fritillaria (*Fritillaria cirrhosa* [*huan¹ bei⁴ mu³*]) is round, and pointed at one end, with numerous fibrous roots sprouting from its base. It is about 0.5–1 cm in diameter. The exterior layer comprises two scales that interlock. The interior comprises a number of scales with a stalk in the center. It is white or yellow in color, and pure white on the inside. It is brittle, and when broken the ruptured edge has a farinaceous appearance. Zhejiang fritillaria (*F. verticillata* var. *thunbergii* [*zhe⁴ bei⁴ mu³*]) is bunshaped, 2–3.5 cm in diameter and 1–1.5 cm high. It has 2 thick scales on the exterior enveloping numerous small ones. It is often sold in the form of separated scales, which are white on the outer surface and pale brown on the inner surface. These are often cut into 2 mm thick slices.

Quality: Dry, neatly shaped, heavy, pure-white, farinaceous bulbs are the best.

Production areas: *Fritillaria cirrhosa:* China (Sichuan, Xizang, Yunnan, Gansu, Qinghai). *F. verticillata* var. *thunbergii:* China (Zhejiang, Jiangsu).

Properties and actions: Slightly cold; bitter. Enters the lung and heart channels. Suppresses cough and dispels phlegm; clear heat and dissipates binds.

Indications: Cough; blood ejection; thirst; throat bi; scrofulous lumps; mammary yong; dorsal effusions; painful, swollen sores. Daily dosage: 5–10 g. Contraindicated in spleen-stomach vacuity cold. Used in *bai³-he² gu⁴ jin¹ tang¹* (Lily Bulb Metal-Securing Decoction, 20), *jie²-geng³ bai² san³* (Platycodon White Powder, 146), *bei⁴-mu³ tang¹* (Fritillaria Decoction, 27).

Remarks: Constituents: Alkaloids (0.1–0.4%): verticine (peimine, ca. 0.1%), verticinone (peiminine), peimiphine, peimidine, peimitidine, verticilline, isoverticine, propeimine, peiminoside.

Allied drug: Bulb of *Fritillaria thunbergii* Miq. (Japan).

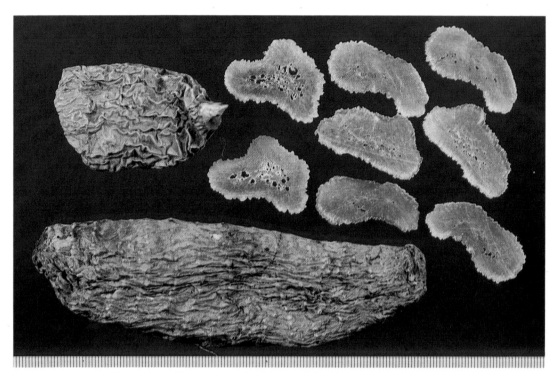

Gastrodiae Rhizoma: crude (left) and sliced treated with ginger juice (right). (× 5/6)

86 GASTRODIAE RHIZOMA

天麻 *tian¹ ma²*. English: gastrodia rhizome Japanese: *tenma*.

Alternate names: 赤箭 *chi⁴ jian⁴*, 明天麻 *ming² tian¹ ma²*.

Origin: Orchidaceae family. *Gastrodia elata* Blume.

Characters: This is an oval rhizome, 7-10 cm long, and 2-3 cm in diameter. At one end are the remains of the stem. The exterior is pale brown in color, and slightly translucent, with irregular wrinkles due to shrinkage. It is hard and horny, and not easily broken. If crushed it breaks into pieces that reveal the glossy, dark brown interior. The decocting pieces are extremely fine, semitranlucent slices, on which vascular bundles appear as speckles or streaks.

Quality: The best quality cuts into clear, bright slices.

Production areas: China (Yunnan, Sichuan, Guizhou).

Properties and actions: Warm; sweet. Extinguishes wind and calms fright. Treats dizziness, head wind and headache, numbness of the limbs, hemiplegia, impeded speech, child fright epilepsy.

Indications: Dizziness and blackouts; head wind and headache; wind stroke with hemiplegia and speech difficulty; child fright epilepsy; wind, cold, and damp bi. Daily dosage: 3-5 g. Contraindicated in yin vacuity. Used in *ban⁴-xia⁴ bai²-zhu² tian¹-ma² tang¹* (Pinellia, Atractylodes Ovata, and Gastrodia Decoction, 24), *chen²-xiang¹ tian¹-ma² tang¹* (Aquilaria and Gastrodia Decoction, 40).

Remarks: Constituents: Phenylpropanoids: vanillyl alcohol, vanillin, benzyl alcohol, 4-hydroxybenzaldehyde, gastrodin. Steroids: β-sitosterol, daucosterol. Saccharides: sucrose.

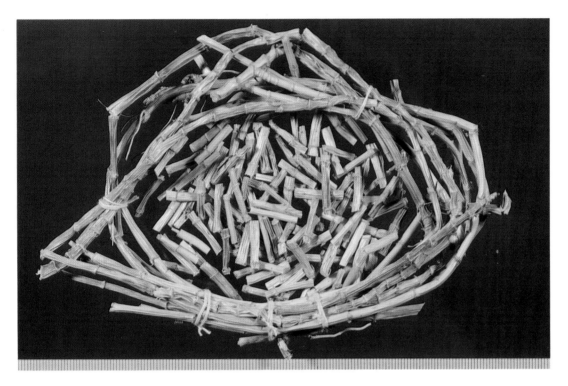

Imperatae Rhizoma: crude and cut. (×5/6)

87   IMPERATAE RHIZOMA

白茅根 *bai² mao² gen¹*. English: imperata (or cogon) rhizome. Japanese: *hakubōkon, bōkon*.
Alternate names: 白茅 *bai² mao²*, 茅根 *mao² gen¹*.
Origin: Gramineae family. *Imperata cylindrica* (L.) P. Beauv. var. *major* (Nees) C.E. Hubb.
Characters: This is a long, thin, cylindrical rhizome that sometimes has branches. It varies in length and is 2–4 mm thick. It has nodes, at which there are scaly leaf sheaths and fine roots or their remains. The outer surface is pale yellow, and has longitudinal wrinkles. The decocting pieces are sections 2–5 mm long, which are pale yellow on the cut edge.
Quality: Thick, dry, sparsely noded, pure white rhizomes without fibrous roots are the best.
Production areas: China (most parts, but Qingyuan and Yangshan in Guangdong produce the best).
Properties and actions: Cold; sweet; nontoxic. Enters the lung, stomach, and small intestine channels. Cools the blood and staunches bleeding; clears heat; disinhibits urine.
Indications: Internal heat; vexation; inhibited urination; heat strangury; blood in the urine; blood ejection; spontaneous external bleeding. Daily dosage: 10–15 g. Contraindicated in vacuity cold and the absence of repletion heat. Used in *mao²-gen¹ tang¹* (Imperata Decoction, 183).
Remarks: Constituents: Triterpenoids: cylindrin (0.01%), arundoin (0.01%), fernenol, simiarenol, isoborinol. Acids: citric acid, malic acid. Saccharides (18.8%): sucrose.
Allied drug: Rhizome of *Imperata cylindrica* (L.) P. Beauv. var. *koenigii* Durand. et Schinz. (Japan).

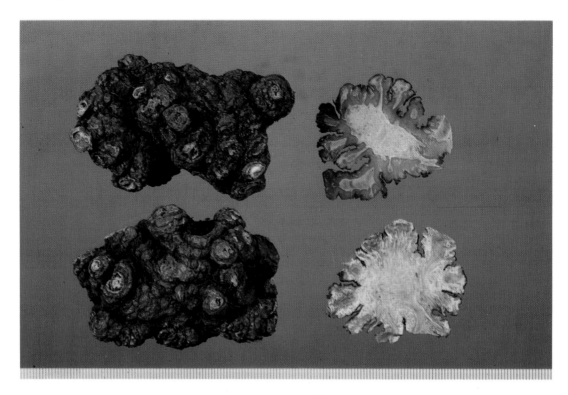

Ligustici Rhizoma: crude (left) and treated with wine (right). (×5/6)

88   LIGUSTICI RHIZOMA

川芎 *chuan¹ xiong¹*. English: ligusticum (or chuanxiong, Sichuan lovage) rhizome. Japanese: *senkyu*.

Alternate names: 川藭 *chuan¹ qiong²*, 芎藭 *xiong¹ qiong²*.

Origin: Umbelliferae family. *Ligusticum chuanxiong* Hort. [= *L. striatum* DC., and *L. wallichi* Franch.].

Characters: This is an irregular fist-shaped noded rhizome, 3–10 cm long and 2–5 cm in diameter. The exterior surface is brown, with numerous ringed nodes, each with a large depression marking the place where the stem was attached. The nodes also have many protuberant scars where the roots were attached. This rhizome is firm and solid, and has a distinct aroma. It is cut in longitudinal slices, which on the cut edge appear yellow brown, or paler at the medulla, and have darker brown speckles (oil sacs). Slices are darker in color when stir-fried with wine.

Quality: Large, fat, heavy rhizomes with white interiors and a strong aroma are the best.

Production areas: China (Sichuan, Yunnan, Hubei).

Properties and actions: Warm; acrid. Enters the liver and gallbladder channels. Moves qi and relieves depression; expels wind and dries damp; quickens the blood and relieves pain. Stir-frying in wine enhances the blood-quickening and channel-freeing action.

Indications: Wind-cold headache and dizziness; abdominal and lateral costal pain; hypertonicity of the sinews in cold bi; dizziness; menstrual block; postpartum stasis obstruction; yong, ju, and sores. Daily dosage: 3–5 g. Contraindicated in effulgent yin vacuity fire. Used in *si⁴ wu⁴ tang¹* (Four Agents Decoction, 256), *chuan¹-xiong¹ cha²-tiao² san³* (Tea-Blended Ligusticum [Cnidium] Powder, 42), *sheng¹ hua⁴ tang¹* (Engendering Transformation Decoction, 235).

Remarks: Constituents: Phthalides: ligustilide, 3-butylidene-7-hydroxyphthalide, *cis-* and *trans*-6,7-dihydroxyligustilides, wallichilide, butylphthalide, butylidenephthalide, senkyunolide A, neocnidilide.

Allied drug: *Cnidium officinale* Makino (Japan).

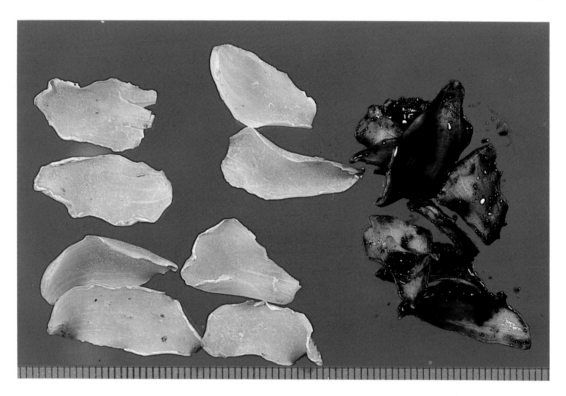

Lilii Bulbus: crude scales (left) and mix-fried with honey (right). (×5/3)

89 LILII BULBUS

百合 *bai³ he²*. English: lily bulb. Japanese. *byakugo.*

Alternate names: 白百合 *bai² bai³ he²*, 白花百合 *bai² hua¹ bai³ he².*

Origin: Liliaceae family. *Lilium brownii* F.E. Brown var. *colchestri* Wils., *L. pumilum* DC.,* *L. longiflorum* Thunb.*

Characters: The scales of this bulb are about 2–3.5 cm long and 1–1.5 cm wide. They are about 1–5 mm thick in the middle, and thinner at the edges, where they curl inward slightly. They are wide at the base and pointed at the ends. They are yellowish white, and semitranslucent, and have longitudinal streaks (vascular bundles). They are hard and horny, and break cleanly.

Quality: Heavy, white wild-grown bulbs with small scales and bitter flavor are the best.

Production areas: China (Hunan, Sichuan, Zhejiang, Hubei, Jiangsu, Shaanxi, Guangdong, Huabei, Manchuria).

Properties and actions: Cold; sweet and slightly bitter; nontoxic. Enters the heart and lung channels. Moistens the lung and suppresses cough; clears the heart and quiets the spirit; disinhibits water. Mix-frying with honey enhances the lung-moistening action.

Indications: Taxation cough; blood ejection; vacuity vexation; fright palpitation; water swelling; hysteria. Daily dosage: 5–10 g. Not suitable for wind-cold or phlegm cough. Used in *bai³-he² gu⁴ jin¹ tang¹* (Lily Bulb Metal-Securing Decoction, 20), *bai³-he² zhi¹-mu³ tang¹* (Lily Bulb and Anemarrhena Decoction, 21), *bai³ hua¹ gao¹* (Lily Bulb and Tussilago Paste, 22).

Remarks: Constituents: starch, protein, anthocyanin, mannan, liliosterin. Similar plants: *Lilium dahuricum* Kel-Gawl., *L. concolor* Salisb.

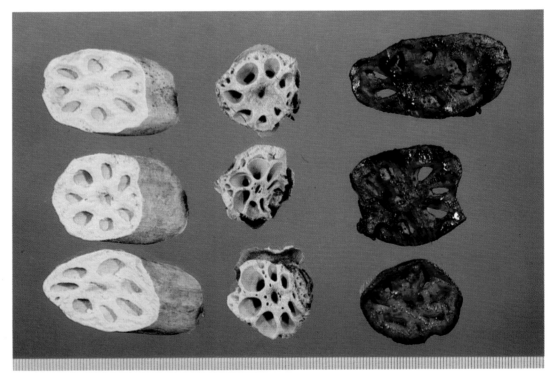

Nelumbinis Rhizoma: sliced (left); Rhizomatis Nodus
crude (middle) and mix-fried with honey (right). (×5/6)

90 NELUMBINIS RHIZOMATIS NODUS

藕節 *ou³ jie²*. English: lotus rhizome node. Japanese: *gusetsu.*

Alternate names: 光藕節 *guang¹ ou³ jie²*, 藕節疤 *ou³ jie² ba¹*.

Origin: Nymphaeaceae family. *Nelumbo nucifera* Gaertn.

Characters: Lotus rhizomes may be spheroid or cylindrical in shape, 7–20 cm long and 5–8 cm thick, and are joined together in linear array. The exterior surface is pale yellow-brown. On the transverse cross section is a distinct configuration of eight holes, one in the center and seven encircling it. The node, which joins two rhizomes, is solid, sometimes with fibrous roots still attached, and scars left by the leafstalk bases. It is cut in such a way that a little of the rhizome, with its distinctive holes, is still attached.

Quality: Black nodes with white rhizomes are the best.

Production areas: China (Zhejiang, Jiangsu, Anhui, Hubei, Hunan, Shandong, Jiangxi, Fujian, Hebei).

Properties and actions: Balanced; sweet, astringent; nontoxic. Enters the lung, stomach, and liver channels. Staunches bleeding and dissipates stasis. Use crude to clear blood heat, allay thirst, and transform stasis. Char-fry to staunch bleeding.

Indications: Blood ejection; spontaneous external bleeding; blood in the urine; blood in the stool; blood dysentery; profuse uterine bleeding. Daily dosage: 5–10 g. Used in *bai²-ji² pi²-pa² wan²* (Bletilla and Loquat Pills, 13).

Remarks: Constituents: tannin, asparagine.

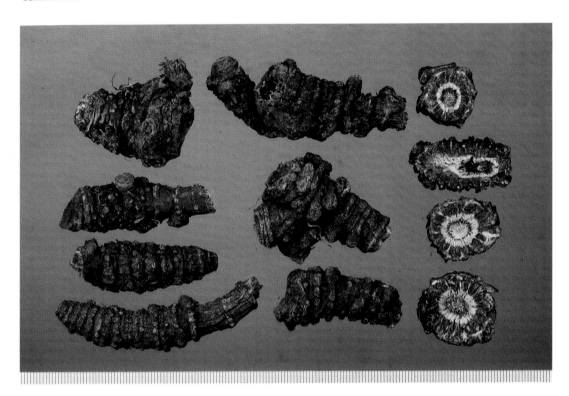

Notopterygii Rhizoma: crude (left) and sliced (right). (×5/6)

91 NOTOPTERYGII RHIZOMA

羌活 qiang¹ huo². English: notopterygium rhizome. Japanese: *kyokatsu.*

Alternate names: 竹節羌 zhu² jie² qiang¹, 蠶羌 can² qiang¹.

Origin: Umbelliferae family. *Notopterygium incisum* Ting, *N. forbesii* Boiss., *N. franchetii* Boiss.

Characters: This is a roughly cylindrical rhizome or varying length, 1–3 cm in diameter. It bears scars left by branch roots, and at the top has a scar left by the stalk. The exterior surface is a blackish brown, and is covered with annular nodes, dense at the top and growing scarce further down, that are covered with numerous tumorous shoot scars. This rhizome is light and breaks cleanly. It is cut into thin transverse or oblique slices roughly 1 mm thick. On the cut surface, which is broken by radial fissures, the cortex is brown, the wood is whitish yellow, and the central medulla is a blackish brown.

Quality: Fat rhizomes that have annular protuberances, and have a pattern on the cross section resembling a chrysanthemum flower are the best. A strong odor is also a mark of good quality.

Production areas: China (Sichuan, Gansu, Qinghai, Shaanxi, Yunnan, Xinjiang, Tibet).

Properties and actions: Warm; acrid, bitter; nontoxic. Enters the kidney and bladder channels. Dissipates exterior cold, dispels wind-damp, and disinhibits the joints.

Indications: Contraction of wind-cold with headache and absence of sweating; wind, cold, and damp bi; stiffness of the neck; wind water swelling; yong, ju, and sore-toxin. Daily dosage: 3–10 g. Contraindicated in blood vacuity. Used in *jiu³ wei⁴ qiang¹-huo² tang¹* (Nine-Ingredient Notopterygium Decoction, 152), *qiang¹-huo² bai²-zhi³ san³* (Notopterygium and Angelica Powder, 202) *qiang¹-huo² sheng⁴ shi¹ tang¹* (Notopterygium Dampness-Overcoming Decoction, 204), *chuan¹-xiong¹ cha² tiao² san³* (Tea-Blended Ligusticum [Cnidium] Powder, 42).

Remarks: Constituents: Coumarins: angelical.

Similar drugs: Root of *Aralia cordata* Thunb. (China), *Angelica pubescens* Maxim. (Japan), and *A. koreana* Maxim. (Korea).

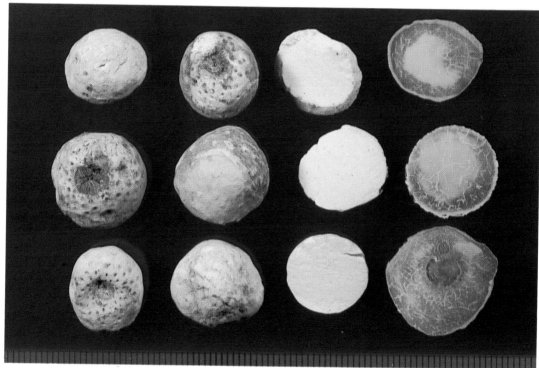

Pinelliae Tuber: crude (left), pro formula (middle), and boiled in
ginger juice (right). (× 5/3)

92 PINELLIAE TUBER

半夏 *ban⁴ xia⁴*. English: pinellia tuber. Japanese: *hange.*
Alternate names: 水玉 *shui³ yu⁴*, 珠半夏 *zhu¹ ban⁴ xia⁴.*
Origin: Araceae family. *Pinellia ternata* (Thunb.) Breitenbach.
Characters: Crude pinellia is usually sold with its cortex already removed. It is hard, spheroid
in shape, and about 5–14 mm in diameter. The exterior surface bears fine wrinkles, and is pale
gray in color, and yellowish where the cork has not been completely removed. At the fatter end
is a depression where the shoot was removed, and around it are many small pits where the roots
were once attached. It is sold in ready prepared in slices, either prepared according to a complex
procedure (pro formula), or boiled in ginger juice. Pro formula pinellia (*fa³ ban⁴ xia⁴*) slices are
white and farinaceous, while ginger pinellia slices are semitranslucent and horny.
Quality: Dry, firm, round, farinaceous tubers with the skins completely removed are the best.
Production areas: China (Sichuan, Hubei, Anhui, Jiangsu, Henan, Zhejiang).
Properties and actions: Warm; acrid; toxic. Enters the spleen and stomach channels. Dries
damp and transforms phlegm; downbears counterflow and suppresses vomiting; disperses glomus
and dissipates binds. Use crude for topical application only. Use the ginger–treated kind, which
is warm and dry in nature, to check vomiting. Use the other processed forms to dry damp and
transform phlegm.
Indications: Phlegm-damp and water rheum; cough and dyspnea; dizziness. Daily dosage: 5–10
g. Contraindicated in all blood patterns, in pregnancy, and yin vacuity and damage to fluids. Used in *er⁴ chen² tang¹* (Double Vintage Decoction, 80), *gan¹-jiang¹ ren²-shen¹ ban⁴-xia⁴ wan²* (Dried
Ginger, Ginseng, and Pinellia Pills, 95), *ban⁴-xia⁴ hou⁴-po⁴ tang¹* (Pinellia and Magnolia Bark
Decoction, 25), *xiao³ ban⁴-xia⁴ jia¹ fu²-ling² tang¹* (Minor Pinellia Decoction Plus Poria, 297), *da⁴
ban⁴-xia⁴ tang¹* (Major Pinellia Decoction, 43), *ban⁴-xia⁴ xie⁴ xin¹ tang¹* (Pinellia Heart-Draining
Decoction, 26).
Remarks: Constituents: Phenylpropanoids: homogentisic acid, homogentisic acid glucoside,
3,4-dihydroxybenzaldehyde, 3,4-dihydroyxybenzaldehyde diglucoside.
Similar drug: *Pinellia pedatisecta* Schott.

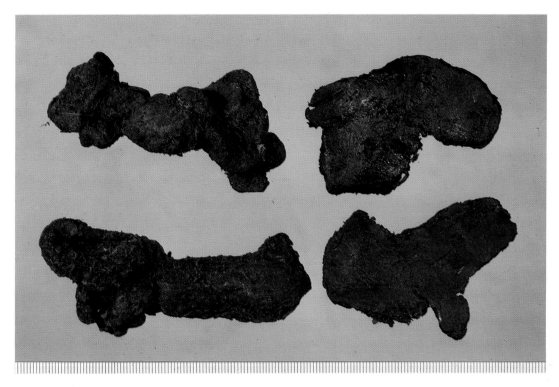

Polygonati Rhizoma: crude (left); steamed nine times and sliced (right). (×5/6)

93 POLYGONATI RHIZOMA

黄精 *huang² jing¹*. English: polygonatum rhizome . Japanese: *osei.*

Alternate names: 薑形黃精 *jiang¹ xing² huang² jing¹*, 雞頭黃精 *ji¹ tou² huang² jin¹.*

Origin: Liliaceae family. *Polygonatum sibiricum* Redoute, *P. multiflorum* L., *P. cyrtonema* Hua,* *P. macropodium* Turcz.,* *P. kingianum* Coll. et Hemsl.,* *P. cirrhifolium* (Wall.) Royle*.

Characters: This rhizome is lumpy and irregularly shaped. It is about 6–18 cm long, and 1–3 cm thick. The exterior surface is varying shades of brown and semitranslucent. It has longitudinal wrinkles, protuberant annular nodes, and scars left by leafstalks and fibrous roots. It is usually sold in pre-treated form—steamed nine times, stir-fried with wine, or boiled with black beans, and is dark brown or black. It is sliced before decocting.

Quality: Large, soft, fat, yellow rhizomes with a sweet taste are the best.

Production areas: *Polygonatum sibiricum:* China (Hebei, Inner Mongolia). *P. multiflorum:* China (Hubei, Guizhou, Sichuan).

Properties and actions: Slightly cold; sweet; nontoxic. Enters the spleen, lung, and kidney channels. Supplements the center and boosts qi; moistens the lung; strengthens the sinews and bones. The commercial processing enhances the supplementing action.

Indications: Fever and chills in vacuity detriment; pulmonary consumption; coughing of blood; weak constitution after disease; weak sinews and bones; wind lai and xian. Daily dosage: 10–15 g. Contraindicated in splenic vacuity with exuberant damp and food accumulations, and unsuitable for patients with thin stool diarrhea. Used in *man⁴-jing¹-zi³ san³* (Daikon Seed Powder, 182).

Remarks: Constituents: Saccarides: mucilage. Starch.

Allied drug: Dried rhizome of *Polygonatum falcatum* A. Gray (Japan).

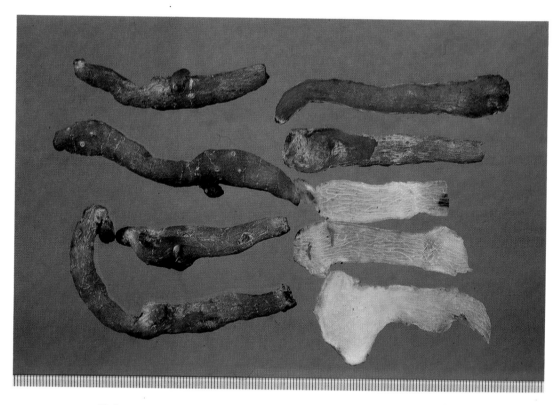

Polygonati Officinalis Rhizoma: crude (left) and sliced (right). (×5/6)

94 POLYGONATI OFFICINALIS RHIZOMA

玉竹 *yu⁴ zhu²*. English: Solomon's seal rhizome. Japanese: *gyokuchiku.*

Alternate names: 明玉竹 *ming² yu⁴ zhu²*, 萎蕤 *wei¹ rui²*.

Origin: Liliaceae family. *Polygonatum officinale* All., *P. odoratum* (Mill.) Druce var. *pluriform* (Miq.) Ohwi*, *P. macropodium* Turcz.,* *P. involucratum* Maxim.,* *P. inflatum* Komar.*

Characters: The dry rhizome is cylindrical and slightly shrunken, with sparse branches of differing length. Its overall length can be as much as 40 cm, but is usually sold broken into 5–15 cm lengths. The diameter is about 1 cm. The exterior surface is a pale, yellowish brown, and has distinct fine annular nodes 0.3–1 cm apart, and bears the scars left by fibrous roots. It is hard when dry, but when affected by damp it softens and becomes supple. It is cut into longitudinal slices, which are pale yellow, horny, and semitranslucent.

Quality: Long, soft, fat rhizomes pale in color, with a sweet flavor are the best.

Production areas: China (Jiangsu, Zhejiang, Anhui, Hunan, Guangdong, Guangxi, Yunnan, Sichuan).

Properties and actions: Slightly cold; sweet; nontoxic. Enters the lung and stomach channels. Nourishes yin; moistens dryness; eliminates vexation; allays thirst. Use crude to clear heat and nourish yin. Use processed forms to supplement the center and boost qi, and to enrich yin and moisten dryness.

Indications: Damage to yin in febrile disease; cough, vexation, and thirst; vacuity taxation with fever; swift digestion with rapid hungering; frequent urination. Daily dosage: 5–10 g. Contraindicated in debilitation of yang and exuberance of yin, in spleen vacuity with thoracic oppression, and stagnant phlegm-damp. Used in *yu⁴-zhu² yin³* (Solomon's Seal Beverage, 330).

Remarks: Constituents: Glycosides: convallamarin, convallarin.

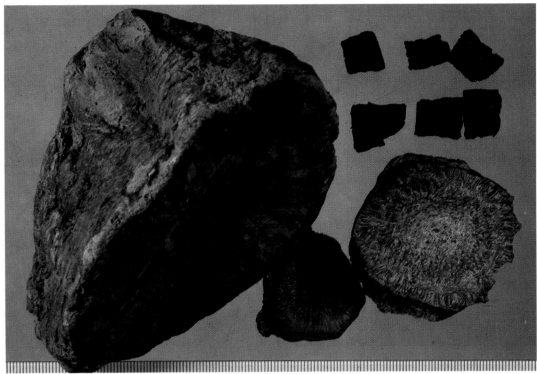

Rhei Rhizoma: crude (left); prepared with wine and sliced (top right); steamed with wine (bottom right). (× 5/6)

95 RHEI RHIZOMA

大黃 da⁴ huang². English: (Chinese) rhubarb rhizome. Japanese: *daio*.

Alternate names: 將軍 *jiang¹ jun¹*, 錦紋 *jin³ wen²*.

Origin: Polygonaceae family. *Rheum palmatum* L., *R. officinale* Baill., *R. tanguticum* Maxim.

Characters: This rhizome is roughly ovate in shape, and is a yellow brown in color with paler reticular markings. *R. palmatum* is 5–10 cm long and 4–8 cm in diameter and is heavy. *R. officinale* is larger, being anything up to 15 cm in diameter. It is lighter and spongier, and bears pale reticular markings. The decocting pieces are slices 2–4 mm thick, that are crude, cooked (steamed or stir-fried), or prepared in wine.

Quality: Firm, heavy, oleaceous, mottled or speckled, yellow-brown rhizomes that are bitter, but not astringent to the taste are best.

Production areas: *Rheum palmatum:* Tongde area of Qinghai and the Quanshui and Xili areas of Gansu. *R. officinale:* Sichuan.

Properties and actions: Cold; bitter. Enters the stomach, large intestine, and liver channels. Drains heat toxin; breaks accumulation and stagnation; moves static blood. It has a milder precipitating effect when cooked, and bears upward when treated with wine (head and eye disorders).

Indications: Repletion heat constipation; delirious mania; food accumulation glomus and fullness; initial stage of dysentery; abdominal urgency and rectal heaviness; menstrual block; concretions and gatherings; seasonal heat toxin; blood ejection; spontaneous external bleeding; fulminant reddening and swelling of the eyes; yang jaundice; water swelling; turbid strangury; dark-colored urine; yong, ju, sores, burns, scalds. Daily dosage: 3–10 g. Contraindicated in the absence of depressed heat in the blood aspect or absence of food stagnation. Used in *da⁴-huang² fu⁴-zi³ tang¹* (Rhubarb and Aconite Decoction, 47), *da⁴ cheng² qi⁴ tang¹* (Major Qi-Infusing Decoction, 46), *xie⁴ xin¹ tang¹* (Heart-Draining Decoction, 304), *da⁴-huang² gan¹-cao³ tang¹* (Rhubarb and Licorice Decoction, 48), *tao²-he² cheng² qi⁴ tang¹* (Peach Kernel Qi-Infusing Decoction, 260), *xiao³ cheng² qi⁴ tang¹* (Minor Qi-Infusing Decoction, 299), *tiao² wei⁴ cheng² qi⁴ tang¹* (Stomach-Regulating Qi-Infusing Decoction, 263).

Remarks: Constituents: Dianthrones (0.5–2%): sennosides A, B, C, D, E, F, rheinosides A, B, C, D; sennidins A, C. Anthraquinones (free 0.1–1.3%, as glycosides 0.8–4.4%, total 1.0–5.2%).

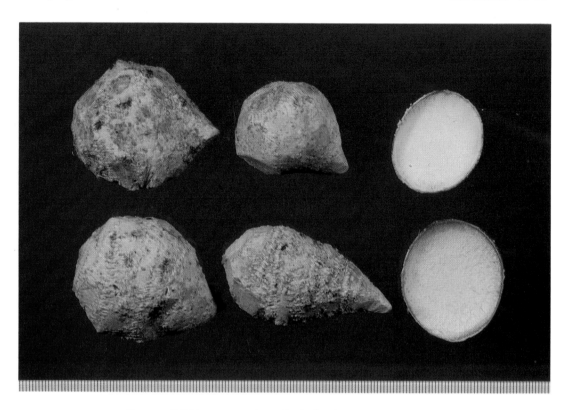

Sparganii Rhizoma: crude and stir-fried in vinegar. (×5/6)

96 SPARGANII RHIZOMA

三稜 *san¹ leng²*. English: sparganium (or bur-reed). Japanese: *sanryo*.

Alternate names: 光三稜 *guang¹ san¹ leng²*, 京三稜 *jing¹ san¹ leng²*.

Origin: Sparganiaceae family. *Sparganium stoloniferum* Buch.-Ham., *S. simplex* Huds., *S. stenophyllum* Maxim.

Characters: This is a spheroid rhizome about 5 cm long and 3 cm in diameter, with a slightly twisted point at the base. There is the scar left by the stalk at the top. The exterior surface is brown, and is relatively smooth, with numerous straight longitudinal wrinkles. It is encircled by 5–8 annular node scars, and toward the lower extremity has numerous small tumorous spots, which are the scars left by fibrous roots. It is hard and light. The decocting pieces are thin transverse slices, revealing the creamy white interior, which turns darker after processing with vinegar.

Quality: Firm rhizomes with the outer skin completely removed, and a pale yellow outer surface are the best.

Production areas: China (Jiangsu, Henan, Shandong, Jiangxi, Liaoning, Anhui, Zhejiang, Sichuan, Hubei).

Properties and actions: Balanced; bitter and acrid. Moves qi and breaks blood; disperses accumulations and relieves pain; promotes menstruation. Stir-fry with vinegar to promote contraction or to disperse accumulations and relieve pain. Stir-fry with bran to disinhibit water. Stir-fry with bran and wine to move qi and break blood.

Indications: Menstrual block; concretions and conglomerations; pain in the abdomen and region of the heart; postpartum stasis and stagnation. Daily dosage: 5–10 g. Contraindicated in qi vacuity without stasis accumulation, and in pregnancy. Used in *san¹-leng² wan²* (Sparganium Pills, 219).

Remarks: Constituents: Volatile oil (0.05%).

Similar drug: Dried rhizome of *Scirpus yagara* Ohwi (Japan).

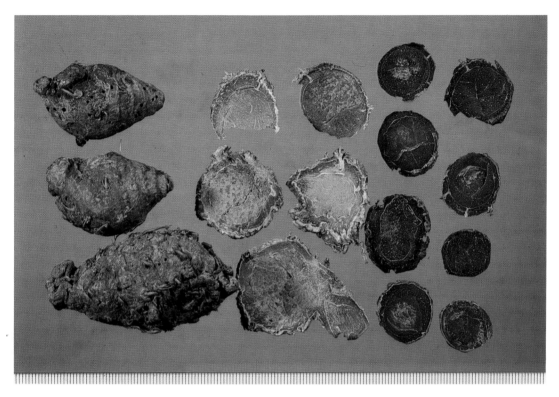

Zedoariae Rhizoma: crude (left); crude slices (middle); treated in vinegar (right). (× 5/6)

97 ZEDOARIAE RHIZOMA (CURCUMAE ZEDOARIAE RHIZOMA)

莪朮 e^2 zhu^2. English: zedoary. Japanese: *gajutsu*.

Alternate name: 蓬莪朮 $peng^2$ e^2 zhu^2.

Origin: Zingiberaceae family. *Curcuma zedoaria* (Berg.) Rosc.

Characters: This is a fat, pear-shaped rhizome, 1–4 cm in diameter. The exterior surface is a yellowish brown, and is rough in texture. It has prominent annular notes about 5–8 mm apart, and the scars of lateral roots. It is firm and hard. The decocting pieces are transverse slices, about 2–8 mm thick, revealing a brown cut edge with yellow speckles at the core. Slices treated with vinegar are much darker, and less yellow in color.

Quality: Large, firm, smooth rhizomes, that have are yellow-green on the cut edge are best.

Production areas: China (Guangxi, Sichuan, Fujian, Guangdong, Zhejiang, Yunnan, Taiwan).

Properties and actions: Warm; sour, sweet, slightly bitter; nontoxic. Enters the lung, heart, and small intestine channels. Dispels wind and clears heat; breaks blood and disperses accumulation; disperses swelling and resolves toxin. Used crude to break blood and disperse accumulation. Used mix-fried with vinegar to harmonize the liver, resolve toxin, and relieve pain.

Indications: Distention and pain in the abdomen and region of the heart; concretions and gatherings; food stagnation; menstrual block due to blood stasis; impact injuries pain. Daily dosage: 5–10 g. Contraindicated in dual vacuity of qi and blood, and in spleen-stomach vacuity without stagnation. Used in mu^4-$xiang^1$ bin^1-$lang^2$ wan^2 (Saussurea and Areca Pills, 190), e^1-wei^4 hua^4 pi^3 gao^1 (Asafoetida Glomus-Transforming Paste, 77), san^1-$leng^2$ wan^2 (Sparganium Pills, 219).

Remarks: Constituents: Monoterpenoids and sesquiterpenoids (volatile oil, 1–1.5%): 1,4-cineole, (+)-camphene, (+)-α-pinene, zederone, curculone, curdione, curcumol, zingiberene, curchromone, furanodiene. Curcuminoids: curcumin.

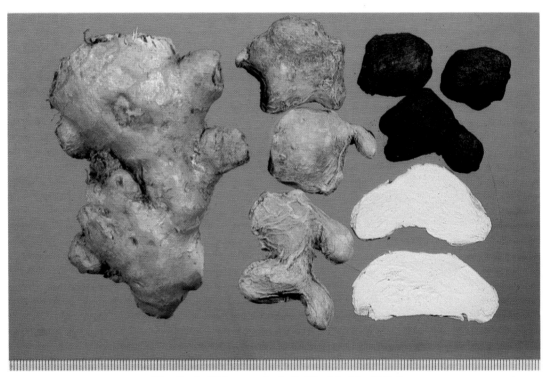

**Zingiberis Rhizoma: fresh (left); dried (middle);
blast-fried (top right); dried (bottom right). (× 5/6)**

98 ZINGIBERIS RHIZOMA

薑 *jiang[1]*. English: ginger root (fresh and dried). Japanese: *kyo (shokyo, kankyo)*.
Origin: Zingiberaceae family. *Zingiber officinale* Rosc.
Characters: The fresh rhizome is a long, knobbly, slightly flat rhizome with finger-like branches,
that have depressed scars at the ends, where shoots have been removed. It is 4–10 cm long, and
about 1–2 cm thick. The exterior surface is a grayish brown, with distinct annular nodes. It breaks
easily, revealing a pale yellow or brown fracture that is granular and fibrous in texture. It is cut
into slices 1–2 mm thick after the skin is removed. The dried rhizome is smaller, having undergone
shrinkage. It is hard, and breaks with difficulty to leave a fibrous, farinaceous fracture.
Quality: The fresh rhizome is best if large, fat, and tender. The dried form should be pale in col-
or, farinaceous in texture, and have a strong pungent flavor.
Production areas: China (Sichuan, Guangdong, Shandong, Shaanxi, Taiwan).
Properties and actions: Warm; acrid; nontoxic. Enters the lung, stomach, and spleen channels. Effuses the exterior, dissipates cold, checks retching and vomiting, and frees phlegm. Fresh
ginger effuses the exterior. Crude dried ginger warms the center. Blast-fried dried ginger warms
the center and staunches bleeding.
Indications: Wind-cold colds and flu; retching and vomiting; phlegm-rheum; cough and dyspnea;
fullness and dyspnea; diarrhea; resolves toxin of Pinelliae Tuber, Arisaematis Rhizoma,
fish, crabs, animals, birds. Daily dosage: 3–10 g. Contraindicated in yin vacuity heat. Used in
sheng[1]-jiang[1] ban[4]-xia[4] tang[1] (Fresh Ginger and Pinellia Decoction, 237), *xiao[3] ban[4]-xia[4] jia[1]
fu[2]-ling[2] tang[1]* (Minor Pinellia Decoction Plus Poria, 297), *ju[2]-pi[2] tang[1]* (Tangerine Peel Decoction,
153), *da[4] jian[4] zhong[1] tang[1]* (Major Center-Fortifying Decoction, 51), *tong[1] mai[4] si[4] ni[4] tang[1]*
(Vessel-Freeing Counterflow Frigidity Decoction, 264).
Remarks: Constituents: Sesquiterpenoids, monoterpenoids, and alkanes (volatile oil, 0.053–0.15%)
in the fresh rhizome, 0.25–2% in the dried rhizome: (–)-zingiberene (main). Arylalkanoids: [6]-
shogaol (0–0.6%), zingerone, [6]-gingerol.

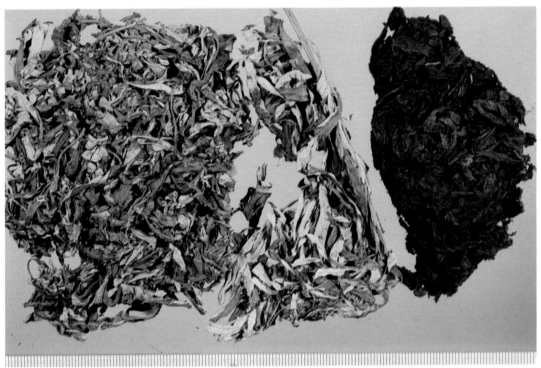

Artemisiae Argyi Folium: stir-fried with vinegar (left); crude (middle); char-fried (right). (×5/6)

99 ARTEMISIAE ARGYI FOLIUM

艾葉 ai⁴ ye⁴. English: mugwort leaf, moxa. Japanese: gaiyō.

Alternate name: 艾蒿 ai⁴ hao¹.

Origin: Compositae family. *Artemisia argyi* Levl. et Vant., *A. vulgaris* L.*

Characters: This leaf is feather-shaped with deep incisions. When dried for pharmaceutical use, it becomes shrunken and broken. It is yellowish green on the upper surface with scant white down and a grayish white on the lower surface with dense down. The short leafstalk is sometimes still attached. This product turns a brownish green when stir-fried and blackish when char-fried.

Quality: Leaves that are gray-white on the under side and have a thick downy covering and a strong odor are the best.

Production areas: China (Anhui, Shandong).

Properties and actions: Warm; bitter and acrid; nontoxic. Enters the spleen, liver, and kidney channels. Rectifies qi and the blood; expels cold-damp; warms the channels; staunches bleeding; quiets the fetus. Use crude to dissipate cold and relieve pain, and stir-fried with vinegar to relieve abdominal pain and staunch bleeding. Char for enhanced blood-staunching action.

Indications: Abdominal cold pain; frigid dysentery; menstrual block; uterine bleeding in pregnancy; blood ejection or nosebleed; vaginal discharge; stirring fetus; yong, jie, and xian. Daily dosage: 3–5 g. Contraindicated in yin vacuity and blood heat. Used in *xiong¹ gui¹ jiao¹ ai⁴ tang¹* (Ligusticum [cnidium], Tangkuei, Ass Hide Glue, and Mugwort Decoction, 307).

Remarks: Constituents: Volatile oil: *d*-α-phellandrene, cadinene, 1,8-cineole.

Similar drugs: *Artemisia princeps* Pamp. (Japan); *A. montana* Pamp. (Japan).

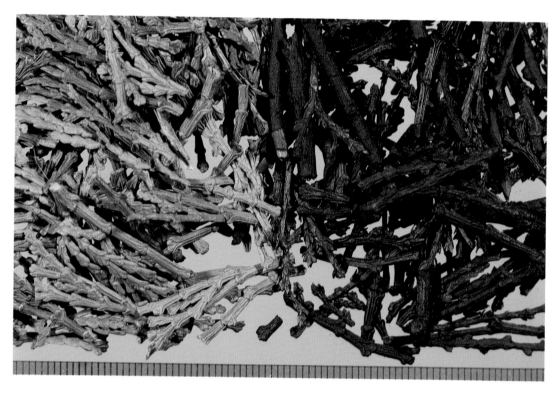

Biotae Folium et Ramulus: crude (left); charred (right), (× 5/3)

100 BIOTAE FOLIUM ET RAMULUS

側柏葉 *ce⁴ bo² ye⁴*. English: biota (or arborvitae) leaf. Japanese: *sokuhakuyō*.

Alternate names: 扁柏葉 *bian³ bo² ye⁴*, 側柏 *ce⁴ bo²*.

Origin: Cupressaceae family. *Biota orientalis* (L.) Endl. [= *Thuja orientalis* L.].

Characters: These twigs vary in length, and have numerous branches. The leaves take the form of fine deep green scales that are densely interlocked and lie tightly against the flat stem. The twigs are brittle and break easily.

Quality: Green, unbroken twigs are the best.

Production areas: China, Korea, and Japan.

Properties and actions: Cold; bitter, astringent. Enters the heart, liver, and large intestine channels. Cools the blood, staunch bleeding, dispels wind-damp, dissipates swelling toxin. Use crude to cool the blood and staunch bleeding. Use charred to staunch bleeding.

Indications: Blood ejection; spontaneous external bleeding; blood in the urine; blood dysentery; intestinal wind; profuse uterine bleeding; wind-damp bi pain; bacillary dysentery; hypertension; cough; cinnabar toxin; mumps; burns and scalds. Daily dosage: 5–10 g. Contraindicated in the absence of damp-heat. Used in *si⁴ sheng¹ wan²* (Four Raw Agents Pills, 255), *bo²-ye⁴ tang¹* (Biota Leaf Decoction, 28), *huai²-hua¹ san³* (Sophora Flower Powder, 125).

Remarks: Allied drug: Ramulus of *Cupressus funebris* Endl.

Constituents: Volatile oil (0.26%). Wax: juniperic acid, sabinic acid.

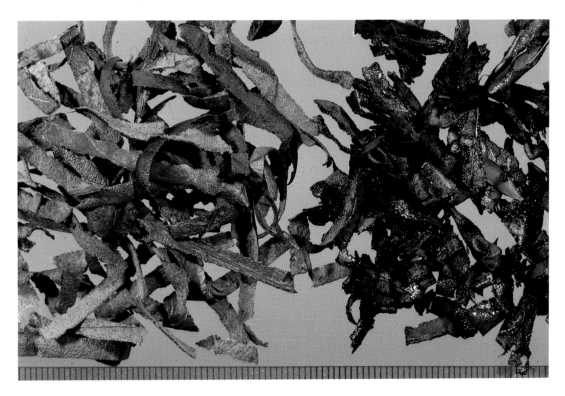

Eriobotryae Folium: crude (left); mix-fried with honey (right). (×5/6)

101 ERIOBOTRYAE FOLIUM

枇杷葉 *pi² pa² ye⁴*. English: loquat (or eriobotrya) leaf. Japanese: *biwayo*.

Alternate name: 杷葉 *pa² ye⁴*.

Origin: Rosaceae family. *Eriobotrya japonica* (Thunb.) Lindl.

Characters: These are oval leaves 12–25 cm long and 4–9 cm wide. They are quill-shaped with a gentle point and short leafstalks, and are veined with a midrib that bulges on the lower surface. They are brittle, and have a grayish, yellowish, or reddish green, shiny upper surface, and a brown lower surface.

Quality: Large, unbroken, gray-green leaves are the best.

Production areas: China (Jiangsu, Zhejiang, Hubei, Fujian, the best quality coming from Guandong's limited production), Japan, and Korea.

Properties and actions: Balanced; bitter; nontoxic. Enters the lung and stomach channels. Clears the lung and harmonizes the stomach; downbears qi and transforms phlegm. Has a strong lung-moistening effect when mix-fried with honey. It is usually stir-fried with ginger juice when used to treat stomach disorders.

Indications: Heat cough; copious phlegm; thirst; coughing of blood; spontaneous external bleeding; vomiting due to stomach heat. Daily dosage: 5–10 g. Use with care in vacuity vexation and vomiting, and cold cough. Used in *bai²-ji² pi²-pa² wan²* (Bletilla and Loquat Pills, 13).

Remarks: Allied drugs: Leaf of *Eriobotrva deflexa* Hemsley (Taiwan), and *E. bengalensis* Hook. (Yunnan).

Constituents: Saponins: ursolic acid, oleanolic acid. Cyanophore glycosides: amygdalin..

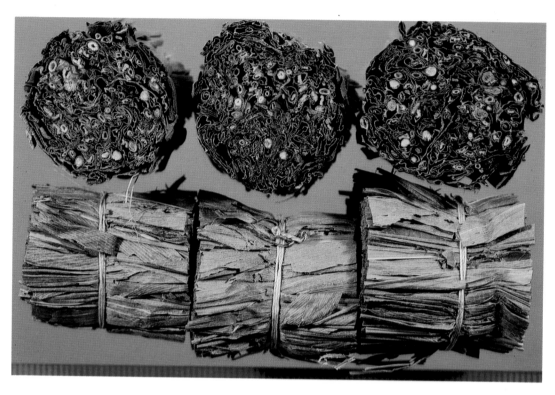

Lophatheri Folium: bundled (bottom) and cut (above). (×5/3)

102 LOPHATHERI FOLIUM

淡竹葉 *dan⁴ zhu² ye⁴*. English: bamboo (or lophatherum) leaf. Japanese: *tanchikuyo*.
Alternate name: 淡竹米 *dan⁴ zhu² mi³*.

Origin: Gramineae family. *Lophatherum gracile* Brongn.

Characters: This leaf is 5–20 cm long, and 2–3.5 cm wide. It is green or yellowish green in color and may or may not have soft hair on both its surfaces. It has parallel veins with distinct transverse venules. It is soft and supple in texture. The stalk is 1–2 mm in diameter. Leaves are sold with stalks, usually bound in neat bundles and cut into 2–3 cm lengths.

Quality: Clean, dry, green leaves without flowers are the best.

Production areas: China (Zhejiang, Jiangsu, Hunan, Hubei, Guangdong, Anhui, Jiangxi, Sichuan, Fujian, Henan).

Properties and actions: Cold; sweet, bland; nontoxic. Enters the heart and kidney channels. Clears heart fire, eliminates vexation heat, and disinhibits urine.

Indications: Thirst in febrile disease; vexation; inhibited voidings of dark-colored urine; turbid strangury; oral putrescence; tongue sores; sore, swollen gums. Daily dosage: 6–12 g. Contraindicated in pregnancy. Used in *dao³ chi⁴ san³* (Red-Abducting Powder, 64), *zhu²-ye⁴ shi²-gao¹ tang¹* Bamboo Leaf [Lophatherum] and Gypsum Decotion, 349).

Remarks: Similar plant: *Phyllostchys nigra* Munro var. *henonis* Stapf. (Japan).
Constituents: Triterpenoids: arundoin, cylindrin, friedelin.

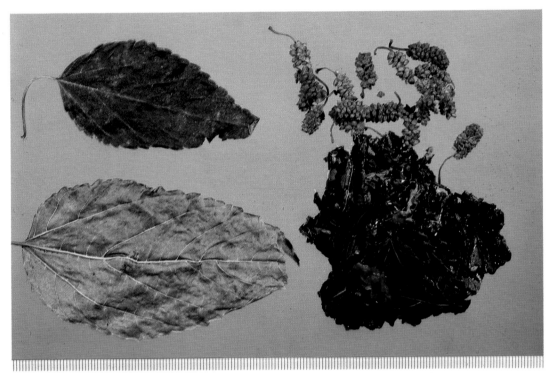

Mori Folium: crude (left); mix-fried with honey (bottom right).
Mori Fructus (top right). (×5/6)

103 MORI FOLIUM

桑葉 *sang¹ ye⁴*. English: (white) mulberry leaf. Japanese: *soyo*.

Alternate name: 桑樹葉 *sang¹ shu⁴ ye⁴*.

Origin: Moraceae family. *Morus alba* L.

Characters: The dried leaves are usually shrunken and broken. Those in tact are ovate or wide ovate, 8–13 cm long and 7–11 cm wide. The tip and margins are serrated, sometimes with irregular incisions. The base is truncated, rounded, or heart-shaped. The upper surface is yellow green with a slight sheen, and fine down along the veins. On the paler under surface, the protuberant veins form a reticular pattern.

Quality: Clean, unbroken leaves that are yellow green in color are the best.

Production areas: China (Jiangsu, Zhejiang).

Properties and actions: Cold; sweet, bitter. Enters the lung and liver channels. Dispels wind and clears heat; cools the blood and brightens the eyes. It is mix-fried with honey to moisten the lung, and steamed to brighten the eyes. The fruit, Mori Fructus (*sang¹ shen⁴*), supplements the liver and boost the kidney, extinguishes wind and enriches humor.

Indications: Wind warmth fever; headache; reddening of eyes; thirst; lung heat cough; wind bi; dormant papules; elephantiasis of the lower limbs. The fruit treats liver-stomach depletion, wasting thirst, dim vision, tinnitus, scrofulous lumps, and inhibited movement of the joints. Daily dosage: 5–10 g. Used in *sang¹ ju² yin³* (Mulberry Leaf and Chrysanthemum Beverage, 225), *sang¹ ma² wan²* (Mulberry Leaf and Sesame Pills, 226), *sang¹ xing⁴ tang¹* (Mulberry Leaf and Apricot Kernel Decoction, 227).

Remarks: Constituents: Flavonoids: rutin, quercetin, isoquercitrin. Steroids: β-sitosterol, campesterol.

Allied drug: Leaf of *Morus bombycis* Koidz. (Japan, Korea).

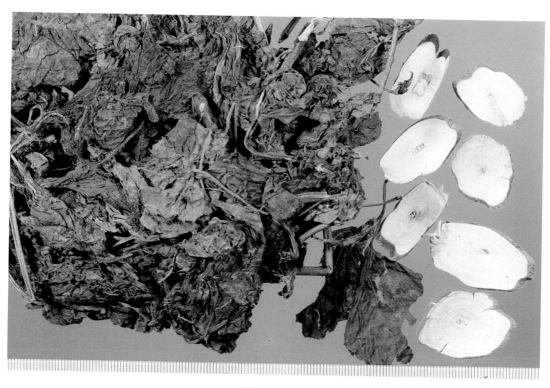

Perillae Folium (left). Perillae Caulis (right). (×5/6)

104 PERILLAE FOLIUM

紫蘇葉 zi^3 su^1 ye^4. English: perilla leaf. Japanese: *shisoyo*.

Alternate name: 蘇葉 su^1 ye^4.

Origin: Labiatae family. *Perilla frutescens* (L.) Britt. var. *crispa* (Thunb.) Hand.-Mazz., *P. frutescens* (L.) Britt. var. *acuta* (Thunb.) Kudo.

Characters: These are long or round ovate leaves, 4–11 cm long, with long pointed tips and serrated margins. Their upper surface is green or purple, and their under surface is purple, the color deepening when they dry. Both surfaces are covered with downy hair, which is densest on the veins of the lower surface.

Quality: Dry, purple leaves of even thickness are the best.

Production areas: China (Jiangsu, Hubei, Guangdong, Hubei, Shandong, Shanxi, Zhejiang, Sichuan), and Japan.

Properties and action: Warm; acrid; nontoxic. Enters the lung and spleen channels. Effuses the exterior, dissipates cold, rectifies qi, and harmonizes nutrition. Char-fry to staunch bleeding.

Indications: External wind-cold; aversion to cold and fever; cough and dyspnea; distention and fullness in the chest and abdomen; stirring fetus. Daily dosage: 5–10 g. Contraindicated in qi vacuity and exterior vacuity. Used in *xiang¹ su¹ san³* (Cyperus and Perilla Powder, 294), *shen¹ su¹ yin³* (Ginseng and Perilla Beverage, 232), *xing⁴ su¹ san³* (Apricot Kernel and Perilla Powder, 306).

Remarks: Constituents: Monoterpenoids, sesquiterpenoids, alkanes, and phenylpropanoids (volatile oil, 0.4–1.8%): (–)-perillaldehyde (55-68%), (–)-limonene (10–30%); elscholziaketone (up to 45%), naginataketone (up to 53%); dillapiol (up to 77%). Flavonoids: shisonin. Phenylpropanoids: rosmarinic acid (1.0–1.2%).

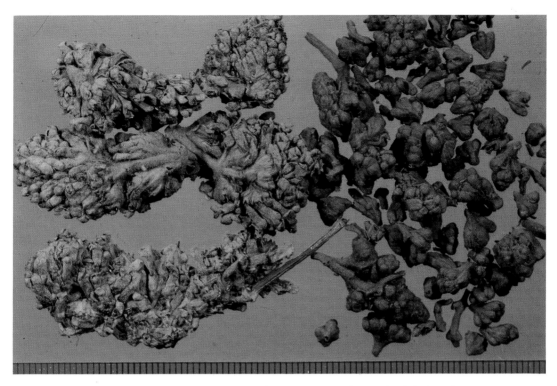

Buddleiae Flos: crude (left) and mix-fried with honey (right). (×5/6)

105 BUDDLEIAE FLOS

密蒙花 *mi⁴ meng² hua¹*. English: buddleia flower. Japanese: *mitsumoka*.
Alternate names: 老蒙花 *lao³ meng² hua¹*, 蒙花 *meng² hua¹*.
Origin: Loganiaceae family. *Buddleia officinalis* Maxim.
Characters: This inflorescence comprises numerous small clustered buds, ocher in color, and covered with a dense pile. It varies in shape and size. The individual buds are club-shaped with a bell-shaped calyx, 3–6 mm long and about 1.5 mm in diameter. They have four fissures and their corolla is tubular. The whole inflorescence is soft and breaks easily to reveal a blackish interior.
Quality: Dense buds and a pronounced velvet texture are the marks of good quality.
Production areas: China (Hubei, Sichuan, Shaanxi, Henan, and less importantly in Yunnan, Guangxi, Hunan).
Properties and actions: Cool; sweet; nontoxic. Enters the liver channels. Dispels wind, cools the blood, moistens the liver, and brightens the eyes.
Indications: Red, sore, and swollen eyes; copious tears; aversion to light; clear-eye blindness; eye screens; wind ulceration of the eyes. Daily dosage: 3–5 g. Used in *mi⁴-meng²-hua¹ san³* (Buddleia Powder, 185).
Remarks: Allied drug: Flower of *Edgeworthia chrysantha* Lindl. (Thymelaeaceae).
Constituents: Flavonoids: buddleo-glucoside, acacetin.

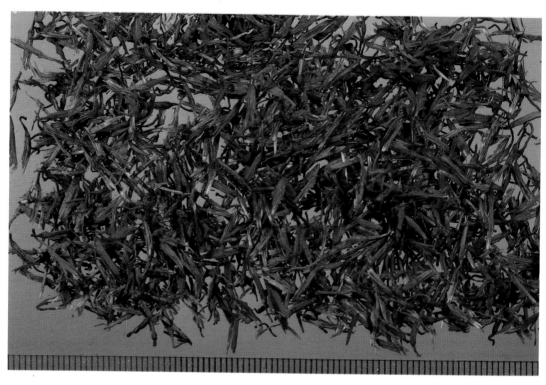

Carthami Flos. (×5/3)

106 CARTHAMI FLOS

紅花 *hong² hua¹*. English: carthamus flower, safflower. Japanese: *koka*.
Alternate names: 刺紅花 *ci⁴ hong² hua¹*, 紅藍花 *hong² lan² hua¹*.
Origin: Compositae family. *Carthamus tinctorius* L.
Characters: This is a tubular flower without ovaries, about 1.5 cm long, and orangy red or brown in color. The corolla is long and narrow, and has five incisions, each lobe being 5–7 mm long. There are five stamens. The anthers are yellow and form a tubular shape that projects beyond the lobes, within which is a stigma.
Quality: Large, brightly colored flowers that are soft to the touch and do not contain any stalks are the best.
Production areas: China (Henan, Zhejiang, Sichuan), Japan, and India.
Properties and actions: Warm; acrid; nontoxic. Enters the heart and liver channels. Quickens the blood and promotes menstruation; eliminates stasis and relieves pain. Use crude to quicken the blood and dispel stasis. Boil with wine to break blood. Boil in water to nourish the blood. Triturate for topical application.
Indications: Menstrual block; concretions and conglomerations; difficult delivery; dead fetus; retention of the lochia; stasis pain; swollen yong; impact injuries. Daily dosage: 3–5 g. Contraindicated in the absence stasis and stagnation and in pregnancy. Used in *hong²-hua¹ san³* (Carthamus Powder, 119), *ge²-gen¹ hong²-hua¹ tang¹* (Pueraria and Carthamus Decoction, 99).
Remarks: Constituents: Phenylpropanoids: carthamin (0.3–0.6%), carthamone, safflor yellow (safflomins A, B, 20–30%). Flavonoids: carthamidin, neocarthamin. Fixed oil (safflower oil): glycerides of linoleic acid (ca. 70%). Saccharides: glycans.

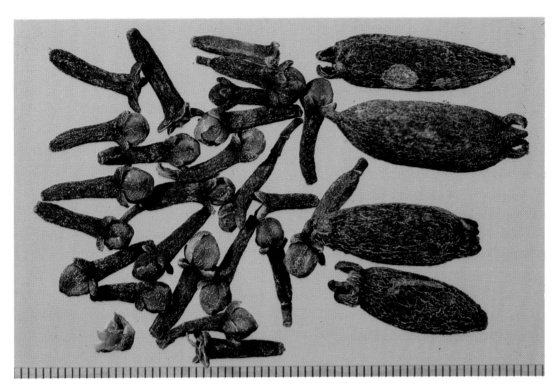

Caryophylli Flos (left) and Caryophylli Fructus (right). (× 2)

107 CARYOPHYLLI FLOS

丁香 *ding¹ xiang¹*. English: clove. Japanese: *choko*.

Alternate names: 丁子 *ding¹ zi³*, 公丁香 *gong¹ ding¹ xiang¹*.

Origin: Myrtaceae family. *Syzygium aromaticum* (L.). Merr. et Perry [= *Eugenia caryophyllata* Thunberg].

Characters: This is a short, club-shaped bud, about 1.5–2 cm long, and reddish brown in color. The lower part is a slightly squared cylindrical calyx about 1–1.3 cm long, 5 mm wide and 3 mm thick, that tapers at the base and exudes oil when scratched. At the top of the calyx are four fat sepals, each 3 mm long. The upper part is a sphere roughly 6 mm in diameter, comprising four petals folded around each other. The bud cuts open to reveal numerous stamens curled toward the center, in which there is a thick, straight style. It is oily in substance.

Quality: Best are large, dry, unopened buds that have no stalk, are oily in substance, and sink in water.

Production areas: China (Guangdong), Indonesia, Malaysia (Penang), the Moluccas, Zanzibar, and Madagascar.

Properties and actions: Warm; acrid; nontoxic. Enters the stomach, spleen, and kidney channels. Warms the center, warms the kidney, and downbears counterflow.

Indications: Hiccough; vomiting; stomach reflux; diarrhea; cold pain in the abdomen and region of the heart; elusive and bowstring masses; shan qi. Daily dosage: 1–3 g. Contraindicated in yin vacuity heat and other heat patterns, hyperchlorhydria, acute gastroenteritis, and gastric hemorrhage. Used in *ding¹-xiang¹ shi⁴-di⁴ tang¹* (Clove and Persimmon Decoction, 70), *zi³ xue³ dan¹* (Purple Snow Elixir, 354), *zhu² han² dang⁴ jing¹ tang¹* (Cold-Dispelling Fright-Assuaging Decoction, 348), *hei¹ hu³ dan¹* (Black Tiger Elixir, 118).

Remarks: Constituents: Phenylpropanoids, sesquiterpenoids, and alkanes (volatile oil, clove oil, 14–23%): eugenol (64–95%), eugenyl acetate (3–17%), α-, and β-caryophyllenes. Chromones: eugenosides I, II. Tannoids (10–22%): eugeniin. Fixed oil (5–10%).

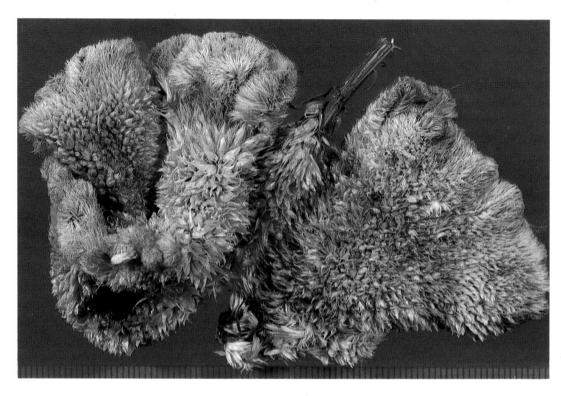

Celosiae Cristatae Flos. (× 5/3)

108 CELOSIAE CRISTATAE FLOS

雞冠花 *ji¹ guan¹ hua¹*. English: cockscomb flower. Japanese: *keikanka*.

Alternate name: 雞冠頭 *ji¹ guan¹ tou²*.

Origin: Amaranthaceae family. *Celosia cristata* L.

Characters: This is a short-stemmed inflorescence, which has the appearance of a cock's crest. The upper part, usually reddish brown in color, is composed of glandular hairs, which are small buds. The lower part comprises dense flowers, each with gray-white membranous bracts and perianths. The capsules are split and the seeds are kidney-shaped, black, and shiny.

Quality: Thin, flat, bright, white inflorescences are the best. The red ones are inferior.

Production areas: China (most parts), and Japan.

Properties and actions: Cool; sweet; nontoxic. Enters the liver channels. Staunches bleeding and cools the blood. Char-fry to staunch bleeding.

Indications: Bleeding from hemorrhoids; red and white dysentery; blood ejection; coughing of blood; blood strangury; profuse uterine bleeding; red and white vaginal discharge. Daily dosage: 5–10 g. Contraindicated in accumulation and stagnation. Used in *ji-guan¹ san³* (Cockscomb Powder, 138).

Remarks: Constituents: unknown.

Similar drug: Spike of *Celosia argentea* L.

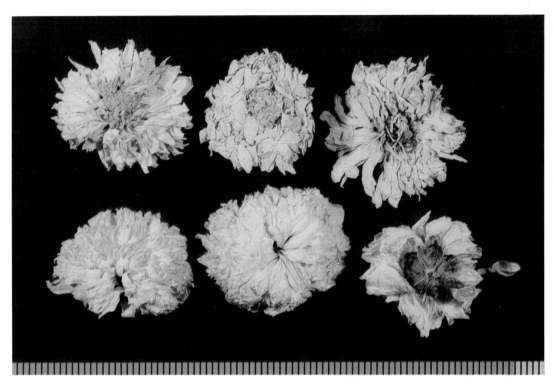

Chrysanthemi Flos: Sichuanese (top); Taiwanese cultivated (bottom). (×5/3)

109 CHRYSANTHEMI FLOS

菊花 *ju² hua¹*. English: chrysanthemum flower. Japanese: *kikka*.

Alternate names: 眞菊 *zhen¹ ju²*, 藥菊 *yao⁴ ju²*.

Origin: Compositae family. *Chrysanthemum morifolium* Ramat. [= *C. sinense* Sabine].

Characters: These are button-shaped inflorescences, comprising an outer layer of about 15–20 shrivelled, ligulate, pale yellow, male flowers, and a center of numerous tubular yellow flowers of both genders and each with five lobes and brown ovaries. At the base is the involucre composed of 3–4 layers of bracts.

Quality: Bright colored flowers that are in tact are best.

Production areas: China.

Properties and actions: Cool; sweet, bitter; nontoxic. Enters the lung and liver channels. Courses wind-heat, calms the liver and brightens the eyes. Use crude to course wind-heat. Char-fry to clear heat and resolve toxin.

Indications: Headache; dizziness; reddening of the eyes; vexation heat in the heart and chest; clove sores; toxins swelling. Daily dosage: 3–10 g. used in *sang¹ ju² yin³* (Mulberry Leaf and Chrysanthemum Beverage, 225), *qi³ ju² di⁴-huang² wan²* (Lycium, Chrysanthemum and Rehmannia Pills, 198).

Remarks: Allied drugs: Flower of *Chrysanthemum lavandulaefolium* Mak., *C. boreale* Mak., and *C. indicum* L.

Constituents: 2,2,4-trimethyl- cyclohexene-(3)-1-carboxylic acid, chrysanthenone.

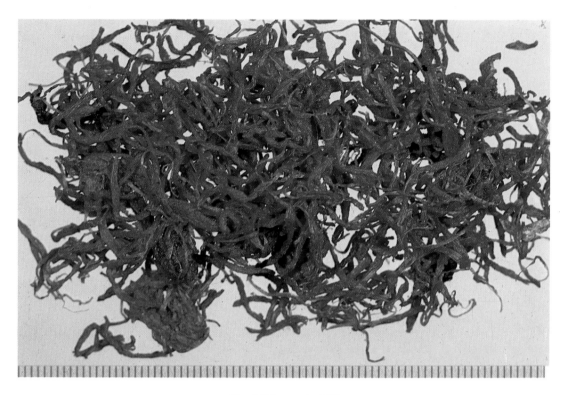

Croci Stigma. (×5/3)

110 CROCI STIGMA (CROCUS)

藏紅花 *zang⁴ hong² hua¹*. English: saffron. Japanese: *zokoka, safuran*.
Alternate names: 泊夫藍 *ji⁴ fu¹ lan²*, 番紅花 *fan¹ hong² hua¹*.
Origin: Iridaceae family. *Crocus sativus* L.
Characters: The product comprises many flat red-brown stigmas pressed together. It gives off an unusual smell. Undamaged stigmas are about 2.5 cm in length, and are slightly funnel-shaped and have a short split. At the top, they have irregularly serrated margins and have a downy surface. Stigmas placed in water float, and exude a yellow coloring.
Quality: Soft, oily, bright red stigmas with a sheen are best. When placed in water, the coloring should sink vertically, and then gradually diffuse, creating a trumpet of color.
Production areas: Spain, Greece, China, and Japan.
Properties and actions: Balanced; sweet; nontoxic. Enters the heart and liver channels. Quickens the blood and transforms stasis; dissipates depression and frees binds.
Indications: Binding depression due to excessive sorrow or thought; glomus and oppression in the chest and diaphragm; blood ejection; cold damage mania; fright and shock; abstraction; menstrual block; postpartum abdominal pain due to blood stasis; impact injury. Daily dosage: 1.5–3 g. Contraindicated in pregnancy. Croci Stigma can be mixed with congee to treat glomus, or with wine to treat all types of blood ejection.
Remarks: Constituents: Carotenoids (ca. 2%) crocin (crocetin digentiobiose ester, main). Monoterpenoids: picrocrocin. Volatile oil (0.4–1.3%): safranal, dihydrosafranal, cineole.

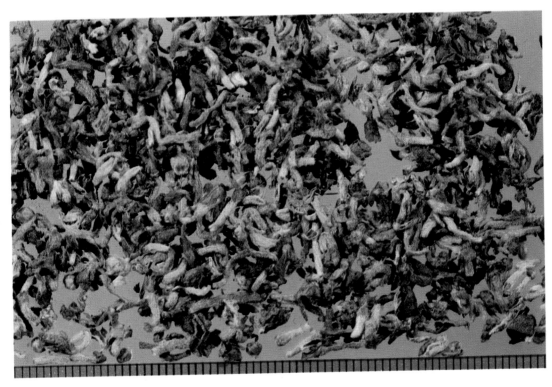

Daphnes Genkwa Flos: steamed with vinegar. (×2)

111 DAPHNES GENKWA FLOS

芫花 *yuan² hua¹*. English: genkwa (or daphne) flower. Japanese: *genka*.

Alternate names: 悶頭花 *men¹ tou² hua¹*, 頭痛花 *tou² tong⁴ hua¹*.

Origin: Tymelaeaceae family. *Daphne genkwa* Sieb. et Zucc.

Characters: This product comprises 3–7 flowers on a short axis, with 1–2 bracts at the base, which are covered with dense yellow down. The calyx is contorted, about 1–1.7 cm long, yellowish brown, or less commonly pale purple, on the outside, with short dense down. The upper part, which accounts for about one third of the total length, is made up of four supple, light brown lobes.

Quality: Small, fine, unopened flowers with a purple hue are best.

Production areas: China (Anhui, Jiangsu, Zhejiang, Shandong, Sichuan, Fujian, Hubei).

Properties and actions: Warm; acrid, bitter; toxic. Enters the lung and spleen channels. Expels water and flushes phlegm. Stir-fry with vinegar for milder action.

Indications: Phlegm-rheum; elusive masses; dyspnea and cough; water swelling; lateral costal pain; distention and fullness in the abdomen and heart; food poisoning; mother of malaria, swollen yong. Daily dosage: 1.5–3 g. Contraindicated in original qi vacuity and pregnancy. Used in *shi² zao³ tang¹* (Ten Jujubes Decoction, 245).

Remarks: Constituents: Flavonoids: genkwanin, apigenin.

Allied drug: Flower of *Wikstroemia chamaedaphne* Meissn.

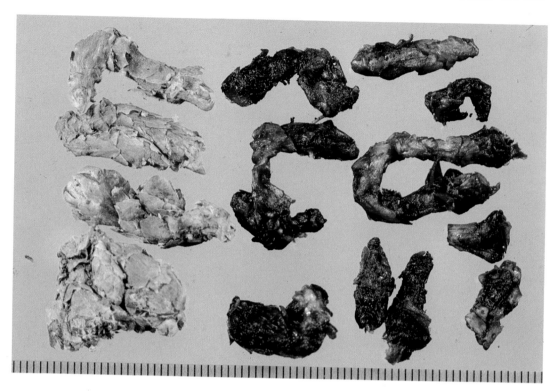

Farfarae Flos: crude (left); mix-fried with honey (right). (× 2)

112 FARFARAE FLOS (TUSSILAGINIS FLOS)

款冬花 *kuan³ dong¹ hua¹*. English: tussilago (or farfara, coltsfoot) flower. Japanese: *kantoka*.
Alternate names: 款花 *kuan³ hua¹*, 款冬 *kuan³ dong¹*.
Origin: Compositae family. *Tussilago farfara* L.
Characters: The dry flower buds form an irregular club shape, 1–2.5 cm long and 6–10 mm thick. Sometimes 2–3 efflorescences are joined together. They are full at the tip, and taper toward the often still attached stalk. The outer layer is composed of scaly mauve or pink bracts bearing a fine white down.
Quality: Large mauve buds without stalks are the best.
Production areas: China (Shaanxi, Shanxi, Henan, Gansu, Qinghai, Sichuan, Inner Mongolia).
Properties and actions: Warm; acrid; nontoxic. Enters the lung channels. Moistens the lung and precipitates qi; transforms phlegm and suppresses cough. Use crude to warm the lung. Stir-fry with honey to moisten the lung and suppress cough.
Indications: Counterflow cough; dyspnea; throat bi. Daily dosage: 5–10 g. Contraindicated in yin vacuity lung heat. Used in *kuan³-dong¹-hua¹ tang¹* (Tussilago Decoction, 161), *zi³-wan³ san³* (Aster Powder, 353), *bai³ hua¹ gao¹* (Lily Bulb and Tussilago Paste, 22), *bu³ fei⁴ tang¹* (Lung-Supplementing Decoction, 30), *ding⁴ chuan³ tang¹* (Dyspnea-Stabilizing Decoction, 71).
Remarks: Allied drug: Flower of *Petasites japonicus* Maxim. (Japan).
Constituents: Tannoid. Flavonoid.

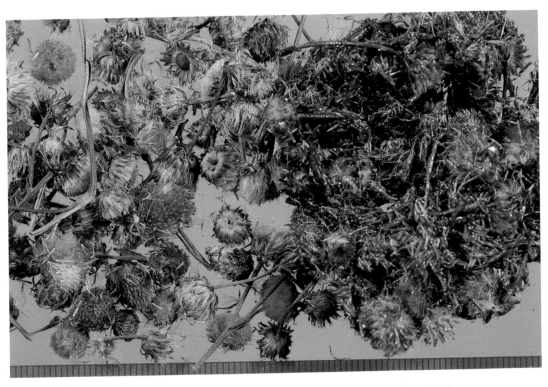

Inulae Flos: crude (left) and mix-fried with honey (right). (× 5/3)

113 INULAE FLOS

旋覆花 xuan[2] fu[4] hua[1]. English: inula (or elecampane) flower. Japanese: *senpukuka*.
Alternate name: 金沸花 jin[1] fei[4] hua[1].
Origin: Compositae family. *Inula britannica* L. var. *chinensis* (Rupr.) Reg., *I. linariaefolia* Turcz., *I. britannica* L., *I. chrysantha* Diels,* *I. helianthus-aquatilis* C.Y. Wu ex Ling,* *I. helianthus-aquatilis* C.Y. Wu ex Ling subsp. *hupehensis* Ling.*
Characters: These flowers are spherical, with a diameter of 1–2 cm. The involucre is composed of numerous lanceolate or linear imbricate bracts in five layers. The flowers are dull yellow-green. The outer layer is a ring of ligulate flowers.
Quality: Large, golden flowers with white hairs and without stalks are the best.
Production areas: China (Henan, Jiangsu, Heibei, Zhejiang, Anhui, Heilongjiang, Jilin, Liaoning).
Properties and actions: Warm; salty; nontoxic. Enters the lung, liver, and stomach channels. Disperses phlegm, precipitates qi, softens hardness, and moves water. Mix-fry with honey to moisten the lung and suppress cough.
Indications: Phlegm bind in the chest; distention and fullness in the lateral costal region; cough and dyspnea; hiccough; sticky spittle; hard thoracic glomus; persistent belching; water swelling; of the upper abdomen. Daily dosage: 5–10 g. Contraindicated in diarrhea. Used in xuan[2]-fu[4] dai[4]-zhe[3] tang[1] (Inula and Hematite Decoction, 311), jin[1]-fei[4]-cao[3] san[3] (Inula Powder, 148).
Remarks: Constituents: inusterol A, B, C, britianin, inulicin, quercetin, caffeic acid.

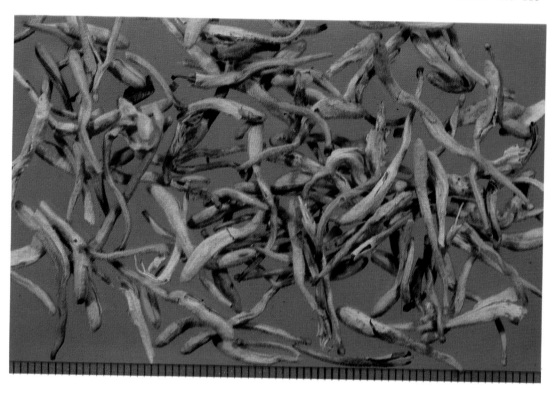

Lonicerae Flos. (×2)

114 LONICERAE FLOS

金銀花 *jin¹ yin² hua¹*. English: lonicera or (Japanese)honeysuckle flower. Japanese:*kinginka*.
Alternate names: 雙花 *shuang¹ hua¹*, 忍冬花 *ren³ dong¹ hua¹*.
Origin: Caprifoliaceae family. *Lonicera japonica* Thunb., *L. henryi* Hemsl., *L. lanceolata* Wall.,*
L. confusa DC.,* *L. hypoglauca* Miq., *L. dasystyla* Rehd.,* *L. similis* Hemsl.,* *L. fuchsioides* Hemsl.*
Characters: The dried flower buds ar clavate, slightly contorted, 2–3 cm long, and 2–3 mm thick.
Their exterior surface is yellow or light brown, and is covered with short soft hairs and glandular
hairs. At the base is a small, thin, green calyx. The bud can be cut open to reveal five stamens
and one pistil.
Quality: Large, yellow-white, unopen buds are the best.
Production areas: China (most places, with production highest in Shandong, and the best quality produced in Henan).
Properties and actions: Cold; sweet; nontoxic. Enters the lung and stomach channels. Clears
heat and resolves toxin. Distillate of Lonicerae Flos resolves summerheat and clears heat.
Indications: Initial-stage warm disease with heat in the upper burner; swelling and toxin of sores.
Char-fry to treat blood dysentery and blood in the stool. Stir-fry to treat diarrhea. Daily dosage:
10–15 g. Contraindicated in spleen-stomach vacuity cold. Used in *yin² qiao² san³* (Lonicera and
Forsythia Powder, 323), *tuo¹ li³ xiao¹ du² yin³* (Internal Expulsion Toxin-Dispersing Beverage,
265), *ba¹ wei⁴ dai⁴ xia⁴ fang¹* (Eight-Ingredient Discharge Formula, 5).
Remarks: Constituents: Flavonoids: luteolin, lonicerin (= luteolin-7-rhamnoglucoside). Tannoid.
Wax.

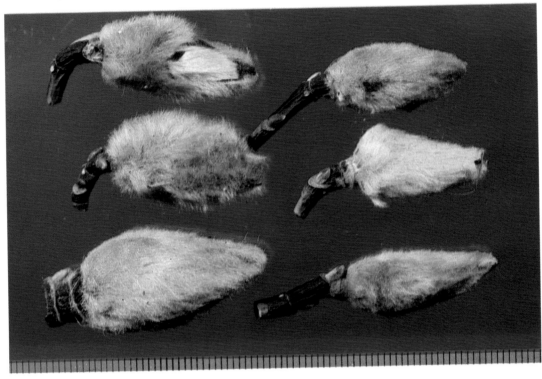

Magnoliae Flos. (× 5/3)

115 MAGNOLIAE FLOS

辛夷 *xin¹ yi²*. English: magnolia flower. Japanese: *shin'i*.

Alternate names: 木筆花 *mu⁴ bi³ hua¹*, 辛黃 *xin¹ yi²*.

Origin: Magnoliaceae family. *Magnolia liliflora* Desr., *M. denudata* Desr., *M. fargesii* Cheng.

Characters: Attached to a short woody twig, the dried buds are ovate in shape, like the end of an artist's paint brush. They are 1–4 cm long, and 0.7–2 cm in diameter. The outer layer comprises 2 bracts in 2 layers, whose outer surface is covered with soft, long whitish brown hairs 5 mm in length, and whose inner surface is brown and smooth. The bracts can be removed to reveal 3 calyces, and 6–12 tightly wrapped brown petals, amidst which are numerous brownish yellow stamens and a brown pistil. The buds are brittle and break easily.

Quality: Dry, unopened buds that are green in color and have no stalks are the best.

Production areas: China (Henan, Sichuan, Anhui, Shaanxi, Hubei).

Properties and actions: Warm; acrid; nontoxic. Enters the lung and stomach channels. Dispels wind and frees the portals.

Indications: Headache; deep-source nasal congestion; nasal obstruction; toothache. Daily dosage: 3–5 g. Contraindicated in effulgent yin vacuity fire. Used in *cang¹-er³ san³* (Xanthium Powder, 34), *ge²-gen¹ tang¹ jia¹ chuan¹-xiong¹ xin¹-yi²* (Pueraria Decoction Plus Liguisticum [Cnidium] and Magnolia Flower, 102).

Remarks: Constituents: *M. liliflora:* Monoterpenoids and phenylpropanoids (volatile oil, 0.26–1%): α-pinene, citral, cineole, safrole, methyl eugenol, eugenol.
M. denudata: Monoterpenoids and phenylpropanoids (volatile oil): 1) 1,8-cineole (34–57%), sabinene, α-terpineol, 2) α-pinene, cineole, methyl chavicol.

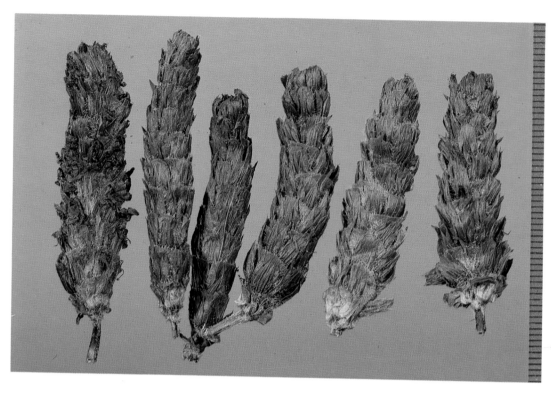

Prunellae Spica. (×5/3)

116 PRUNELLAE SPICA

夏枯草 *xia⁴ ku¹ cao³*. English: prunella (or self-heal, heal-all) spike. Japanese: *kagoso*.
Alternate names: 麥夏枯 *mai⁴ xia⁴ ku¹*, 枯草穗 *ku¹ cao³ sui⁴*.
Origin: Labiatae family. *Prunella vulgaris* L.
Characters: This product is cylindrical or pagoda-shaped, 2.5–6.5 cm long, and 1–1.5 cm in diameter. It is mid-brown in color, and is attached to a stalk. It comprises up to or over ten whorls of persistent calyces 5–7 mm apart. Each whorl comprises 5–6 persistent calyces, and has below it two brown, opposite-growing, kidney-shaped bracts with a pronounced midrib, sharply pointed tip, and rough hair on the outer surface. The calyces are ligulate, the upper lip being broaod with three lobes, and the lower lip having only two lobes. The obles are triangular with hair on the outside. The corollas and stamens have usually all fallen off. Within each calyx are four shiny, brown seeds. This spike is light, and has a faint odor.
Quality: Large purplish spikes are the best.
Production areas: China (Jiangsu, Anhui, Zhejiang, Hunan), and Japan.
Properties and actions: Cold; acrid, bitter; nontoxic. Enters the liver and gallbladder channels. Clears the liver, and dissipates binds.
Indications: Scrofulous lumps; goiter; mammary yong; nocturnal eyeball pain; tearing and aversion to light; dizziness of the head and eyes; deviated mouth and eyes; sinew and bone pain; pulmonary tuberculosis; acute icteric infectious hepatitis; uterine bleeding. Daily dosage: 3–10 g. Use with care in spleen-stomach vacuity. Used in *xia⁴-ku¹-cao³ tang¹* (Prunella Decoction, 285), *bu³ gan¹ san³* (Liver-Supplementing Powder, 31).
Remarks: Constituents: Triterpenoids: (saponins) prunellin; oleanolic acid, ursolic acid. Carotenoids: caroten. Monoterpenoids (volatile oil): (+)-camphor, (+)-fenchone. Flavonoids: rutin, hyperin; delphinidin, cyanidin. Phenylpropanoids: *trans*-caffeic acid, *cis*-caffeic acid; rosmarinic acid (0.3–1.9%). Tannoids. Potassium chloride, potassium sulfate.
Similar drugs: Spike of *Prunella hispida* Benth., and herb of *Ajuga decumbens* Thunb.

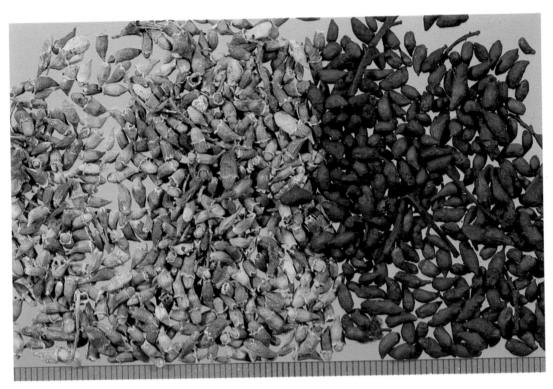

Sophorae Flos: Immaturus crude (left); charred (right). (×5/3)

117 SOPHORAE FLOS IMMATURUS

槐花 *huai² hua¹*. English: sophora (or pagoda tree, Chinese scholartree) flower. Japanese: *kaika*.

Alternate name: 槐米 *huai² mi³*.

Origin: Leguminosae family. *Sophora japonica* L.

Characters: These small buds are oval in shape, 4–8 mm long, and 2–3 mm thick, and sharply pointed at one end. The calyx, which accounts for two thirds of the total length, is gray-brown, with longitudinal furrows, and with five shallow, lighter-colored lobes at the extremity. The unopened corolla is a flattened sphere about 2 mm long, and reddish brown in color. There is a short stalk at the base of the bud.

Quality: The best buds are the size of grains of rice, are a greenish yellow in color, and when soaked in water, color it bright yellow.

Production areas: China (Hebei, Shandong, Henan, Jiangsu, Guangdong, Guangxi).

Properties and actions: Cool; bitter; nontoxic. Enters the liver and large intestine channels. Clears heat, cools the blood and staunches bleeding. Mix-fry with honey to moisten the lung. Char-fry to staunch bleeding.

Indications: Intestinal wind hemafecia; bleeding hemorrhoids; blood in the urine; blood strangury; uterine bleeding; spontaneous external bleeding; red and white dysentery; wind-heat reddening of the eyes; yong, ju and other sores. The crude drug treats hypertension. The stir-fried drug treats throat bi, blood ejection, nosebleed, and uterine bleeding. The char-fried drug is effective for red and white dysentery. Daily dosage: 5–10 g. Contraindicated in vacuity cold diarrhea and qi vacuity uterine bleeding. Used in *huai²-hua¹ san³* (Sophora Flower Powder, 125), *huai²-xiang¹ san³* (Sophora and Musk powder 127).

Remarks: Constituents: Flavonoids: rutin (10–30%), quercetin. Triterpenoids: betulin, sophoradiol. Saponins: kaikasaponins I, II, III, soyasaponins I, III azukisaponins I, II, III.

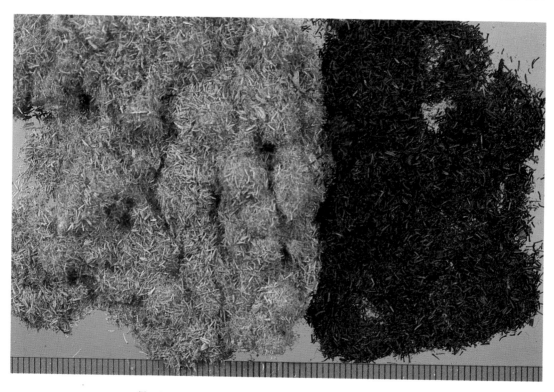

Typhae Pollen: crude (left); char-fried (right). (×5/3)

118 TYPHAE POLLEN

蒲黃 *pu² huang²*. English: typha (cat-tail) pollen. Japanese: *hoō*.
Alternate names: 蒲花 *pu² hua¹*, 蒲草花 *pu² cao³ hua¹*.
Origin: Typhaceae family. *Typha angustifolia* L. [= *T. angustata* Bory et Chaub.], *T. latifolia* L.
Characters: This bright yellow pollen is light; it is easily blown around, and floats on water. It sticks to the fingers but not together in lumps. Under a microscope it appears spheroid grains bearing fine hairs.
Quality: Clean, lustrous, bright yellow pollen is the best.
Production areas: China (Jiangsu, Shandong).
Properties and actions: Balanced; sweet acrid; nontoxic. Enters the liver and heart channels. Cools the blood and staunches bleeding; quickens the blood and disperses stasis. Use crude to quicken the blood and dispel stasis, to disinhibit urine, and to disperse swelling. Use stir-fried to staunch bleeding and supplement the blood. Char-fry (or stir-fry with vinegar) to staunch bleeding. Treat with wine to move the blood.
Indications: Use crude for treating abdominal pain due to menstrual block, postpartum stasis pain, impact injury, swelling and toxin of sores and boils. Char-fry for treating blood ejection, spontaneous external and uterine bleeding, blood in the urine, blood dysentery, vaginal discharge. Apply topically to purulent ear, mouth sores, and genital damp itch. Daily dosage: 5–10 g. Contraindicated in yin vacuity and pregnancy. Used in *shi¹ xiao⁴ san³* (Sudden Smile Powder, 240), *er⁴ shen² wan²* (Two Spirits Pills, 81).
Remarks: Constituents: Flavonoid: isorhamnetin glucoside. Volatile oil. Fixed oil.
Similar plants: *Typha orientalis* Presl.; *T. davidiana* Hand.-Mazz.; *T. minima* Funk.

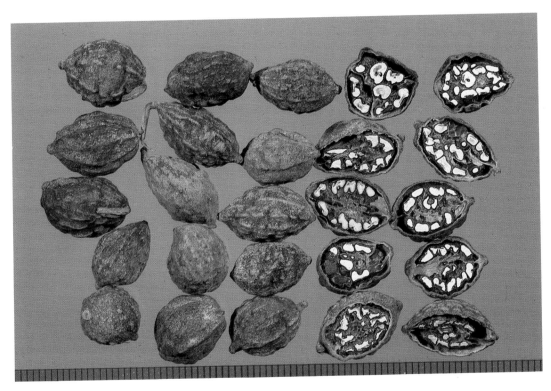

Alpiniae Oxyphyllae Fructus. (×5/3)

119 ALPINIAE OXYPHYLLAE FRUCTUS

益智仁 yi⁴ zhi⁴ ren². English: alpinia fruit, bitter cardamom. Japanese: *yakuchinin*.
Alternate names: 益智 yi⁴ zhi⁴, 益智子 yi⁴ zhi⁴ zi³.
Origin: Zingiberaceae family. *Alpinia oxyphylla* Miq.
Characters: This fruit is oval, about 1.5 cm long, 1–1.2 cm thick, and pointed at each end. The outer skin is reddish or grayish brown, with 13–18 discontinuous protuberant lines. The interior is divided into three segments that are separated in the center by a thin membrane, and that each contain 6–11 seeds pressed together. The seeds are irregularly shaped, grayish brown or yellow, about 3 mm in diameter, with the hilum located in a slight depression on the ventral side.
Quality: Large, full fruits with a high oil content are best.
Production areas: China (Guangdong, Guangxi, Fujian).
Properties and actions: Warm; acrid; nontoxic. Enters the spleen and kidney channels. Warms the spleen and kidney, secures qi, astringes essence. Stir-fry to reduce dryness and prevent damage to the kidney. Stir-fry with brine to warm the spleen and check diarrhea.
Indications: Frigid qi pain in the abdomen; vomiting and diarrhea due to cold stroke; profuse sleeping; seminal emission; dribbling urination; nocturia.
Daily dosage: 3–10 g. Contraindicated in dryness and heat patterns. Used in *yi⁴-zhi⁴ san³* (Alpinia Fruit Powder, 320).
Remarks: Constituents: Monoterpenoids and sesquiterpenoids (volatile oil, 0.6–2%): 1,8-cineole, α-pinene, *p*-cymene, camphor; nootkatone (main), nootkatol, β-selinene, (+)-α-copaene, β-caryophyllene, zingiberene, zingiberol. Diarylheptanoids: yakuchinones A, B.

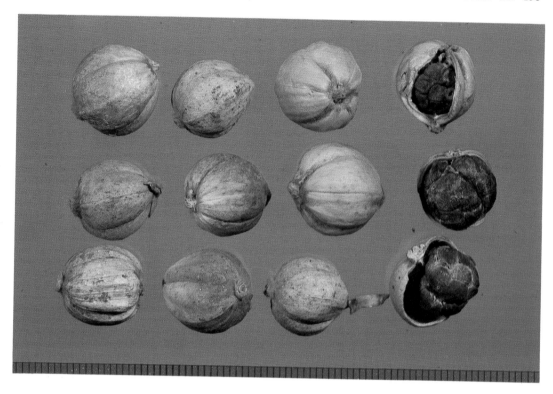

Amomi Cardamomi Fructus. (× 5/3)

120 AMOMI CARDAMOMI FRUCTUS

白豆蔻 *bai² dou⁴ kou⁴*. English: cardamon fruit. Japanese: *byakuzuku.*
Alternate names: 白蔻 bai² kou⁴, 白蔻仁 *bai² kou³ ren².*
Origin: Zingiberaceae family. *Amomum cardamomum* L.
Characters: These fruits are spheroid, yellowish or brownish white, and about 1.5 cm in diameter. They have three equidistant longitudingal furrows, numerous shallower longitudingal furrows, and fine longitudinal veins. The seeds are packed together in a globular mass, which is easily broken into three portions, each comprising 7–10 irregular, many-sided, light to dark brown seeds.
Quality: Large, full, unbroken fruits are the best.
Production areas: Vietnam, Thailand, India, and Sri Lanka.
Properties and actions: Warm; acrid; nontoxic. Enters the lung and spleen channels. Moves qi; warms the stomach; disperses food; loosens the center.
Indications: Stomach pain; abdominal distention; oppression in the venter and belching; stomach reflux; alcohol poisoning. Daily dosage: 1.5–3 g. Contraindicated in retching, vomiting, stomach reflux, and abdominal pain attributable to depressed fire. Used in *san¹ ren² tang¹* (Three Kernels Decoction, 220), *xiang¹ sha¹ yang³ wei⁴ tang¹* (Saussurea and Amomum Stomach-Nourishing Decoction, 292).
Remarks: Allied drug: Fruit of *Elettaria cardamomum* White et Maton.
Constituents: Volatile oil (ca 2-4%): *d*-borneol, *d*-camphor.

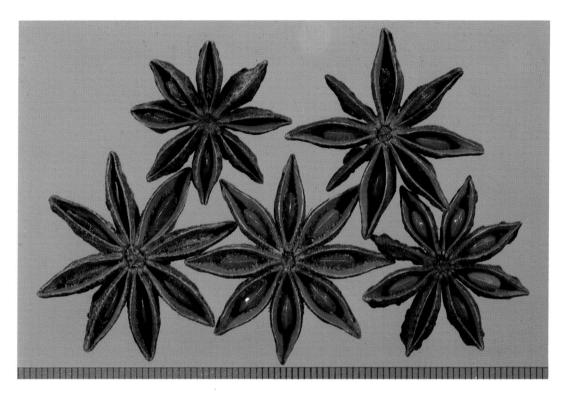

Anisi Stellati Fructus. (×5/3)

121 ANISI STELLATI FRUCTUS (ILLICII VERI FRUCTUS)

八角茴香 *ba¹ jiao³ hui² xiang¹*. English: star anise. Japanese: *hakkakuuikyo.*

Alternate names: 八角 *ba¹ jiao³*, 大茴香 *da⁴ hui² xiang¹*.

Origin: Magnoliaceae family. *Illicium verum* Hook. f.

Characters: This fruit is composed of eight reddish brown follicles, 0.5–2 cm long and 0.5–1.2 cm high, radiating from a common axis. Each follicle bears irregular wrinkles on the outside, and has a suture along one edge that is often split open, revealing the smoother interior surface, and shiny ovate seed of the same color contained within. The seed is very brittle, and breaks open to reveal a white interior.

Quality: Strong smelling, large, unbroken, reddish fruits with a high oil content are the best.

Production areas: China (Guangxi, Guangdong, Yunnan).

Properties and actions: Warm; acrid and sweet; nontoxic. Enters the spleen and kidney channels. Warms yang, dissipates cold, and rectifies qi.

Indications: Cold strike; counterflow retching; cold shan; abdominal pain; kidney vacuity; lumbar pain; dry and damp leg qi. Stir-fry lightly for lumbar pain and leg qi. Daily dosage: 3–5 g. Contraindicated in effulgent yin vacuity fire. Used in *hui¹-xiang¹ wan²* (Star Anise Pills, 136).

Remarks: Constituents: Phenylpropanoids, monoterpenoids, and sesquiterpenoids (volatile oil, star anise oil, 2.5–5%): anethole (80–95%), methyl chavicol, anisaldehyde, anisic acid, anisylacetone (*p*-methoxyphenylacetone), safrole; fenchone, (+)-α-pinene, farnesol. Acids: shikimic acid. Fixed oil (ca. 22%).

Similar plant: *Illicium lanceolatum* A. C. Smith.

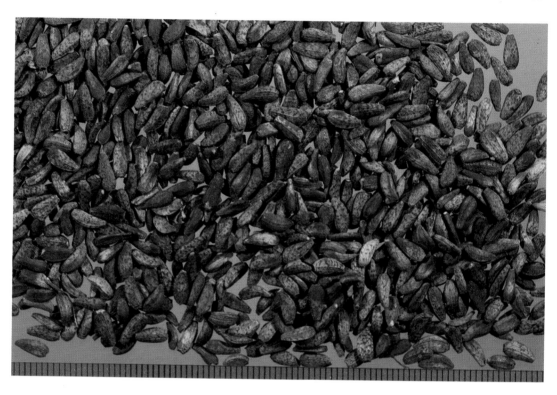

Arctii Fructus (stir-fried) (×5/3)

122 ARCTII FRUCTUS

牛蒡子 *niu² bang⁴ zi³*. English: arctium (or burdock) fruit. Japanese: *goboshi.*
Alternate names: 大力子 *da⁴ li⁴ zi³*, 惡實 *e⁴ shi².*
Origin: Compositae family. *Arctium lappa* L.
Characters: This fruit is ovate, but slightly twisted, in shape, and roughly 6 mm long. The diameter in the middle is about 3 mm. The exterior surface is gray-brown with a slightly paler spot at the tip, and a small indentation at the other, broader end. It bears protuberant longitudinal wrinkles. The outer skin is hard, and contains two white, oleaceous seeds.
Quality: The best ones come from Zhejiang.
Production areas: China (Hebei, Jilin, Liaonin, Zhejiang, Helongjiang, Sichuan, Henan, Hubei, Shaanxi), Korea, and Japan.
Properties and actions: Cold; acrid and bitter; nontoxic. Enters the lung and stomach channels. Courses wind and dissipates heat; diffuses the lung and outthrusts papules; disperses swelling and resolves toxin.
Indications: Wind-heat cough; sore, swollen throat; non-outthrust macules and papules; itchy wind papules; swollen yong and toxin of sores. Daily dosage: 5–10 g. Contraindicated in spleen-stomach vacuity with diarrhea. Used in *yin² qiao² san³* (Lonicera and Forsythia Powder, 323), *niu²-bang⁴-zi³ san³* (Arctium Powder, 191).
Remarks: Allied drug: Fruit of *Onopordon acanthium* L. (Compositae).
Constituents: Lignoids: arctiin. Volatile oil (25–30%).

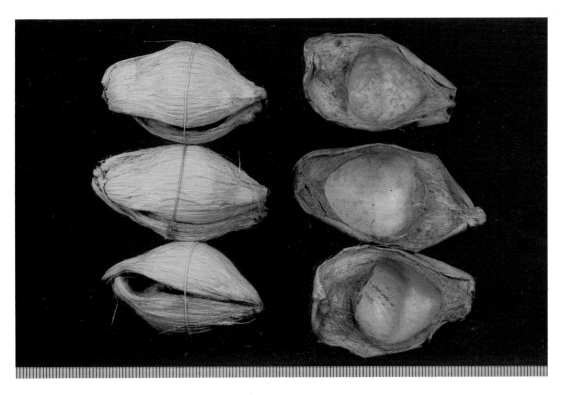

Arecae Pericarpium. (×1)

123 ARECAE PERICARPIUM

大腹皮 *da⁴ fu⁴ pi²*. English: areca (or betel) husk. Japanese: *daifukuhi.*

Alternate names: 大腹絨 *da⁴ fu⁴ rong²*, 檳榔皮 *bin¹ lang² pi²*.

Origin: Palmae family. *Areca catechu* L.

Characters: This is a oval pericarp is sold in two halves with the seed (Arecae Semen, see No. 161) removed. It is 6 cm long, and about 8 mm in diameter. It is white in color, and, apart from the endocarp, is highly fibrous and pliable.

Quality: Dry, supple, whitish yellow ones are the best.

Production areas: China (Hainandao, Guangdong, Guangxi, Yunnan, Taiwan), Philippines, and Indonesia.

Properties and actions: Slightly warm; acrid; nontoxic. Enters the spleen, stomach, large and small intestines channels. Precipitates qi and loosens the center; moves water. Wash in wine or licorice water to reduce toxicity.

Indications: Abdominal glomus and distention; leg qi; water swelling. Daily dosage: 5–10 g. Contraindicated for weak patients with qi vacuity. Used in *dao³ shui³ fu²-ling² tang¹* (Water-Abducting Poria Decoction, 66), *wu³ pi² san³* (Five Cortices Powder, 281), *fen¹ xiao¹ tang¹* (Separating and Dispersing Decoction, 87).

Remarks: Allied drug: Pericarp of *Areca dicksonii* Roxb.

Constituents: Tannoids.

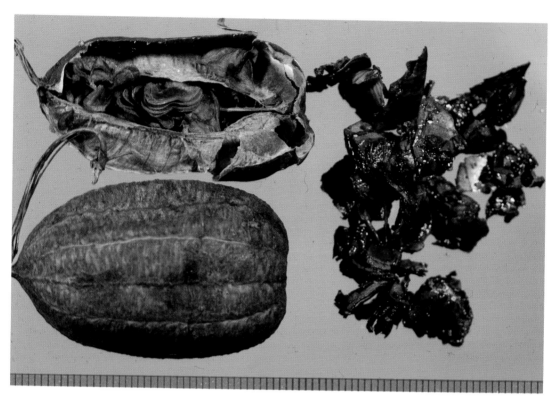

Aristolochiae Fructus: crude (left); mix-fried with honey (right). (× 5/3)

124 ARISTOLOCHIAE FRUCTUS

馬兜鈴 *ma³ dou¹ ling²*. English: aristolochia (or birthwort) fruit. Japanese: *batorei*.
Alternate name: 水馬香果 *shui³ ma³ xiang¹ guo³*.
Origin: Aristolochiaceae family. *Aristolochia contorta* Bge., *A. debilis* Sieb. et Zucc., *A. kaempferi* Willd.*
Characters: The dried fruit is ovate, 3–5 cm long, and 2–22.5 cm in diameter. The exocarp is gray green or gray yellow, and has six undulating ridges separated by six creases and bearing fine transverse veins. The exocarp is light and brittle, and easily breaks into six portions, the stalk thus breaking too. Inside, there are six tiers of seeds. The seeds are triangular or fan-shaped, and are brown in the center and pale brown at the edges, and have a thin membrane on one side. On the inside they are white and oleaceous.
Quality: Large, unbroken, gray-green fruits are the best.
Production areas: China (Hebei, Shandong, Shaanxi, Shanxi, Henan, Helongjiang).
Properties and actions: Cold; bitter; nontoxic. Enters the lung channel. Clears the lung and downbears qi; transforms phlegm and suppresses cough. Mix-fried with honey, it has a stronger lung-moistening function.
Indications: Lung heat dyspnea and cough; expectoration of blood; loss of voice; hemorrhoids and fistulae with pain and swelling. Daily dosage: 3–5 g. Contraindicated in vacuity cold cough and dyspnea, and in spleen vacuity diarrhea. Used in *ma³-dou¹-ling² san³* (Aristolochia Fruit Powder, 179).
Remarks: Constituents: volatile oil, aristolochic acid.

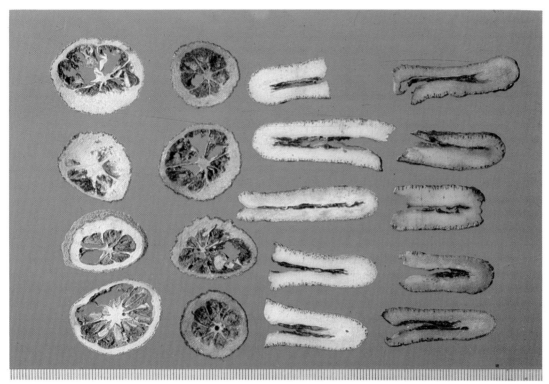

Aurantii Fructus Immaturus: crude and stir-fried (left). Aurantii Fructus: crude and stir-fried (right). (×5/6)

125 AURANTII FRUCTUS IMMATURUS (CITRI AURANTII FRUCTUS IMMATURUS)

枳實 *zhi³ shi²*. (Including Aurantii Fructus 枳殼 *zhi³ ke²*). English; unripe bitter orange fruit. Japanese: *kijitsu*.

Origin: Rutaceae family. *Poncirus trifoliata* (L.) Raf., *Citrus aurantium* L., *C. wilsonii* Tanaka.

Characters: *Poncirus trifoliata:* spherical, 0.5–1.5 cm in diameter, with green yellow skin, and 7–12 segments. *Citrus wilsonii:* spherical or obovate, 0.5–6.5 cm in diameter, with reddish brown skin, and 10–12 segments. *C. aurantium:* spherical, 0.8–3 cm in diameter, with grayish or blackish green skin, and 7–12 segments. The ripe fruit, Aurantii Fructus, is supplied with the flesh removed, squashed flat and cut into slices. All three varieties are supplied pre-cut.

Production areas: *Poncirus trifoliata:* China (Fujian, Shaanxi, Shanxi, Guangxi, Taiwan). *Citrus wilsonii:* China (Jiangxi, Sichuan). *C. aurantium:* China (Sichuan, Jiangxi, Zhejiang).

Properties and actions: Cold; bitter; nontoxic. Enters the spleen and stomach channels. Breaks qi, dissipates glomus, drains phlegm, and disperses accumulation. Use crude to break qi and disperse accumulations, stir-fried with bran to produce a milder effect and strengthen the spleen, and scorch-fried to staunch bleeding and to loosen the center. The ripe fruit, Aurantii Fructus, is milder in action, and is therefore more suitable for weaker patients.

Indications: Distention and fullness in the chest and abdomen; thoracic bi; glomus pain; phlegm pi; water swelling; food accumulation; constipation; gastroptosis (downward displacement of the stomach); prolapse of the uterus and rectum. Daily dosage: 3–5 g. Contraindicated in spleen-stomach vacuity. Used in *zhi³ zhu² tang¹* (Unripe Bitter Orange and Atractylodes Ovata Decoction, 344), *zhi³-shi² dao³ zhi⁴ wan²* (Unripe Bitter Orange Stagnation-Abducting Pills, 341), *zhi³-shi² zhi¹-zi³ chi³ tang¹* (Unripe Bitter Orange, Gardenia, and Fermented Soybean Bean Decoction, 342).

Remarks: Constituents: *C. aurantium:* Monoterpenoids, phenylpropanoids, and alkanes (volatile oil, orange oil 1.2–2.5%): (+)-limonene (main). Coumarins: umbelliferone, aurapten. Flavonoids: hesperidin, neohesperidin, naringin, poncirin. Limonoids: limonin. Alkaloids: (–)-synephrine (0.024–0.18 %).

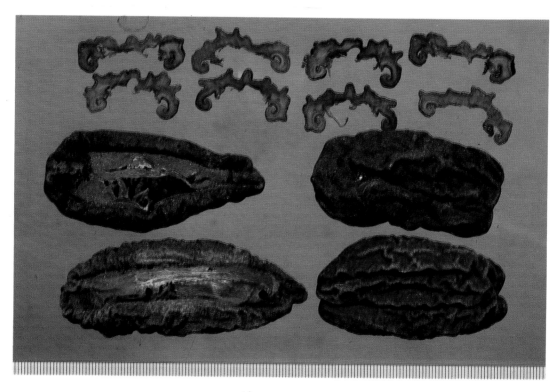

Chaenomelis Fructus: sliced (top); crude (bottom). (×7/8)

126 CHAENOMELIS FRUCTUS

木瓜 *mu⁴ gua¹*. English: chaenomeles (or Japanese quince) fruit. Japanese: *mokka*.

Alternate names: 木瓜實 *mu⁴ gua¹ shi²*, 宣木瓜 *xuan¹ mu⁴ gua¹*.

Origin: Rosaceae family. *Chaenomeles lagenaria* (Loisel.) Koidz., *C. sinensis* (Thouin) Koehne,* *C. lagenaria* (Loisel.) Koidz. var. *cathayensis* Rehd.,* *C. lagenaria* (Loisel.) Koidz. var. *wilsonii* Rehd.,* *C. thibetica* Yu.*

Characters: The dry fruit is oval, 4–8 cm long, and 3.5–5 cm in diameter, with a purple red, 2–8 mm thick exocarp that has a slight sheen and deep wrinkles. It is often sold cut in half, the pieces curling at the edges. Inside are flat or depressed ovaries, with reddish brown seeds, which are often missing. The fruit is soaked, steamed, and cut into slices 1–2 mm thick.

Quality: Large, wrinkled, reddish fruits are the best.

Production areas: China (Anhui, Zhejiang, Hubei, Sichuan).

Properties and actions: Warm; sour; nontoxic. Enters the liver and spleen channels. Calms the liver and harmonizes the stomach; eliminates damp and soothes the sinews.

Indications: Choleraic cramp; leg qi; damp bi. Daily dosage: 5–10 g. Contraindicated in gastrointestinal stagnation. Used in *mu⁴ gua¹ wan²* (Chaenomeles Pills, 189), *ji¹ ming² san³* (Cockcrow Powder, 139).

Remarks: Constituents: Organic acids: malic acid. Saponins (2%). Tannoids.

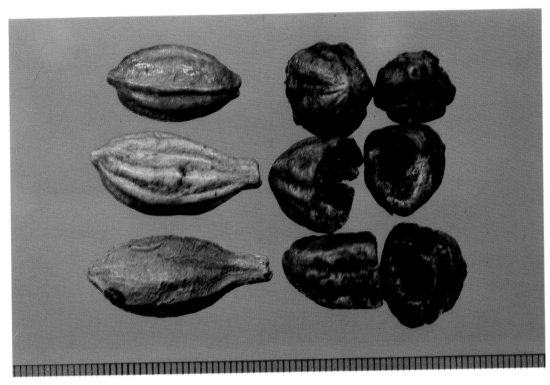

Chebulae Fructus: crude (left); roasted (right). (×5/3)

127 CHEBULAE FRUCTUS (TERMINALIAE FRUCTUS)

訶子 *he¹ zi³*. English: chebule, myrobalan. Japanese: *kashi.*

Alternate names: 訶子肉 *he¹ zi³ rou⁴*, 訶黎勒 *he¹ li² le⁴*.

Origin: Combretaceae family. *Terminalia chebula* Retz., *T. chebula* Retz. var. *gangetica* Roxb.*

Characters: The dried fruit is elliptical or flask-shaped, 3–5 cm long, 1.5–2.2 cm wide. Its exterior surface is a grayish yellow and bears longitudinal wrinkles, and five longitudinal ridges. It is hard and dense, and does not easily break. It is yellow inside.

Quality: Hard, yellow-brown fruits with a pronounced sheen are the best.

Production areas: India, Burma, Malaysia, Thailand, and China (Yunnan, Guangdong, Guangxi).

Properties and actions: Warm; bitter, sour, astringent; nontoxic. Enters the lung, stomach, and large intestine channels. Contracts the lung, astringes the intestines and precipitates qi. Roasting, stir-frying with bran, and scorch-frying strengthen the intestine-astringing action.

Indications: Enduring cough and loss of voice; enduring diarrhea and dysentery; prolapse of the rectum; blood in the stool; uterine bleeding; vaginal discharge; seminal emission; frequent urination. Daily dosage: 3–5 g. Contraindicated in the initial stages of cough and dysenteric disease. Used in *he¹-zi³ yin³* (Chebule Beverage, 116).

Remarks: Constituents: Tannoids (23–37%): chebulinic acid, chebulagic acid, ellagic acid, gallic acid, luteoic acid.

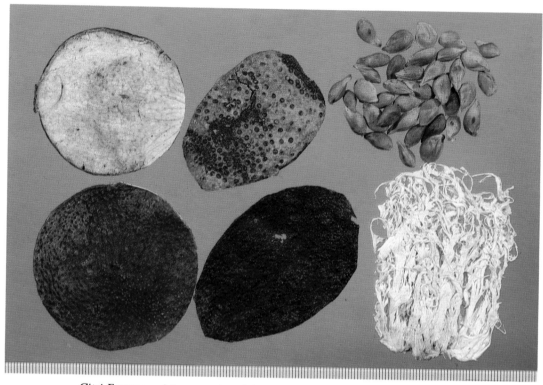

Citri Fructus: white part of peel (top left), whole peel (bottom left), red part of peel (middle), seeds (top right), and vascular bundles (bottom right)(× 5/6)

128 CITRI EXOCARPIUM (CITRI RETICULATAE EXOCARPIUM)

陳皮 *chen² pi²*. (Including Citri Exocarpium Album 橘白 *ju² bai²*, Citri Exocarpium Rubrum 橘紅 *ju² hong²*, Citri Semen 橘核 *ju² he²*, and Citri Fasciculus Vascularis 橘絡 *ju² luo⁴*). English: tangerine (or mandarin) peel. Japanese: *chinpi*.

Alternate name: 橘皮 *ju² pi²*.

Origin: Rutaceae family. *Citrus tangerina* Hort. et Tanaka, *C. erythrosa* Tanaka, *C. grandis* Osbeck. var. *tomentosa* Hort., *C. chachiensis* Hort., *C. unshiu* Marcor. [=*C. aurantium* L. subsp. nobilis Makino],* *C. ponki* Tanaka.*

Characters: The dried skin is 1–2 mm thick. The exterior surface is reddish brown and wrinkled, and bears numerous oil spots. The inside is white and spongy. The red and white layers may be cut apart before drying to be used separately. Stir-fry to stimulate the appetite.

Quality: Thin, red, oleaceous, strong-smelling peel in large pieces is the best quality.

Production areas: China (Guangdong, Guangxi, Fujian, Zhejiang, and Sichuan).

Properties and actions: Warm; acrid and bitter; nontoxic. Enters the lung and stomach channels. Rectifies qi; regulates the center; dries damp; transforms phlegm; resolves fish and crab toxin. The red part of the peel, Citri Exocarpium Rubrum, is stronger in its drying, warming, and qi-rectifying effect, while the white part, Citri Exocarpium Album, is milder in its effect. The seeds, Citri Semen, rectify qi and relieve pain, while the vascular bundles (i.e., the pith), Citri Fasciculus Vascularis, free the connecting vessels.

Indications: Distention and fullness in the chest and abdomen; no thought of food or drink; retching, vomiting, and hiccough; cough with copious phlegm. Daily dosage: 3–10 g. Contraindicated in yin vacuity with thirst. Used in *er⁴ chen² tang¹* (Double Vintage Decoction, 80), *ping² wei⁴ san³* (Stomach-Calming Powder, 196), *ju²-pi² zhi³-shi² sheng¹-jiang¹ tang¹* (Tangerine Peel, Unripe Bitter Orange, and Fresh Ginger Decoction, 154), *ju²-pi² tang¹* (Tangerine Peel Decoction, 153), *ju²-pi² zhu²-ru² tang¹* (Tangerine Peel and Bamboo Shavings Decoction, 155).

Remarks: Constituents: Monoterpenoids (volatile oil): limonene (main), α-, β-pinenes. Flavonoids: hesperidin, nobiletin.

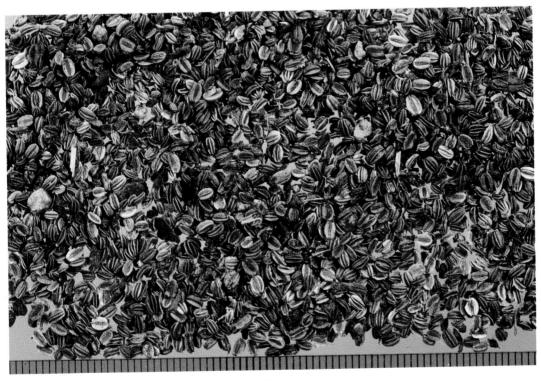

Cnidii Monnieri Fructus. (×5/3)

129 CNIDII MONNIERI FRUCTUS

蛇床子 *she² chuang² zi³*. English: cnidium fruit. Japanese: *jashoshi*.

Alternate names: 蛇床仁 *she² chuang² ren²*, 蛇床實 *she² chuang² shi²*.

Origin: Umbelliferae family. *Cnidium monnieri* (L.) Cusson.

Characters: These fruits are oval in shape, 2 mm long and 1 mm in diameter, and yellow-gray in color. They comprise two schizocarps, each with the remains of their styles, which are curled, and turned outward. On the two sides that touch, they are smooth but for two slightly protuberant, longitudinal lines. On the outward facing sides of each schizocarp, there are 5 distinct ridges. The exocarp is light and brittle. The seeds within are small, brown and oily, and are cool, pungent, and numbing to the taste.

Quality: Full, yellow fruits with a strong taste and smell are best.

Production areas: China (Hebei, Shandong, Jiangsu, Zhejiang, and less importantly in Guangxi, Sichuan, Shaanxi, and Shanxi).

Properties and actions: Warm; acrid, bitter. Enters the kidney and spleen channels. Warms the kidney and assists yang; dispels wind, dries damp, and kills worms.

Indications: Impotence; infertility due to uterine cold; wind-damp bi. Apply topically to damp scrotal itch, genital itch (e.g., trichomonal vaginitis), jie, xian, and damp sores. Daily dosage: 3–10 g. Contraindicated in lower burner damp-heat and in insufficiency of kidney yin. Used in *she²-chuang²-zi³ san³* (Cnidium Fruit Powder, 230), *yi¹ sao³ guang¹* (Gone-In-One-Sweep, 314).

Remarks: Constituents: Volatile oil (ca. 1.3%): *ℓ*-pinene, *ℓ*-camphene, bornylisovalerate. Coumarins: columbianadin, O-acetyl-columbianetin, columbianetin, O-isovalerylcolumbianetin, cnidiadin, archangelicin, osthol, isopimpinellin.

Allied drugs: Fruit of *Cnidium formosanum* Yabe (Taiwan), and *Torilis japonica* DC. (Japan).

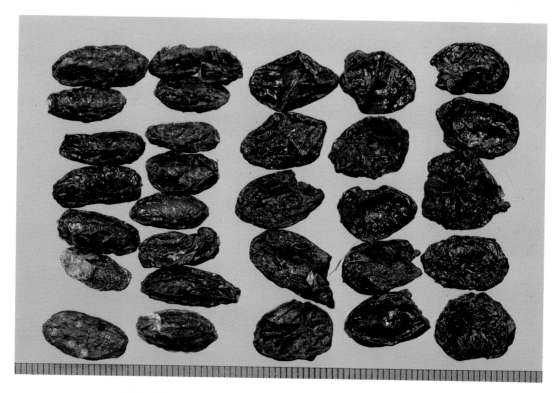

Corni Fructus: crude (left); steamed in wine (right). (×5/3)

130 CORNI FRUCTUS

山茱萸 *shan¹ zhu¹ yu²*. English: cornus (or Asiatic cornelion cherry, Japanese dogwood) fruit. Japanese: *sanshuyu.*

Alternate names: 山萸肉 *shan¹ yu² rou⁴*, 肉棗 *rou⁴ zao³*.

Origin: Cornaceae family. *Cornus officinalis* Sieb. et Zucc.

Characters: The dried fruit is 1–1.6 cm long and has shrunken flesh and wrinkled glossy blackish or purplish red translucent skin, through which the light-colored seed can be seen. At one end there is a small round scar left by the persistent calyx. The flesh is soft and sticky.

Quality: Fat, shiny, red fruits with a strong sour taste and no bloom are the best.

Production areas: China (Zhejiang, Henan, Anhui, Shaanxi, Shanxi, and Sichuan).

Properties and actions: Slightly warm; sour; nontoxic. Enters the liver and kidney channels. Supplements the liver and kidney; astringes essential qi and checks vacuity desertion.

Indications: Lumbar and knee pain; dizziness; tinnitus; impotence; seminal emission; frequent urination; fever and chills due to liver vacuity; incessant vacuity sweating; weak heart with scattered pulse. Daily dosage: 5–10 g. Contraindicated in intense life gate fire usually due to insufficiency of kidney yin, with signs such as inhibited urination, insomnia, and profuse dreaming. Used in *liu⁴ wei⁴ di⁴-huang² wan²* (Six-Ingredient Rehmannia Pills, 168).

Remarks: Constituents: Iridoids: loganin, sweroside, morroniside, verbenalin (cornin). Triterpenoids: oleanolic acid, ursolic acid: (saponins, ca 13%). Tannoids: cornus-tannins I, II, III, cornusiins A, B, C. Acids: gallic acid; malic acid. Saccharides: glycans.

Similar drug: Fruit of *Elaeagnus crispa* Thunb. (Elaeagnaceae) (Japan).

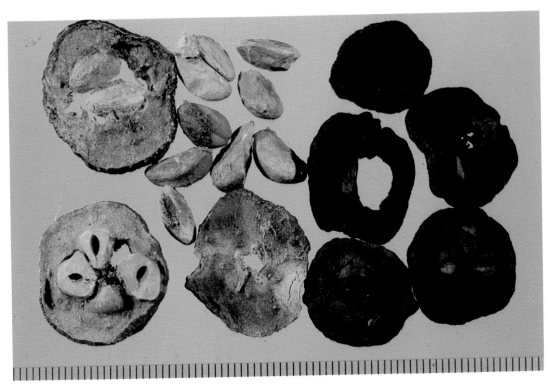

Crataegi Fructus: crude (left); charred (right). (× 5/3)

131 CRATAEGI FRUCTUS

山楂 shan[1] zha[1]. English: crataegus (or redhaw) fruit. Japanese: *sanza, sanzashi.*

Alternate names: 山楂片 shan[1] zha[1] pian[4], 山楂肉 shan[1] zha[1] rou[4], 山楂乾 shan[1] zha[1] gan[1].

Origin: Rosaceae family. *Crataegus pinnatifida* Bunge var. *major* N.E. Brown, *C. cuneata* Sieb. et Zucc., *C. pinnatifida* Bunge.,* *C. hupensis* Sarg.,* *C. sanguinea* Pall.,* *C. scabrifolia* (Franch.) Rehd.*

Characters: *Crataegus pinnatifida* var. *major* is spherical or pear-shaped (changing into a small cake shape after pressure has been applied), 1.2 cm in diameter. It has a round depression at the tip, which is black inside, with the remains of sepals at its margins. The exterior surface is red or reddish brown. Within are five earth-colored seeds. *C. cuneata* is nearly spherical in shape, and about 2 cm in diameter. When ripe, it is bright red with a sheen, and pale speckles. Within are 3–4 seeds. It is soft. It is sweeter than the other variety, and has a stronger scent. The decocting pieces are 3–5 mm thick slices. The cut edge shows the yellow seeds surrounded by the yellow-brown flesh of the fruit.

Quality: Large, dry, red-skinned, and thick-fleshed fruits are the best.

Production areas: *Crataegus pinnatifida* var. *major:* China (Liaoning, Jilin, Heilongjiang, Shandong, Henan, Hebei, Shanxi). *C. cuneata:* China (Zhejiang, Jiangsu, Anhui, and Sichuan).

Properties and actions: Slightly warm; sour and sweet; nontoxic. Enters the spleen, stomach, and liver channels. Disperses food accumulations; dissipates static blood; expels tapeworm. When charred, its astringent quality is enhanced, making it more effective for blood dysentery.

Indications: Concretions and conglomerations; phlegm-rheum; lump glomus; acid regurgitation; diarrhea; intestinal wind; lumbar pain; shan qi; afterpains; persistent flow of the lochia; stagnation of milk in suckling infants. Daily dosage: 5–10 g. Contraindicated in spleen-stomach vacuity. Used in qi[3] pi[2] tang[1] (Spleen-Arousing Decoction, 199), jia[1] wei[4] ping[2] wei[4] san[3] (Supplemented Stomach-Calming Powder, 142).

Remarks: Constituents: amygdalin, quercetin, chlorogenic acid, ursolic acid, tartaric acid.

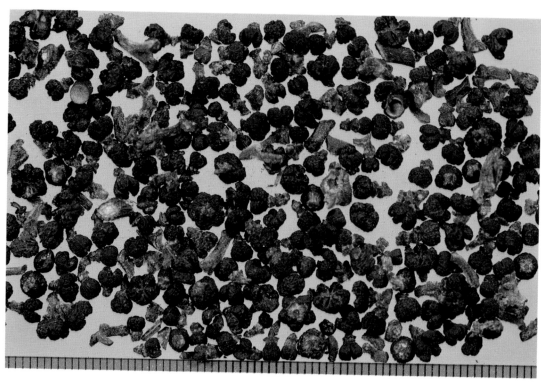

Evodiae Fructus, treated with licorice water. (× 2)

132 EVODIAE FRUCTUS

吳茱萸 *wu² zhu¹ yu²*. English: evodia fruit. Japanese: *goshuyu*.

Alternate names: 吳萸 *wu² yu²*, 茱萸 *zhu¹ yu²*.

Origin: Rutaceae family. *Evodia rutaecarpa* (Juss.) Benth.

Characters: This fruit is spherical, 2–5 cm in diameter, with stalk. The outside is dark brown or black in color, and hard in substance. It splits into five loculi, each containing one globular, brown seed.

Quality: Full, hard, strong smelling, acrid tasting fruits without stalks are the best.

Production areas: China (Guizhou, Guangxi, Hunan, Yunnan, Shaanxi, Zhejiang, Sichuan).

Properties and actions: Warm: acrid and bitter; toxic. Enters the liver and stomach channels. Warms the center and relieves pain; rectifies qi and dries damp. Treated with licorice water, its harsh, pungent quality is reduced. Stir-fried with wine, it quickens the blood. Stir-fried with vinegar, it calms the liver. Stir-fried with brine, it enters the kidney and treats shan pain. Stir-fried with Coptidis Rhizoma *(huang² lian²)* it treats vomiting. Stir-fried with ginger juice, it expels cold and relieves pain. Stir-fried without additives, it precipitates qi and downbears counterflow.

Indications: Counterflow retching; acid vomiting; jue yin headache; vomiting and diarrhea due to visceral cold; distention pain in the venter and abdomen; leg qi; shan qi; mouth sores and ulcers; toothache; eczema; yellow water sores. Daily dosage: 1.5–3 g. Contraindicated in yin vacuity and cold-damp. Used in *wu²-zhu¹-yu² tang¹* (Evodia Decoction, 274), *si⁴ shen² wan²* (Four Spirits Pills, 254), *ji¹ ming² san³* (Cockcrow Powder, 139), *wen¹ jing¹ tang¹* (Channel-Warming Decoction, 269), *zuo³ jin¹ wan²* (Metal-Assisting Pills, 356), *dang¹-gui¹ si⁴ ni⁴ jia¹ wu²-zhu¹-yu² sheng¹-jiang¹ tang¹* (Tangkuei Counterflow Frigidity Decoction Plus Evodia and Fresh Ginger, 61).

Remarks: Constituents: Alkaloids: evodiamine, hydroxyevodiamine (rhetsinine), dehydroevodiamine, carboxyevodiamine, rutaecarpine, dihydrorutaecarpine. Limonoids: limonin (evodin), evodol, obakunone. Acids. goshuynic acid, palmitic acid, linoleic acid.

Allied drug: Dried fruit of *Evodia officinalis* Dode [= *E. rutaecarpa* Benth. var. *officinalis* (Dode) Huang].

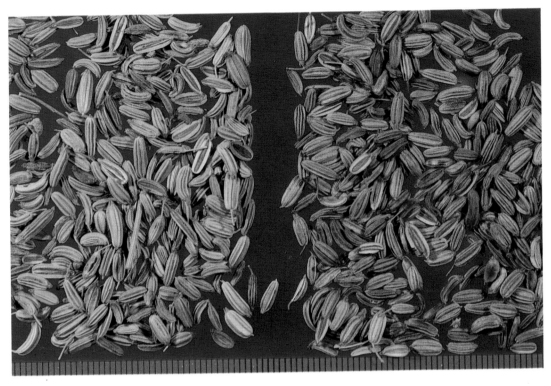

Foeniculi Fructus: crude (left); stir-fried (right). (×5/3)

133 FOENICULI FRUCTUS

茴香 *hui² xiang¹*. English: fennel fruit. Japanese: *uikyo.*

Alternate name: 小茴香 *xiao³ hui² xiang¹*.

Origin: Umbelliferae family. *Foeniculum vulgare* Mill.

Characters: This is a cylindrical cremocarp, 3–5 mm long. The outside is yellow-green or gray-black, sometimes with a 3–10 mm stalk attached. At the tip are the 1 mm long remains of the two cylindrical styles. Each schizocarp is a broad ellipse, up to 2 mm wide, with a rounded dorsum bearing 5 distinct ribs. The touching sides have a furrow, and are dark in the middle and light at the edges.

Quality: The best quality is dry, greenish yellow, and fragrant.

Production areas: China (Northwest, Inner Mongolia, Shanxi, Shaanxi, Manchuria), Japan, India, and Southern Europe.

Properties and actions: Warm; acrid; nontoxic. Enters the kidney, bladder, and stomach channels. Warms the kidney and dissipates cold; harmonizes the stomach and rectifies qi.

Indications: Cold shan; frigid pain in the lower abdomen; kidney vacuity lumbar pain; stomach pain; vomiting; dry and damp leg qi. Use stir-fried for pain in the bladder, and stir-fried in brine to treat kidney vacuity lumbar pain. Daily dosage: 3–10 g. Contraindicated in yin vacuity fire. Used in *dao³ qi⁴ tang¹* (Qi-Abducting Decoction, 65), *an¹ zhong¹ san³* (Center-Quieting Powder, 3).

Remarks: Constituents: Phenylpropanoids and monoterpenoids (volatile oil, 1–8%): anethole (50–85%), methyl chavicol (ca. 3%), anisaldehyde, anisic acid; (+)-fenchone (10–20%), (+)-limonene, (+)-α-pinene. Fixed oil (10–18%): glycerides of pteroselinic acid, linoleic acid.

Similar drugs: Fruits of *Foeniculum dulce* DC., *F. piperitum* DC., and *Illicium verum* Hook. f. (Magnoliaceae).

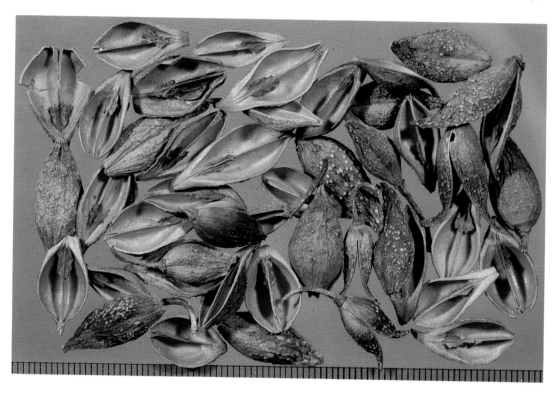

Forsythiae Fructus. (×5/3)

134 FORSYTHIAE FRUCTUS

連翹 *lian² qiao²*. English: forsythia (or weeping golden bell) fruit. Japanese: *rengyō*.
Alternate name: 連翹殼 *lian² qiao² ke²*.
Origin: Oleaceae family. *Forsythia suspensa* (Thunb.) Vahl.
Characters: This fruit is ovate with acute points at each end. It is 0.7–2.5 cm long, and 0.5–1 cm wide, splitting into two points at the tip. The exterior surface of the exocarp is yellow-brown and bears irregular protuberant lines and speckles. Its interior surface is paler in color, and smooth, and has a distinct septum. The seeds are usually missing.
Quality: Dry, yellowish fruits with thick shells, and copious seeds are the best.
Production areas: China (Shanxi, Henan, Shanxi, Hubei, Shandong).
Properties and actions: Slightly cold; bitter; nontoxic. Enters the heart, liver, and gallbladder channels. Clears heat, resolves toxin, dissipates binds, and disperses swelling. Use crude to clear heat and resolve toxin. Blend with cinnabar to clear the heart and quiet the spirit in febrile diseases.
Indications: Warm heat; cinnabar toxin; maculopapular eruption; swelling and toxin of yong; scrofulous lumps; dribbling urinary block. Can be applied topically to jie and xian. Daily dosage: 5–10 g. Contraindicated in yin vacuity blood heat, gastric vacuity diarrhea, and burst yong exuding light green pus. Used in *yin² qiao² san³* (Lonicera and Forsythia Powder, 323), *jing¹-jie⁴ lian²-qiao² tang¹* (Schizonepeta and Forsythia Decoction, 151), *fang²-feng¹ tong¹ sheng⁴ san³* (Ledebouriella Sage-Inspired Powder, 83), *jing¹ fang² bai⁴ du² san³* (Schizonepeta and Ledebouriella Toxin-Vanquishing Powder, 150).
Remarks: Constituents: Lignoids: phillygenin, (+)-pinoresinol, phillyrin, (+)-pinoresinol-D-glucoside. Phenylpropanoids: forsythoside A (forsythiaside), C (suspensaside), D, E, cornoside, rengyosides A, B, C. Monoterpenoids: α-, β-pinenes, terpinen-4-ol, p-cymene.
Allied drugs: Dried fruit of *Forsythia koreana* Nakai and *F. viridissima* Lindl.

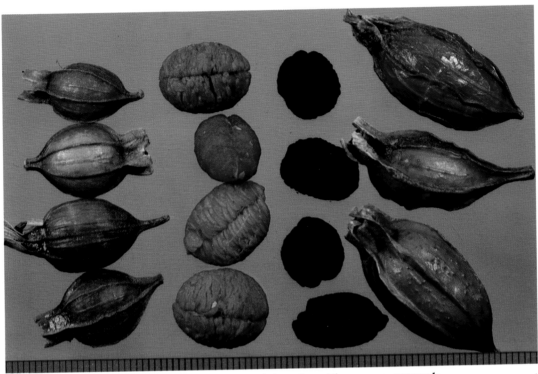

Gardeniae Fructus: (left to right) crude; with exocarp removed;
charred; Gardeniae Grandiflorae Fructus. (×5/3)

135 GARDENIAE FRUCTUS

栀子 *zhi¹ zi³*. English: gardenia (or Cape jasmine) fruit. Japanese: *shishi, sanshishi*.
Origin: Rubiaceae family. *Gardenia jasminoides* Ellis.
Characters: This fruit is elliptical, 3.5–4.5 cm long, and 1.2–2 cm wide. The outer surface is reddish or yellowish brown, and glossy. It has 6 wing-like longitudinal ridges, with a rib between each. At the tip of the fruit are the remains of the sepals, and a scar left by the fruit stalk. The exocarp is thin, and is bright yellow and smooth on the inner surface. It contains numerous reddish brown oval seeds with protuberant markings, packed tightly together in a solid mass. The decocting pieces are fine slices of the seed mass.
Quality: The small, dry, unbroken fruits containing red seeds are the best.
Production areas: China (Zhejiang, Jiangxi, Hunan, Fujian, and less importantly Sichuan, Hubei, Yunnan, Guizhou, Jiangsu, Anhui, Guangdong, Guangxi, and Henan), and Japan.
Properties and actions: Cold; bitter; nontoxic. Enters the heart, liver, lung, and stomach channels. Clears heat, drains fire, and cools the blood. Use crude to clear heat and drain fire. Stir-fry or scorch-fry for an additional blood-cooling action. Char to treat blood ejection, nosebleed, and blood dysentery. Stir-fry with ginger juice to check vexation and vomiting. Stir-fry with brine to clear vacuity fire. Remove the skin to drain heart fire, but leave it on to drain lung fire.
Indications: Vacuity vexation and sleeplessness in febrile disease; jaundice and strangury; wasting thirst; reddening of the eyes; sore throat and blood ejection; spontaneous external bleeding and blood dysentery; blood in the urine; heat toxin sores; sprains. Daily dosage: 3–10 g. Contraindicated in spleen-stomach vacuity cold. Used in *zhi¹-zi³ da⁴-huang² tang¹* (Gardenia and Rhubarb Decoction, 339), *zhi¹-zi³ chi³ tang¹* (Gardenia and Fermented Soybean Decoction, 338), *zhi³-shi² zhi¹-zi³ chi³ tang¹* (Unripe Bitter Orange, Gardenia, and Fermented Soybean Bean Decoction, 342), *jia¹ wei⁴ gui¹ pi² tang¹* (Supplemented Spleen-Returning Decoction, 140).
Remarks: Constituents: Iridoids: geniposide (3.9–7.5%), genipin-1-β-gentiobioside, 10-acetylgeniposide, geniposidic acid, gardenoside, shanzhiside, genipin. Monoterpenoids: jasminoids A, B, C. Yellow pigment: crocin.

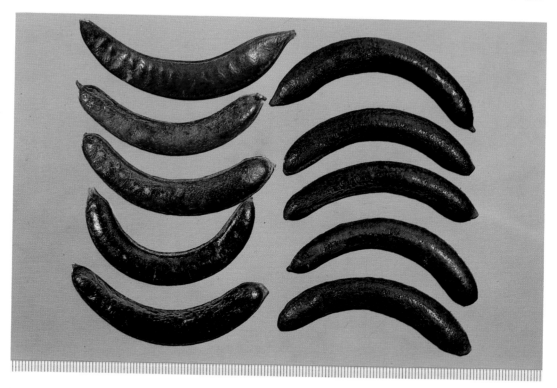

Gleditsiae Fructus: crude (left); stir-fried (right). (×7/8)

136 GLEDITSIAE FRUCTUS

皂荚 *zao⁴ jia²*. English: gleditsia (or Chinese honeylocust) fruit. Japanese: *sokyo.*
Alternate name: 皂角 *zao⁴ jiao³.*
Origin: Leguminosae family. *Gleditsia sinensis* Lam.
Characters: The dried pod is a long, flat cylinder, usually slightly curved and sometimes fatter at one end. It is 12–25 cm long, 2–3.5 cm wide, and 0.8–1.4 cm thick. The surface is smooth, and dark brown with a red or purple hue. It is covered in a gray-white bloom, which can be wiped away to leave a shiny surface. Both ends are pointed. At the base is the stalk or what remains of it. The dorsal suture protrudes to form a ridge-like spine. It is hard, and rattles when shaken. It can be broken open to reveal a light yellow interior, sometimes with seeds.
Quality: Hard, fat pods are the best.
Production areas: China (Sichuan, Shandong, and less importantly Hubei, Guizhou, Yunnan, Henan, and Zhejiang).
Properties and actions: Warm; acrid; slightly toxic. Enters the lung and large intestine channels. Dispels wind-phlegm (especially when roasted or stir-fried), eliminates damp toxin, and kills worms. Boil and remove the yellow skin to treat constipation.
Indications: Deviation of eyes and mouth in wind stroke; head wind headache; phlegm dyspnea and cough; intestinal wind hemafecia; dysentery; trismus; swollen yong; inguinal lumps; sores, xian, jie, and lai. Daily dosage: 1–3 g. Contraindicated in vacuity and pregnancy. Used in *zao⁴ jia² wan²* (Gleditsia Fruit Pills, 332).
Remarks: Constituents: Seed: saponins (5–8%): gleditsia saponin, gledigenin.
Allied drugs: Fruit of *Gleditsia officinalis* Hemsley and *G. japonica* Miq. (Japan).

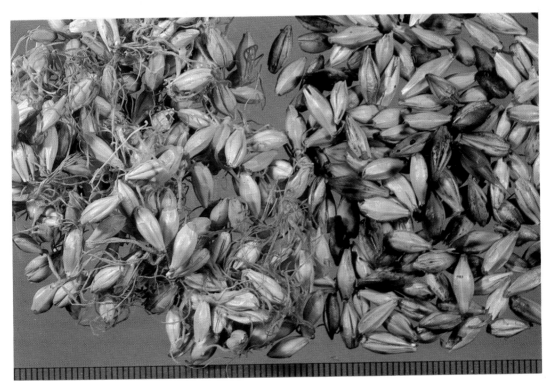

Hordei Fructus Germinatus: crude (left); stir-fried (right). (×5/3)

137 HORDEI FRUCTUS GERMINATUS

麥芽 *mai⁴ ya²*. English: (dried) barley sprout, malt. Japanese: *bakuga.*

Alternate names: 大麥芽 *da⁴ mai⁴ ya²*, 大麥蘗 *da⁴ mai⁴ nie⁴.*

Origin: Gramineae family. *Hordeum vulgare* L.

Characters: This is a ridged fruit tapering to a point at both ends. It is 8–12 mm long, and 2.5–3.5 mm in diameter. From the upper end spring yellow-brown young shoots roughly 3 mm long, while from the lower end grow contorted fibrous roots, 0.2–2 cm long. The exterior is pale brown. The dorsum has five veins and is protected by an outer glume, while the ventral aspect bears a furrow, and is covered by an inner glume.

Quality: Large, full fruits with shoots intact are best.

Production areas: China, Japan, Korea.

Properties and actions: Slightly warm; sweet; nontoxic. Enters the spleen and stomach channels. Disperses food, harmonizes center, and precipitates qi. Used crude, it promotes lactation and disperses food, while stir-fried it fortifies the spleen and disperses stagnation.

Indications: Food accumulation; distention and fullness in the venter and abdomen; loss of appetite; vomiting and diarrhea; persistent distention of the breasts. Daily dosage: 10–12 g. Used in *ban⁴-xia⁴ bai²-zhu² tian¹-ma² tang¹* (Pinellia, Atractylodes Ovata, and Gastrodia Decoction, 24).

Remarks: Similar plant: *Hordeum vulgare* L. var. *nudum* Hook. f.

Constituents: Enzymes: diastase, invertase, lipase, peptidase, protease. Starch.

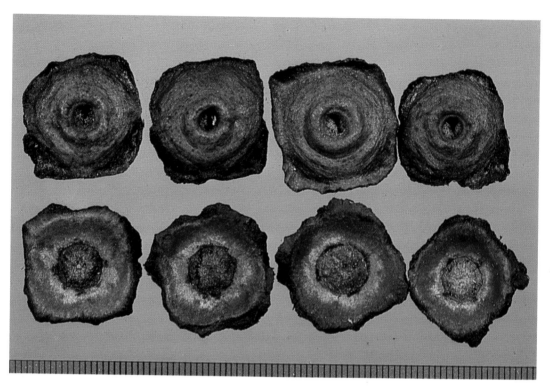

Kaki Calyx. (× 5/3)

138 KAKI CALYX (DIOSPYRORIS KAKI CALYX)

柿蒂 *shi⁴ di⁴*. English: persimmon calyx. Japanese: *shitei*.

Alternate names: 柿萼 *shi⁴ e⁴*, 柿子把 *shi⁴ zi³ ba³*.

Origin: Ebenaceae family. *Diospyros kaki* L. f.

Characters: The dried calyx is lid-shaped, with a stalk at the tip, or a hole if it is missing. The central part is thicker, and the margin, which is thinner, comprises four triangular lobes, which often curl upward and easily break. The base is saucer-shaped, 1.5–2.5 cm, and 1–4 mm thick. The outer surface is a reddish brown. When closely observed, it is seen to have sparse fine short rust-colored hairs on the inner surface. It is hard and brittle in substance, and has no smell.

Quality: Thick, brown calyces with a bloom are the best.

Production areas: China (Henan, Shandong, Fujian, Hebei, Shandong), and Japan.

Properties and actions: Warm; bitter and astringent; nontoxic. Enters the lung channel. Downbears counterflow qi. Used char-fried to staunch bleeding.

Indications: Counterflow cough; lower esophageal qi constriction; stomach reflux. Daily dosage: 5–10 g. Used in *ding¹-xiang¹ shi⁴-di⁴ tang¹* (Clove and Persimmon Decoction, 70), *shi⁴-di⁴ tang¹* (Persimmon Decoction, 247).

Remarks: Similar plant: *Diospyros moriciana* Hance (Taiwan).

Constituents: Triterpenoids: betulinic acid, oleanolic acid, ursolic acid. Tannoids.

Allied drugs: Kaki Saccharum, and Kaki Siccatus Succus.

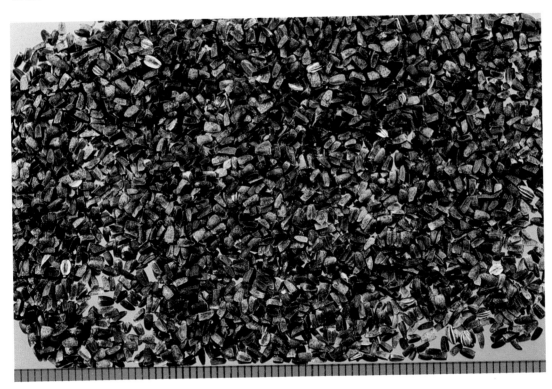

Leonuri Fructus. (×2)

139 LEONURI FRUCTUS

茺蔚子 *chong¹ wei⁴ zi³*. English: leonurus (or Chinese motherwort) fruit. Japanese: *juishi*.
Alternate names: 茺玉子 *chong¹ yu⁴ zi³*, 益母子 *yi⁴ mu³ zi³*.
Origin: Labiatae family. *Leonurus heterophyllus* Sweet [= *L. sibiricus* L.].
Characters: The dried fruit is truncated at one end and bluntly pointed at the other. It has three sides, two of which are flat and stand at 90 degrees to each other, while the third is rounded. It is about 2–3 mm long and 1.5 mm wide. The exterior surface is a dark gray-brown, with darker flecks. It has no sheen, and may be rough.
Quality: Clean, large, full fruits are the best.
Production areas: China, Korea, and Japan.
Properties and actions: Slightly warm; sweet, acrid, nontoxic. Enters the liver and pericardium channels. Quickens the blood and promotes menstruation; courses wind and clears heat.
Indications: Menstrual irregularities; profuse uterine bleeding; postpartum static blood with pain; liver heat headache; reddening, soreness, and swelling of the eyes; eye screens. Daily dosage: 5–10 g. Contraindicated in insufficiency of liver blood with dilated pupils, and in pregnancy. Used in *yi⁴-mu³ sheng⁴ jin¹ dan¹* (Leonurus Metal-Overcoming Elixir, 316).
Remarks: Similar plants: *Leonurus heterophyllus* Sweet f. *leucanthus* C.Y. Wu et H.W. Li; *L. turkestanicus* V. Krecz. et Kuprian.
Constituents: Alkaloids: leonurinine. Fixed oil (ca. 40%): oleic acid (64%), linoleic acid (21%).

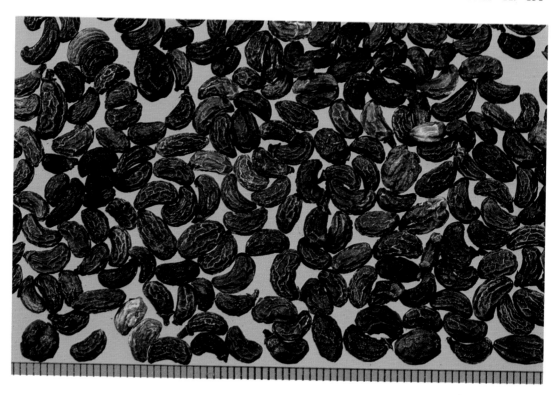

Ligustri Fructus: steamed. (×2)

140 LIGUSTRI FRUCTUS

女貞子 *nu³ zhen¹ zi³*. English: ligustrum (or glossy privet) fruit. Japanese: *joteishi*.
Alternate name: 白臘樹子 *bai² la⁴ shu⁴ zi³*.
Origin: Oleaceae family. *Ligustrum lucidum* Ait.
Characters: The dried fruit is ovate or oval, sometimes bent or twisted. It is 5–10 mm long, and 3–4 mm in diameter. The exterior surface is blue-black, with wrinkles. Both ends are rounded, and at the base is the scar left by the stalk. This fruit is hard and light. Inside is a single seed, or two seeds isolated in the fruit pulp. The seeds are elliptical, and pointed at each end. They are black on the outside and white on the inside.
Quality: Large, full, hard, blue-black fruits are the best.
Production areas: China (Zhejiang, Jiangsu, Hunan, Fujian, Guangxi, Jiangxi, Sichuan).
Properties and actions: Balanced; bitter and sweet. Enters the liver and kidney channels. Supplements the liver and kidney, strengthens the lumbus and knees. Steaming with vinegar or brine eliminates the side effect of diarrhea.
Indications: Internal heat due to yin vacuity; dizziness; flowery vision; tinnitus; weak, aching lumbus and knees; premature graying. Daily dosage: 5–10 g. Contraindicated in spleen-stomach vacuity diarrhea, and yang vacuity. Used in *nü³-zhen¹ tang¹* (Ligustrum Decoction, 195).
Remarks: Constituents: nuezhnide, α-mannitol, oleanolic acid, anthocyan. Seed: fixed oil (14.9%).
Similar plant: *Ligustrum japonicum* Thunb. (Japan).

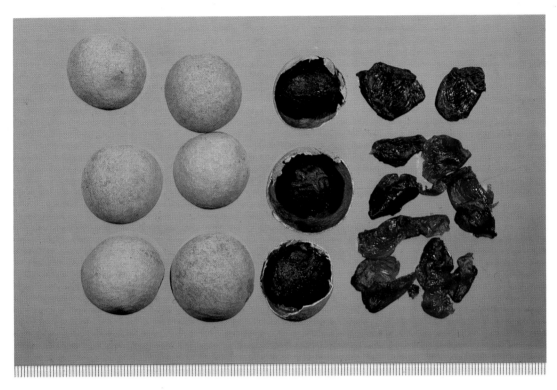

Longanae Arillus: crude (left); with shell and pit removed (right). (× 7/8)

141 LONGANAE ARILLUS (EUPHORIAE LONGANAE ARILLUS)

龍眼肉 *long² yan³ rou⁴*. English: longan aril flesh. Japanese: *ryuganniku*.

Alternate names: 桂圓肉 *gui⁴ yuan² rou⁴*, 龍眼 *long² yan³*.

Origin: Sapindaceae family. *Euphoria longana* (Lour.) Steud.

Characters: The dried fruit is spherical, and about 1.5 cm in diameter. The exterior surface is smooth, and a gray-yellow in color. The skin, about 1 mm thick, is brittle, and breaks easily to reveal the interior flesh, which through drying has turned from white to dark brown, and shrunken to a sticky, semitranslucent mass, detaching itself from the skin. Amid the flesh is a single, dark brown pit.

Quality: Large fruits with thick, soft, semi-translucent brown flesh that has a strong sweet flavor are the best.

Production areas: China (Guangxi, Fujian, Guangdong, Sichuan, Taiwan).

Properties and actions: Warm; sweet; nontoxic. Enters the heart and spleen channels. Boosts the heart and spleen, supplements qi and quiets the spirit.

Indications: Vacuity taxation; marked emaciation; insomnia; impaired memory; fright palpitations and racing of the heart. Daily dosage: 6–15 g. Contraindicated in phlegm-fire patterns and vomiting. Used in *gui¹ pi² tang¹* (Spleen-Returning Decoction, 108).

Remarks: Constituents: Aril: Water soluble (79.77%): glucose (24.91%), sucrose (0.22%), tartaric acid (1.26%). Ash: 2.36%. Protein 5.6%.

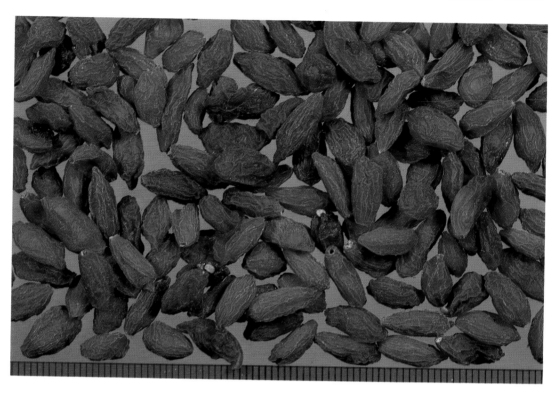

Lycii Fructus. (×5/3)

142 LYCII FRUCTUS

枸杞子 *gou³ qi³ zi³*. English: lycium (or Chinese matrimony vine) berry. Japanese: *kukoshi*.
Alternate names: 甘枸杞 *gan¹ gou³ qi³*, 地骨子 *di⁴ gu³ zi³*.
Origin: Solanaceae family. *Lycium chinense* Mill., *L. barbarum* L. [= *L. halimifolium* Mill.].*
Characters: The dried fruit is ovate, spindle-shaped, or elliptical. It is 1–1.6 cm long, and 5–7 mm thick. The skin is bright or dark red with a good sheen, turning black and dull when stored for a long time. At one end there is stalk trace, appearing as a white fleck, and at the other there is a small, nipple-like protuberance. Amid the soft, moist, semitranslucent flesh are 10 kidney-shaped seeds, 2.5 mm long, and 2 mm wide, and 0.5 mm thick. These are earth color, sometimes darker at the edges, and bear fine depressions on the surface, and hilum on the indented side.
Quality: Large, red fruits with few seeds and sweet flesh are best.
Production areas: China (Hebei, and less importantly Henan, Shaanxi, Sichuan, and Jiangsu).
Properties and actions: Balanced; sweet; nontoxic. Enters the liver and kidney channels. Enriches the kidney, moistens the lung, supplements the liver, and brightens the eyes.
Indications: Liver-kidney yin depletion; weak, aching knees and lumbus; dizziness; copious tears; vacuity taxation cough; wasting thirst; seminal emission. Daily dosage: 5–10 g. Contraindicated in externally contracted repletion heat, and in spleen vacuity with damp. Used in *qi³ ju² di⁴-huang² wan²* (Lycium, Chrysanthemum, and Rehmannia Pills, 198).
Remarks: Constituents: Amino acids: betaine (0.09%). Sesquiterpenoids: (–)-1,2-dehydro-α-cyperone, solavetivone. Tetraterpenoids (0.0034%): zeaxanthin, physalien (zeaxanthin dipalmitate). Steroids: β-sitosterol. Acids: linoleic acid. Fixed oil.

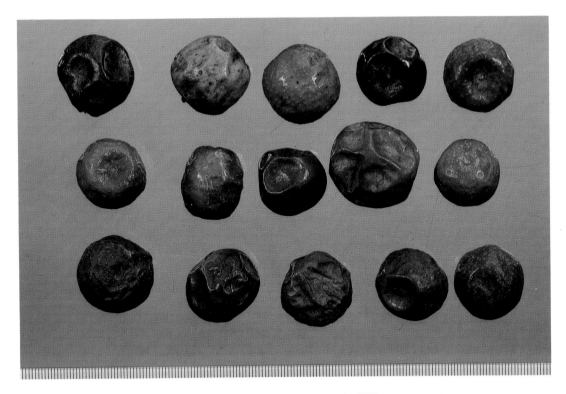

Meliae Toosendan Fructus. (× 7/8)

143 MELIAE TOOSENDAN FRUCTUS (TOOSENDAN FRUCTUS)

川楝子 *chuan¹ lian⁴ zi³*. English: toosendan fruit. Japanese: *senrenshi*.

Alternate names: 楝子 *lian⁴ zi³*, 苦楝子 *ku³ lian⁴ zi³*.

Origin: Meliaceae family. *Melia toosendan* Sieb. et Zucc.

Characters: The dried fruit is spherical or oval, 1.7–3 cm long and 1.7–2.3 cm in diameter. The exterior surface is yellow-brown, with a slight sheen, and with indentations due to shrinkage. At one end is the stalk trace, and at the other is an indented stele trace. The exocarp is leathery, and often separated from the thick, light yellow, soft flesh contained within. Amidst the flesh is an earth-colored spheroid or ovate drupe, truncated at both ends, and bearing 6–8 longitudinal ridges. Inside, this is divided into 6–8 loculi, each containing 6–8 seeds. The endosperm of the seeds is cream-colored and oleaceous.

Quality: Golden fruits with thick, light-colored flesh are the best.

Production areas: China (Sichuan, Hubei, Guizhou, and Henan).

Properties and actions: Cold; bitter; toxic. Enters the liver, stomach, and small intestine channels. Eliminates damp-heat; clears liver fire; relieves pain; and kills worms. Used crude to clear liver fire.

Indications: Heat inversion; heart pain; lateral costal pain; shan pain; abdominal pain due to worm accumulation. Stir-fry to treat shan pain. Daily dosage: 5–10 g. Contraindicated in spleen-stomach vacuity cold. used in *dao³ qi⁴ tang¹* (Qi-Abducting Decoction, 65).

Remarks: Similar drug: Fruit of *Melia azedarach* L. (Japan).

Constituents: toosendanin, margosine.

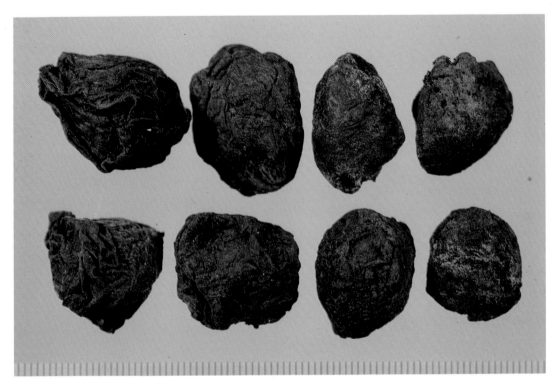

Mume Fructus: steamed (left); charred (right). (×5/3)

144 MUME FRUCTUS (PRUNI MUME FRUCTUS)

烏梅 *wu¹ mei²*. English: mume (or Japanese apricot) fruit. Japanese: *ubai.*

Alternate names: 梅實 *mei² shi²*, 熏梅 *xun¹ mei²*.

Origin: Rosaceae family. *Prunus mume* (Sieb.) Sieb. et Zucc.

Characters: The dried, shrunken fruit is oblate or irregular in shape, with a diameter of 1.5–3 cm. The exterior surface is dark brown or black, and highly wrinkled. The flesh is soft and pliable. Within is a hard, light brown pit.

Quality: Large, thick, unbroken flesh fruits with black skin, small pits, and a strong sour taste are the best.

Production areas: China (Sichuan, Zhejiang, Fujian, Hunan, and Guizhou), and Japan.

Properties and actions: Warm; sour; nontoxic. Enters the liver, lung, spleen, and large intestine channels. Promotes contraction and engenders liquid; kills worms. Used char-fried, it checks diarrhea.

Indications: Vacuity heat, vexation and thirst; enduring diarrhea and dysentery; blood in the stool and urine; profuse uterine bleeding; roundworm with abdominal pain and vomiting; hookworm infestation; oxhide xian; outcrop. Daily dosage: 3–5 g. Contraindicated in pathogen repletion. Used in *wu¹-mei² wan²* (Mume Pills, 272), *jiao¹ mei² tang¹* (Zanthoxylum and Mume Decoction, 145).

Remarks: Constituents: Organic acids. Triterpenoid: oleanolic acid. Steroid: sitosterol.

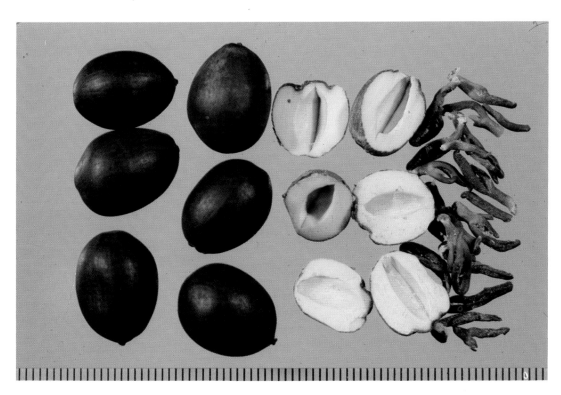

Nelumbinis Fructus (left), Semen (middle), and Embryo (right). (×5/3)

145 NELUMBINIS FRUCTUS

石蓮子 *shi² lian² zi³*. (Including Nelumbinis Semen 蓮肉 *lian² rou⁴*, (Including Nelumbinis Embryo 蓮芯 *lian² xin¹*). English: lotus fruit. Japanese: *sekirenshi*.

Alternate names: 殼蓮子 *ke² lian² zi³*.

Origin: Nymphaeaceae family. *Nelumbo nucifera* Gaertn.

Characters: This fruit is removed from the receptacle of the lotus after the plant has been subjected to frost. It is elliptical in shape and 1.5–2 cm long. Its exterior surface is smooth and dark brown, and has on it a powdery gray-white substance. At one end is the round scar left by the stigma, and at the other are residual traces of the hard fruit stalk. The brown pericarp can be removed leaving the seed (Nelumbinis Semen [*lian² rou⁴*]), which has a yellow brown seed-coat. The seed itself consists of two fat, cream-colored cotyledons with a plumule (Nelumbinis Embryo [*lian² xian¹*]), radicle, and tender leaf, which are yellow-green in color. The cotyledons are sweet to the taste, but bitter in the green parts.

Quality: Firm elliptical fruits are the best.

Production areas: China (Hunan, Hubei, Fujian, Jiangsu, Zhejiang, Jiangxi).

Properties and actions: Whole fruit: cold; bitter; nontoxic. Enters the heart and spleen channels. Clears the heart and eliminates vexation. Seed: balanced; astringent and sweet; nontoxic. Astringes the intestines; nourishes the stomach; secures essence. Plumule: cold; bitter. Resolves heat and quiets the heart.

Indications: The whole fruit treats chronic dysentery. The seed treats spleen diarrhea and enduring diarrhea, uterine bleeding, vaginal discharge, and seminal emission. The plumule treats vexation, thirst, and blood ejection. Daily dosage: 5–10 g (plumule 1.5–3 g). Used in *kai¹ jin⁴ san³* (Food Denial Powder, 158), *qing¹ xin¹ lian² zi³ yin³* (Heart-Clearing Lotus Seed Beverage, 211), *qing¹ gong¹ tang¹* (Palace-Clearing Decoction, 206).

Remarks: Constituents: Nelumbinis Embryo: Alkaloids: liensinine, isoliensinine, neferine, lotusine chloride.

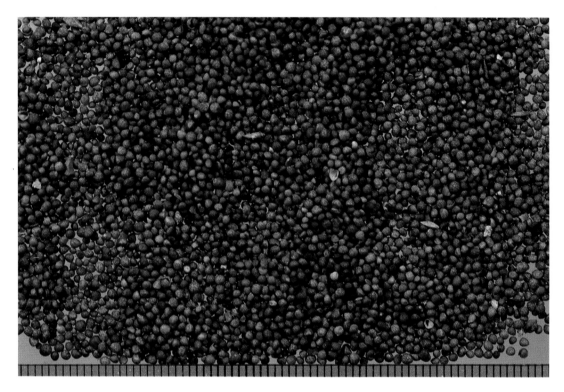

Perillae Fructus: stir-fried. (×2)

146 PERILLAE FRUCTUS

紫蘇子 zi^3 su^1 zi^3. English: perilla fruit. Japanese: *shisoshi*.

Alternate names: 黑蘇子 hei^1 su^1 zi^3, 蘇子 su^1 zi^3.

Origin: Labiatae family. *Perilla frutescens* (L.) Britt. var. *crispa* (Thunb.) Hand.-Mazz., *P. frutescens* (L.) Britt. var. *acuta* Kudo.

Characters: The dried fruit is ovate or spherical, 0.6–2 mm long, and 0.5–1.5 mm in diameter. Cultivated fruits are larger than wild ones. The exterior surface is brown, with raised reticular makings. At the more pointed end is the scar of the fruit stalk. The exocarp is thin, hard and brittle, and is easily broken. The seed is yellow-white and oily. Stir-frying turns this fruit a dark, golden brown.

Quality: Full, uniform, gray-brown fruits are the best.

Production areas: China (Hubei, Jiangsu, Henan, Shandong, Jiangxi, Zhejiang, Sichuan), and Japan.

Properties and actions: Warm; acrid; nontoxic. Enters the lung and large intestine channels. Precipitates qi, disperses phlegm, moistens the lung, and loosens the intestines. Used stir-fried, it has a milder effect, and a strong qi-moving effect. Mix-fry with honey for a strong lung-moistening effect.

Indications: Counterflow cough; phlegm dyspnea; qi stagnation; constipation. Daily dosage: 5–10 g. Contraindicated in diarrhea due to intestinal qi vacuity. Used in su^1-zi^3 $jiang^4$ qi^4 $tang^1$ (Perilla Fruit Qi-Downbearing Decoction, 258), $ding^4$ $chuan^3$ $tang^1$ (Dyspnea-Stabilizing Decoction, 71).

Remarks: Constituents: Seed: volatile oil (45.30%): linolenic acid (main).

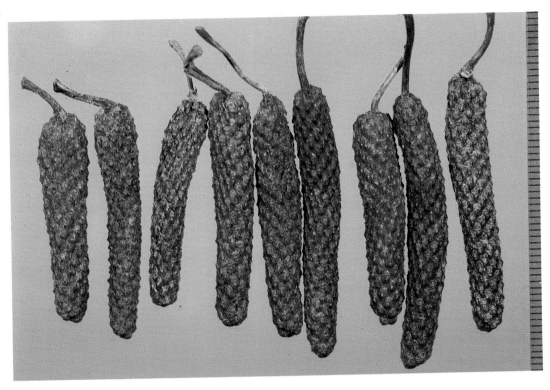

Piperis Longi Fructus. (×5/3)

147 PIPERIS LONGI FRUCTUS

蓽茇 *bi⁴ ba²*. English: long pepper, long fruit. Japanese: *hihatsu.*

Alternate names: 畢撥 *bi⁴ bo¹*, 蓽撥 *bi⁴ bo¹*.

Origin: Piperaceae family. *Piper longum* L.

Characters: This is a slightly curved cylindrical fruit spike, 2–5 cm long, and 0.5–0.8 cm in diameter, usually with the main fruit stalk missing. It is composed of many small round fruits neatly arranged to form a diagonal crisscross pattern. The individual seeds, each covered with a bract, are 1 mm in diameter. They break open with difficulty to expose a reddish interior, with white endosperm. This fruit has an unusual aroma and a hot, acrid taste.

Quality: Large, hard fruits with a strong smell are the best.

Production areas: China (Yunnan and Guangdong), Indonesia, Philippines, and Vietnam.

Properties and actions: Warm; acrid; nontoxic. Enters the spleen and kidney channels. Warms the center, dissipates cold, precipitates qi and relieves pain. Soaking in vinegar can prevent it from damaging the lung.

Indications: Frigid pain in the abdomen and region of the heart; vomiting and acid regurgitation; rumbling intestines and diarrhea; frigid dysentery; yin shan; headache; deep-source nasal congestion; toothache. Daily dosage: 1.5–3g. Contraindicated in lung-spleen repletion heat or depressed heat. Used in *er⁴ shen² wan²* (Two Spirits Pills, 81).

Remarks: Similar drug: Cubebae Fructus (fruit of *Piper cubeba* L.) .

Constituents: Alkaloids: piperine, chavicine, piperlongumine, piperlonguminine. Volatile oil (ca. 0.1%): sesamin.

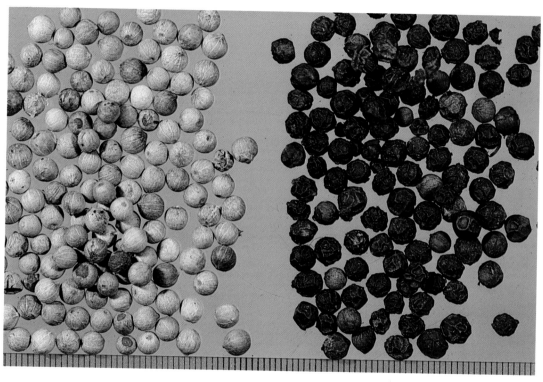

Piperis Fructus Immaturus (right) and Piperis Fructus Albicatus (left). (×5/3)

148 PIPERIS FRUCTUS

胡椒 *hu² jiao¹*. English: pepper (black and white). Japanese: *kosho.*
Alternate names: 玉椒 *yu⁴ jiao¹*, 古月 *gu³ yue⁴*.
Origin: Piperaceae family. *Piper nigrum* L.
Characters: Black pepper (Piperis Fructus Immaturus) [*hei¹ hu² jiao¹*] is the dried immature fruit. It is spherical, 3.5–6 mm in diameter, black in color, with a wrinkles forming a reticular pattern. At the head is the slightly protuberant scar of the stigma. At the base is the scar of the fruit axis. Inside the fruit is one white colored seed. When broken open, it has gives of a strong smell, and is hot and acrid to the taste. White pepper (Piperis Fructus Albicatus [*bai² hu² jiao¹*]) is the processed ripened fruit. It is slightly larger than black pepper, and has a smooth light brown surface. It is slightly flat at the top, and slightly pointed at the base, with 10–16 pale lines running between the two.
Quality: Large hard fruits with a strong flavor are best. Black pepper should be dark in color.
Production areas: China (Guangdong, Guangxi, Yunnan), Malaysia, Indonesia, Southern India, Thailand, and Vietnam.
Properties and actions: Hot; acrid. Enters the stomach and large intestine channels. Warms the center, precipitates qi, disperses phlegm, and resolves toxin.
Indications: Cold phlegm; food accumulation; frigid pain in the venter and abdomen; stomach reflux; vomiting of clear fluid; diarrhea; frigid dysentery. Daily dosage: 1.5–3 g. Contraindicated in upflaming yin vacuity fire.
Remarks: Similar plants: *Piper longum* L.; *P. cubeba* L.
Constituents: Alkaloids (5–13%): piperine (5–9%), chavicine, piperyline, piperanine, piperoleines A, B, piperidine, N-(2,4-dodecadien-landrene. Lignoids: (-)-cubebin. Fixed oil (6–13%).

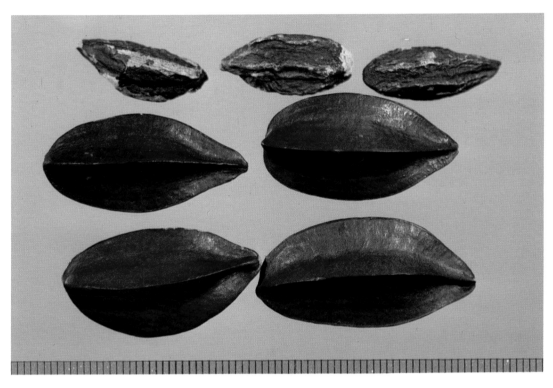

Quisqualis Fructus: stir-fried in brine. (×5/3)

149 QUISQUALIS FRUCTUS

使君子 *shi³ jun¹ zi³*. English: quisqualis (or Rangoon creeper) fruit. Japanese: *shikunshi*.
Alternate names: 使君子肉 *shi³ jun¹ zi³ rou⁴*, 使君子仁 *shi³ jun¹ zi³ ren²*.
Origin: Combretaceae family. *Quisqualis indica* L.
Characters: This fruit is elliptical in shape with pointed ends. It is about 4 cm long and 1.5–2 cm in diameter. It is dark brown in color and has 5 sharp longitudinal ridges. It is hard, and cannot be broken with the fingers. The transverse section appears as a five-pointed star shape. This fruit contains one seed, which has a purple-black seed-coat bearing longitudinal wrinkles.
Quality: Dry, large fruits with full, oleaceous fruits are the best.
Production areas: China (Sichuan, Guangdong, Guangxi, and less importantly Fujian, Jiangxi, Yunnan, and Guizhou).
Properties and actions: Warm; sweet; toxic. Enters the spleen and stomach channels. Kills worms, disperses stagnation, fortifies the spleen.
Indications: Abdominal pain due to roundworm; child gan accumulations; stagnation of milk and food in infants; abdominal distention; diarrhea. Daily dosage: 5–10 g. Tea is contraindicated when taking this drug. Used in *shi³-jun¹-zi³ wan²* (Quisqualis Pills, 246).
Remarks: Similar plants: *Quisqualis indica* L. var. *villosa* Clark.
Constituents: Volatile oil (ca. 2.5%): glycerides of palmitic acid and oleanic acid. Organic acids: malic acid, citric acid, succinic acid. Alkaloids: trigonelline. quisqualic acid, potassium quisqualate.

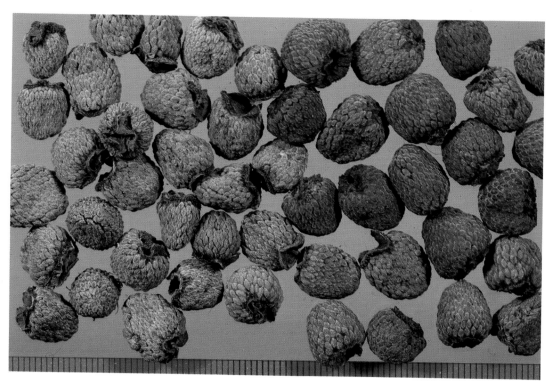

Rubi Fructus: crude (left); stir-fried (right). (×5/3)

150 RUBI FRUCTUS

覆盆子 *fu⁴ pen² zi³*. English: rubus fruit, Chinese raspberry. Japanese: *fukubonshi*.
Alternate names: 小托盤 *xiao³ tuo¹ pan²*, 覆盆 *fu⁴ pen²*.
Origin: Rosaceae family. *Rubus chingii* Hu, *R. coreanus* Miq.*
Characters: This unripened aggregate fruit is spheroid or spherical shape, 4–9 mm in diameter and 5–12 mm high. It is truncated at the bottom with a five-lobed brown involucre, covered with brown hairs. The fruit stalk is often attached, and is easily removed. The little fruits are densely covered with gray-white hairs on the their dorsal surface, and have reticular markings on the inner surface. Each contains one seed.
Quality: Large, firm, unbroken, green-gray fruits without petioles are the best.
Production areas: China (Zhejiang, Fujian, and Hubei).
Properties and actions: Warm; sweet, sour; nontoxic. Enters the liver and kidney channels. Supplements the liver and kidney, assists yang, secures essence and brightens the eyes.
Indications: Impotence; seminal emission; urinary frequency; enuresis; vacuity taxation; dark vision. Daily dosage: 5–10 g. Contraindicated in of exuberance of yang and in difficult urination. Used in *wu³ zi³ yan³ zong¹ wan²* (Five Seeds Procreation Pills, 283).
Remarks: Similar drugs: Fruit of *Rubus carchorifolius* L.f., *R. foliolosus* D. Don, and *R. idaeopsis* Focke.
Constituents: Organic acids. Saccharides.

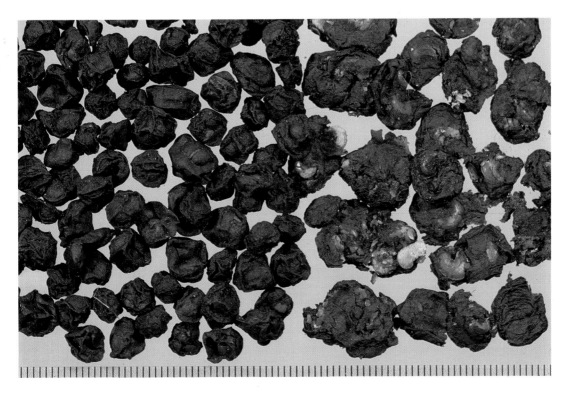

Schisandrae Fructus: unflattened (left); flattened (right). (×5/3)

151 SCHISANDRAE FRUCTUS

五味子 *wu³ wei⁴ zi³*. English: (Chinese) schisandra fruit. Japanese: *gomishi*.

Alternate name: 北五味子 *bei³ wu³ wei⁴ zi³*.

Origin: Schisandraceae family. *Schisandra chinensis* (Turcz.) Baill.

Characters: This is a ripe, spherical berry, 5-7 mm in diameter. It is usually flat and wrinkled, and irregular in shape. The pericarp is soft and fleshy, red or purple in color, and semitranslucent. It contains a white oleaceous kidney-shaped seed, roughly 4.5 mm long, and 3.5 mm wide, with a hard, yellow, shiny, seed-coat.

Quality: Large, fat, shiny, purple-red berries with marked wrinkles are the best.

Production areas: China (Liaoning, Jilin, Heilongjiang, Hebei), and the Korean Peninsula.

Properties and actions: Warm; sour; nontoxic. Enters the lung, and kidney channels. Constrains the lung; enriches the kidney; engenders liquid; constrains sweating; astringes essence. Use crude to clear vacuity fire and suppress cough. Treat with wine to enrich the kidney, or with vinegar to constrain the lung. Mix-fry with honey to moisten the lung.

Indications: Lung vacuity dyspnea and cough; thirst and dry mouth; spontaneous sweating; taxation emaciation; dream emissions; enduring dysentery or diarrhea. Daily dosage: 1.5–3g. Contraindicated in the presence of exterior pathogens and internal repletion heat. Used in *xiao³ qing¹ long² tang¹* (Minor Green-Blue Dragon Decoction, 302), *sheng¹ mai⁴ san³* (Pulse-Engendering Powder, 239), *si⁴ shen² wan²* (Four Spirits Pills, 254), *qing¹ shu³ yi⁴ qi⁴ tang¹* (Summerheat-Clearing Qi-Boosting Decoction, 210), *ling² gan¹ jiang¹ wei⁴ xin¹ xia⁴ ren² tang¹* (Poria, Licorice, Ginger, Schisandra, Pinellia, and Apricot Kernel Decoction, 163).

Remarks: Constituents: Lignoids: deoxyschizandrin (wuweizisu A, schizandrin A; 0.41%), gomisin A, B, C, D, E, F, G, H, N, O, R. Monoterpenoids and sesquiterpenoids (volatile oil, 0.3% in sarcocarp, 2% in seed): *p*=cymene, γ-terpinene; (+)-α-ylangene, δ-cadinene, cuparene. Acids: citric acid, malic acid, tartaric acid. Fixed oil (30–33% in seed).

Similar drugs: Dried fruit of *S. sphenanthera* Rehd. et Wils., and *Kadsura japonica* L. (Japan).

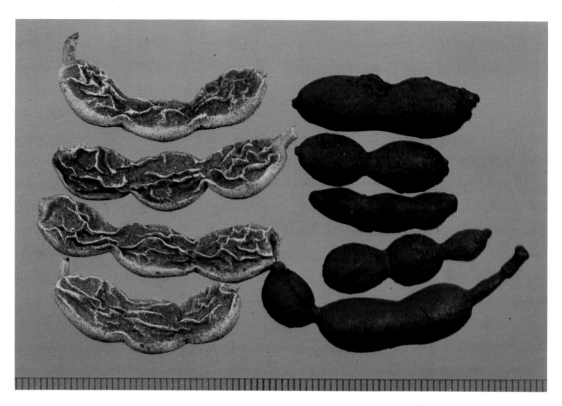

Sophorae Fructus: crude (left); charred (right). (×5/3)

152 SOPHORAE FRUCTUS

槐角 *huai² jiao³*. English: sophora (or pagoda tree, Chinese scholar tree) fruit. Japanese: *kaikaku*.

Alternate names: 槐豆 *huai² dou⁴*, 槐實 *huai² shi²*.

Origin: Leguminosae family. *Sophora japonica* L.

Characters: The dried pod is cylindrical, and twisted. It is shrunken between the seeds, creating a pearl-string appearance. It is 1–6 cm long, with a diameter of 0.6–1 cm. The exterior surface is yellow-green to dark brown, with a marked yellow coloring along the dorsal suture on one side. There is often a fruit stalk at the base. The flesh is soft and sticky, and shrinks with drying. There are 1–6 kidney-shaped seeds within, 8–10 mm long, 5–8 mm wide, and 5 mm thick. They are dark brown to black, and shiny, with an elliptical hilum on one edge, with a round micropyle to one side and a protuberant raphe to the other. The leathery seed-coat covers two green-yellow cotyledons.

Quality: Large, firm, fat, yellow-green fruits are the best.

Production areas: China (Hebei, Shandong, Jiangsu, Liaoning, and other parts of the country).

Properties and actions: Cold; bitter; nontoxic. Enters the liver and large intestine channels. Clears heat, moistens the liver, cools the blood, and staunches bleeding. Charring enhances the blood-staunching effect and ability to treat hemorrhoids. Mix-frying gives it an intestine-moistening action.

Indications: Intestinal wind bleeding; hemorrhoidal bleeding; uterine bleeding; blood strangury and dysentery; vexation and oppression in the chest and heart; wind dizziness with difficulty in keeping balance; itching genital sores. Daily dosage: 6–15 g. Contraindicated spleen-stomach vacuity cold and pregnancy. Used in *huai²-jiao³ wan²* (Sophora Fruit Pills, 126).

Remarks: Constituents: Flavonoids: rutin, genistein, sophoricoside, sophorabioside, kaempferol glycoside-C, sophoraflavonoloside.

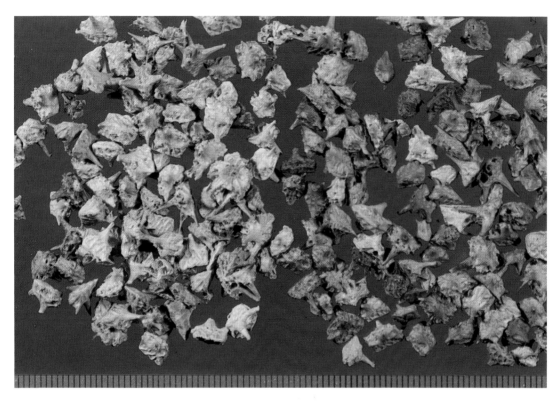

Tribuli Fructus: crude (left); stir-fried (right). (×5/3)

153 TRIBULI FRUCTUS

刺蒺藜 ci^4 ji^2 li^2. English: tribulus fruit. Japanese: *shishitsuri*.

Alternate names: 白蒺藜 bai^2 ji^2 li^2, 蒺藜子 ji^2 li^2 zi^3.

Origin: Zygophyllaceae family. *Tribulus terrestris* L.

Characters: This dried fruit is made up of 5 capsules. It is 6–10 mm in diameter, star-shaped with radiating points. Each capsule has a green-white or gray-white exterior surface, with a protuberant dorsum. It has reticular markings and a number of small thorns, including one pair of long thorns and one pair of short thorns, or the scars left after these have been mechanically removed. They are hard, and prick the fingers. The cross section is white or yellow white, and reveals the oleaceous endosperm.

Quality: Evenly sized, full, firm, white fruits are the best.

Production areas: China (Henan, Hebei, Shandong, Anhui, and less importantly Sichuan, Jiangsu, Yunnan, Shaanxi, Xinjiang, Qinghai, Jilin, Liaoning, and Shanxi).

Properties and actions: Warm; bitter, acrid; nontoxic. Enters the liver and lung channels. Dissipates wind, brightens the eyes, precipitates qi, moves the blood. Stir-fry in brine for extra kidney-supplementing action.

Indications: Headache (use crude form): generalized itchy; red swollen eyes; thoracic fullness; counterflow cough; concretions and conglomerations; mammary yong; yong and ju; scrofulous lumps. For eye diseases stir-fry till yellow. Daily dosage: 10–12 g. Contraindicated in blood and qi vacuity, and pregnancy. Used in bai^2-ji^2 san^3 (Tribulus Powder, 12), $dang^1$-gui^1 yin^3 zi^3 (Tangkuei Drink, 63).

Remarks: Constituents: Flavonoids: kaempferol-3-glucoside, kaempferol-3-rutinoside. Volatile oils. Fixed oil. Alkaloids.

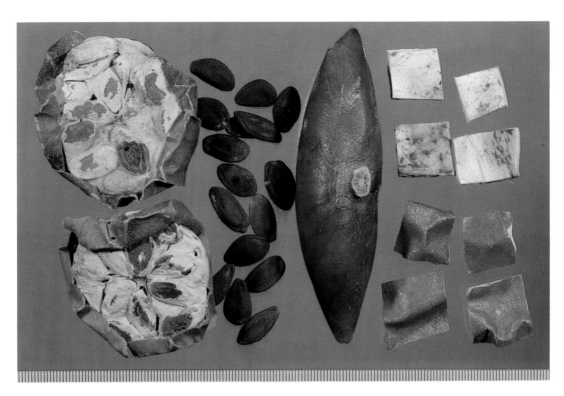

Left to right: Trichosanthis Fructus, Semen (stir-fried), and Pericarpium (×5/6)

154 TRICHOSANTHIS FRUCTUS

栝樓 *gua¹ lou²*. English: trichosanthes fruit. Japanese: *karo*.

Alternate names: 瓜蔞 *gua¹ lou²*, 栝蔞 *gua¹ lou²*.

Origin: Cucurbitaceae family. *Trichosanthes kirilowii* Maximowicz, *T. hylonoma* Hand.-Mazz.,* *T. sinopunctata* C.Y. Cheng et C.H. Yueh.*

Characters: Trichosanthis Pericarpium is shell-like in appearance, with the scar of the fruit stalk. It is usually cut into 2 or more portions. It is wrinkled and shrunken, curling at the edges. It is a yellow brown, and shiny like tanned leather. It is earth brown inside, with fibers. It is brittle, and has a mild sour taste. Trichosanthis Semen, the seed of the fruit, is flat and elliptical, 1.8 cm long, 1 cm wide, and about 4 mm thick. It is brown in color, has a round hilum, and a distinct trough running around the periphery. It is hard, and breaks open to reveal a lighter-colored interior with two fat, oily, sweet-tasting cotyledons.

Quality: Large fruits with undamaged, golden yellow pericarps and fat, oleaceous seeds are the best.

Production areas: China (Anhui, Shandong, Henan, Sichuan, and less importantly Jiangsu, Zhejiang, Hebei, Shanxi, Shaanxi, Fujian, and Guangdong).

Properties and actions: Whole fruit: cold; sweet and bitter. Enters the lung, stomach, and large intestine channels. Moistens the lung, transforms phlegm, and dissipates binds. Pericarp: cold; bitter and sweet. Clears heat, transforms phlegm, and disinhibits qi. Stir-fried it suppresses cold and transforms phlegm, while mix-fried with honey it loosens the center, clears heat, and moistens the intestines. Seed: cold; sweet. Moistens the lung, transforms phlegm, and moistens the intestines.

Indications: Whole fruit: phlegm-heat cough; thoracic bi; chest bind; pulmonary atony; coughing of blood; wasting thirst. Pericarp: phlegm-heat cough, sore throat, and blood ejection. Seed: phlegm-heat cough; constipation, and yong and ju. Daily dosage: 10–12 g. Contraindicated in spleen-stomach vacuity cold with diarrhea, and in cold phlegm or damp phlegm. Used in *gua¹-lou² zhi³-shi² tang¹* (Trichosanthes and Unripe Bitter Orange Decoction, 105).

Remarks: Constituents: Fatty oil (ca 26%). Triterpenoids: 11-oxo-cucurbit-5-ene-3β, 24, 25-triol. Allied drug: Dried fruit of *T. japonica* Regel. (Japan).

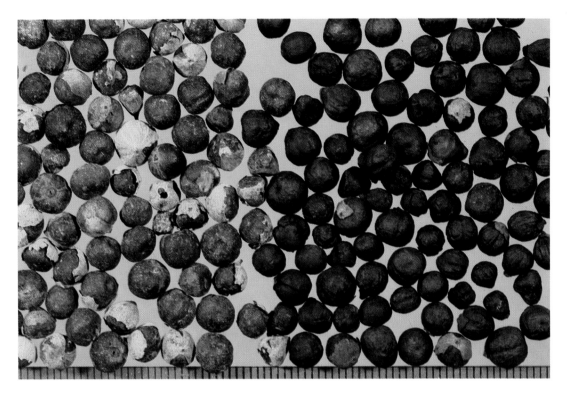

Viticis Fructus: crude (left); stir-fried (right). (×5/3)

155 VITICIS FRUCTUS

蔓荆子 *man⁴ jing¹ zi³*. English: vitex fruit. Japanese: *mankeishi*.

Alternate names: 萬荆子 *wan⁴ jing¹ zi³*, 蔓青子 *man⁴ qing¹ zi³*.

Origin: Verbenaceae family. *Vitex rotundifolia* L., *V. trifolia* L.

Characters: The dried fruit is spherical, with a diameter of 4–6 mm. The exterior surface is black, or brown-black, and slightly rough. It has four shallow equidistant longitudinal furrows. At the tip is a depression, and close to the fruit stalk is a white persistent calyx. The exocarp is thin, the mesocarp is spongy, and the endocarp is light yellow. In the center are four seed chambers, each with one seed. The fruit as a whole is light and hard, and its oiliness is seen when it is cut open. It has a bitter taste and an unusual smell.

Quality: Clean, full, dark-colored, aromatic fruits are the best.

Production areas: China (Shandong, Zhejiang, Jiangxi, and Fujian, Shandong being the biggest producer), Japan, and Korea.

Properties and actions: Slightly cold; bitter, acrid. Enters the liver, stomach, and bladder channels. Courses wind-heat; clears the head and eyes. Stir-frying reduces the pungent, dissipating quality and helps it to ascend to clear the head and eyes.

Indications: Wind-heat colds; ambilateral and hemilateral headache; toothache; reddening of the eyes; inner eye pain; clouded vision; tearing; damp bi and hypertonicity. Daily dosage: 5–10 g. Contraindicated in headache or dizziness in patterns of blood vacuity with heat, and in stomach vacuity. Used in *qiang¹-huo² bai²-zhi³ san³* (Notopterygium and Angelica Powder, 202), *yi⁴ qi⁴ cong¹ ming² tang¹* (Qi-Boosting Sharp and Bright Decoction, 317).

Remarks: Constituents: Volatile oil: α-pinene, camphene 50%, terpineol-acetylester 10%, diterpene alchohol 20%. Flavonoids: vitexicarpin.

Similar plants: *Vitex cannabifolia* Sieb. et Zucc., and *V. negundo* L.

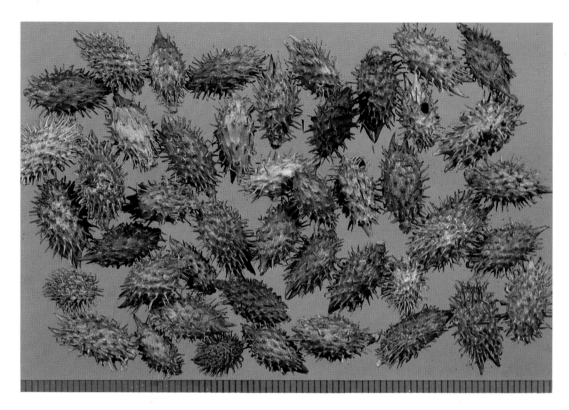

Xanthii Fructus: stir-fried. (× 5/3)

156 XANTHII FRUCTUS

蒼耳子 *cang¹ er³ zi³*. English: xanthium (or cocklebur) fruit. Japanese *sojishi.*

Alternate names: 蒼子 *cang¹ zi³*, 枲耳子 *xi³ er³ zi³*.

Origin: Compositae family. *Xanthium sibiricum* Patr. ex Widd. [*X. strumarium* L.].

Characters: The dried fruit with involucre is spindle-shaped or elliptical. It is 1–1.7 cm long, and 4–7 mm in diameter. The exterior surface is yellow-green, or brown green, and is covered with hooked thorns roughly 2 mm long. At one end are two larger and thicker thorns joined or separate. The involucre (outer skin) is tough and supple. Within are two chambers, each with one achene that is spindle-shaped, flat on one side, and black in color. The seed is light gray and comprises two cotyledons with a radicle at the tip.

Quality: Full, yellow fruits are the best.

Production areas: China (Shandong, Jiangxi, Hubei, and Jiangsu).

Properties and actions: Warm; sweet; toxic. Enters the lung and liver channels. Dissipates wind, relieves pain, dispels damp, and kills worms. The toxin is removed by stir-frying.

Indications: Wind-cold headache; deep-source nasal congestion; toothache; wind, cold, and damp bi; hypertonicity of the limbs; jie and lai. Daily dosage: 5–10 g. Contraindicated in blood vacuity, and in bi disease. Used in *cang¹-er³ san³* (Xanthium Powder, 34).

Remarks: Constituents: Xanthostrumarin (1.2%). Resin (3.3%). Fixed oil (9.2%): oleic acid, palmitic acid. Alkaloid.

Allied drug: Fruit of *Xanthium canadense* Mill. (Japan).

Similar plants: *X. pennsylvanicum* Wallr.

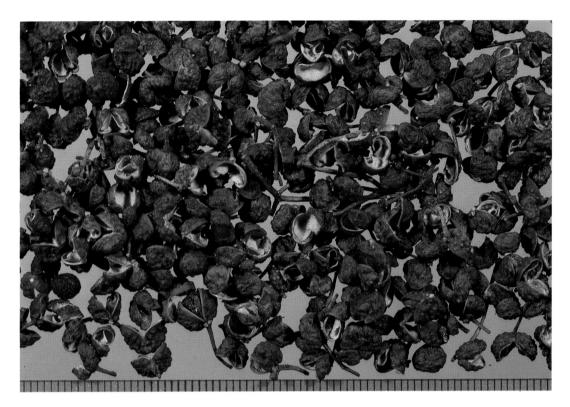

Zanthoxyli Fructus: stir-fried. (×5/3)

157 ZANTHOXYLI FRUCTUS

花椒 *hua¹ jiao¹*. English: zanthoxylum (xanthoxylum) fruit. Japanese: *kasho.*

Alternate names: 紅椒 *hong² jiao¹*, 蜀椒 *shu³ jiao¹*.

Origin: Rutaceae family. *Zanthoxylum bungeanum* Maxim., *Z. schinifolium* Sieb. et Zucc.*

Characters: The fruit of *Zanthoxylum bungeanum* is a spherical, 3.5–4 mm in diameter. The pericarp is split open on the ventral side into two hemispherical portions, which remain joined at the base. The exterior surface is a rusty red in color, and rough and warty in texture. At the tip are the remains of the stigma, and at the base is a small fruit stalk, and 1–2 undeveloped carpels.

Quality: Clean, bright red, lustrous, thin-skinned, uniform fruits are the best.

Production areas: China (Hebei, Shanxi, Shaanxi, Gansu, Henan).

Properties and actions: Warm; acrid; toxic. Enters the spleen, lung, and kidney channels. Warms the center and dissipates cold; eliminates damp, relieves pain, kills worms, and resolves fish toxin.

Indications: Food accumulation; frigid pain in the abdomen and heart; vomiting; belching and hiccough; cough and qi counterflow; wind, cold, and damp bi; diarrhea; dysenteric disease; shan pain; toothache; roundworm and pinworm infestation; genital itch; jie. Daily dosage: 1.5–5 g. Contraindicated in effulgent yin vacuity fire. Used in *da⁴ jian⁴ zhong¹ tang¹* (Major Center-Fortifying Decoction, 51), *jiao¹ mei² tang¹* (Zanthoxylum and Mume Decoction, 145), *wu¹-mei² wan²* (Mume Pills, 272).

Remarks: Constituents: *Z. bungeanum:* Monoterpenoids, alkanes, and arenes (volatile oil, 0.7–9%): α-pinene, sabinene, 1,8-cineole, limonene, myrcene.
Alkaloids: kokusaginine, skimmianine, haplopine. Coumarins: herniarin.

Z. schinifolium: Phenylpropanoids (volatile oil, 4–9%): methylchavicol (ca. 90%), anisaldehyde, bennoic acid. Coumarins: bergapten.

Allied drug: Dried fuit of *Z. piperitum* DC. (Japan).

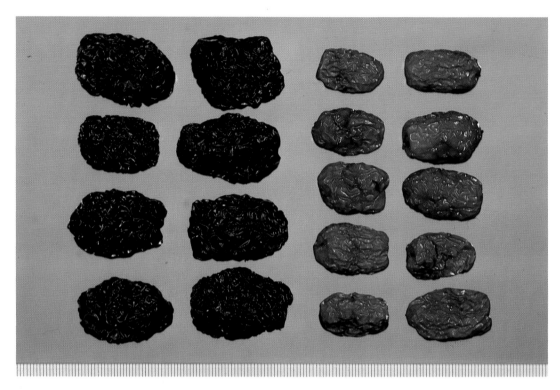

Zizyphi Fructus: Black jujube (left) and red jujube (right). (×7/8)

158 ZIZYPHI FRUCTUS

大棗 *da⁴ zao³*. English: jujube, Chinese date. Japanese: *taiso*.

Alternate names: 紅棗 *hong² zao³*, 棗 *zao³*.

Origin: Rhamnaceae family. *Zizyphus jujuba* Miller var. *inermis* (Bge.) Rehd. [=*Z. vulgaris* Lamarck var. *inermis* Bge.].

Characters: This fruit is ovate or elliptical, 2–3 cm in length and 1–2 cm in diameter. The red ones (Zizyphi Fructus Rubrus [*hong² zao³*]), the type usually used in medicine, are rust red with large wrinkles. The black ones (Zizyphi Fructus Ater [*hei¹ zao³*]), which are usually only used in cooking, are blackish red with fine wrinkles. Both types have a luster. There are depressions at each end, usually with the remains of the style at one end, and the fruit stalk at the other. The exocarp is thick and leathery. The mesocarp is dark gray-brown, fat, sticky, and spongy. The endocarp is hard and spindle-shaped, and sharply pointed at one end. Within are two chambers each containing a flat, oveate seed.

Quality: Fruits with thick, sweet flesh and small seeds are the best.

Production areas: China (Hebei, Henan, Shandong, Sichuan, Guizhou).

Properties and actions: Warm; sweet; nontoxic. Enters the spleen and stomach channels. Supplements the spleen and harmonizes the stomach; reinforces qi and engenders liquids; regulates construction-defense; resolves drug toxins.

Indications: Stomach vacuity; low food intake; thin stool due to spleen vacuity; insufficiency of qi, blood and fluids; construction-defense disharmony; palpitations and racing of the heart; visceral agitation in women. Daily dosage: 10–15 g. Contraindicated in phlegm-heat. Used in *shi² zao³ tang¹* (Ten Jujubes Decoction, 245), *gan¹ mai⁴ da⁴-zao³ tang¹* (Licorice, Wheat, and Jujube Decoction, 97), *xiao³ jian⁴ zhong¹ tang¹* (Minor Center-Fortifying Decoction, 300).

Remarks: Constituents: Triterpenoids: oleanolic acid, maslinic acid; (saponins) zizyphus saponins I, II, III, jujuboside. Nucleotides: cyclic AMP, cyclic GMP. Saccharides: zizyphus-arabinan, zizyphus-pectin A.

Similar drug: Dried fruit of *Z. mauritiana* Lam.

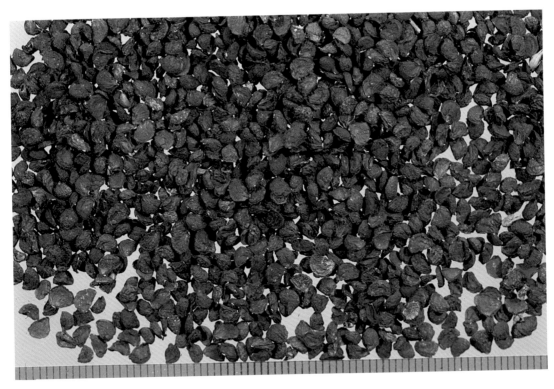

Allii Tuberosi Semen. (×5/3)

159 ALLII TUBEROSI SEMEN

韭子 *jiu³ zi³*. English: Chinese leek seed. Japanese: *kyushi, kyusaishi.*

Alternate names: 韭菜仁 *jiu³ cai⁴ ren²*, 韭菜子 *jiu³ cai⁴ zi³.*

Origin: Liliaceae family. *Allium tuberosum* Rottler.

Characters: This seed is triangular or irregularly shaped, 3–4 mm long. Its exterior is black with reticular wrinkles. One end is slighty pointed while the other end is dull.

Quality: Dry, black seeds without pericarp are the best.

Production areas: China (all provinces, with production highest in Hebei, Shanxi, Jilin, Jiangsu, Shandong, Anhui, and Henan).

Properties and actions: Warm; salty, acrid; nontoxic. Enters the liver channel. Supplements the liver and kidney, warms lumbus and knees, strengthens yang and secures essence. Has a more moderate effect when scorch-fried.

Indications: Impotence; dream emissions; frequent urination; enuresis; limp, aching, cold lumbus and knees; diarrhea; vaginal discharge; turbid strangury. Daily dosage: 5–10 g. Contraindicated in effulgent yin vacuity fire. Used in *mi⁴ jing¹ wan²* (Essence-Containing Pills, 184).

Remarks: Constituents: Alkaloids. Saponins.

Similar plant: *Allium fistulosum* L.

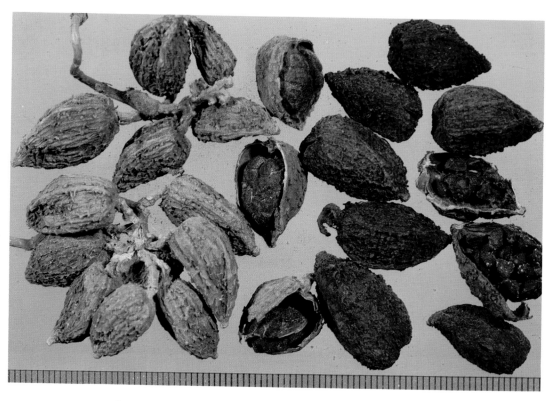

Amomi Semen: crude (left); stir-fried in ginger (right). (×5/3)

160 AMOMI SEMEN

砂仁 *sha¹ ren²*. English: amomun seed. Japanese: *shajin (shanin), shukusha*.
Alternate names: 縮砂 *suo¹ sha¹*, 縮砂仁 *suo¹ sha¹ ren²*.
Origin: Zingiberaceae family. *Amomum villosum* Lour., *A. xanthioides* Wall.
Characters: The dried fruit is ovate or elliptical, 1–1.5 cm long, and 0.8–1 cm in diameter. The pericarp is brown, with soft thorns. Within are three chambers, each containing 12–18 seeds formed together in a mass. The seeds are about 5 mm long, and 3 mm in diameter, many-cornered in shape, and brown in color. They are hard, and when bitten open, they release aroma and pungent flavor.
Quality: Large, full seeds with with a strong smell are the best.
Production areas: *Amomum villosum:* China (Guangdong, Guangxi), Burma, Vietnam, Thailand, and Indonesia. *A. xanthioides:* China (Guangdong).
Properties and actions: Warm; acrid; nontoxic. Enters the spleen and stomach channels. Moves qi and harmonizes the center, harmonizes stomach, and arouses the spleen. Stir-fry with brine to treat yin vacuity. Steam with the juice of Rehmanniae Radix Conquita (*shou² di⁴ huang²*) to rectify kidney qi.
Indications: Abdominal pain; glomus and distention; torpid stomach; food stagnation; esophageal constriction; vomiting; cold diarrhea and frigid dysentery; pregnancy fetus. Stir-fry with ginger juice for glomus and distention, and for vomiting. Daily dosage: 1.5–3 g. Contraindicated in yin vacuity with heat. Used in *xiang¹ sha¹ liu⁴ jun¹ zi³ tang¹* (Cyperus and Amomum Six Gentlemen Decoction, 290), *xiang¹ sha¹ zhi³ zhu² wan²* (Saussurea, Amomum, Unripe Bitter Orange, and Atractylodes Ovata Pills, 293).
Remarks: Constituents: *A. xanthioides:* Monoterpenoids and sesquiterpenoids (volatile oil 1.5–3.5%): (+)-bornylacetate (48.9%), (+) camphor (23%), camphene (8.4%), limonene (7.3%), β-pinene (5.9%), α-pinene (1.6%). Flavonoids: liquiritin. Phenylpopanoids: glucovanillic acid. *A. villosum:* Volatile oils: borneol, bornylacetate, camphor, limonene.
Similar drugs: Fruit of *Alpinia japonica* Miquel (Japan) and *A. speciosa* K. Schum. (Taiwan).

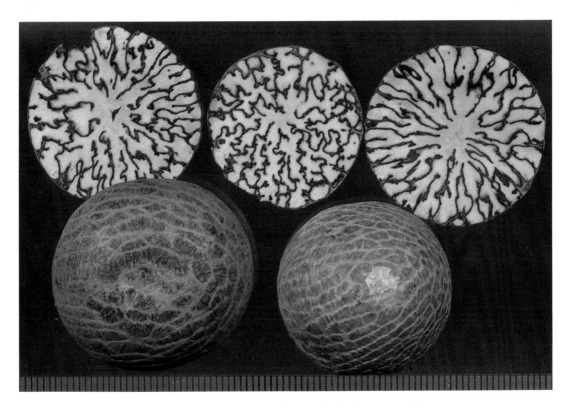

Arecae Semen: crude (below); sliced (above). (×5/3)

161 ARECAE SEMEN

檳榔 *bin¹ lang².* English: areca (or betel) nut. Japanese: *binro.*

Alternate name: 檳榔子 *bin¹ lang² zi³.*

Origin: Palmae family. *Areca catechu* L.

Characters: This seed is spheroid or conical in shape, 4 cm in length, and 3 cm in diameter at the base. The base bears a slight depression in which there is a small embryo and large scar-like hilum. The exterior surface is a pale red-brown, with a distinct reticular formation of shallow, light-colored grooves. Sometimes the silvery, brittle endocarp and fibrous mesocarp are partly exposed. The fruit is hard. The decocting pieces are 1–2 mm slices, revealing a marble-patterned cross section created by the maroon of the seed-coat folds amid the endosperm. The center of the seed is often hollow.

Quality: Large, hard, unbroken fruits are the best.

Production areas: China (Guangdong, Guangxi, Fujian, and Taiwan), and Indonesia, India, Sri Lanka, and Philippines.

Properties and actions: Warm; bitter, acrid; nontoxic. Enters the spleen, stomach, and large intestine channels. Kills worms, breaks accumulation, precipitates qi, and moves water. Use crude to kill worms. Scorch-fry for a stronger dispersing and abducting action.

Indications: Worm accumulation; food stagnation; distention pain in the venter and abdomen; diarrhea with rectal heaviness; malarial disease; water swelling; leg qi; phlegm pi; concretions and conglomerations. Char-fry to treat malarial disease. Daily dosage: 5–10 g. Contraindicated in qi vacuity fall and the absence of food stagnation. Used in *mu⁴-xiang¹ bin¹-lang² wan²* (Saussurea and Areca Pills, 190), *fei² er² wan²* (Chubby Child Pills, 86), *shu¹ zao² yin³ zi³* (Coursing and Piercing Beverage, 250), *jie² nüe⁴ qi³ bao³ yin³* (Malaria-Terminating Seven-Jewel Beverage, 147).

Remarks: Constituents: Alkaloids (0.3–0.7%): arecoline (0.1–0.5%), arecaidine, guvacine, isoguvacine, homoarecoline, arecaine, arecolidine. Tannoids: procyanidins A-1, B-1 (main), B-2, B-7, C-3. Fixed oil (14-18%): glycerides of lauric acid (20–50%).

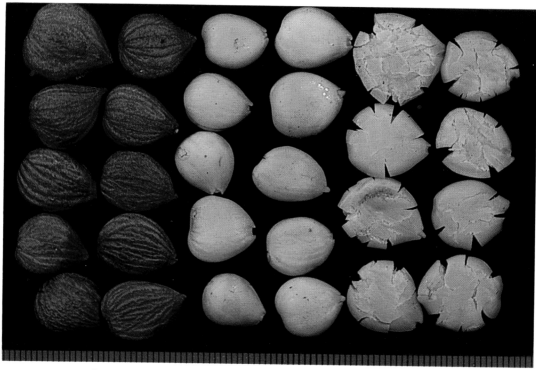

Armeniacae Semen: crude (left); stir-fried with seed-coat removed (middle); crushed (right). (×5/3)

162 ARMENIACAE SEMEN (PRUNI ARMENIACAE SEMEN)

杏仁 *xing⁴ ren²*. English: apricot kernel. Japanese: *kyonin*.

Alternate names: 杏核仁 *xing⁴ he² ren²*, 苦杏仁 *ku³ xing⁴ ren²*.

Origin: Rosaceae family. *Prunus armeniaca* L., *P. armeniaca* L. var. *ansu* Maxim.

Characters: This is a flat, heart-shaped seed, 1–1.7 cm long, 1.2 cm wide, and 0.5–0.8 cm thick. The top is pointed and the base is rounded. The seed-coat is light red-brown, with irregular longitudinal wrinkles. The seed has a micropyle at its tip. The raphe runs along the edge of the seed from the hilum to the chalaza. The thin seed-coat covers two broad, thin, oleaceous, yellow-white cotyledons, between which the radicle is located at the tip.

Quality: Large, full seeds, with white cotyledons are the best.

Production areas: China (Manchuria, Huabei).

Properties and actions: Warm; bitter; toxic. Enters the lung and large intestine channels. Dispels phlegm and suppresses cough; calms dyspnea and lubricates the intestines. Steaming or stir-frying reduces toxicty. Apricot kernel frost (Armeniacae Seminis Pulvis [*xing⁴ ren² shuang¹*]), i.e., the kernels crushed with the oil removed, moves the connecting vessels, diffuses the lung, dispels phlegm, and settles dyspnea.

Indications: External contraction cough; dyspnea and fullness; throat bi; constipation due to dryness intestines. Daily dosage: 5–10 g. Contraindicated in yin vacuity cough. Used in *ma² xing⁴ gan¹ shi² tang¹* (Ephedra, Apricot Kernel, Licorice, and Gypsum Decoction, 176), *ma²-huang² tang¹* (Ephedra Decoction, 175), *da⁴ qing¹ long² tang¹* (Major Green-Blue Dragon Decoction, 53), *gui⁴-zhi¹ jia¹ hou⁴-po⁴ xing⁴-ren² tang¹* (Cinnamon Twig Decoction Plus Magnolia and Apricot Kernel, 110), *xing⁴ su¹ san³* (Apricot Kernel and Perilla Powder, 306), *ren²-shen¹ ge²-jie⁴ san³* (Ginseng and Gecko Powder, 215), *san¹ ren² tang¹* (Three Kernels Decoction, 220), *sang¹ ju² yin³* (Mulberry Leaf and Chrysanthemum Beverage, 225).

Remarks: Constituents: Cyanophore glycosides (3–5%): amygdalin, neoamygdalin. Fixed oil (apricot kernel oil, 30–50%): olein. Enzymes: emulsin (amygdalase, prunase).

Similar plants: *P. sibirica* L.; *P. mandshurica* Koehne.

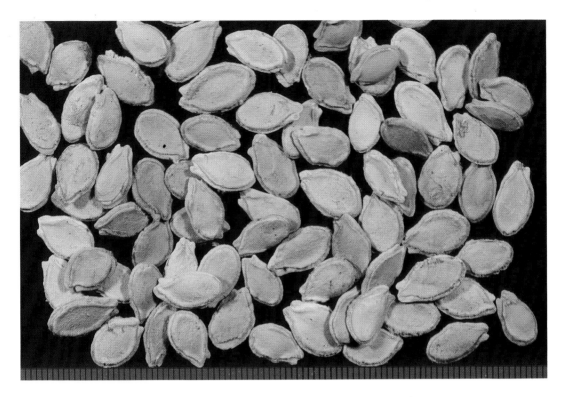

Benincasae Semen. (×5/3)

163 BENINCASAE SEMEN

冬瓜子 *dong¹ gua¹ zi³*. English: wax (or white) gourd seed. Japanese: *tokashi*.

Alternate names: 瓜子 *gua¹ zi³*, 冬瓜仁 *dong¹ gua¹ ren²*.

Origin: Cucurbitaceae family. *Benincasa cerifera* Savi [= *B. hispida* (Thunb.) Cogn.].

Characters: The dried seed is flat, and ovate or elliptical, about 1 cm long and 6 mm wide. The exterior surface is a brownish white, sometimes with fissures. One end is pointed and the other blunt, and at the pointed end are two small protuberances, the smaller one being the hilum, and the larger one bearing the micropyle. The margin is smooth or has a protruding rim on either side. When the seed-coat is peeled off, the white interior of the seed can be seen.

Quality: The best quality seeds are clean, large, and white.

Production areas: China (most parts of the country, with production highest in Sichuan, Zhejiang, Jiangsu, Henan, Hebei, Anhui).

Properties and actions: Cool; sweet; nontoxic. Enters the liver channels. Moistens the lung; transforms phlegm; disperses yong, and disinhibits water. Stir-fry with bran to harmonize the stomach.

Indications: Phlegm-heat cough; pulmonary and intestinal yong; strangury; water swelling; leg qi; hemorrhoids; drinker's nose. Daily dosage: 3–12 g. Contraindicated in diarrhea in enduring disease. Used in *da⁴-huang² mu³-dan¹-pi² tang¹* (Rhubarb and Moutan Decoction, 50), *qian¹ jin¹ wei³ jing¹ tang¹* (Thousand Gold Pieces Phragmites Decoction, 200).

Remarks: Similar plants: *Benincasa cerifera* Savi forma *emarginata* K. Kimura et Sugiyama. Constituents: Saponins (10%). Fixed oil.

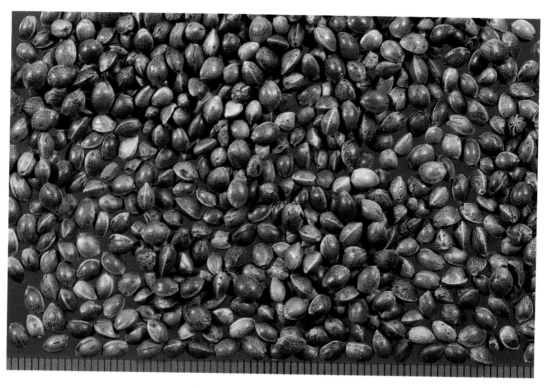

Cannabis Semen. (×5/3)

164 CANNABIS SEMEN

火麻仁 *huo³ ma² ren²*. English: cannabis (or hemp) seed. Japanese: *kamanin, mashinin*.
Alternate names: 大麻仁 *da⁴ ma² ren²*, 麻子仁 *ma² zi³ ren²*.
Origin: Moraceae family. *Cannabis sativa* L.
Characters: The dried seed is flat and ovate, 4–5 mm long, and 3–4 mm thick. The exterior surface is smooth, and gray-green or gray-yellow in color, with fine white, brown, or black markings. The marginal ridge on both sides is paler in color. One end is dull, while the other end has a depression where the fruit stalk was attached. The exocarp is extremely thin, and the endocarp is hard and brittle. The green seed-coat is often stuck to the mesocarp, and is hard to remove. The endosperm is gray white, and very thin. There are two thick, oleaceaous cotyledons.
Quality: Fat, yellowish seeds without shells are the best.
Production areas: China (Heilongjiang, Liaoning, Jilin, Sichuan, Gansu, Yunnan, Jiangsu, Zhejiang).
Properties and actions: Balanced; sweet; nontoxic. Enters the spleen, stomach, and large intestine channels. Moistens dryness; lubricates the intestine; frees strangury; quickens the blood.
Indications: Constipation due to intestinal dryness; wasting thirst; heat strangury; wind bi; dysenteric disease; menstrual irregularities; jie and xian. Daily dosage: 10–15 g. Contraindicated in diarrhea. Used in *ma²-zi³-ren² wan²* (Cannabis Pills, 178), *zhi⁴-gan¹-cao³ tang¹* (Honey-Fried Licorice Decoction, 345), *run⁴ chang² tang¹* (Intestine-Moistening Decoction, 218).
Remarks: Constituents: Fixed oil (ca. 30%): glycerides of linoleic acid (53%), linolenic acid (25%), oleic acid (12%). Amines: muscarine, trigonelline, choline. Cannabinoids.
Similar plant: *Cannabis sativa* L. var. *indica* Lamark (India).

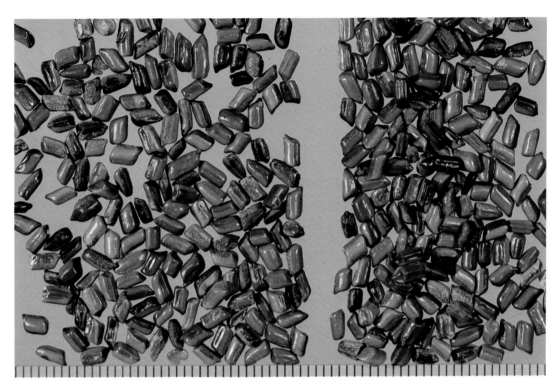

Cassiae Torae Semen: crude (left); stir-fried (right). (×2)

165 CASSIAE TORAE SEMEN

决明子 *jue² ming² zi³*. English: fetid cassia seed. Japanese: *ketsumeishi*.
Alternate name: 馬蹄决明 *ma³ ti² jue² ming²*.
Origin: Leguminosae family. *Cassia tora* L.
Characters: The dried seed is rhomboid in shape, like a horse's hoof, pointed at one end and truncated at the other. It is 5–8 mm long, and 2.5–3 mm wide. The exterior surface is yellowish or greenish brown, smooth and shiny, with a protuberant brown ridge line on each face that has an indented paler line either side of it. From here the seed cracks open when it swells after soaking in water. This seed is hard, and not easily broken. The cross section shows the seed-coat to be thin, the endosperm to be gray-white or pale yellow, the cotyledons to be yellow or brown, heavily pleated and wrinkled.
Quality: Fat, evenly sized, yellow-brown seeds are the best.
Production areas: China (all parts, with principal production in Anhui, Guangxi, Sichuan, Zhejiang, and Guangdong).
Properties and actions: Cool; bitter, sweet; nontoxic. Enters the liver and kidney channels. Clears liver fire, brightens the eyes, disinhibits water, and frees the stool. Stir-fry to disinhibit urine and dispel summerheat.
Indications: Wind-heat reddening of the eyes; clear-eye blindness; night blindness; hypertension; hepatitis; ascites due to cirrhosis; habitual constipation. Daily dosage: 5–10 g. Contraindicated in diarrhea. Used in *jue²-ming²-zi³ san³* (Cassia Powder, 157).
Remarks: Allied drug: Seed of *C. obtusifolia* L. (Japan).
Similar plants: *C. occdentalis* L.; *C. torosa* Cav.; *C. sophera* L.
Constituents: Anthraquinones: free (0.0–0.3%), bound (0.84–1.3%): chrysophanol, physicion, obtusin, aurantio-obtusin, emodin, aloe-emodin, rhein and their glucosides, emodinanthrone.
Naphthalenes: rubrofusarin, nor-rubrofusarin. Fixed oil (4.6–5.8%): glycerides of palmitic acid.

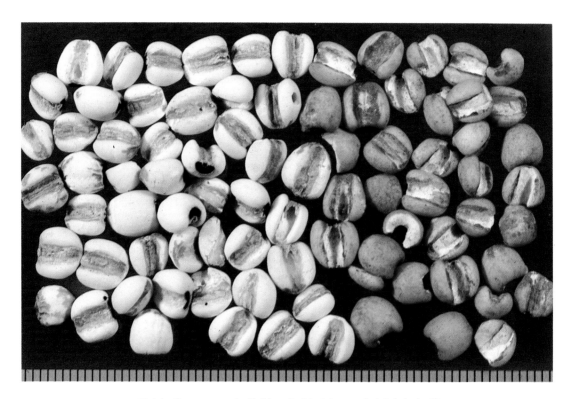

Coicis Semen: crude (left); stir-fried in earth (right). (×2)

166 COICIS SEMEN

薏苡仁 *yi⁴ yi³ ren²*. English: coix (or Job's tears) seed. Japanese: *yokuinin*.
Alternate names: 苡仁米 *yi³ ren² mi³*, 薏米仁 *yi⁴ mi³ ren²*.
Origin: Gramineae family. *Coix lachryma-jobi* var. *ma-yuen* (Roman.) Stapf [= *C. ma-yuen* Roman.].
Characters: This is a spheroid or ovate seed with a wide, flat base, and a dull rounded tip. It is 5–7 mm long and 3–5 mm thick. It is white or yellow-white in color, smooth, sometimes with longitudinal markings. There is a broad, deep longitudinal groove, whose surface is brown and rough. At the base is a depression with a dark brown spot. This seed is hard, and when broken open, the white, farinaceous inside can be seen.
Quality: Unbroken, large, fat, white seeds are the best.
Production areas: China (most parts of the country, and notably Fujian, Hebei, and Liaoning).
Properties and actions: Cold; sweet, bland; nontoxic. Enters the spleen, lung, and kidney channels. Fortifies the spleen and supplements the lung; clears heat and disinhibits damp. Use crude to disinhibit water-damp, and stir-fried with earth for better spleen-fortifying and diarrhea-checking action.
Indications: Diarrhea; damp bi; hypertonicity of the limbs; water swelling; leg qi; pulmonary atony and yong; intestinal yong; turbid strangury; vaginal discharge. Daily dosage: 10–30 g. Use with care in pregnancy. Used in *yi⁴-yi³-ren² tang¹* (Coix Decoction, 319), *yi⁴-yi³ fu⁴-zi³ bai⁴-jiang⁴ san³* (Coix, Aconite, and Baijiangcao Powder, 318), *qian¹ jin¹ wei³ jing¹ tang¹* (Thousand Gold Pieces Phragmites Decoction, 200), *ma² xing⁴ yi⁴ gan¹ tang¹* (Ephedra, Apricot Kernel, Coix, and Licorice Decoction, 177), *san¹ ren² tang¹* (Three Kernels Decoction, 220).
Remarks: Constituents: Fatty acids: coixenolide (0–0.25%). Fixed oil (5–7%). Proteins (18%): coicin. Saccharides: coixans A, B, C, glycans CA-1, CA-2; starch (52%). Steroids: feruloyl stigmasterol, feruloyl campesterol.
Similar drug: Dried fruit of *Coix lachryma-jobi* L.

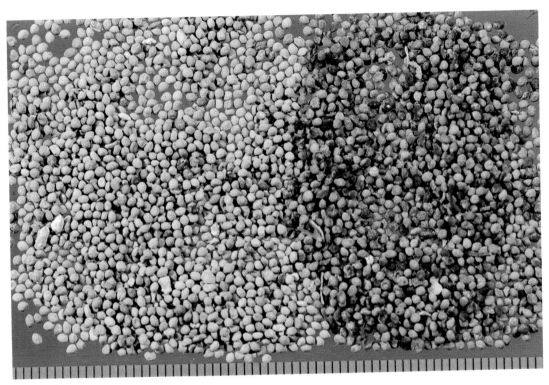

Cuscutae Semen: crude (left); steamed (right). (×2)

167 CUSCUTAE SEMEN

菟絲子 *tu⁴ si¹ zi³*. English: cuscuta (or Chinese dodder) seed. Japanese: *toshishi*.

Alternate names: 吐絲子 *tu⁴ si¹ zi³*, 兎絲子 *tu⁴ si¹ zi³*.

Origin: Convolvulaceae family. *Cuscuta chinensis* Lam.

Characters: This seed is spheroid or ovate, often with a depression on each side. It is 1.5 mm long and 1 mm thick, and has a light reddish brown seed-coat. It is hard and does not easily break. It is often comes in the form of cakes made by crushing and steaming the seeds.

Quality: Clean, fat seeds are the best.

Production areas: China (Liaoning, Jilin, Hebei, Henan, Shandong, Shanxi, Jiangsu).

Properties and actions: Balanced; acrid, sweet; nontoxic. Enters the liver and kidney channels. Supplements the kidney and liver, boosts essence and brightens the eyes. Stir-fry with brine to supplement the kidney, with wine to warm the flesh, and with wine and rice to treat diarrhea.

Indications: Aching pain in the lumbus and knees; seminal emission; wasting thirst; dribble after voiding; dark vision. Daily dosage: 10–12 g. Contraindicated in pregnancy, uterine bleeding, prolonged erection, bound stool, fire in the kidney, and fire stirring from yin vacuity. Used in *fu² tu⁴ wan²* (Poria and Cuscuta Pills, 91).

Remarks: Constituents: Resin glycosides. Saccharides. Vitamin A.

Similar plants: *C. japonica* Choisy, *C. maritima* Mak., *C. australis* R. Br.

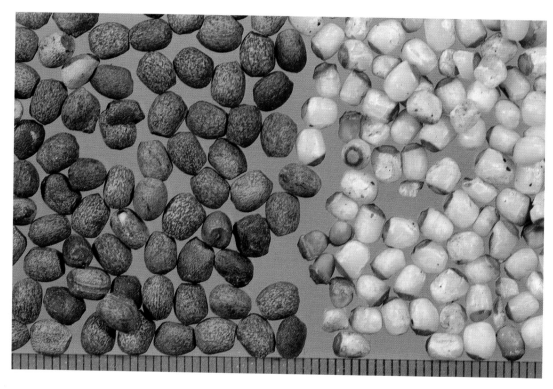

Euphorbiae Lathyridis Semen: crude (left); stir-fried (right). (× 2)

168 EUPHORBIAE LATHYRIDIS SEMEN

千金子 *qian¹ jin¹ zi³*. English: caper spurge (or mole plant) seed. Japanese: *senkinshi*.
Alternate name: 續隨子 *xu⁴ sui² zi³*.

Origin: Euphorbiaceae family. *Euphorbia lathyris* L.

Characters: This seed is elliptical, 5–6 mm long, and 3–4 mm in diameter. The exterior surface is mid-brown. One end is rounded, while the other has a small pointed tip, or the round scar left behind if it has been knocked off. The raphe is distinct. The seed-coat can be removed, to reveal a brittle oleaceous seed that is gray-white in color and darker at one end.

Quality: Clean large, full, firm seeds are the best.

Production areas: China (Hebei, Henan, Zhejiang, and less importantly Sichuan, Liaoning, Jilin, Hunan, Guangxi).

Properties and actions: Warm; acrid; toxic. Enters the lung, stomach, and bladder channels. Expels water and disperses swelling; breaks concretions and kills worms. Remove oil for milder action.

Indications: Water swelling and distention; phlegm-rheum; food stagnation; stomach pain; concretions and gatherings; menstrual block; jie, xian, and sores; insect bites; warts. Daily dosage: 0.3–1.5 g. Contraindicated in insufficiency of center qi, spleen vacuity diarrhea, and pregnancy. Used in *xu⁴-sui²-zi³ wan²* (Caper Spurge Pills, 310).

Remarks: Similar plant: *Euphorbia amygdaloides* L.

Constituents: Fixed oil (40–46%): epoxylathyrol, ingenol-3-hexadecanoate. Coumarins: esculetin, euphorbetin.

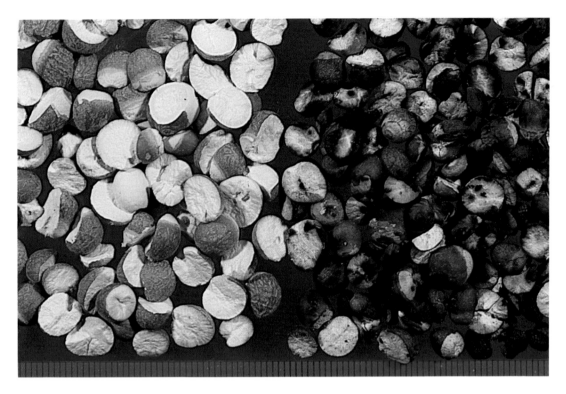

Euryales Semen: crude (left); stir-fried (right). (×5/3)

169 EURYALES SEMEN

芡實 *qian⁴ shi²*. English: euryale seed. Japanese: *kenjitsu*.

Alternate names: 刀芡 *dao¹ qian⁴*. 蘇芡 *su¹ qian⁴*.

Origin: Nymphaeaceae family. *Euryale ferox* Salisb.

Characters: The dry seed is spherical, with a diameter of 6 mm. A third of the length from one end is white in color, with a round depression, while the rest is reddish brown. The exterior surface is smooth with irregular wrinkles. This seed is dry and brittle, breaking open to reveal an uneven, farinaceous, white fracture. It has a faint, unoffensive odor.

Quality: Clean, full, farinaceous seeds are the best.

Production areas: China (Jiangsu, Hunan, Hubei, Shandong, and less importantly in Fujian, Hebei, Henan, Jiangxi, Zhejiang, and Sichuan).

Properties and actions: Balanced; sweet, astringent; nontoxic. Enters the spleen and kidney channels. Secures the kidney and astringes essence; supplements the spleen and checks diarrhea. Stir-frying without additives enhances the sweet and astringent properties. Stir-frying in bran gives it a distinct spleen-fortifying effect.

Indications: Seminal emission; turbid strangury; vaginal discharge; urinary incontinence; diarrhea. Daily dosage: 5–10 g. Contraindicated in inhibited stool and urine. Used in *jin¹ suo³ gu⁴ jing¹ wan²* (Golden Lock Essence-Securing Pills, 149).

Remarks: Constituents: starch, catalose, vitamin B₂.

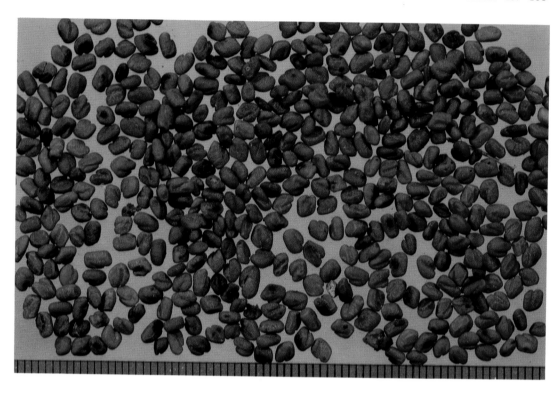

Foeni-Graeci Semen, stir-fried. (× 2)

170 FOENI-GRAECI SEMEN (TRIGONELLAE FOENI-GRAECI SEMEN)

胡蘆巴 *hu² lu² ba¹*. English: fenugreek seed. Japanese: *koroha*.

Origin: Leguminosae family. *Trigonella foenum-graecum* L.

Characters: This seed is rhomboid or rectangular in shape, 3–5 mm long, 2–3 mm wide, and 2 mm thick. The exterior surface is yellow-brown or red-brown, and smooth. The two faces each have a diagonal furrow that meets the other at the hilum and micropyle. This seed is hard, and is not easily broken. The seed-coat is thin. The longitudinal section shows a circle of endosperm, which turns sticky after soaking in water. The cotyledons are slightly asymmetrical, and pale yellow in color. The radicle is long, fat, and crooked. On the transverse section, the endosperm is seen to account for the larger part of the total area, while the two cotyledons appear round, with the radicle at one end.

Quality: The best seeds are large, full, and without impurities.

Production areas: India, Southern Europe, North Africa, and China (cultivated in Henan, Anhui, and Sichuan).

Properties and actions: Warm; bitter; nontoxic. Enters the kidney and liver channels. Supplements kidney yang, and dispels cold-damp. Soak in wine to warm the kidney. Steam to increase the enriching effect. Stir-fry to invigorate original yang.

Indications: Cold shan; distention and fullness in the abdomen and lateral costal region; cold-damp leg qi; aching lumbus due to kidney vacuity; impotence. Daily dosage: 3–5 g. Contraindicated in effulgent yin vacuity fire. Used in *hu²-lu²-ba¹ san³* (Fenugreek Powder, 121).

Remarks: Constituents: Mucilage (ca. 28%). Aromatic Fixed oil (6%). Proteins (ca. 22%).

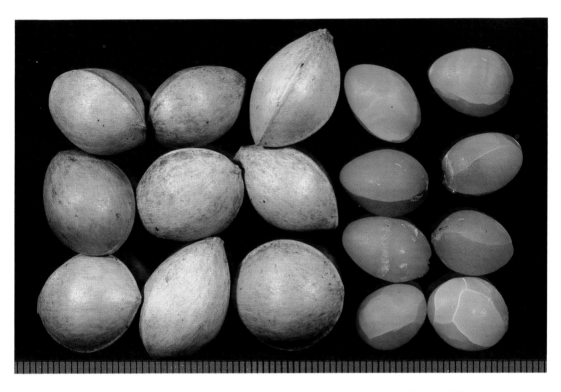

Ginkgo Semen: crude (left); with seed coat removed (right). (×5/3)

171 GINKGO SEMEN

白果 *bai² guo³*. English: ginkgo nut. Japanese: *byakuka, hakka. ginkyo.*
Alternate name: 銀杏肉 *yin² xing⁴ rou⁴.*
Origin: Ginkgoaceae family. *Ginkgo biloba* L.
Characters: The dried seed is obovate or elliptical, and slightly flat. It is 1.5–2.5 cm long, and 1–1.5 cm thick. The seed-coat is white or pale gray, smooth, and hard, with a ridge running around the margins. At the tip is the scar of the funiculus. The actual seed is spheroid, pale yellow, or yellow-green, with a white, farinaceous interior and a hollow core. Close to the tip are two cotyledons or more.
Quality: White seed-coats and full seeds that are white on the inside are best.
Production areas: China (most areas, with principal production in Guangxi, Sichuan, Henan, Shandong, Hubei, and Liaoning), Japan, and Korea.
Properties and actions: Balanced; sweet, bitter, and astringent; nontoxic. Enters the lung and kidney channels. Constrains lung qi, calms cough and dyspnea, checks vaginal discharge, and reduces urine flow. Use crude to downbear phlegm, disperse toxin, and kill worms. Use prepared to warm the lung and boost qi, suppress cough and calm dyspnea, and to reduce urination and check vaginal discharge.
Indications: Wheezing dyspnea; phlegm cough; white turbidity; vaginal discharge; seminal emission; strangury; frequent urination. Daily dosage: 5–10 g. Contraindicated in pathogen repletion. Used in *ding⁴ chuan³ tang¹* (Dyspnea-Stabilizing Decoction, 71).
Remarks: Constituents: gibberellin, ginkgolic acid, bilobol, hydroginkgolinic acid.

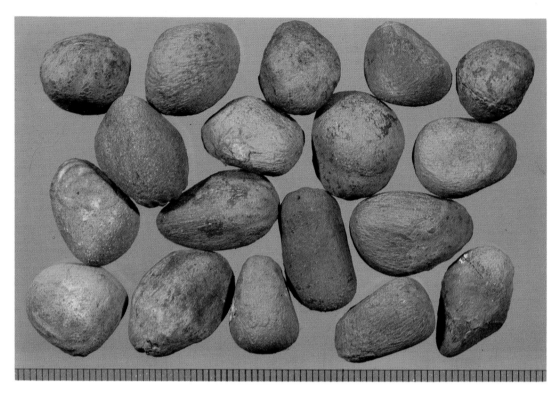

Hynocarpi Semen. (×5/3)

172 HYDNOCARPI SEMEN

大風子 *da⁴ feng¹ zi³*. English: hydnocarpus (or chaulmoogra) seed. Japanese: *daifushi*.
Alternate name: 大楓子 *da⁴ feng¹ zi³*.
Origin: Flacourtiaceae family. *Hydnocarpus anthelmintica* Pier.
Characters: The dried mature seed is an irregular ovate or many-sided body, 1–2.5 cm long and 1–2 cm in diameter. The exterior surface is gray-brown with fine wrinkles. At the smaller end is a distinct trough 1.5–2 mm thick, shiny on the inside, and light yellow-brown in color. The seed is separated from the shell. The two endosperms are gray-white in color, and oleaceous. The seed-coat is a thin red-brown or dark purple membrane.
Quality: Large, full, white, oleaceous seeds are the best.
Production areas: China (Guangxi, Guangdong, Taiwan), Vietnam, Thailand, and Malaysia.
Properties and actions: Hot; acrid; toxic. Enters the liver, spleen, and kidney channels. Dispels wind and dries damp; attacks toxin and kills worms.
Indications: Leprosy; jie and xian; red bayberry (syphilitic) sores. Daily dosage: 1.5–3 g. Contraindicated in yin vacuity blood heat. Used in *yi¹ sao³ guang¹* (Gone-In-One-Sweep, 314).
Remarks: Allied drugs: Dried seed of *Hydnocarpus alpina* Wight, grown in southern China, southeast Asia, and India, and *H. wightiana* Blume, grown in southwestern India, contain similar constituents and are used for the same purposes.
Constituents: Fixed oil (hydnocarpus oil, 45% in kernel): glycerides of hydnocarpic acid, chaulmoogric acid, deydrochaulmoogric acid, gorlic acid, oleic acid, and palmitic acid.

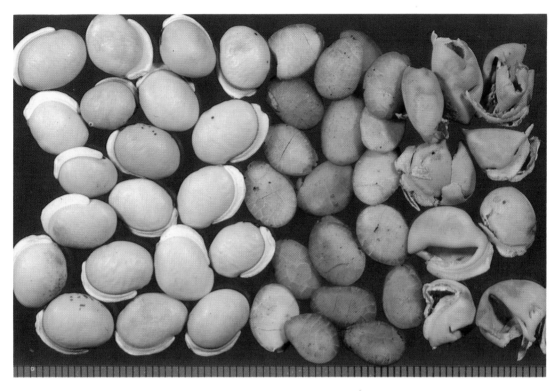

Lablab Semen: crude (left); stir-fried (middle); seed coat (right), (×5/3)

173 LABLAB SEMEN

扁豆 *bian³ dou⁴*. English: lablab seed, hyacinth bean. Japanese: *henzu, byakuhenzu.*
Alternate name: 白扁豆 *bai² bian³ dou⁴.*
Origin: Leguminosae family. *Lablab vulgaris* Savi [= *Dolichos lablab* L.].
Characters: The dry seed is elliptical or ovate in shape, 8–12 mm in length, 6–9 mm wide, and 4–7 mm thick. The exterior surface is yellow-white, smooth and shiny. There is a protruding, crescent-shaped caruncle lying around the edge, taking up a third to a half of the total periphery. If removed, an indented hilum can be seen. Close to one end of the caruncle is the micropyle. At the other end is a short raphe. This seed is hard, and the thin, brittle seed-coat that covers it can be removed to reveal two fat, white cotyledons. This product gives off the characteristic odor of beans.
Quality: Fat, white beans are the best.
Production areas: China (most parts, especially Hunan, Anhui, Henan, Zhejiang), and Japan.
Properties and actions: Slightly warm; sweet; nontoxic. Enters the spleen and stomach channels. Fortifies qi and harmonizes the center; dispels summerheat and transforms damp. Use crude to dispel summerheat. Stir-fry without additives to fortify the spleen and check diarrhea. Stir-fry with earth to check diarrhea. Stir-fry with vinegar to treat vomiting with diarrhea.
Indications: Summerheat-damp vomiting and diarrhea; spleen vacuity counterflow retching; low food intake; enduring diarrhea; wasting thirst; red and white vaginal discharge; child gan accumulation. Daily dosage: 5–12 g. Contraindicated in disease cold-heat complexes. Used in *xiang¹-ru² san³* (Elsholtzia Powder, 288), *shen¹ ling² bai²-zhu² san³* (Ginseng, Poria, and Atractylodes Ovata Powder, 231), *liu⁴ wei⁴ xiang⁴-ru² yin³* (Six-Ingredient Elsholtzia Beverage, 169).
Remarks: Constituents: Proteins (22.7%). Fat (1.8%).

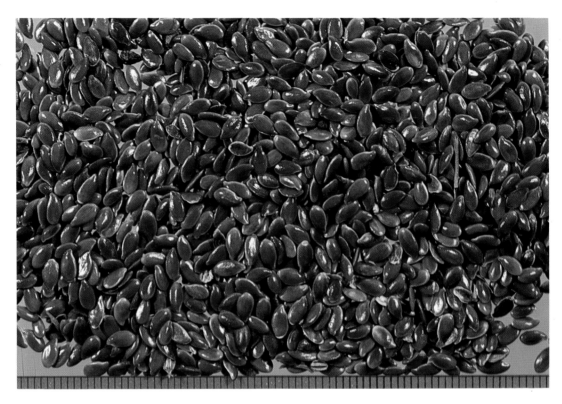

Lini Semen. (×5/3)

174 LINI SEMEN

亞麻仁 ya³ ma² ren². English: flax (or linum) seed. Japanese: *amanin.*
Alternate name: 亞麻子 ya³ ma² zi³.
Origin: Linaceae family. *Linum usitatissimum* L.
Characters: This seed is ovate, flat, with one side thinner than the other. One end is rounded, while the other tapers to a point that is slightly bent to one side. It is 4–6 mm long, 2–3 mm wide, and 1.4 mm thick. The exterior surface is maroon-brown, smooth, and shiny. Inside, there is a membranous brown endosperm, within which there are two yellow, oleaceous cotyledons, each with a flat and a rounded side. The radicle points toward the tip of the seed. When soaked in water, the mucus of the exterior coating swellings and to provide a mucous shield that surrounds the whole of the seed. This seed feels slimy in the mouth when chewed, and has no smell.
Quality: Clean, fat, shiny, maroon seeds are the best.
Production areas: China (Inner Mongolia, Heilongjiang, Liaoning, Jilin, and less importantly Sichuan, Hubei, Shaanxi, Shanxi, Yunnan), Korea, Japan, and other parts of the world.
Properties and actions: Warm; sweet; nontoxic. Enters the liver channels. Frees the stool and kills worms.
Indications: Leprosy; itchy skin; alopecia; dry stool. Daily dosage: 5–10 g. Contraindicated vomiting due to a weak stomach. Flax seed oil works as a mild laxative (1–25 ml at a time).
Remarks: Constituents: Fixed oil (lini oleum, 20–40%): linoleic acid, linolenic acid, oleic acid, glycerides of stearic acid, palmitic acid. Porteins (25%). Mucilage. (6%)

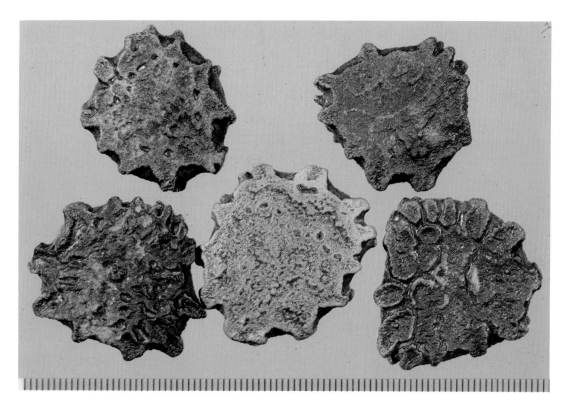

Momordicae Semen (×5/3)

175 MOMORDICAE SEMEN

木鼈子 *mu⁴ bie¹ zi³*. English: momordica seed. Japanese: *mokubesshi*.

Alternate name: 土木鼈 *tu³ mu⁴ bie¹*.

Origin: Cucurbitaceae family. *Momordica cochinchinensis* (Lour.) Spr.

Characters: This seed is round and flat, bulging slightly in the middle. It is about 2–2.5 cm in diameter, 1.5–2.5 cm wide, and 4–6 mm thick. The exterior is gray-brown or gray-black, with an irregular reticular formation of depressions. Around the edges are ten or more dull spikes. The episperm is hard and brittle, while the endotesta is membranous and gray-green on the surface with down. Within there are two large, fat, yellow-white cotyledons that are oleaceous in substance and bitter in taste.

Quality: Unbroken, full, heavy seeds, with yellow-white cotyledons that do not exude oil are the best.

Production areas: China (Guangxi, Sichuan, Hubei, and less importantly Hunan, Guizhou, Yunnan, Guangdong, and Anhui).

Properties and actions: Warm; bitter and slightly sweet; toxic. Enters the liver, spleen, and stomach channels. Disperses swelling and bind; dispels toxin.

Indications: Swollen yong; clove sores; scrofulous lumps; hemorrhoids; innominate swollen toxin sores; xian; wind-damp bi pain; hypertonicity of the sinews. Use crude for topical treatment of sores. Make into a frost to moderate the effect. Bake or stir-fry to treat gan accumulation and diarrhea. Daily dosage: 0.5–1 g. Contraindicated in pregnancy and debilitation. Used in *yi¹ sao³ guang¹* (Gone-In-One-Sweep, 314), *xiao³ jin¹ dan¹* (Minor Golden Elixir, 301), *mu⁴-bie¹-zi³ wan²* (Momordica Pills, 188).

Remarks: Constituents: pipecolic acid, momordic acid. Oil (35.72%), Proteins (30.59%).

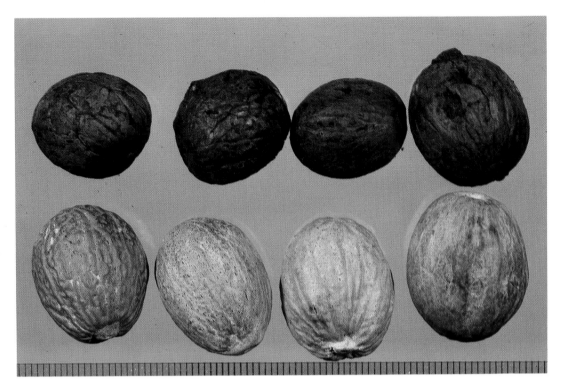

Myristicae Semen: crude (below); roasted (above), (×5/3)

176 MYRISTICAE SEMEN

肉豆蔻 *rou⁴ dou⁴ kou⁴*. English: nutmeg. Japanese: *nikuzuku*.

Alternate name: 肉果 *rou⁴ guo³*.

Origin: Myristicaceae family. *Myristica fragrans* Houttuyn.

Characters: The dried seed is ovate or elliptical, 2–3.5 cm long, and 1.5–2.5 cm wide. The exterior surface is mid-brown to dark brown, with indistinct, broken longitudinal ridges. On one side is a distinct furrow marking the raphe. At the wider end is a round protuberance that marks the hilum, and at the narrow end is a faint indentation that marks the chalaza. On the longitudinal section, the perisperm that forms the superficial layer stretches inward to intermesh with the white endosperm creating a marble pattern. At the broader end is an indentation in which the dried shrunken embryo can be seen. This seed is hard and has a strong aroma.

Quality: Large, firm, heavy seeds with strong aroma are the best.

Production areas: Malaysia and Indonesia.

Properties and actions: Warm; acrid; nontoxic. Enters the spleen and large intestine channels. Warms the center; precipitates qi; disperses food; secures the intestines (especially when roasted).

Indications: Pain and distention in the abdomen and region of the heart; cold and vacuity diarrhea; retching and vomiting; retention of food. Daily dosage: 3–5 g. Contraindicated in hot diarrhea or dysentery. Used in *si⁴ shen² wan²* (Four Spirits Pills, 254).

Remarks: Constituents: Monoterpenoids and phenylpropanoids (volatile oil, nutmeg oil, 5–15%): (+)-camphene (60–80%), (+)-, (–)-α-pinenes, (+)-limonene (2.6–8%), geraniol (ca. 6%), (+)-linalool (5%), β-pinene (3%), myristicin (4–12%), safrole (0.6–3%), eugenol (0.2%). Fixed oil (nutmeg or banda soap, 30–45%): myristin (35–70%), olein (3%). Saccharides: starch.

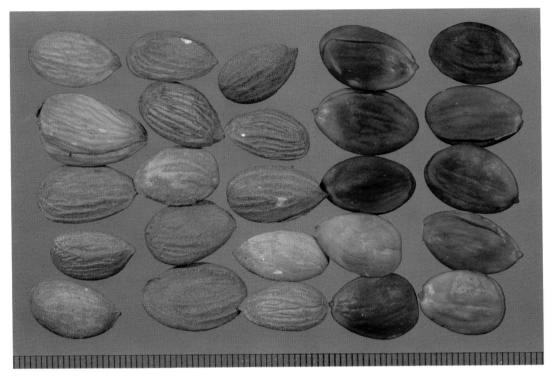

Persicae Semen: crude (left); stir-fried in bran (right). (×5/3)

177 PERSICAE SEMEN

桃仁 *tao² ren²*. English: peach kernel. Japanese *tonin*.

Alternate names: 光桃仁 *guang¹ tao² ren²*, 桃核仁 *tao² he² ren²*.

Origin: Rosaceae family. *Prunus persica* (L.) Batsch., *P. persica* (L.) Batsch. var. *davidiana* (Carr.) Maximowicz.

Characters: The dry seed is flat and ovate, 1–1.6 cm long, and 0.8–1 cm wide. The exterior surface is a reddish or yellowish brown, with longitudinal wrinkles spreading from the base. The tip is pointed and the base is rounded, and slightly skew. The linear hilum at the base is brown in color, and protrudes slightly. The thin, brittle seed-coat covers a cream-colored, oleaceous seed, that comprises two cotyledons with a fissure between. The seed has only a faint smell.

Quality: Unbroken, neat, fat seeds of even size are the best.

Production areas: China (Sichuan, Yunnan, Shaanxi, Shandong, Hebei, Shanxi, and Henan), and Japan.

Properties and actions: Balanced; bitter, sweet; nontoxic. Enters the heart, liver, and large intestine channels. Breaks the blood and moves stasis; moistens dryness and lubricates the intestines.

Indications: Menstrual block; concretions and conglomerations; blood amassment in febrile disease; wind bi; malarial disease; bruises due to impact injury (static blood); constipation due to dryness blood. Daily dosage: 5–10 g. Contraindicated in pregnancy and in the absence of stasis and stagnation. Used in *gui⁴-zhi¹ fu²-ling² wan²* (Cinnamon Twig and Poria Pills, 109), *tao²-he² cheng² qi⁴ tang¹* (Peach Kernel Qi-Infusing Decoction, 260), *da⁴-huang² mu³-dan¹ tang¹* (Rhubarb and Moutan Decoction, 50).

Remarks: Constituents: Cyanophore glycosides: amygdalin (2.3–3.7%), prunasin (0.38%). Triterpenoids: 24-methylene cycloartanol; squalene. Steroids: β-sitosterol, campesterol. Phospholipids: phosphatidylcholine (44–55%). Fixed oil (40–50%). Enzymes: emulsin (β-glycosidase).

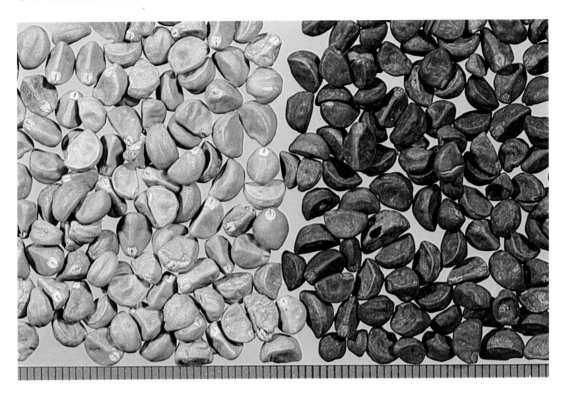

Pharbitidis Semen Album (left) and Atrum (right). (×2)

178 PHARBITIDIS SEMEN

牵牛子 *qian¹ niu² zi³*. English: morning glory (or pharbitidis) seed. Japanese: *kengoshi*.
Alternate names: 二丑 *er⁴ chou³*, 黑白丑 *hei¹, bai² chou³*.
Origin: Convolvulaceae family. *Pharbitis nil* (L.) Choisy.
Characters: The dried, ripe fruit is ovate and three-sided. Two of the sides are flat, while the third, the dorsal face, bows outward, with a wide longitudinal furrow. At the lower end of the ventral ridge that separates the two flat sides is a round, light-colored hilum. The seed is 4–8 mm long, while the sides are about 3–5 mm wide. The external surface is either black (Pharbitidis Semen Atrum [*hei¹ chou³*]) or pale brown (Pharbiditis Semen Album [*bai² chou³*]). The seed-coat is hard. The transverse section shows two heavily folded, pale yellow cotyledons. When soaked in water, the seed-coat splits along the ventral ridge, and becomes mucous. This seed has no smell.
Quality: Ripe, full seeds of mixed coloration, with no impurities are the best.
Production areas: China (most parts), and Japan.
Properties and actions: Cold; acrid, bitter; toxic. Enters the lung, kidney, large and small intestines channels. Drains water, precipitates qi, and kills worms.
Indications: Water swelling; dyspnea and fullness; phlegm-rheum; leg qi; worm accumulation; food stagnation; bound stool. Daily dosage: 3–6 g. Contraindicated in pregnancy and stomach qi vacuity. Used in *yu³ gong¹ san³* (Hallowed Ancient Yu Powder, 324), *qian¹-niu² wan²* (Morning Glory Pills, 201).
Remarks: Constituents: Resin glycosides (Pharbitis resin): pharbitin (2–3%). Acids: nilic acid, gallic acid. Tannoids. Fixed oil (10–11%): glycerides of oleic acid, palmitic acid.

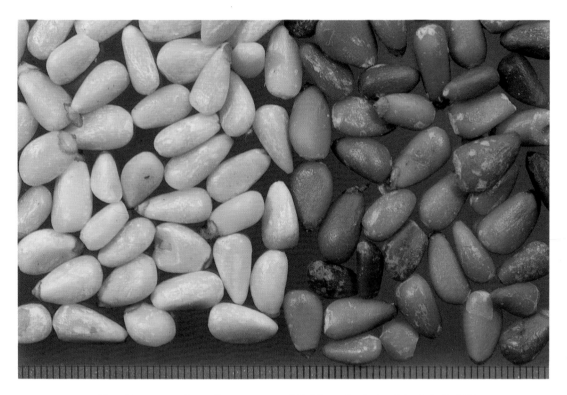

Pini Semen: with seed-coat removed (left); and stir-fried (right). (×5/3)

179 PINI SEMEN

海松子-*hai³ song¹ zi³*. English: pine nut. Japanese: *kaishoshi, shoshinin.*
Alternate names: 松子*song¹ zi³*, 松子仁 *song¹ zi³ ren².*
Origin: Pinaceae family. *Pinus koraiensis* Sieb. et Zucc.
Characters: This is a long, oval seed bluntly pointed at one end. It is 10 mm long and 5 mm in diameter. The thin seed-coat is a reddish brown, while the endosperm is cream-colored.
Quality: Large seeds with cream-colored endosperm and a strong smell are the best.
Production areas: China (Manchuria), and Korea.
Properties and actions: Warm; sweet; nontoxic. Enters the lung, liver, and large intestine channels. Nourishes humor, extinguishes wind, moistens the lung, and lubricates the intestines.
Indications: Wind bi; dizziness; dryness cough; blood ejection; constipation. Daily dosage: 5–10 g. Contraindicated in loose bowels or in damp phlegm disorders. Make a congee with pine nuts and rice to moisten the heart and lung, and free the stool. Make a paste with 30 g pine nuts and 60 g walnuts, and blend with honey to treat lung dryness cough (take 6 g at a time mixed with water).
Remarks: Constituents: Fixed oil (74%). Proteins. Volatile oil.

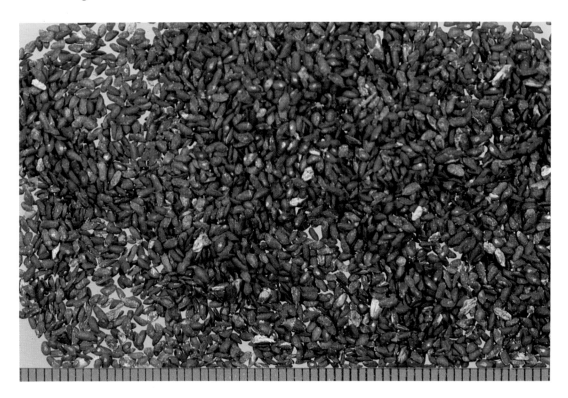

Plantaginis Semen: stir-fried in brine. (×2)

180 PLANTAGINIS SEMEN

車前子 *che¹ qian² zi³*. English: plantago seed. Japanese: *shazenshi.*

Alternate name: 車前實 *che¹ qian² shi².*

Origin: Plantaginaceae family. *Plantago asiatica* L. [= *P. major* L. var. *asiatica* Decaisne.]

Characters: This seed is elliptical, slightly flat, 2–3 mm long, and 1 mm wide. The exterior surface is pale brown, with black speckles. It is shiny, and has linear markings. The hilum is white, the dorsum bulges, and the base is flat. The cross section is gray-white or pale yellow. It has little smell, and has a glutinous quality most clearly observed when it is boiled.

Quality: Dry, plump, black seeds without shells are the best.

Production areas: China (Jiangxi and Henan).

Properties and actions: Cold; sweet; nontoxic. Clears heat (especially when used crude); disinhibits water (especially when stir-fried in brine); brightens the eyes; dispels phlegm.

Indications: Urinary stoppage; turbid strangury; vaginal discharge; blood in the urine; jaundice; water swelling; heat dysentery; diarrhea; nosebleed; reddening, soreness, and swelling of the eyes; throat bi; throat moth; cough; ulcers. Daily dosage: 5–10 g. Contraindicated in profuse urination with constipation, and in the absence of damp-heat. Used in *ba¹ zheng⁴ san³* (Eight Corrections Powder, 7), *niu² che¹ shen⁴ qi⁴ wan²* (Achyranthes and Plantago Kidney Qi Pills, 192).

Remarks: Constituents; Saccharides: plantago-mucilage A, plantasan; disaccharide I (O-β-D-xylopyranosyl-(1→2)-D-xylopyranose). Iridoids: aucubin, geniposidic acid. Flavonoids: plantagoside (5,7,3′,4′,5′-pentahydroxyflavanone-3′-O-glucoside). Phenylpropanoids: syringin, acteoside.

Allied drug: Plantaginis Herba.

Similar drug: Dried ripe seed of *Plantago depressa* Willd.

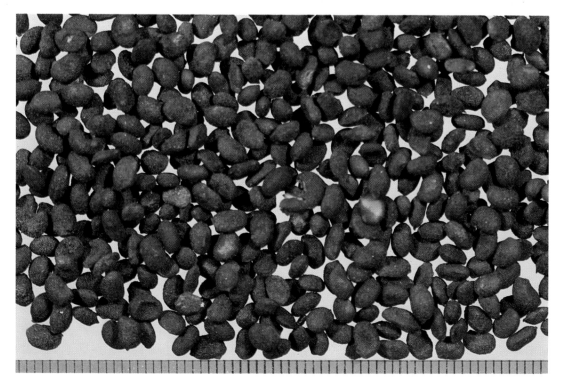

Psoraleae Semen: stir-fried in brine. (×2)

181 PSORALEAE SEMEN

補骨脂 *bu³ gu³ zhi¹*. English: psoralea (or scurfy pea) seed. Japanese: *hokotsushi*.
Alternate names: 破固脂 *po⁴ gu⁴ zhi¹*, 破故脂 *po⁴ gu⁴ zhi³*.
Origin: Leguminosae family. *Psoralea corylifolia* L.
Characters: This seed is elliptical or kidney shaped, 3–5 mm long, 2–4 mm in diameter, and about 1.5 mm thick, with a depression in the center. The exterior surface is blackish brown, and bears fine reticular wrinkles and dense glandular points. A small proportion of fruits have a persistent calyx on the outside. The exocarp is thin, and difficult to separate from the seed-coat. Inside are two seeds, each with two cotyledons, which are oleaceous and light brown or yellow in color. This seed has no smell.
Quality: Large, clean, hard, full, black fruits are the best.
Production areas: China (Sichuan, Henan, Shaanxi, Anhui).
Properties and actions: Warm; acrid. Enters the kidney channel. Supplements the kidney and assists yang. Stir-frying in brine enhances the kidney-supplementing effect.
Indications: Frigid diarrhea due to kidney vacuity; enuresis; seminal efflux; frequent urination; impotence; frigid pain in the lumbus and knees; cough and dyspnea due to vacuity cold. Applied topically to white patch wind. Daily dosage: 5–10 g. Contraindicated in effulgent yin vacuity fire, blood in the urine, and constipation. Used in *si⁴ shen² wan²* (Four Spirits Pills, 254), *bu³-gu³-zhi¹ wan²* (Psoralea Pills, 32).
Remarks: Constituents: Furano coumarins: psoralen, angelicin. Flavanones: bavachin, bavachinin, isobavachin. Chalcones: isobavachalcone, bakuchiol.

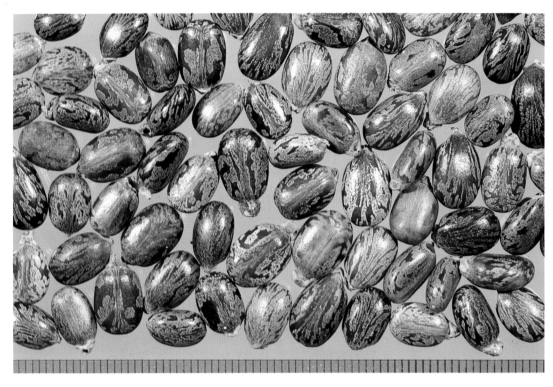

Ricini Semen. (×2)

182 RICINI SEMEN

蓖麻子·*bi⁴ ma² zi³*. English: castor bean. Japanese: *himashi.*

Alternate names: 草麻子*bi⁴ ma² zi³*, 蓖麻仁*bi⁴ ma² ren².*

Origin: Euphorbiaceae family. *Ricinus communis* L.

Characters: The dried seeds are broad ovate, 8–18 mm long, and 6–9 mm in diameter. The ventral side is flat, and the dorsal is rounded. At the smaller end there is a spongy caruncle and hilum. At the other end is the chalaza. Running between the hilum and chalaza is a distinct raphe. The smooth, shiny surface is maroon with cloudlike yellow-brown patches.

Quality: Large, plump, shiny, maroon seeds are the best.

Production areas: China (most parts), and Japan.

Properties and actions: Balanced; sweet, acrid; toxic. Enters the large intestine and lung channels. Disperses swelling and draws out pus; lubricates the intestines and frees stagnation.

Indications: Swelling and toxin of yong and ju; scrofulous lumps; throat bi; jie, lai, and xian; water swelling and abdominal fullness; dry, bound stool. Daily dosage: 4–16 cc at a time taken orally. Contraindicated in pregnancy. Used in *e¹-wei⁴ hua⁴ pi³ gao¹* (Asafetida Glomus-Transforming Daste, 77).

Remarks: Constituents: Fixed oil (castor oil, 40–50%): triricinolein (triglyceride of ricinoleic acid (12-hydroxy-octadeca-9-enoic acid), esters of diricinoleoglyceride with isoricinoleic acid, oleic acid, linolenic acid, linoleic acid. Alkaloids: ricinine. Proteins (ca. 20%): ricin. Enzyme: lipase. Allergens: castor bean allergen.

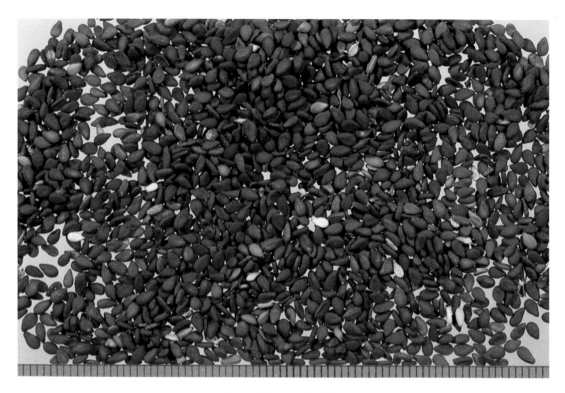

Sesami Semen. (×5/3)

183 SESAMI SEMEN

黑脂麻 *hei¹ zhi¹ ma²*. English: sesame seed. Japanese: *kokushima*.

Alternate name: 黑芝麻 *hei¹ zhi¹ ma²*.

Origin: Pedaliaceae family. *Sesamum indicum* L.

Characters: This seed is flat and ovate in shape, with one end pointed, and the other rounded. It is 2–4 mm long, 1–2 mm wide, and 1 mm thick. The exterior surface is black, sometimes with reticular markings. Under a magnifying glass, tiny wart-like protuberances can be seen on the surface. The edges are smooth, and ridge-shaped. At the pointed end is a round brown spot that marks the hilum. The seed-coat is thin and papery. The longitudinal section shows a membranous endosperm. The embryo stands erect. There are two oleaceous, large, white cotyledons. This seed normally has a mild smell, but gives off a strong aroma when stir-fried.

Quality: Large, clean, plump, black seeds are the best.

Production areas: South East Asia (cultivated), and China (Sichuan, Shandong, Shanxi, Henan).

Properties and actions: Balanced; sweet. Enters the liver and kidney channels. Supplements the liver and kidney and moistens the five viscera. Stir-fried to bring out the aroma, it promotes lactation. Steamed with wine, it expels wind and supplements.

Indications: Insufficiency of the liver and kidney; vacuity wind dizziness; wind bi; paralysis; vacuity marked emaciation after disease; premature graying; scant breast milk. Daily dosage: 5–10 g. Contraindicated in spleen vacuity with thin stool. Used in *sang¹ ma² wan²* (Mulberry Leaf and Sesame Pills, 226).

Remarks: Constituents: Fixed oils (sesame oil, 40–60%): glycerides of oleic acid (37–49%), linoleic acid (35–48%), palmitic acid (7–9%), stearic acid (4–5%). Lignoids: sesamin (1%), sesamolin, Phenols: sesamol (0.1%).

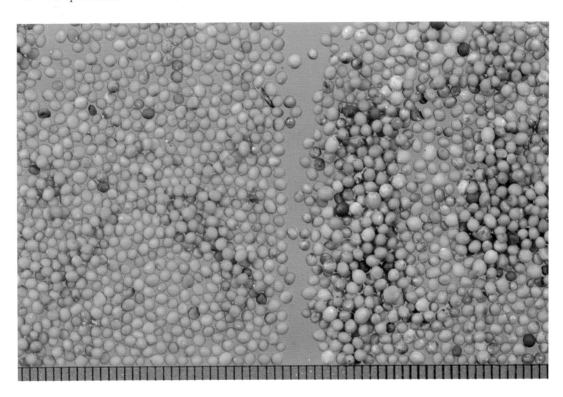

Sinapis Semen: crude (left); stir-fried (right). (×2)

184 SINAPIS SEMEN (BRASSICAE JUNCEAE SEMEN)

芥子 *jie⁴ zi³*. English: white mustard (or Indian mustard) seed. Japanese: *gaishi*.

Alternate names: 芥菜子 *jie⁴ cai⁴ zi³*, 黃芥子 *huang² jie⁴ zi³*.

Origin: Cruciferae family. *Brassica juncea* (L.) Czern. et Coss. [= *Sinapis juncea* L.].

Characters: This seed is round, with a diameter of 1–1.6 mm. The seed-coat is deep yellow or light brown, some having a red tinge. Under a magnifying glass, the surface has faint reticular markings, and the hilum appears as a distinct spot. When soaked in water this seed swells, allowing the seed-coat to be removed to reveal two cotyledons.

Quality: Full, evenly sized seeds that are yellow or red-brown in color are best.

Production areas: China (most parts, Henan and Anhui being the biggest producers).

Properties and actions: Warm; acrid; nontoxic. Enters the lung channel. Warms the center and dissipates cold; disinhibits qi and sweeps phlegm; frees the channels and the connecting vessels, disperses swelling. Stir-frying enhances the phlegm-transforming action.

Indications: Vomiting of food due to stomach cold; pain in the abdomen and region of the heart; lung cold cough; painful bi; throat bi; yin ju; cold phlegm; impact injuries. Daily dosage: 3–5 g. Contraindicated in lung vacuity cough and in effulgent yin vacuity fire. Used in *kong⁴ xian² dan¹* (Drool-Controlling Elixir, 159).

Remarks: Constituents: Glucosinolates (mustard glycosides, ca. 4%): sinigrin (potassium myrosinate). Phenylpropanoids: sinapine. Enzymes: myrosinase. Fixed oil (30–37%): glycerides of erucic acid, arachidonic acid, linoleic acid.

Allied drug: Sinapis Albae Semen, the seed of *Brassica alba* Boiss.

Similar drug: Sinapis Nigrae Semen, the seed of *B. nigra* Koch.

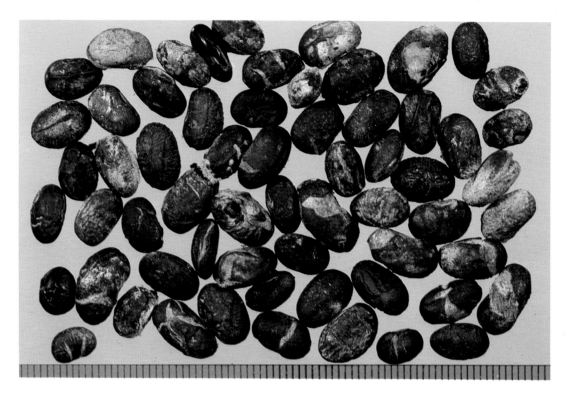

Sojae Semen Praeparatum (×5/3)

185 SOJAE SEMEN PRAEPARATUM

淡豆豉 *dan⁴ dou⁴ chi³*. English: unsalted fermented soybean. Japanese: *tantoshi*.
Alternate name: 香豉 *xiang¹ chi³*.
Origin: Leguminosae family. *Glycine max* (L.) Merr. [= *G. soja* Benth.].
Characters: The dried product is elliptical, slightly flat, 0.6–1 cm long, and 3–6 mm wide. The outer skin is black with irregular, yellowish wrinkles and a thin, gray-brown coating. It is loose, and in some cases has been stripped away to reveal the seed. This product is easily broken, exposing a cross section that is lighter in color than the skin. It has a the smell of rot and a sweet flavor.
Quality: The best quality is black with a membranous coating.
Production areas: China (all parts, Shandong being the biggest producer).
Properties and actions: Cold; bitter; nontoxic. Enters the lung and stomach channels. Resolves the exterior, eliminates vexation, diffuses depression, and resolves toxin.
Indications: Cold damage febrile disease; fever and chills; headache; vexation and agitation; thoracic oppression. Daily dosage: 10–12 g. Contraindicated in the absence of external contraction of wind-cold. Used in *zhi¹-zi³ chi³ tang¹* (Gardenia and Fermented Soybean Decoction, 338), *zhi¹-zi³ gan¹-cao³ chi³ tang¹* (Gardenia, Licorice, and Fermented Soybean Decoction, 340).
Remarks: Constituents: Proteins.

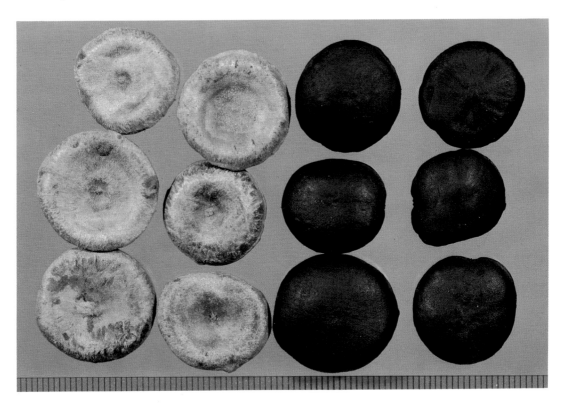

Strychnotis Nux-Vomicae Semen: crude (left); processed (right). (× 5/3)

186 STRYCHNOTIS NUX-VOMICAE SEMEN

馬錢子 *ma³ qian² zi³*. English: nux vomica. Japanese: *machinshi, homika.*
Alternate name: 番木鼈 *fan¹ mu⁴ bie¹.*
Origin: Loganiaceae family. *Strychnos nux-vomica* L., *S. pierriana* A.W. Hill.*
Characters: The dried, mature fruit is round and flat like a button, thicker at the edge, and often with a distinct depression in the middle of one side. It is 1–3 cm in diameter, and 3–6 mm thick. The external surface is brown or green-gray. It is densely covered with fine, silver gray, surface-running hairs that radiate from the center. In the middle of the undersurface is a ridge line. This seed is hard, and difficult to break. Inside is a slightly translucent, pale yellow-white horny endosperm. The longitudinal section shows a heart-shaped cotyledon. It has a bitter flavor, but care should be taken when tasting it since it is highly toxic. It is usually prepared by frying in sesame seed oil and grinding to a powder.
Quality: Large, thick, hard seeds are the best.
Production areas: India, Vietnam, Burma, and China (Yunnan, Tibet).
Properties and actions: Cold; bitter; toxic. Dissipates blood heat, disperses swelling and relieves pain.
Indications: Throat bi; swelling and toxin of yong and ju; wind bi pain; bone fractures; facial paralysis; myasthenia gravis. Daily dosage: 0.3–0.6 g. Contraindicated in pregnancy and in vacuity. Used in *ba¹ li² san³* (Eight Pinches Powder, 4).
Remarks: Constituents: Alkaloids (strychnos alkaloids, 1.8–5.3%): strychnine:(1–2%), brucine (1.6%) strychnicine, vomicine, α-, β-colubrines. Iridoids: loganin (4–5%). Acid: chlorogenic acid (as salts). Fixed oil (2.5–4.2%): glycerides of oleic acid, palmitic acid, arachidic acid, butyric acid.

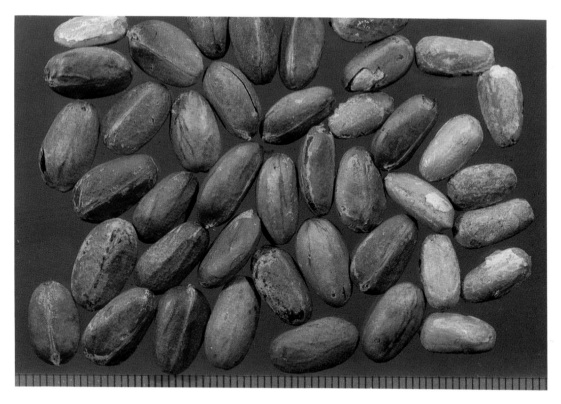

Tiglii Semen. (× 5/3)

187 TIGLII SEMEN (CROTONIS SEMEN)

巴豆 $ba^1 dou^4$. English: croton (or tiglium) seed. Japanese: *hazu*.

Alternate names: 川江子$chuan^1 jiang^1 zi^3$, 巴豆仁$ba^1 dou^4 ren^2$.

Origin: Euphorbiaceae family. *Croton tiglium* L.

Characters: This seed is elliptical or ovate, and slightly flat. It is about 1–1.5 cm long, 6–9 mm in diameter, and 4–7 mm thick. The exterior surface is brown or dark brown and smooth, with a faint luster. The caruncle is at one end of the hilum, appearing as a small protuberance that easily breaks off. The chalaza is at the other end, joined to the hilum by a slightly protruding longitudinal raphe. The transverse section appears slightly squared. The seed-coat is thin, and brittle and can be easily peeled away to reveal the seed, which has a membranous silver white perisperm. The endosperm is thick, pale yellow, and oleaceous. In the center are two thin cotyledons. The radicle is small, and points to the end where the caruncle is.

Quality: is. Large, plump seeds with white endosperm are the best. Empty seeds or ones that have exuded oil and changed color are inferior.

Production areas: China (Sichuan, Guangxi, Yunnan, and Guizhou, the biggest producer being Sichuan).

Properties and actions: Hot; acrid; toxic. Enters the stomach and large intestine channels. Drains cold accumulations; free the jaw and portals; expels phlegm; moves water; kills worms. Use frost (Tiglii Seminis Pulvis [$ba^1 dou^4 shuang^1$]) for milder precipitating action.

Indications: Frigid accumulations; distention and acute pain in the chest and abdomen; blood conglomerations; phlegm pi; diarrhea; water swelling;. Applied externally to throat wind, throat bi, malign sores, jie and xian. Daily dosage: 0.15–0.3 g. Contraindicated in pregnancy, general weakness, and in the absence of repletion cold accumulation and stagnation. Used in $san^1 wu^4 bei^4 ji^2 wan^2$ (Three Agents Emergency Pills, 223).

Remarks: Constituents: Fixed oil (croton oil, 30–60%): glycerides of oleic acid (37%), linolic acid (19%), arachidic acid (1.5%), palmitic acid (0.9%). Diterpenoids: phorbolesters A_1, A_2, A_3, A_4, B_1, B_2 B_3, B_4, B_5, B_6, B_7.

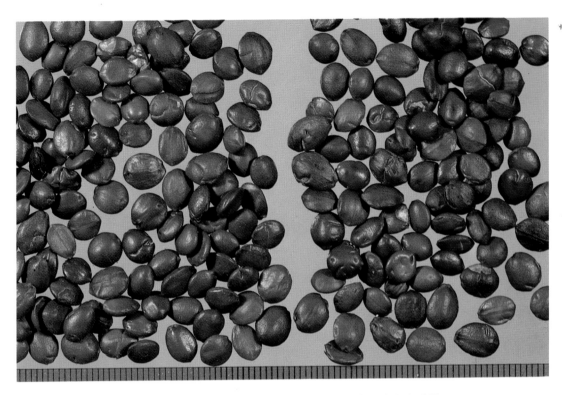

Zizyphi Spinosi Semen: crude (left); stir-fried (right). (×5/3)

188 ZIZYPHI SPINOSI SEMEN

酸棗仁 *suan¹ zao³ ren²*. English: spiny jujube kernel. Japanese: *sansonin*.

Alternate names: 棗仁 *zao³ ren²*, 酸棗核 *suan¹ zao³ he²*.

Origin: Rhamnaceae family. *Zizyphus jujuba* Miller [= *Z. vulgaris* Lamarck var. *spinosus* Bunge, and *Z. spinosus* Hu].

Characters: The dried ripe seed is elliptical and flat, 5–9 mm long, 5–7 mm wide, and 3 mm thick. The exterior surface is reddish brown or maroon, and shiny. If unripe, it is lighter and more yellow in color. One side is flatter than the other, and has protruding line running longitudinally down the center. The other side bulges in the middle. The hilum is distinctly visible at one end, and a protuberant chalaza is visible at the other end. An indistinct raphe runs along one side. The white endosperm sticks to the seed-coat when the latter is removed. Beneath are two elliptical, yellow-white, oleaceous cotyledons. The seed has only a faint smell.

Quality: Large, fat, maroon seeds without epicarp are the best.

Production areas: China (Hebei, Shaanxi, Liaoning, Henan, and less importantly Inner Mongolia, Gansu, Shanxi, Shandong, Anhui, and Jiangsu).

Properties and actions: Balanced; sweet; nontoxic. Enters the heart, spleen, liver, and gallbladder channels. Nourishes the liver, quiets the heart, calms the spirit and contains sweating. Use crude to drain the liver and gallbladder and to quiet the spirit. Use stir-fried to nourish liver blood and quiet the spirit.

Indications: Vacuity vexation and sleeplessness; fright palpitation; racing of the heart; vexation and thirst; vacuity sweating. Daily dosage: 5–10 g. Contraindicated in pathogen repletion and depressed fire. Used in *suan¹-zao³-ren² tang¹* (Spiny Jujube Decoction, 259), *gui¹ pi² tang¹* (Spleen-Returning Decoction, 108), *tian¹ wang² bu³ xin¹ dan¹* (Celestial Emperor Heart-Supplementing Elixir, 262).

Remarks: Constituents: Triterpenoids: (saponins, 2.5%) jujubosides A, B, C; betulic acid (betulinic acid), betulin. Steroids: β-sitosterol. Alkaloids: frangufoline (sanjoinine-A), sanjoinines-B, C, D, F, G_1, G_2, (+)-coclaurine, nuciferine.

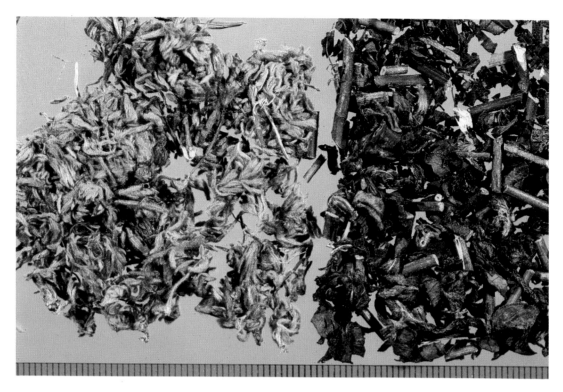

Artemisiae Capillaris Herba (left) and Origani Vulgaris Herba (right). (×5/3)

189 ARTEMISIAE CAPILLARIS HERBA

茵陳蒿 *yin¹ chen² hao¹* (Including Origani Vulgaris Herba 土茵陳 *tu³ yin¹ chen²*) English: artemisia, capillaris. Japanese: *inchinkō.*

Alternate names: 茵陳 *yin¹ chen²*, 綿茵陳 *mian² yin¹ chen².*

Origin: Compositae family. *Artemisia capillaris* Thunb.

Characters: The dried new shoots, gray-green in color, form a loose, soft mass. They are completely covered with soft, white down. The stems, which are often broken, are slender, tortuous, and branching, measuring 6 to 10 cm in length 1.5 mm in diameter at the base. When the white hair is removed from the stalks, longitudinal markings can be seen. Leaves that are intact are usually attached to leafstalks, which are joined to the fine stems. This product gives off an unusual smell. Oregano (*Origanum vulgare*), often used as a substitute for this drug, is distinguished by its darker color.

Quality: The best quality is soft, green, with a strong aroma.

Production areas: China (Shaanxi, Shanxi, Anhui, and less importantly Shandong, Jiangsu, Hubei, Henan, Sichuan, Gansu, and Fujian).

Properties and actions: Slightly cold; acrid, bitter; nontoxic. Enters the liver, spleen, and bladder channels. Clears heat and disinhibits damp.

Indications: Damp and heat jaundice; inhibited urination; itchy wind sores and jie. Daily dosage: 10–15 g. Contraindicated in jaundice not caused by damp-heat. Used in *yin¹-chen²-hao¹ tang¹* (Capillaris Decoction, 321), *yin¹-chen² wu³ ling² san³* (Capillaris and Poria Five Powder, 322).

Remarks: Constituents: Polyeynes, monoterpenoids, sesquiterpenoids, and phenylpropanoids (volatile oil 0.1–1%): capillin, capillene, capillone, capillarin. Coumarins: scoparone (6, 7-di-O-methylesculetin, up to 1.98%). Chromones: capillarisin.

Similar drug: Herb of *Origanum vulgare* L.(Labiatae).

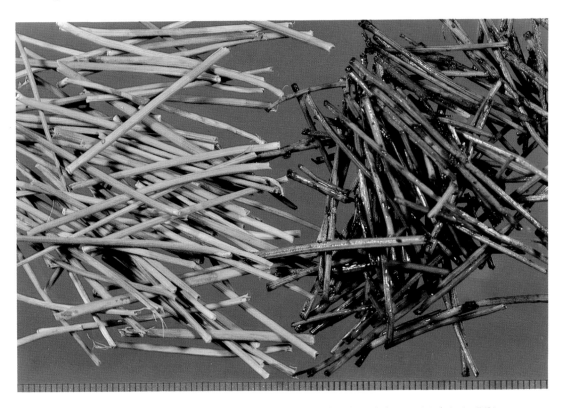

Ephedrae Herba: with nodes removed (left); mix-fried with honey (right). (×5/3)

190 EPHEDRAE HERBA

麻黃 *ma² huang²*. English: ephedra, mahuang. Japanese: *mao.*
Alternate name: 龍沙 *long² sha¹.*
Origin: Ephedraceae family. *Ephedra sinica* Stapf, *E. equisetina* Bge.,* *E. intermedia* Schrenk et Mey.,* *E. distachya* L.*
Characters: Fine, long cylindrical stalks, slightly flat, with few branches, 1–2 mm in diameter, usually cut into 2–3 cm lengths. The outer surface is light green, or light yellow green, with fine longitudinal ridges rough to the touch, and nodes 2.5–6 cm apart. At the nodes are two, or rarely three, membranous scaly leaves, which are 3–4 mm long, brown-red in color, triangular with a sharp, slightly bent tip. The stalks are brittle, and break easily, leaving a fibrous fracture that is light green in the surface layer, and brown red in the central medulla. They give off a slight fragrance. The roots and nodes are removed before use.
Quality: Dry, fat, light-green stalks with solid cores and a bitter, astringent taste are the best.
Production areas: China (Hebei, Henan, Shaanxi, Inner Mongolia, Liaoning, Shanxi).
Properties and actions: Warm; acrid and bitter. Enters the lung and bladder channels. Promotes sweating, calms dyspnea, and disinhibits water. Honey mix-frying reduces the diaphoretic action, making it suitable for debilitated patients with qi vacuity.
Indications: Exterior repletion cold damage patterns with aversion to cold, adiaphoretic fever, headache and nasal congestion, generalized joint pain; cough and dyspnea; wind water swelling; inhibited urination; stubborn wind bi; wind numbness; wind papules. Daily dosage: 1.5–6 g. Contraindicated in general weakness with spontaneous or night sweats and dyspnea. Used in *ma²-huang² tang¹* (Ephedra Decoction, 175), *ma² xing⁴ gan¹ shi² tang¹* (Ephedra, Apricot Kernel, Licorice, and Gypsum Decoction, 176), *ma²-huang² fu⁴-zi³ xi⁴-xin¹ tang¹* (Ephedra, Aconite, and Asarum Decoction, 174).
Remarks: Constituents: Alkaloids (ephedra alkaloids, 0.3–2%): (–)-ephedrine, (+)-pseudoephedrine, (–)-methylephedrine.

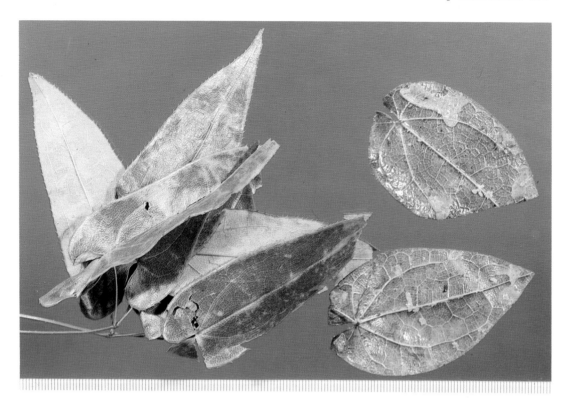

Epimedium sagittatum (left); *Epimedium grandiflorum*, mix-fried with sheep fat (right). (×5/6)

191 EPIMEDII HERBA

淫羊藿 *yin² yang² huo⁴*. English: epimedium. Japanese: *inyokaku*.
Alternate names: 仙靈脾 *xian¹ ling² pi²*, 羊藿 *yang² huo⁴*.
Origin: Berberidaceae family.
Epimedium grandiflorum Merr. [= *E. macranthum* Morr. et Decne.], *E. brevicornum* Maxim.,* *E. sagittatum* (Sieb. et Zucc.) Maxim.,* *E. acuminatum* Franch.*
Characters: The dried stalks of *E. grandiflorum*, are long, fine, and cylindrical, and hollow. They are 20–30 cm long, and brown in color, with longitudinal ridges and no hairs. Each stalk usually has three branches, each of which has 3 leaves at its extremity. The leaves are ovate, with pointed tips, cordate bases, and finely serrate margins. They are yellow-green and shiny on the upper surface, and gray-green on the lower undersurface, with a main central rib and finer, branching ribs. The leaves are paper thin and supple. *E. brevicornum* has cordate leaves, but is otherwise the same. The leaves of *E. sagittatum*, are arrow-shaped, i.e., they are longer, taper gradually to the apex, and have pointed lobes.
Quality: The best quality product has many, unbroken leaves and few stalks.
Production areas: China (Heilongjiang, Jilin, Liaoning, Shandong, Jiangsu, Jiangxi, Hunan, Guangxi, Sichuan, Guizhou, Shaanxi, and Gansu).
Properties and actions: Warm; acrid, sweet; nontoxic. Enters the liver and kidney channels. Supplements the kidney and fortifies yang; dispels wind and eliminates damp. Used mix-fried in sheep fat to enhance the yang-invigorating action.
Indications: Impotence; dribbling urination; hypertonicity of the sinews and bones; hemiplegia; lack of strength in lumbus and knees; wind-damp bi pain; insensitivity of the extremities. Daily dosage: 3–10 g. Contraindicated in yin vacuity and stirring ministerial fire. Used in *er⁴ xian¹ tang¹* (Two Immortals Decoction, 82).
Remarks: Constituents: *E. grandiflorum*: Flavonoids: icariin, icarisids I,II, epimedins A, B, C. Lignoids: (+)-syringaresinol-O-β-D-glucoside. Sesquiterpenoids: roseoside. Alkanes (volatile oil): cerylalcohol, hentriacontane.

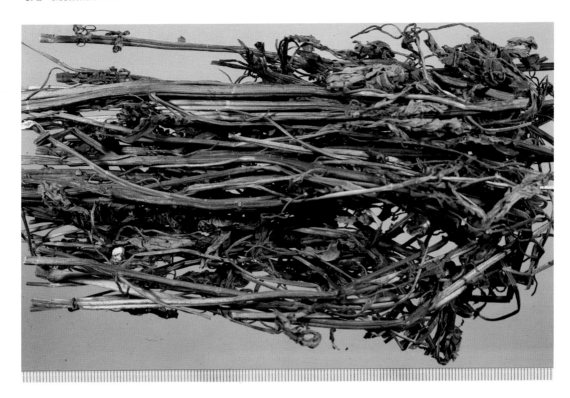

Menthae Herba. (×6/7)

192 MENTHAE HERBA

薄荷 *bo⁴ he²*. English: mint. L. Japanese: *hakka*.

Alternate name: 薄荷草 *bo⁴ he² cao³*

Origin: Labiatae family. *Mentha arvensis* L. var. *piperascens* Malinvaud,ᵉ *M. piperita* L.,• *M. spicata* L.,• *M. arvensis* L.•

Characters: The squared cylindrical stem of the dried herb is 15–35 cm long, and 2–4 mm thick, with opposite branches on the upper part, and nodes 3–7 cm apart. It is yellow-brown with a purple hue, or green in color, and is covered with white down that is densest at the ridges. It is brittle, breaking easily to show a white hollow interior. The leaves are shriveled, and often broken. Their upper surface is dark green, while their undersurface is pale green. They are brittle, and are covered with white down. At the ends of the branches are often yellow-brown verticillate inflorescences with multiple corollas.

Quality: Green, leafy plants with a strong scent and no roots are the best.

Production areas: China (cultivated in most parts, the main producers being Jiangsu, Zhejiang, and Jiangxi).

Properties and actions: Cool; acrid. Enters the lung and liver channels. Courses wind, dissipates heat, repels foulness and resolves toxin. Used crude to dissipate wind-heat, and mix-fried with honey to produce a stronger cough-suppressing action.

Indications: External wind-heat; headache; reddening of the eyes; sore, swollen throat; food stagnation and qi distention; mouth sores; toothache; sores; dormant papules. Daily dosage: 1.5–5 g. Contraindicated in yin vacuity and blood dryness, and in exterior vacuity with copious sweating. Used in *chuan¹-xiong¹ cha² tiao² san³* (Tea-Blended Ligusticum [Cnidium] Powder, 42), *qing¹ shang⁴ fang² feng¹ tang¹* (Upper-Body-Clearing Ledebouriella Decoction, 208).

Remarks: Constituents: Monoterpenoids, sesquiterpenoids, and alkanes (volatile oil, 0.65–2%); (–)-menthol (65–90%). Phenylpropanoids: rosmarinic acid (0.3–0.7%).

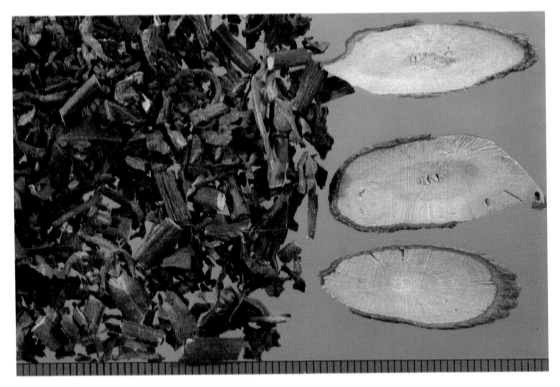

Postogemi Herba: stalks and leaves (left); thicker stems (right). (× 5/3)

193 POGOSTEMI (SEU AGASTACHES) HERBA

藿香 *huo⁴ xiang¹*. English: Patchouli. Japanese: *kakko*.

Alternate name: 土藿香 *tu³ huo⁴ xiang¹*.

Origin: Labiatae family. *Pogostemon cablin* (Blanco) Benth., *Agastache rugosa* (Fisch. et Mey.) O. Ktze.*

Characters: The dried herb *Pogostemon cablin* is 30–60 cm long, with opposite branches. The older stems, cylindrical and slightly squared, 4–10 mm in diameter, are grayish green or brown, with scant down. The younger stems are covered with dense down, and snap easily to reveal a greenish interior. The leaves, which are shriveled and torn, are soft and pliable, grayish or yellowish green and covered with hairs on each side. *Agastache rugosa* is similar, but has only scant hair on the stalks, and sometimes has a cylindrical inflorescence.

Quality: A strong aroma is a sign of superior quality.

Production areas: China (Guangdong) and Philippines.

Properties and actions: Slightly warm; acrid. Enters the lung, spleen, and stomach channels. Normalizes qi, harmonizes the center, repels foulness and dispels damp. The stems regulate qi and loosen the chest.

Indications: Summerheat-damp colds and flu; fever and chills; headache; glomus and oppression in the chest and venter; vomiting and diarrhea; malarial disease; dysenteric disease; bad breath. Daily dosage: 5–10 g. Contraindicated in effulgent yin vacuity fire, and stomach vacuity with desire to vomit. Used in *huo⁴-xiang¹ zheng⁴ qi⁴ san³* (Agastache/Patchouli Qi-Correcting Powder, 137), *bu² huan⁴ jin¹ zheng⁴ qi⁴ san³* (Satisfaction Guaranteed Qi-Correcting Powder, 29).

Remarks: Constituents: Volatile oil (pachouli oil 4–5%): pachoulic alcohol, pogostol.

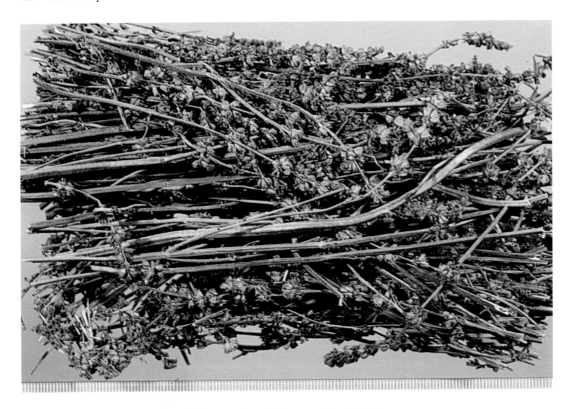

Schizonepetae Herba seu Flos. (×5/3)

194 SCHIZONEPETAE HERBA SEU FLOS

荆芥 *jing¹ jie⁴*. English: schizonepeta. Japanese: *keigai*.

Origin: Labiatae family. *Schizonepeta tenuifolia* (Benth.) Briq., *S. multifida* (L.) Briq.*

Characters: The stem of the dried herb is squared with a longitudinal furrow on each face, and branches on the upper part. It is about 45–90 cm long, and 3–5 mm in diameter. The exterior surface has a purple hue, and is covered in short hairs. It is light, and snaps easily, revealing a yellow, white fibrous transverse section with a white medulla in the center. The leaves, which are opposite-growing, with deep incisions forming long lobes, are brittle and break off easily. At the top of the stalk is a verticillate cylindrical, green inflorescence, 7–10 mm in diameter, with green calyx tubes from which the corollas have fallen and which contain four black seeds.

Quality: Herbs with a pale purple hue, fine stems, and numerous inflorescences are the best.

Production areas: China (Jiangsu, Zhejiang, Jiangxi, Hubei, and Hunan).

Properties and actions: Warm; acrid. Enters the lung and liver channels. Effuses the exterior, dispels wind, and rectifies the blood; staunches bleeding when used char-fried.

Indications: Colds and fever; headache; sore, swollen throat; wind stroke with clenched jaws; spontaneous external bleeding; blood in the stool; uterine bleeding; postpartrum blood dizziness; yong, jie, and sores; scrofulous lumps. Daily dosage: 5–10 g. Contraindicated in exterior vacuity with spontaneous sweating, and in yin vacuity headache. Used in *jing¹-fang² bai⁴ du² san³* (Schizonepeta and Ledebouriella Toxin-Vanquishing Powder, 150), *jing¹-jie⁴ lian² ian²-qiao² tang¹* (Schizonepeta and Forsythia Decoction, 151), *shi² wei⁴ bai⁴ du² tang¹* (Ten-Ingredient Toxin-Vanquishing Decoction, 244).

Remarks: Constituents: Volatile oil (0.5–1.8%): (+)-menthone (43%), (±)-menthone, (–)-isomenthone, (–)-pulegone (34%), (+)-limonene. Monoterpenoids: schizonepetosides A, B, C, D, E. Flavonoids: luteolin, hesperetin, hesperidin.

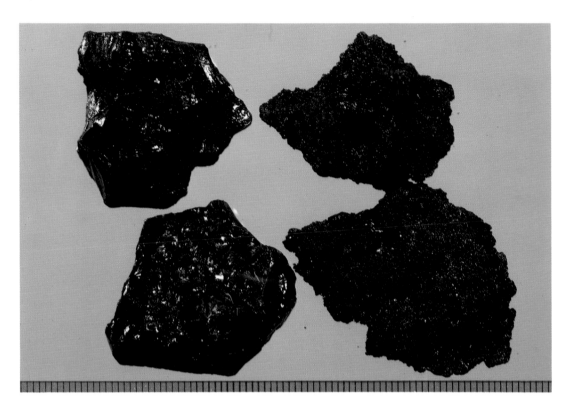

Aloe: crude (left); calcined (right). (×5/3)

195 ALOE

蘆薈 *lu² hui⁴*. English: aloe. Japanese: *rokai, aroe.*

Alternate names: 訥會 *na⁴ hui⁴*, 盧會 *lu² hui⁴*.

Origin: Liliaceae family. *Aloe vera* L., *A. ferox* Mill., *A. vera* L. var. *chinensis* (Haw.) Berger.

Characters: Lucid aloe (Aloe Lucide [*tou⁴ ming² lu² hui⁴*] made from *A. ferox*, is a dark reddish brown or black mass, occsionally coated with a yellow powder. Its broken edges are smooth as glass. Liver-colored aloe (Aloe Hepatitis [*gan¹ se⁴*]), made from *A. vera*, is a black, non-translucent mass whose fractures appear like wax.

Quality: Strong flavor and absence of impurities are signs of good quality.

Production areas: *Aloe vera:* Africa and West Indies (also cultivated in China). *A. ferox:* Southern Africa. *A. vera* var. *chinensis:* China (Guangdong, Guangxi, Fujian, Sichuan).

Properties and actions: Cold; bitter. Enters the liver, heart, and spleen channels. Clears heat, frees the stools and kills worms. Usually used calcined to moderate the effect.

Indications: Heat bind constipation; menstrual block; child fright epilepsy; gan heat; worm accumulation; hemorrhoids and fistulae; atrophic rhinitis; scrofulous lumps. Daily dosage: 0.5–1.5g. Contraindicated in spleen-stomach vacuity. Used in *lu²-hui⁴ wan²* (Aloe Pills, 173), *dang¹-gui¹ long² hui⁴ wan²* (Tangkuei, Gentian, and Aloe Pills, 58).

Remarks: Constituents: Anthrones (aloin, 14.8–24.1%): barbaloin, isobarbaloin (aloe-emodin-9-anthrone 10-C-glucopyranosides; aloin A (10R), aloin B(10S). Anthraquinones: chrysophanol, aloe-emodin. Chromones: aloesone, aloesin. Phenylpropanoids: cinnamoyl resinotannol, *p*-coumaroyl resinotannol.

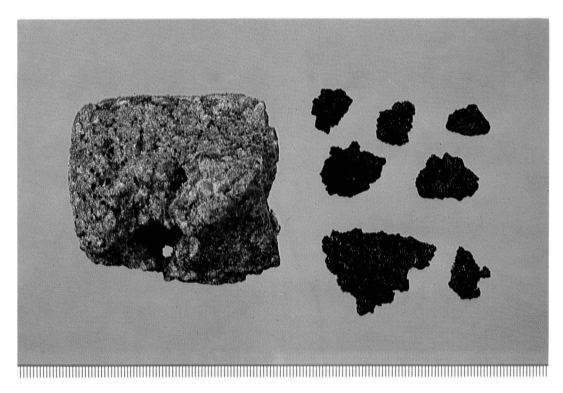

Asafoetida: crude (left); stir-fried (right). (×7/8)

196 ASAFOETIDA

阿魏 e^l wei^4. English: asafetida (asafoetida). Japanese: *agi*.

Alternate name: 阿魏 a^4 wei^4.

Origin: Umbelliferae family. *Ferula assafoetida* L. [=*F. foetida* Regel.], *F. caspica* Marsh.-Bieb.,* *F. conocaula* Eug.*

Characters: This product comes in lumps of different shapes and sizes, and is comprised of fine globular granules. It is dark yellow-brown on the outside, and when stored for a long time, it takes on a reddish hue. Lumps of fresh resin when broken apart, present a cross section that is cream or light brown, sometimes mingled with red. This product is light in weight, and has a powerful fetid odor, and a bitter, acrid taste. It is ground before use.

Production areas: Iran, Afghanistan, and China (Xinjiang).

Properties and actions: Warm; bitter, acrid; nontoxic. Enters the liver, spleen, and stomach channels. Disperses accumulation and kills worms. It is usually stir-fried to moderate the effect.

Indications: Concretions and conglomerations; lump glomus; worm and meat-type food accumulations; frigid pain in the abdomen and region of heart; malarial disease; dysenteric disease. Daily dosage: 0.5–1.5 g. Contraindicated in pregnancy and in spleen-stomach vacuity. Used in e^l-wei^4 hua^4 pi^3 san^3 (Asafetida Glomus-Transforming Powder, 78), e^l-wei^4 wan^2 (Asafetida Pills, 79).

Remarks: Constituents: Volatile oil (6–17%): *sec*-butyl-propenyl-disulfide. Resin (40–60%): ferulic acid ester, farnesiferol A,-B,-C.

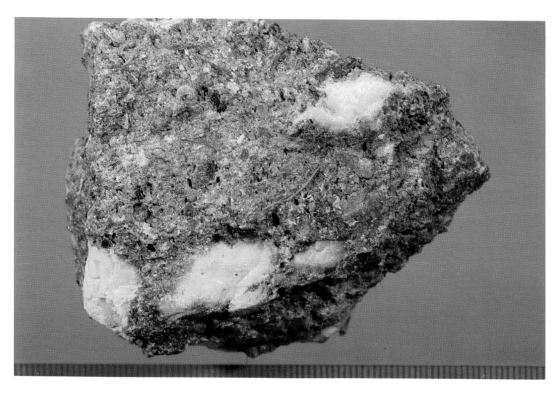

Sumatra benzoin. (× 5/3)

197 BENZOINUM

安息香 an^1 xi^2 $xiang^1$. English: benzoin. Japanese: *ansokuko*.

Alternate name: 安息香脂 an^1 xi^2 $xiang^1$ zhi^1.

Origin: Styracaceae family. *Styrax benzoin* Dryand., *S. tonkinensis* (Pier.) Craib.

Characters: Sumatra benzoin (Benzoinum Sumatrensis [su^1 men^2 da^2 la^4 an^1 xi^2 $xiang^1$]), the dried resin of *Styrax benzoin*, is composed of globular granules compressed into a lumps of varying sizes that are reddish or grayish brown with white or gray-white patches. Siam benzoin (Benzoinum Siamense [yue^4 nan^2 an^1 xi^2 $xiang^1$]), which comes from *Styrax tonkinensis*, takes the form of small lumps or flat tearlike globules that are a few centimeters in diameter, about 1 cm thick, brown on the outside and white on the inside. Both types become hard when low heat is applied for a long time, and melt at high temperatures.

Quality: The best quality has yellow and white granules and a strong aroma.

Production areas: Sumatra benzoin: Indonesia (Sumatra and Java). Siam benzoin: Vietnam, Laos, Thailand, and China (Yunnan, Guangxi).

Properties and actions: Balanced; pungent and bitter; nontoxic. Enters the heart, liver, and spleen channels. Opens the portals; repels foulness; moves qi and the blood.

Indications: Sudden stroke and fulminant inversion; pain in the abdomen and region of the heart; postpartum dizziness; child fright epilepsy; wind bi lumbar pain. Daily dosage: 0.3–1 g. Contraindicated in effulgent yin vacuity fire. Used in an^1-xi^2-$xiang^1$ wan^2 (Benzoin Pills, 2).

Remarks: Constituents: *S. benzoin:* Phenylpropanoids: cinnamyl cinnamate (2–3%), coniferyl cinnamate, phenylpropyl cinnamate. Triterpenoids: sumaresinolic acid (6-hydroxyoleanolic acid or sumaresinol), siaresinolic acid (19-hydroxyoleanolic acid or siaresinol).

S. tonkinensis: coniferylbenzoate (68–75%), cinnamyl benzoate (2.3%), benzoic acid (12%).

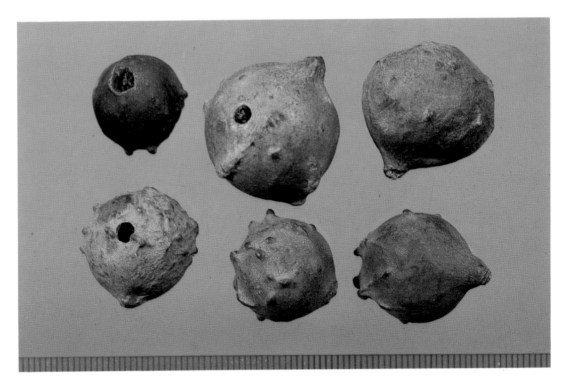

Galla Halepensis. (× 5/3)

198 GALLA HALEPENSIS

没食子 mo^4 shi^2 zi^3. English: Aleppo gall. Japanese: *moshokushi.*

Alternate names: 没石子 mo^4 shi^2 zi^3, 無食子 wu^2 shi^2 zi^3.

Origin: Fagaceae family. *Quercus infectoria* Olivier (host), *Cynips gallae-tinctoriae* Olivier (parasite).

Characters: This gallnut is an excrescence that develops in the tissue of the young branches of the tree *Quercus infectoria* owing to attacks from the parasite *Cynips gallae-tinctoriae.* It is spherical in shape, 1–2.5 cm in diameter. It has a short stem by which it was attached to the tree. It is gray or gray-brown and with wartlike protuberances. It is hard, and does not break cleanly. The cross section is pale yellow and glossy. In the middle is often the body of an insect; if not, there is a hole connecting the center to the exterior, through which the insect escaped. This gallnut is crushed before use.

Quality: Large, heavy galls that are grey in color are the best. Ones perforated by holes are considered inferior.

Production areas: Greece, Turkey, Iran, and India.

Properties and actions: Warm; bitter; nontoxic. Enters the lung, spleen, and kidney channels. Secures qi and astringes essence; constrains the lung and staunches bleeding.

Indications: Large intestinal vacuity efflux; persistent diarrhea; blood in the stool; seminal emission; genital sweating; cough; expectoration of blood; toothache; bleeding due to injury; persistent sores. Daily dosage: 3–5 g. Contraindicated in the initial stages of diarrhea, or when damp-heat or accumulation and stagnation are present. Used in mo^4-shi^2-zi^3 wan^2 (Aleppo Gall Pills, 186).

Remarks: Constituents: Tannoids: (gallotannins) tri-nona-galloyl-D-glucoses (50–70%): gallic acid (2–4%), ellagic acid (ca. 2%), *m*-digallic acid.

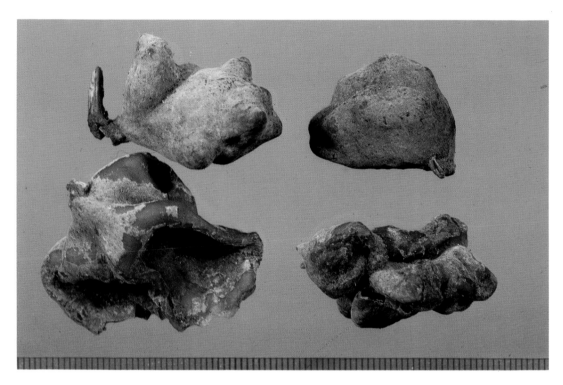

Galla Rhois: Many-horned (left) and Single-horned (right). (×5/3)

199 GALLA RHOIS (RHOIS GALLA)

五倍子 *wu³ bei⁴ zi³*. English: sumac gallnut. Japanese: *gobaishi*.

Alternate names: 百蟲倉 *bai³ chong² cang¹*, 倍子 *bei⁴ zi³*.

Origin: Anacardiaceae family. *Rhus chinensis* Mill. [= *R. javanica* L.] (host), *Melaphis chinensis* (Bell) (parasite), *Rhus paitan* Tsai et Tang (parasite).

Characters: The gall created by the parasite *Melaphis chinensis* is 8 cm long, and 5 cm in diameter. Being rhomboid or ovate in shape with irregular protuberances, it is called the "many-horned" variety (*jiao³ bei⁴*). The exterior surface is a yellowish or grayish brown with gray hairs. The skin is 1–2 cm thick, is hard, and easily broken into pieces. The fracture appears horny, and the inside is hollow, containing the small dead body of the insect and a wax-like substance. The gall of *Rhus paitan* is spindle-shaped or long ovate, without protuberances (single-horned, [*du⁴ bei⁴*]. It has little hair. The shell is 2–3 mm thick. The cross section when broken open appears very horny, and has a brighter luster than the gall of *Melaphis chinensis*.

Quality: Thick-skinned, unbroken gallnuts are the best.

Production areas: China (Sichuan, Guizhou, Yunnan, Shaanxi, Hubei, Guangxi), Japan and Korea.

Properties and actions: Balanced; sour. Enters the lung, stomach, and large intestine channels. Constrains the lung; astringes the intestine; staunches bleeding; resolves toxin.

Indications: Enduring lung vacuity cough; enduring dysentery or diarrhea; prolapse of the anus; spontaneous or night sweating; seminal emission; blood in the stool; spontaneous external or uterine bleeding; bleeding from external injury; sores and boils; ingrown eyelashes. Daily dosage: 1.5–6 g. Contraindicated in cough due externally contracted wind-cold or lung repletion heat, and in diarrhea in which accumulation and stagnation has not been cleared. Used in *wu³-bei⁴-zi³ san³* (Sumac Gallnut Powder, 275), *yu⁴ suo³ dan¹* (Jade Lock Elixir, 328).

Remarks: Constituents: Tannoids (gallotannins, 65–75% (Chinese gall); 60–68% (Japanese gall): mono-dodeca-galloyl-glucoses (main: penta-octa-galloylglucoses); gallic acid (2–4%), *m*-digallic acid.

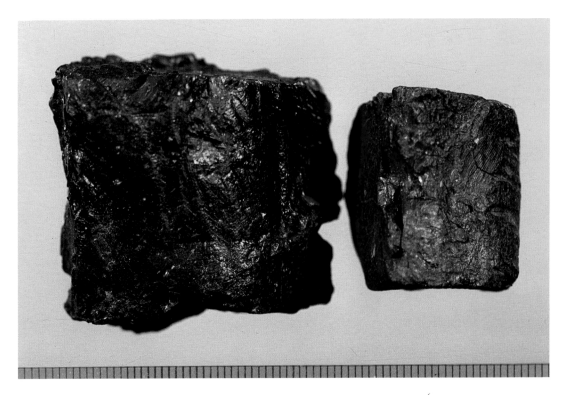

Gambir Catechu. (×2)

200 GAMBIR CATECHU (CATECHU)

孩兒茶 *hai² er² cha²*. English: (black and white) cutch, kutch, catechu. Japanese: *gaijicha*.
Alternate names: 烏爹泥 *wu¹ die¹ ni²*, 兒茶 *er² cha²*.
Origin: *Acacia catechu* (L) willd. (Leguminosae), *Uncaria gambir* Roxb. (Rubiaceae).
Characters: Black cutch (Catechu Atrum [*hei¹ er² cha²*]), which is made from *Acacia catechu* of the Leguminosae family, comes in black lumps, which are hard on the outside, and softer on the inside. The lumps break easily to expose a shiny, porous fracture. The powder is dark brown. White cutch (Catechu Album [*zong¹ er² cha²*]), made from *Uncaria gambir* of the Rubiaceae family, comes in brown, roughly square or rectangular lumps, about 2–3 cm thick. The exterior surface is red-gray or light brown, porous, and without luster. The inside is light brown or orange brown. It only has a faint smell. It is ground before use.
Quality: Products that are gluey in substance, and dark in color with a red hue, and have a strong bitter, astringent taste are best.
Production areas: *Acacia catechu*: China (Yunnan). *Uncaria gambier*: Indonesia and Malaysia.
Properties and actions: Cool; bitter, astringent; nontoxic. Enters the heart and lung channels. Clears heat, transforms phlegm, staunches bleeding, disperses food, engenders flesh, and settles pain.
Indications: Phlegm-heat cough; wasting thirst; blood ejection; spontaneous external bleeding; blood in the urine; blood dysentery; profuse uterine bleeding; child indigestion; gan of the teeth and gums; mouth sores; throat bi. Daily dosage: 1–3 g. Contraindicated in cold-damp patterns. Used in *long¹-gu³ er²-cha² san³* (Dragon Bone and Cutch Powder. 171).
Remarks: Constituents: Tannoids: (+)-catechin (main), (±)-catechin, (+)-epicatechin; gambiriins A_1, A_2, A_3, B_1, B_2, B_3, C; catechutannic acid (22–50%): gallic acid, ellagic acid.

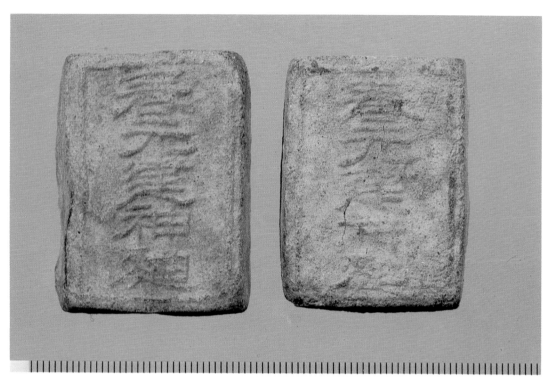

Massa Medicata Fermentata. (× 5/3)

201 MASSA MEDICATA FERMENTATA

神麴 *shen² qu¹*. English: medicated leaven. Japanese: *shinkiku*.

Alternate names: 六神麴 *liu⁴ shen² qu¹*, 神麴 *shen² qu¹*.

Characters: This is a fermented mixture of wheat flour blended with other agents including Phaseoli Calcarati Semen (*chi⁴ xiao³ dou⁴*) Armeniacae Semen (*xing⁴ ren²*), and the juice of Artemisae Apiaceae seu Annuae Herba (*qing¹ hao¹*) and Xanthii Caulis et Folium (*cang¹ er³*). It comes in cakes of different forms and colors depending on the constituents used. If the wheat flour content is higher, the color is light yellow brown. If the bran content is higher, the color is darker. The surface is smooth, and usually bears a brand name molded in relief. It bears a musty, fermented smell.

Quality: Clean, dry, fresh-smelling products are the best.

Production areas: China (Fujian, and other areas), and Japan.

Properties and actions: Warm; acrid, sweet; nontoxic. Enters the spleen and stomach channels. Fortifies the spleen and the stomach; disperses food and harmonizes the center. Used scorch-fried or stir-fried in bran to enhance its effects.

Indications: Food stagnation; thoracic glomus and abdominal distention; vomiting and diarrhea; postpartum stasis and abdominal pain; abdominal distention in children. Daily dosage: 6–12 g. Use with care in excessive stomach acidity and in pregnancy. Used in *hua⁴ shi² yang³ pi² tang¹* (Food-Transforming Spleen-Nourishing Decoction, 124), *shen²-qu¹ san³* (Medicated Leaven Powder, 233), *qu¹ zhu² wan²* (Medicated Leaven and Atractylodes Pills, 213).

Remarks: Constituents: Volatile oil. Yeast. Proteins. Vitamins.

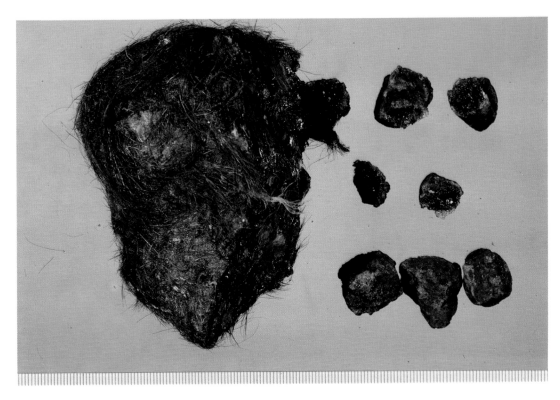

Myrrha: wrapped in dogskin (left) and prepared (right). (×7/8)

202 MYRRHA

沒藥 *mo⁴ yao⁴*. English: myrrh. Japanese: *motsuyaku.*

Alternate name: 末藥 *mo⁴ yao⁴.*

Origin: Burseraceae family. *Commiphora molmol* Engl. [= *C. myrrha* Engl.].

Characters: This resin comes in irregular granules that stick together in lumps of different sizes. The color is red-brown or yellow-brown. The lumps are brittle, and break into semitranslucent granules or thin pieces. It gives off a fine a faint aroma. This product comes wrapped in dog's skin.

Quality: Strong, long-lasting aroma, and few impurities are signs of superior quality. Somalian is usually the best.

Production areas: Somalia, Ethiopia, and the Arabian Peninsula.

Properties and actions: Balanced; bitter; nontoxic. Enters the liver channel. Dissipates the blood and eliminates stasis; disperses swellings and settles pain.

Indications: Impact injury; incised wounds; sinew and bone pain; pain in the abdomen and region of the heart; concretions and conglomerations; menstrual block; painful, swollen yong and ju; hemorrhoids; eye screens. Daily dosage: 3–5 g. Contraindicated in pregnancy. Used in *bu³-gu³-zhi¹ wan²* (Psoralea Pills, 32).

Remarks: Constituents: Resins: α-, β-, γ-commiphoric acid. Volatile oil (2.5–9%): cuminaldehyde, eugenol.

Allied drugs: (1) Somali myrrh: resin of *Commiphora molmol* Engl., (2) Arabian myrrh: resin of *C. abyssinica* Engl., (3) Bissabol myrrh: resin of *C. erythraea* Engl.

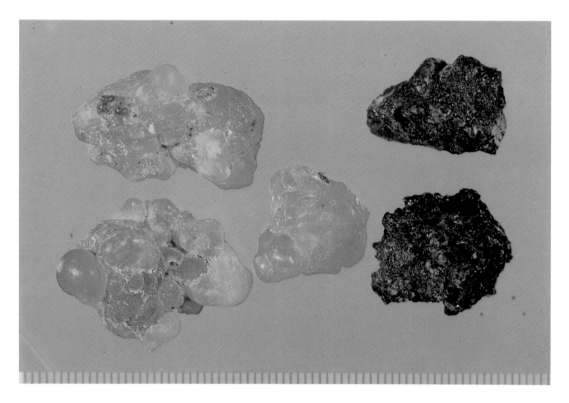

Olibanum: crude (left); processed (right). (×2)

203 OLIBANUM (GUMMI OLIBANUM)

乳香 *ru³ xiang¹*

English: frankincense, olibanum. Japanese: *nyuko.*

Alternate names: 乳頭香 *ru³ tou² xiang¹*, 熏陸 *xun¹ lu⁴.*

Origin: Burseraceae family. *Boswellia carterii* Birdw.

Characters: This resin is in nipple or teardrop shapes, or irregular lumps, 0.5–3 cm long. It is pale yellow with a faint green hue, and is semitranslucent. There is white dust on the surface. It is brittle, and the broken edge usually has a waxlike appearance, though rarely it has a glass-like luster. It has a delicate aroma, and when processed it turns to a blackish brown and glistens.

Quality: Pale yellow, semitranslucent resin in granular form, and with powder that sticks to the finger and a good aroma is best.

Production areas: On the Red Sea coast of Somalia and Ethiopia.

Properties and actions: Warm; bitter, acrid; slightly toxic. Enters the heart, liver, and spleen channels. Regulates qi and quickens the blood; relieves pain, expels toxin. Stir-fry and remove oil, or stir-fry in vinegar for strong blood-quickening and pain-relieving action.

Indications: Qi and blood stagnation; pain in the abdomen and region of the heart; swelling toxin of yong and sores; impact injury; painful menstruation; postpartum blood stasis with stabbing pain. Daily dosage: 3–7 g. Contraindicated in pregnancy. Used in *bu³-gu³-zhi¹ wan²* (Psoralea Pills, 32), *ding¹-xiang¹ shi⁴-di⁴ tang¹* (Clove and Persimmon Decoction, 70), *xiao³ jin¹ dan¹* (Minor Golden Elixir, 301), *juan¹ bi⁴ tang¹* (Bi-Alleviating Decoction, 156), *su¹-he²-xiang¹ wan²* (Liquid Styrax Pills, 257).

Remarks: Constituents: Resins (60–70%): free: α-, β- boswellic acid (ca. 33%), combined: boswellic acid (ca. 1.5%), olibanoresene (ca. 33%). Volatile oil (3–8%): pinene, dipentene, α-, β-phellandrene. Bitter substances: 0.5%.

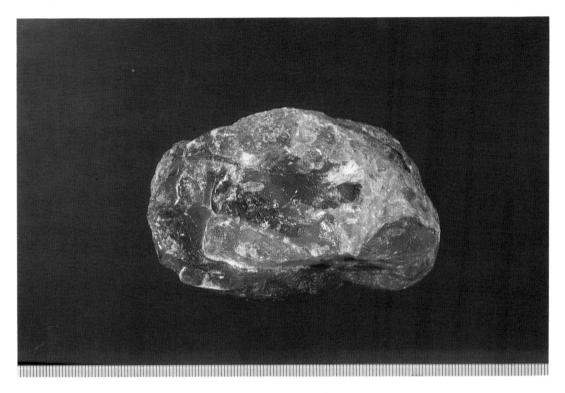

Pini Resina. (×7/8)

204 PINI RESINA

松香 *song¹ xiang¹*. English: rosin. Japanese: *shoko.*
Alternate name: 松脂香 *song¹ zhi¹ xiang¹.*
Origin: Pinaceae family. *Pinus massoniana* Lamb.
Characters: This resin takes the form of semitranslucent irregular lumps of differing sizes. The exterior surface is golden yellow, and often has a lighter yellow powder sticking to it. It becomes harder when subjected to a steady low heat. It is brittle, and the fractures are shiny like glass. When subjected to high temperatures it melts, and burns, giving of a thick brown smoke.
Quality: The best quality comes in neat lumps, and is semitranslucent, oleaceous, and has a strong smell.
Production areas: China (Guangdong, Guangxi, Fujian, Hunan, Jiangxi, Zhejiang, Anhui).
Properties and actions: Warm; bitter, sweet; nontoxic. Enters the liver and spleen channels. Dispels wind, dries damp, expels pus, draws out toxin, engenders flesh, and relieves pain.
Indications: Yong and ju; clove sores; hemorrhoids and fistulae; malign sores; jie and xian; bald white sores; incised wounds; sprains; wind-damp bi pain; itching due to pestilential wind. Daily dosage: Apply topically as a powder. Grind to a powder and apply topically to all types of toxin swellings.
Remarks: Constituents: Diterpenoids (resin acids: ca. 90%): abietic acid (main), neoabietic acid, palustric acid, dihydroabietic acid, dehydroabietic acid, pimaric acid, isopimaric acid.
Rosin is now obtained as a by-product from the kraft pulping process (sulfate rosin or tall oil rosin).
Similar drug: Terbinthina, balsam of *Pinus palustris* Mill.

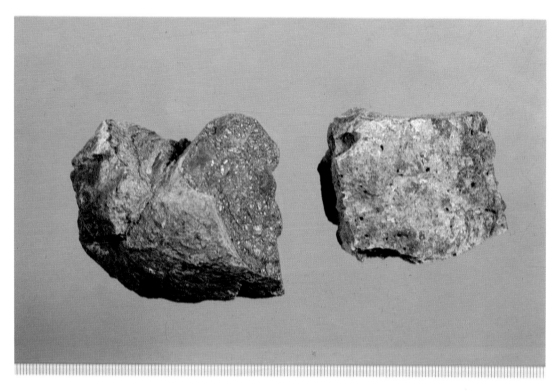

Ambra Grisea. (×7/8)

205 AMBRA GRISEA

龍涎香 *long² xian² xiang¹*. English: ambergris. Japanese: *ryuzenko*.

Alternate name: 龍腹香 *long² fu⁴ xiang¹*.

Origin: Physoteridae family. *Physeter catodon* L.

Characters: Ambergris, found floating in or on the shores of the tropical and semitropical waters, is ash-gray, yellow or black, sometimes variegated, and has the consistency of wax, sticking to the teeth when chewed. It is a pathological secretion that accumulates in the intestines of the sperm whale (*Physeter catodon*). It is crushed before use.

Quality: Black or brown ambergris with a loose consistency is considered the best.

Production areas: China (East and South China Seas).

Properties and actions: Fishy; sweet, sour; nontoxic. Transforms phlegm and opens the portals; moves qi and quickens the blood; dissipates binds and relieves pain; disinhibits water and frees strangury. Has an antispasmodic effect similar to that of Moschus (*she⁴ xiang¹*).

Indications: Cough and dyspnea; qi counterflow; qi bind; concretions and gatherings; pain in the abdomen and region of the heart; strangury. Daily dosage: 0.3–1 g. Contraindicated in wind-cold dyspnea.

Remarks: Constituents: ambrein 25–45%, *epi*-coprostenol 30–40%, coprosterol 1.5%.

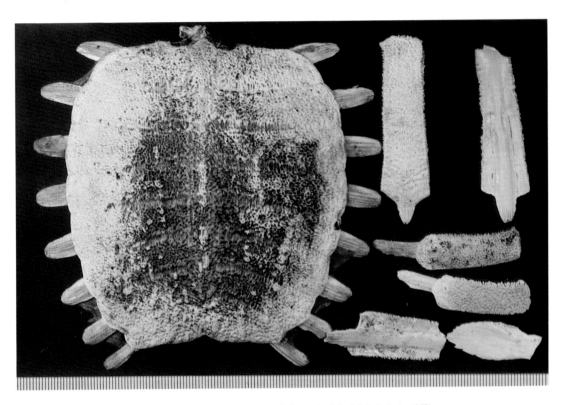

Amydae Carapax: crude (left); stir-fried (right). (×6/7)

206 AMYDAE CARAPAX

鱉甲 *bie¹ jia³*. English: turtle (or amyda) shell. Japanese: *bekko*.

Alternate names: 鱉殼 *bie¹ ke²*, 鱉甲尖 *bie¹ jia³ jian¹*.

Origin: Trionychidae family. *Amyda sinensis* Wiegmann.

Characters: The complete dried shell is ovate or elliptical, 10–20 cm long, 7–15 cm wide, and about 5 mm thick. It gray-brown or blackish green, bulges slightly on the dorsal side, and has wrinkles and protuberant spots. There are distinct protuberances over the ribs, between which are serrated transverse sutures. The inside is white, with the spine running down the middle, and eight ribs transverse ribs that project beyond the edge of the shell. The shell is hard, but is easily broken at the sutures. It gives off a slightly fishy smell.

Quality: Large, thick shells without any remains of the flesh or putrid odor are best.

Production areas: China (Hubei, Anhui, Jiangsu, Henan, Hunan, Zhejiang).

Properties and actions: Cold; salty; nontoxic. Enters the liver and spleen channels. Nourishes yin and clears heat; calms the liver and extinguishes wind; softens hardness and dissipates binds. Used crude to enrich yin and subdue yang, stir-fried for steaming bone fever, and mix-fried with vinegar to soften hardness and dissipate binds.

Indications: Steaming bone taxation fever; stirring wind due to yin vacuity; mother of taxation malaria; concretions and conglomerations; elusive and bowstring masses; menstrual block; scant uterine bleeding; child fright epilepsy. Daily dosage: 10–12 g. Use with care in pregnancy and in spleen-stomach yang debilitation with reduced food intake and thin stool. Used in *qin²-jiao¹ bie¹-jia³ san³* (Macrophylla and Turtle Shell Powder, 205), *huang²-qi² bie¹-jia³ san³* (Astragalus and Turtle Shell Powder, 132).

Remarks: Constituents: Animal gelatin, proteins.

Similar animals: *Amyda maackii* Brandt (Korea); *A. schlegelii* Brandt (northern China); *A. japonica* Temminck et Schlegel (Japan).

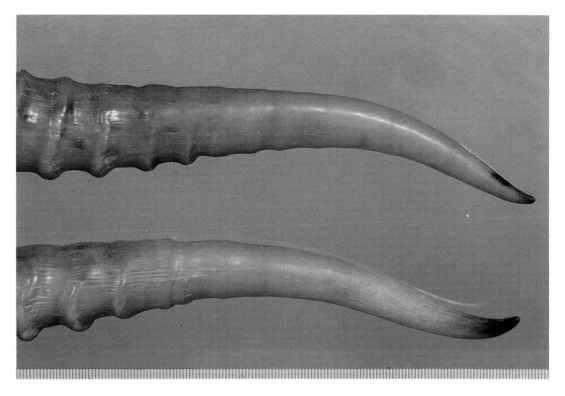

Antelopis Cornu. (×1)

207 ANTELOPIS CORNU

羚羊角 *ling² yang² jiao³*. English: antelope horn. Japanese: *reiyokaku*.
Alternate name: 羚羊角屑*ling² yang² jiao³ xie⁴*.
Origin: Bovidae family. *Saiga tatarica* L.
Characters: The complete horn is funnel-shaped and slightly curved, 25–40 cm long, about 3 cm in diameter at the base. It is a pale smoky yellow, darker at the base. There are 10–20 protuberant rings (fewer in younger horns) evenly distributed over the length of the horn but for the tip. Young horn is translucent and has blood streaks and black speckles. Older horn has no black speckles, and has longitudinal cracks. The transverse section at the base shows a bony plug that forms the core of a third to a half of the length of the horn. The plug has a serrrate edge that meshes tightly with the bone. When it is removed, the horn is left partly hollow, and there is a hole that further penetrates to the end of the horn – a unique feature of antelope horn.
Quality: Young, pale, shiny horn without cracks is best.
Production areas: China (Xinjiang).
Properties and actions: Cold; salty; nontoxic. Enters the liver and heart channels. Calms the liver and extinguishes wind; clears heat and settles fright; resolves toxin.
Indications: Tetany and clouding of the spirit in febrile disease; delirious mania; headache and dizziness; fright epilepsy and spasm; reddening of the eyes; eye screens. Daily dosage: 1.5–3 g. Contraindicated in the absence heat in the liver channel. Used in *ling²-yang²-jiao³ wan²* (Antelope Horn Pills, 165), *zi¹ shou⁴ jie³ yu³ tang¹* (Life-Prolonging Speech-Returning Decoction, 350).
Remarks: Constituents: Proteins.
Similar drugs: Horn of *Gazella gutturosa* Pallas, *Pantholops hodgsonii* Abel, *Naemorhedus goral* Hard., and *Procarpa picticaudata* Hodgson.

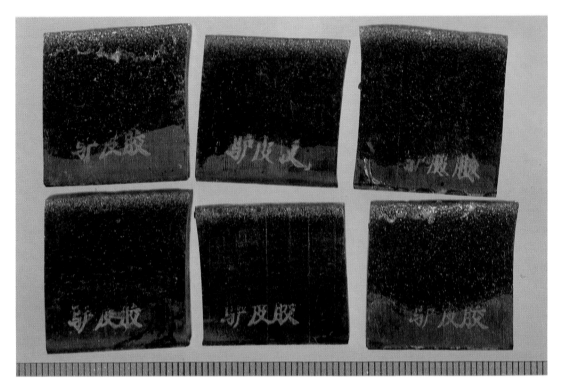

Asini Corii Gelatinum. (×5/3)

208 ASINI CORII GELATINUM

阿膠 *e¹ jiao¹*. English: ass hide glue. Japanese: *akyo.*

Alternate name: 眞阿膠 *zhen¹ e¹ jiao¹.*

Origin: Equidae family. *Equus asinus* L.

Characters: This product takes the form of neat rectangular blocks, usually about 8.5 cm long, 3.7 cm thick, and 0.7 cm or 1.5 cm thick. It is dark brown or black, smooth, shiny, and slightly translucent. It is brittle, and can be easily broken to leave a fracture very similar to the surface of the block. It has only a faint smell.

Quality: Black, shiny, translucent blocks that have no unpleasant odor and do not soften in hot weather are best.

Production areas: China (manufactured in Shandong, Zhejiang, and less importantly Shanghai, Beijing, Tianjin, and Wuhan).

Properties and actions: Balanced; sweet; nontoxic. Enters the lung, liver, and kidney channels. Enriches yin and supplements the blood; quiets the fetus. Stir-fry with clam-shell powder to moisten the lung and transform phlegm, suppress cough and staunch bleeding. Stir-fry with Pollen Typhae (*pu² huang²*) to quicken the blood, staunch bleeding, transform stasis.

Indications: Blood vacuity; vacuity taxation cough; blood ejection; spontaneous external bleeding; blood in the stool; menstrual irregularities; uterine bleeding in or outside pregnancy (stir-fry with Pollen Typhae); insomnia with dry cough and bloody sputum such as in pulmonary tuberculosis). Daily dosage: 5–10 g. Use with care in spleen-stomach vacuity. Used in *e¹-jiao¹ san³* (Ass Hide Glue Powder, 75), *e¹-jiao¹ shao²-yao⁴ tang¹* (Ass Hide Glue and Peony Decoction, 76), *xiong¹ gui¹ jiao¹ ai⁴ tang¹* (Ligusticum [Cnidium], Tangkuei, Ass Hide Glue, and Mugwort Decoction, 307), *huang²-lian² e¹-jiao¹ tang¹* (Coptis and Ass Hide Glue Decoction, 129), *zhi⁴-gan¹-cao³ tang¹* Honey-Fried Licorice Decoction, 345), *zhu¹ ling² tang¹* (Polyporus Decoction, 346).

Remarks: Constituents: collagen, glutin.

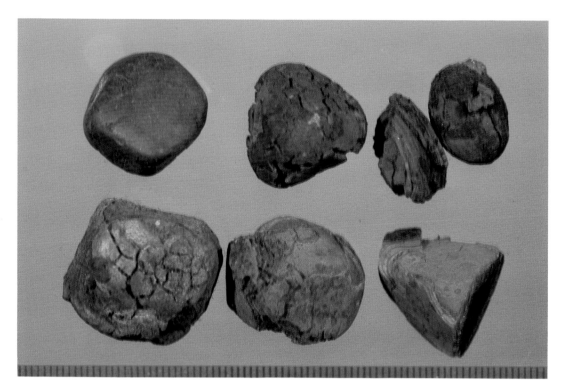

Bezoar Bovis. (× 5/3)

209 BEZOAR BOVIS

牛黃 *niu² huang²*. English: bovine bezoar. Japanese: *goo*.

Alternate name: 犀牛黃 *xi¹ niu² huang²*.

Origin: Bovidae family. *Bos taurus* L. var. *domesticus* Gmelin.

Characters: This product comes is round lumps, or sometimes in a tubular form. The exterior surface is earth brown in color, and has a fine granular texture with a shiny surface that is cracked in places. It is light and brittle. When broken up, the annular layers of the structure can be seen. It is fresh to the taste, and gradually melts without sticking to the teeth. It is ground to a powder before use.

Quality: Chinese bezoar is the best.

Production areas: China (Beijing, Hebei, Inner Mongolia, Liaoning, Heilongjiang, Shaanxi, Gansu, Henan), Canada, U.S.A., Argentina, Uruguay, Chili, Bolivia.

Properties and actions: Balanced; bitter and sweet; slightly toxic. Enters the heart and liver channels. Clears the heart; transforms phlegm; disinhibits the gallbladder; and settles fright.

Indications: Clouding of the spirit and delirious speech in heat diseases; epilipsy and mania; child fright wind; gan of the teeth and gums; swollen throat; mouth sores; yong and ju; clove sores. Daily dosage: 150–400 mg. Use with care in pregnancy. Used in *an¹ gong¹ niu²-huang² wan²* (Peaceful Palace Bovine Bezoar Pills, 1), *niu²-huang² qing¹ xin¹ wan²* (Bovine Bezoar Heart-Clearing Pills, 193).

Remarks: Constituents: Bilirubins (10.6–52%): bilirubin, biliverdin. Steroids: (bile acids) cholic acid (5.6–10.7%), deoxycholic acid (2.0–2.3%), chenodeoxycholic acid (0.6–1.7%); cholesterol, ergosterol; vitamin D. Amino acids: taurine. Peptides: SMC-F, SMC-S.

Similar drugs: Bezoar of *Bos grunniens* L., *B. gaurus* H. Smith, and *Bubalus bubalis* L.

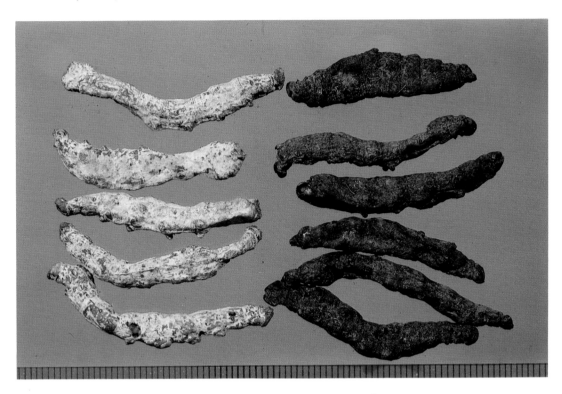

Bombyx Batryticatus: crude (left); stir-fried (right). (× 5/3)

210 BOMBYX BATRYTICATUS

白僵蠶 *bai² jiang¹ can²*. English: (dead infested) silkworm. Japanese: *byakukyosan*.

Alternate names: 僵蠶 *jiang¹ can²*, 殭蠶 *jiang¹ can²*.

Origin: Bombycidae family. *Bombyx mori* L. (host), *Batrytis bassiana* Bals. [= *Beauveria bassiana* (Bals.) Vuill.] (parasite).

Characters: This product is the larva of the silk moth. It is cylindrical, slightly bent or twisted, about 2–5 cm long, and 4–7 mm in thickness. The exterior surface is white or light brown, usually with a white, powdery coating. The spheroid, brown head, and the eight stumpy legs, and the body segments are readily identifiable. The body often has silk wrapped round it, and is easily broken to reveal a transverse fracture that on the outside is white and chalky and on the inside is brown or black, with four shiny circles. It has a slightly putrid odor.

Quality: Fat, hard, white larvae, that are shiny on the cross section are the best.

Production areas: China (Zhejiang, Jiangsu, Sichuan, Guangdong, Shaanxi), Korea, and Japan.

Properties and actions: Balanced; acrid and salty; slightly toxic. enters the liver, lung and stomach channels. Dispels wind and resolves tetany; transforms phlegm and dissipates binds. Stir-frying enhances the power to ''combat toxin with toxin.'' Mix-frying with honey reduces irritation to the stomach.

Indications: Wind stroke loss of voice; fright epilepsy; head wind; throat wind; itchy throat; scrofulous lumps; wind sores; dormant papules (urticaria); cinnabar toxin (erysipelas); mastitis. Daily dosage: 5–10 g. Not suitable for patients suffering from external contractions or uterine bleeding. Used in *bai²-jiang¹-can² san³* (Silkworm Powder, 14).

Remarks: Constituents: Yellow pigment: bassianins.

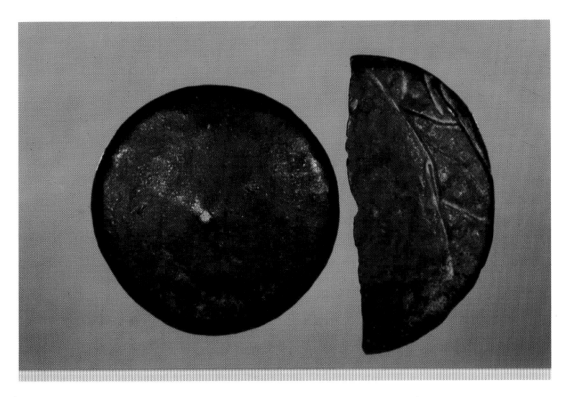

Bufonis Venenum. (×7/8)

211 BUFONIS VENENUM

蟾酥 *chan² su¹*. English: toad venom. Japanese: *senso.*

Alternate name: 蟾蜍眉酥 *chan² chu² mei² su¹*.

Origin: Bufonidae family. *Bufo bufo gargarizans* Cantor, *B. melanostictus* Schneider.

Characters: The secretion of the skin glands of the toad, the animal's only defense, comes in dried form as a round cake or button, slightly thicker in the middle than at the edges. It is about 6–10 cm in diameter, and 2–3 cm thick in the middle. It is purple-brown or brown-black, smooth and shiny on the upper side and rougher on the under side. The best quality is slightly translucent, brittle, has a purple hue, and numbs the tongue when licked.

Quality: The best quality is smooth and shiny on the upper side.

Production areas: China (Hebei, Shandong, Sichuan, Hunan, Jiangsu, Zhejiang, and less importantly Liaoning, Hubei, and Xinjiang).

Properties and actions: Warm; sweet, acrid; toxic. Enters the stomach and kidney channels. Resolves toxin, disperses swelling, strengthens the heart and relieves pain. Its harshness is moderated by stir-frying with vinegar.

Indications: Clove sores; yong and ju; dorsal effusions; scrofulous lumps; chronic osteomyelitis; sore, swollen throat; child gan accumulation; heart failure; toothache due to caries or wind. Daily dosage: 1.5–3mg. Oral administration contraindicated in vacuity and pregnancy. Used in *liu³ shen² wan²* (Six Spirits Pills, 167), *wai⁴ ke¹ chan² su¹ wan²* (External Medicine Toad Venom Pills, 266).

Remarks: Constituents: Steroids: (bufadienolides) cinobufagin (5%), resibufogenin (3.4%), bufalin (1.8%), cinobufotalin (1.6%), bufotalin (1.5%), telocinobufagin (1.4%), gamabufotalin (1.2%), hellebrigenin, cinobufaginol, arenobufagin. Amines: adrenaline, bufotenine.

Allied drug: Dried skin secretion of *Bufo bufo asiaticus* Stein.

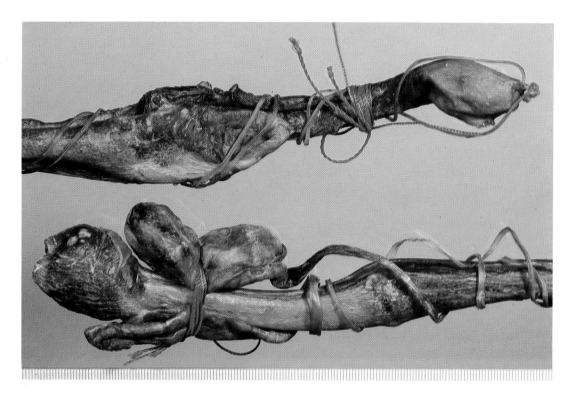

Callorhini Testis et Penis. (×5/6)

212 CALLORHINI TESTIS ET PENIS

海狗腎 *hai³ gou³ shen⁴*. English: seal genitals (testes and penis) Japanese: *kaikujin.*
Alternate name: 膃肭臍 *wen¹ na⁴ qi².*
Origin: Otariidae family. *Callorhinus ursinus* L. [= *Otaria ursinus* Gray].
Characters: This product comes from different sources and varies considerably. It is not always clear what animal it comes from. The penis is cylindrical, about 28–32 cm long and 1.2 cm thick. It thins at the tip and has a bulbous base. It is shrunken, and bears irregular furrows, and 1 single longitudinal protruding sinew. It is yellowish brown in color with black speckles and patches. The testicles are yellow, semitranslucent, and shiny, each with a yellow, semitranslucent sperm duct attached.
Quality: The best quality is long, hard, semitranslucent and without any fishy smell.
Production areas: Canada, Hawaii, and China (Liaoning).
Properties and actions: Hot; salty; nontoxic. Enters the liver and kidney channels. Warms the kidney and strengthens yang; boosts the essence and supplements marrow.
Indications: Vacuity taxation; impotence; atony of the lumbus and knees. Daily dosage: 3–10 g. Contraindicated in effulgent yin vacuity fire and steaming bone tidal fever with cough. Used in *wen¹-na⁴-qi² san³* (Seal Genitals Powder, 270).
Remarks: Constituents: androstenone, proteins.
Allied drug: Dried testis and penis of *Phoca vitulina* L. (Phocidae).

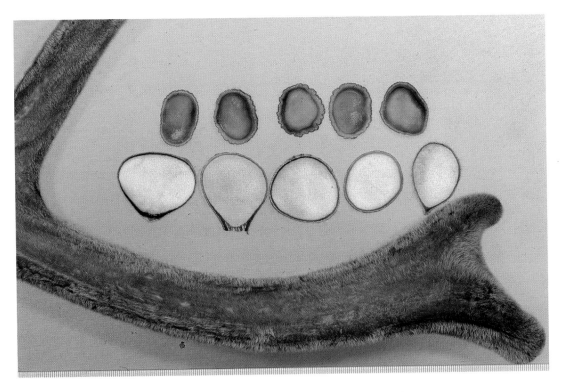

Cervi Cornu Parvum: crude and sliced. (×5/3)

213 CERVI CORNU PARVUM

鹿茸 *lu⁴ rong²*. English: velvet deer antler, velvet deerhorn. Japanese: *rokujo.*

Alternate names: 珠鹿茸 *zhu¹ lu⁴ rong²*, 茸角 *rong² jiao³.*

Origin: Cervidae family. *Cervus nippon* Temminck, *C. elaphus* L.

Characters: This antler comprises a main stem 14–33 cm long, with up to three 1–3 branches. It is gray or brown on the outside with dense short velvety hair that is sparser toward the base. After removing the hair, it is steamed and cut into 2–5 mm slices, which have a small holes in a distinct honey-comb pattern on the transverse section. It has a slight fishy smell.

Quality: Good quality antler should have a red hue and fine, soft hair, and should feel oily.

Production areas: *Cervus nippon:* China (Jilin, Liaoning, Heilongjiang, Hebei, Bejing). *C. elaphus:* China (Heilongjiang, Jilin, Inner Mongolia, Xinjiang, Qinghai, and Gansu).

Properties and actions: Warm; sweet and salty; nontoxic. Enters the liver and kidney channels. Invigorates original yang, supplements qi and blood, boosts essence and marrow, strengthens sinew and bone.

Indications: Vacuity taxation and marked emaciation; exhaustion of essence-spirit; dizziness; deafness; dark vision; aching pain in the lumbus and knees; impotence; seminal efflux; vacuity cold of the uterus; uterine bleeding; vaginal discharge. Daily dosage: 1–3 g. Contraindicated in exuberance of yang due to yin vacuity. Used in *xiang¹ rong² wan²* (Musk and Velvet Deer Antler Pills, 287), *wu³-wei⁴-zi³ wan²* (Schisandra Pills, 282).

Remarks: Constituents: Steroids: cholesterol. Lipids: proteolipids, ganglioside, sphingomyeline. Calcium phosphate, calcium carbonate.

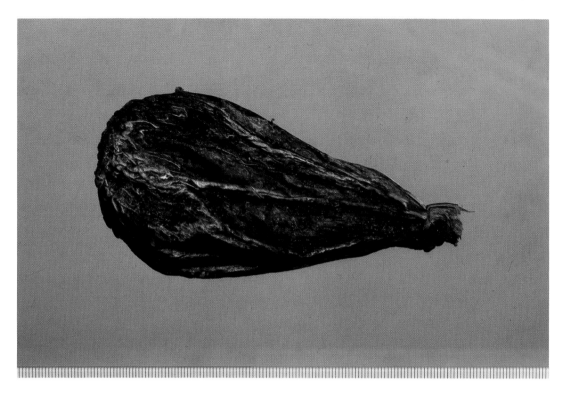

Fel Ursi. (×1)

214 FEL URSI

熊膽 *xiong² dan³*. English: bear's gall. Japanese: *yutan*.

Alternate name: 黑瞎子 *hei¹ xia¹ zi³*.

Origin: Ursidae family. *Selenarctos thibetanus* G. Cuvier, *Ursus arctos* L.

Characters: The dried gallbladder is flat and ovate, narrow at the top, and bulbous at the bottom. It is 10–20 cm long and 5–8 cm wide. The outer surface is gray-black or brown-black, lustrous and with creases. The skin is thin, and looked at against the light, is semitranslucent. This product is hard, and when broken open, the interior appears fibrous with a lump of dried bile that is either powdery, pasty, or shiny like amber. It is ground after the outer skin is removed.

Quality: Large gallbladders with shiny yellow bile lumps are the best.

Production areas: China (Yunnan, Heilongjiang, and Jilin).

Properties and actions: Cold; bitter; nontoxic. Enters the liver, spleen, stomach, and gallbladder channels. Clears heat, settles tetany, brightens the eyes and kills worms.

Indications: Heat jaundice; summerheat diarrhea; child fright epilepsy; gan disease; hookworm infestation; eye screens; throat bi; clove and malign sores; hemorrhoids. Daily dosage: 0.15–0.3 g. Used externally for hemorrhoids. Used in *xiong²-dan³ wan²* (Bear's Gall Pills, 308).

Remarks: Constituents: Steroids (cholic acids, 20%): tauroursodeoxycholic acid (main), taurodeoxycholic acid, glycodeoxycholic acid, taurocholic acid, cholic acid, cholesterol. Bilirubins: bilirubin, biliverdin. The bile acid composition varies significantly depending on the habitat, season, diet , etc.

* Ursodeoxycholic acid is now prepared from cholic acid synthetically and utilized for hepatitis, jaundice, cholelithiasis, cholecystitis, cholepathy, morning sickness, nephrosis, hypercholesterinemia, dyspepsia and anorexia.

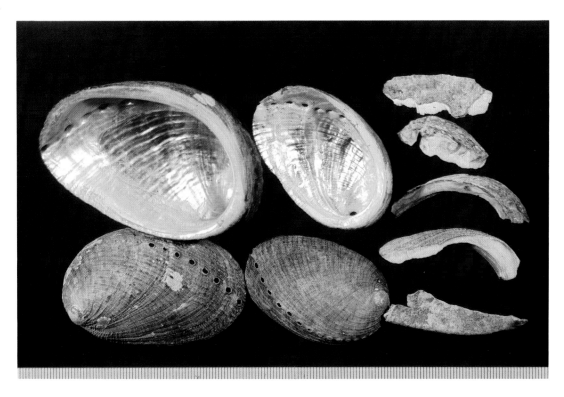

Haliotidis Concha: crude (left); calcined (left). (×5/6)

215 HALIOTIDIS CONCHA

石决明 *shi² jue² ming²*. English: abalone (or haliotis) shell. Japanese: *sekketsumei.*
Alternate names: 鳆魚甲 *fu⁴ yu² jia³*, 九孔决明 *jiu³ kong³ jue² ming²*.
Origin: Haliotidae family. *Haliotis diversicolor* Reeve, *H. gigantea discus* Reeve, *H. ovina* Gmelin.
Characters: This shell is elliptical 3–8 cm long and 2.5–5.5 cm wide. The exterior surface is gray brown and relatively smooth, with distinct growth lines. At the ends of the ridges, there are 8–9 holes that open into the inside of the shell. The interior is shiny like mother of pearl. This shell is hard, and is difficult to break, and the fractures are very sharp. It has no smell. For oral administration, it is calcined until gray white, while for topical application, it is calcined until white. It is crushed before use.
Quality: Large, thick shells with a shiny, pearly inside are the best.
Production areas: *Haliotis diversicolor:* China (Guangdong, Fujian). *H. gigantea discus:* China (Liaoning, Shandong). *H. ovina:* China (Guangdong, Taiwan).
Properties and actions: Balanced; salty; nontoxic. Enters the liver and kidney channels. Calms the liver and subdues yang; eliminates heat; brightens the eyes. Calcined, it helps the active agents to dissolve during decoction, and has an enhanced liver-supplementing action.
Indications: Headache, dizziness, and fright convulsions due to welling up of wind yang; steaming bone tidal fever; clear-eye blindness and internal obstructions of the eye. Daily dosage: 10–15 g. Contraindicated in spleen-stomach vacuity cold. Used in *shi²-jue²-ming² san³* (Abalone Shell Powder, 242).
Remarks: Constituents: Calcium carbonate ($CaCO_3$ up to 90%).
Allied drug: Shell of *Haliotis japonica* Reev. (Japan).

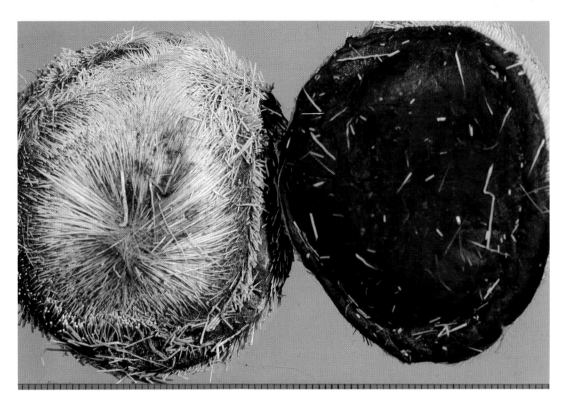

Moschus. (×5/3)

216 MOSCHUS

麝香 *she⁴ xiang¹*. English: musk. Japanese: *jakko.*
Alternate names: 香麝子 *xiang¹ she⁴ zi³*, 元寸香 *yuan² cun⁴ xiang¹*.
Origin: Cervidae family. *Moschus moschiferus* L.
Characters: The gland is elliptical or spheroid, 3–7 cm in diameter. On the side that opens, it is flat, with short dense white or brown hairs in spiral array, with a small hole in the center, about 2–3 mm in diameter. The hair may be removed to reveal a leathery, brown skin. The other side has a brown-black skin and no hair. When cut open with a knife, the cross section shows a semitranslucent silvery outer skin and a red-brown inner skin. Inside is a soft granular or powdery substance with an unusual smell. It is ground to a fine powder before use.
Production areas: China (Manchuria, Huabei, Shaanxi, Gansu, Qinhai, Xinjiang, Sichuan, Tibet, Yunnan, Guizhou, Guangxi, Hubei, Henan, and Anhui).
Properties and actions: Warm; acrid; nontoxic. Enters the heart, spleen, and liver channels. Opens the portals, repels foulness, frees the connecting vessels and dissipates stasis.
Indications: Wind stroke; phlegm inversion; fright epilepsy; malignity sores; vexation and oppression; fulminant pain in the abdomen and region of the heart; concretions and conglomerations; elusive masses; impact injuries; swelling and toxin of yong and ju. Daily dosage: 5–10mg. Contraindicated in pregnancy. Used in *liu⁴ shen² wan²* (Six Spirits Pills, 167)
Remarks: Constituents: Alkanes (volatile oil): muscone (muskone, (–)-3-methylcyclopentadecanone, 0.5–2%), normuscone. Alkaloids: muscopyridine; allantoin (0.0–4.4%). Steroids: androsterone. Fixed oil: olein.
Similar drugs: 1) Umbilical secretion of civet (*Viverra cibetta* Schreber); 2) Artificial musk.

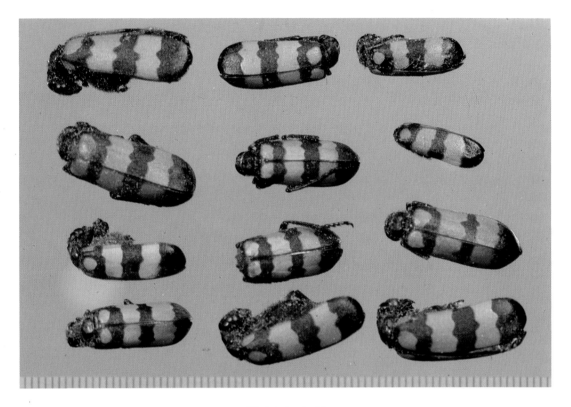

Mylabris. (×2)

217 MYLABRIS (CANTHARIS)

斑蝥 *ban¹ mao²*. English: mylabris, cantharides, Chinese blister fly. Japanese: *hanmyo.*
Alternate name: 斑猫 *ban¹ mao¹.*
Origin: Meloidae family. *Mylabris phalerata* Pallas [= *M. sidae* Fabr.], *M. cichorii* L.
Characters: This insect is oval in shape. *Mylabris phalerata,* is 10–25 mm long, and 5–10 mm wide, while *Mylabris cichorii,* is 10–15 mm long and 5–7 mm wide. In both species, the head is triangular and black, with two large compound eyes. On the dorsum are two black, leathery elytra (wing cases) with three golden brown transverse stripes. The ventral aspect is brown-black, with three pairs of hairy black legs attached to the thorax and a down-covered segmented abdomen. This product has an unusual smell. Large, brightly colored insects that are still intact are the best.
Production areas: China (Henan, Guangxi, Anhui, Sichuan, Guizhou, Hunan, Yunnan, Jiangsu).
Properties and actions: Cold; acrid; toxic. Enters the large intestine, small intestine, liver, and kidney channels. Attacks toxin and expels stasis.
Indications: Applied topically for malign sores; stubborn xian; throat moth. To be taken internally for scrofulous lumps and rabid dog bites. Grind to a powder for external use, and stir-fry before grinding for oral administration. Daily dosage: 0.03–0.05g. Contraindicated in vacuity and in pregnancy. Use with care when administering orally in view of its toxicity. Used in *ban¹-mao² tong¹ jing¹ wan²* (Mylabris Channel-Freeing Pills, 23).
Remarks: Constituents: Monoterpenoids: cantharidin (cantharidic acid anhydride, 0.6–1.9%). Fixed oil (12%).
Allied drugs: Dried body of blister beetle or Spanish fly, *Lytta vesicatoria* Fabricus (Meloidae), distributed over western Asia and central and southern Europe, also contains cantharidin and is employed for the same purposes.

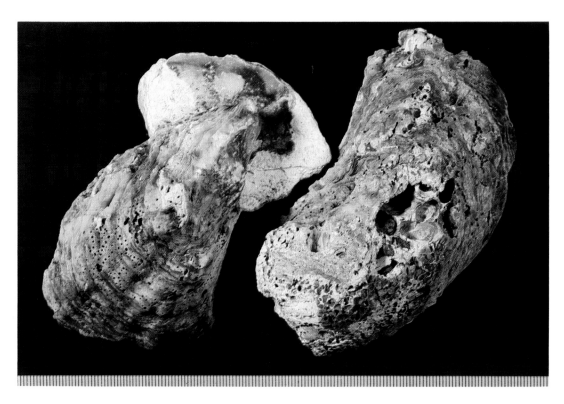

Ostreae Concha: crude (left); calcined (right). (× 7/8)

218 OSTREAE CONCHA

牡蠣 *mu³ li⁴*. English: oyster shell. Japanese: *borei*.

Alternate names: 左牡蠣 *zuo³ mu³ li⁴*, 牡蠣殼 *mu³ li⁴ ke²*.

Origin: Osteridae family. *Ostrea rivularis* Gould., *O. gigas* Thunb., *O. talienwhanensis* Cross.

Characters: This shell is ovate in shape, and made up of two halves that have undulating edges. The top shell is relatively flat, while the bottom shell is trough-shaped. The gray-yellow exterior surface shows the layered structure of its substance. The interior is smooth and shiny, and is cream or yellow-white in color. This shell is hard and not easy to break. It has no smell. It is ground to a very fine powder to facilitate decoction.

Quality: The best quality is large and neatly shaped, with a shiny inside.

Production areas: China (the coast of Jiangsu, Fujian, Guandong, Hebei, Liaoning, Shandong).

Properties and actions: Slightly cold; salt, atringent; nontoxic. Enters the liver and kidney channels. Constrains yin, subdues yang, checks sweating, astringes essence, transforms phlegm, and softens hardness. Used crude, it quiets the spirit and calms the liver. Calcined, it contracts and astringes, and softens hardness.

Indications: Fright epilepsy; dizziness; spontaneous sweating; night sweating; seminal emission; turbid strangury; uterine bleeding; vaginal discharge; scrofulous lumps; goiters and tumors of the neck. Daily dosage: 10–20 g. Contraindicated in kidney vacuity without heat, and spontaneous loss of cold semen. Used in *jin¹ suo³ gu⁴ jing¹ wan²* (Golden Lock Essence-Securing Pills, 149), *mu³-li⁴ san³* (Oyster shell Powder, 187) *chai²-hu² jia¹ long²-gu³ mu³-li⁴ tang¹* (Bupleurum Decoction Plus Dragon Bone and Oyster shell, 38), *gui⁴-zhi¹ jia¹ long²-gu³ mu³-li⁴ tang¹* (Cinnamon Twig Decoction Plus Dragon Bone and Oyster shell, 112), *chai²-hu² gui⁴-zhi¹ gan¹-jiang¹ tang¹* (Bupleurum, Cinnamon Twig, and Dried Ginger Decoction, 36).

Remarks: Constituents: Calcium carbonate (80–95%) with minute amounts of phosphates and sulfates of calcium and magnesium, oxides of iron, aluminum, and silicone. Saccharides: glycans. Proteins: keratin.

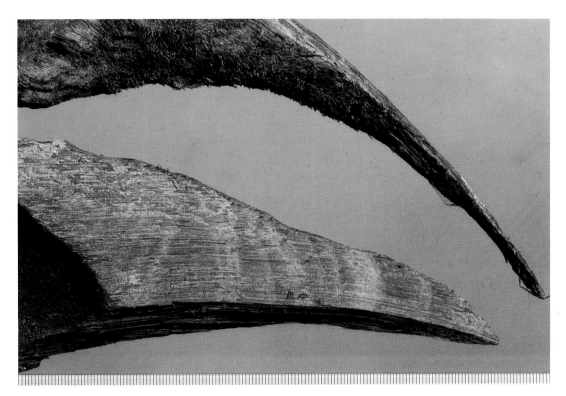

Rhinocerotis Cornu. (× 8/9)

219 RHINOCEROTIS CORNU

犀角 *xi¹ jiao³*. English: rhinoceros horn. Japanese: *saikaku.*

Alternate names: 香犀角 *xiang¹ xi¹ jiao³*, 烏犀角 *wu¹ xi¹ jiao³.*

Origin: Rhinocerotidae family. *Rhinoceros unicornis* L., *R. sondaicus* Desmarest, *R. sumatrensis* Cuvier, *R. bicornis* L., *R. simus* Burchell.

Characters: The horn of the male can be up to 30 cm or more in length. It is curved and tapers to point. It is black, paling to a gray brown at the base. The upper part is speckled and shiny. On the anterior face is a longitudinal groove about 10 cm long and 3 cm deep. The base is oval, and has a 1.5 cm high protrusion where the groove meets it. The base has a cavity 2–6 cm deep, and 33 cm wide. It is symmetrical in shape, has irregular margins, and is smooth.

Quality: Shiny, jet-black horn with a gray-black base and no cracks is best. A fresh odor is also a sign of good quality.

Production areas: India, Nepal, Burma, Thailand, Malaysia, and Indonesia. Horn of *Rhinoceros bicornis* L. and *R. simus* Burchell comes from Africa.

Properties and actions: Cold; sour, salty. Enters the heart and liver channels. Clears heat, cools the blood, settles fright and resolves toxin.

Indications: Heat entering the blood aspect; fright mania; vexation and agitation; delirious frenzy; maculopapular eruptions; yellowing of the skin; blood ejection; spontaneous external bleeding; precipitation of blood; swelling and toxin of yong and ju. Daily dosage: 1–3 g. Contraindicated in preegnancy. Used in *xi¹-jiao³ di⁴-huang² tang¹* (Rhinoceros Horn and Rehmannia Decoction, 284).

Remarks: Constituents: Peptides: cysteic acid-Asp-Ala, cysteic acid-Asp-Val-Thr, Lys-Arg-Glu-Gly. Acids: thio-lactic acid, cysteic acid. Amines: ethanolamine. Steroids: cholesterol. Calcium carbonate, calcium phosphate.

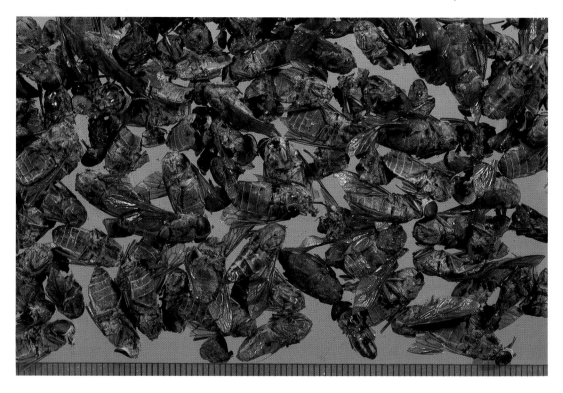

Tabanus (×5/3)

220 TABANUS

虻蟲*meng² chong²*. English: gadfly, tabanus. Japanese: *bochu.*
Alternate names: 牛虻 *niu² meng²*, 蜚虻 *fei³ meng²*.
Origin: Tabanidae family. *Tabanus bivittatus* Mats.
Characters: The dried body of the insect is elliptical, 1.5–2 cm long, and 0.5–1 cm wide. The head is blackish brown, and in most cases the large compound eyes have been lost. The thorax is gray brown, with a shiny shell-like dorsal surface and wings that exceed the length of the tail. The ventral aspect of the thorax protrudes, and has three pairs of legs attached, most of which are broken. The abdomen is brown, and comprises 6 segments. The dried body of the insect is brittle, and gives off an unpleasant odor. The wings and legs are removed before use.
Quality: Large, clean, undamaged insects are the best.
Production areas: China (Guangxi, Sichuan, Zhejiang, Jiangsu, Hunan, Hubei, Shanxi, Henan, Liaoning).
Properties and actions: Slightly cold; bitter; toxic. Enters the liver channel. Expels stasis, breaks accumulations and promotes menstruation.
Indications: Concretions and gatherings; blood amassment in the lower abdomen; blood stagnation and menstrual block; stasis swelling due to impact injury. Daily dosage: 1.5–3 g. Contraindicated in pregnancy. Used in *di³ dang¹ tang¹* (Dead-On Decoction, 67).
Remarks: Allied drugs: *Tabanus yao* Macq.; *T. amaenus* Walker; *T. trigonus* Coquillett; *Hybomitra montana* Meigen.
Constituents: Fat. Proteins.

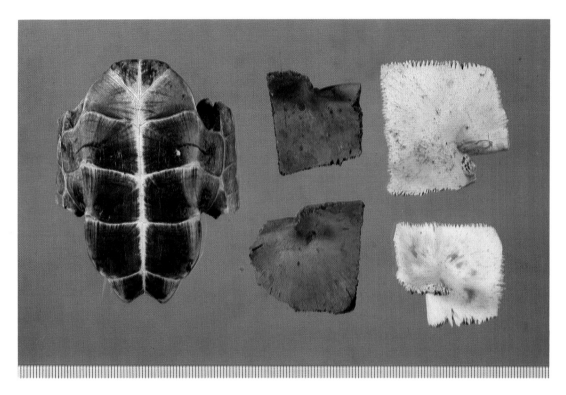

Testudinis Plastrum: crude (left); stir-fried (middle); macerated in water (right). (×6/7)

221 TESTUDINIS PLASTRUM

龜板 *gui¹ ban³*. English: tortoise plastron. Japanese: *kiban.*
Alternate names: 敗龜甲 *bai⁴ gui¹ jia³*, 敗龜板 *bai⁴ gui¹ ban³*.
Origin: Testudinidae family. *Chinemys reevesii* Gray.
Characters: This flat, oval plastron (ventral shell) is 10–20 cm long, and 7–10 cm wide, and about 5 mm thick. It is broad and rounded or truncated at the front, and narrow at the rear, with a V-shaped notch. Its exterior surface is brown with purple-brown markings, while its interior surface is yellow white. It is made up of 12 symmetrically arranged square plates, each having serrated edges that intermesh with those of adjacent plates. At the sides, invariably part of the dorsal shell is attached. This plastron is hard in substance, and gives off a fishy smell.
Quality: Large, clean, undamaged plastrons are the best.
Production areas: China (Hubei, Anhui, Hunan, Jiangsu, Zhejiang, and less importantly Guangdong, Sichuan, Guizhou, Fujian, Shaanxi, and Henan), and Indonesia.
Properties and actions: Cold; sweet, salty. Enters the liver and kidney channels. Enriches yin, subdues yang, supplements the kidney and fortifies the bones. Stir-frying with vinegar improves the yang-subduing action.
Indications: Insufficiency of kidney yin; steaming bone taxation fever; blood ejection; spontaneous external bleeding; enduring cough; seminal emission; uterine bleeding; vaginal discharge; lumbar pain; bone atony; yin vacuity wind; enduring dysentery and malaria; hemorrhoids; non-closure of the fontanels. Daily dosage: 10–20 g. Contraindicated in vacuity patterns without heat signs. Used in *da⁴ bu³ yin¹ wan²* (Major Yin Supplementation Pills, 44), *gui⁴-ban³ tang¹* (Tortoise Plastron Decoction, 106), *gui¹ bo² jiang¹ zhi¹ wan²* (Tortoise Plastron, Phellodendron, Ginger, and Gardenia Pills, 107).
Remarks: Constituents: Calcium salt.

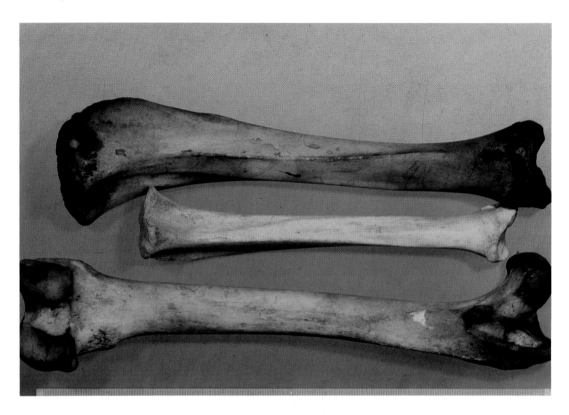

Tibia Tigris. (×1/2)

222 TIGRIS OS

虎骨 *hu³ gu³*. English: tiger bone. Japanese: *kokotsu*.

Origin: Felidae family. *Panthera tigris* L.

Characters: Distinction is made between the limb bones and the skull and spine. The limb bones and skull are the best. On the forelimbs, close to the socket at the lower end of the humerus is a slit called the "phoenix eye." On the back limbs, the fibula is characteristically very thin. The limb bones are yellow brown in color with longitudinal markings, and are smooth to the touch. On the transverse section, the bones are blackish yellow in color and hollow, with reticulate fibers stuck to the cavity wall.

Quality: Heavy, solid bones that saw smoothly, and reveal a small cavity containing luffa-like tissue are the best. The absence of any attached flesh is also a mark of good quality.

Production areas: China (Jilin, Heilongjiang, Hunan, Sichuan, Yunnan, Guizhou).

Properties and actions: Warm; acrid; nontoxic. Enters the liver and kidney channels. Chases wind and settles pain; fortifies the bones, and settles fright. Stir-fry with vinegar or wine, or without additives to dissipate wind-cold and fortify the sinews and bones.

Indications: Articular wind pain, hypertonicity of the limbs, stiff lumbus (use the limb bones); fright palpitation and epilepsy (use the skull); hemorrhoids and fistulae; prolapse of the rectum. Daily dosage: 10–15 g. Use with care in the presence of exuberant fire due to blood vacuity. Used in *hu³ qian² wan²* (Hidden Tiger Pills, 123), *hu³-gu³ mu⁴-gua¹ jiu³* (Tiger Bone and Chaenomeles Wine, 122).

Remarks: Allied drugs: Bone of *Panthera tigris amurensis* Dodge; *P. tigris amoyensis* Hilzheimer; *P. tigris slyani* Pocock.

Constituents: Kalium carbonate.

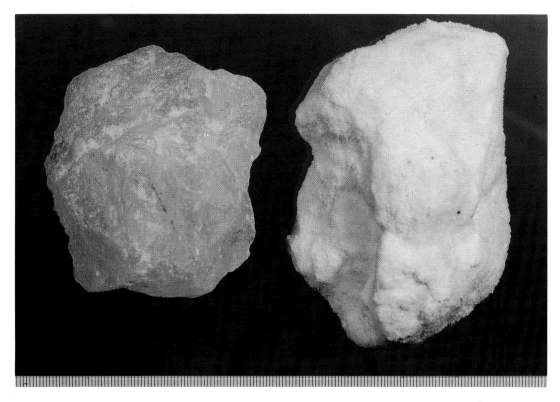

Alumen (left); Alumen Praeparatum (right). (×1)

223 ALUMEN

白礬 *bai² fan²*. English: alum, potash alum. Japanese: *hakuban, myoban*.
Alternate names: 明礬 *ming² fan²*, 礬石 *fan² shi²*.
Origin: Alumitum.
Characters: Potash alum is produced from the mineral alumite. It takes two forms: the regular form (Alumen [*bai² fan²*]) is composed of translucent, colorless octahedral cystals, which have a hardness of 3.5–4, and a specific gravity of 2.6–2.8. Prepared alum (Alumen Praeparatum. [*ku¹ fan²*]) is snow white and opaque. It is light and spongy in substance, and comes in rough, irregularly shaped lumps. Potash alum crystals are apt to be somewhat dirty looking, but on being dissolved and filtered, give a very pure solution of alum.
Production areas: China (Anhui, Zhejiang, Fujian, Shanxi, Hebei, and Hubei).
Properties and actions: Cold; sour and astringent; toxic. Enters the lung, spleen, stomach, and large intestine channels. Disperses phlegm; dries damp; checks diarrhea; staunches bleeding; resolves toxin; kills worms. Alumen can be taken internally to dispel phlegm and resolve toxin (crude), and to engender flesh (calcined), and can be applied topically to astringe and to dry damp. Alumen Praeparatum is used topically as an astringent.
Indications: Epilepsy; throat bi; phlegm-drool; hepatitis, jaundice; yellow swelling; stomach and duodenal ulcers; prolapse of the uterus; white vaginal discharge; diarrrhea; spontaneous external bleeding; mouth and tongue sores; hemorrhoids, jie and xian; scalds and burns. Daily dosage: 0.5–3 g. Contraindicated in yin vacuity. Used in *bai² jin¹ wan²* (Alum and Curcuma Pills, 15).
Remarks: Constituents: $KAl(SO_4)_2 \cdot 12H_2O$.

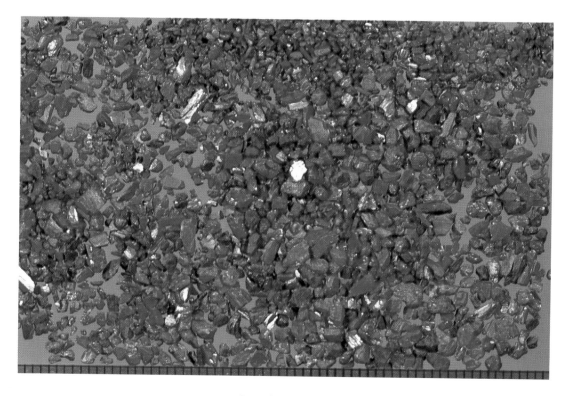

Cinnabaris. (×2)

224 CINNABARIS

朱砂 *zhu¹ sha¹*. English: cinnabar. Japanese: *shusha.*

Alternate names: 丹砂 *dan¹ sha¹*, 辰砂 *chen² sha¹.*

Characters: Cinnabar is naturally occurring red mercuric sulfide (HgS). It is scarlet or red-brown in color, has a metallic sheen, and is either opaque or semitranslucent. It comes in the form of small, irregularly shaped lumps. It is heavy, brittle, but soft in substance. It has a hardness of 2–2.5 and a specific gravity of 8–8.2.

Note: Cinnabar used to be called the "Immortal elixir," and was the equivalent of the Philospher's Stone of Western alchemists.

Quality: Good cinnabar does not leave any stain on paper.

Production areas: China (Guizhou, Hunan, Sichuan, Guangxi, Yunnan).

Properties and actions: Slightly cold; sweet; toxic. Enters the heart channel. Quiets the spirit; calms fright; brightens the eyes; resolves toxin.

Indications: Mania and withdrawal; fright palpitations; vexation; insomnia; dizziness; clouded vision; toxin swellings; jie, xian, sores. Daily dosage: 20–35 mg. Contraindicated in the absence of repletion heat. Used in *zhu¹-sha¹ an¹ shen² wan²* (Cinnabar Spirit-Quieting Pills, 347).

Remarks: Constituents: HgS (Hg 86.2%, S 13.8%).

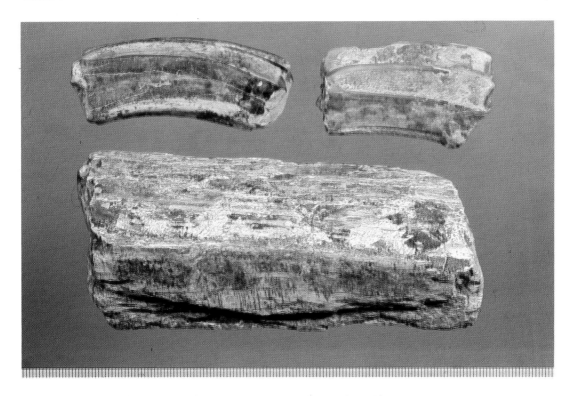

Dragon tooth (top) and flowery dragon bone (bottom). (×1)

225 DRACONIS OS (MASTODI OSSIS FOSSILIA)

龍骨 *long² gu³*. English: dragon bone. Japanese *ryukotsu*.

Alternate names: 化龍骨 *hua⁴ long² gu³*, 花龍骨 *hua¹ long² gu³*.

Origin: Fossilized bones of elephants, rhinoceroses, and sometime cattle, camels, and antelopes.

Characters: Distinction is made between ''flowery'' and ''white'' dragon bone. Flowery dragon bone comes in irregular lumps, 6–10 cm long, 3–5 cm wide and 2–3 cm thick. It is pale gray with red, blue, yellow, and brown markings, and has markings on the fractures like the annual rings of trees. It is hard and brittle, and breaks like slate. White dragon bone is whitish yellow, and comes in larger pieces. It is hard as stone, and chalky in substance. In addition, there is dragon tooth, which is whole or broken fossils of canine teeth or molars.

Quality: Flowery dragon bone with pronounced colored markings is the best.
Sichuan, Yunnan, Guangxi, and Qinghai).

Properties and actions: Balanced; sweet, astringent. Enters the heart, liver, kidney, and large intestine channels. Settles fright and quiets the spirit; constrains sweating and secures essence; staunches bleeding and astringes the intestines; engenders flesh and contracts sores. Use crude to subdue yang and quiet the spirit, calcined to astringe, and coated in cinnabar to quiet the heart spirit.

Indications: Fright epilepsy; mania and withdrawal; racing of the heart; poor memory; insomnia; profuse dreaming; spontaneous and night sweating; seminal emission; turbid strangury; blood ejection; upper portal and uterine bleeding; blood in the stool; diarrhea and prolapse of the anus; open sores that will not heal. Daily dosage: 10–15 g. Contraindicated in damp-heat and other pathogen repletion patterns. Used in *jin¹ suo³ gu⁴ jing¹ wan²* (Golden Lock Essence-Securing Pills, 149), *gui⁴-zhi¹ jia¹ long²-gu³ mu³-li⁴ tang¹* (Cinnamon Twig Decoction Plus Dragon Bone and Oyster shell, 112), *chai²-hu² jia¹ long²-gu³ mu³-li⁴ tang¹* (Bupleurum Decoction Plus Dragon Bone and Oyster shell, 38).

Remarks: Constituents: Calcium carbonate [5–12%, more hydroxyapatite (3 $Ca_3(PO_4)_2 \cdot Ca(OH)_2$) in dense portion; 46–82%, less hydroxyapatite in spongy portion] with minute amounts of calcium phosphate, oxides of silicone, iron, aluminum, manganese, calcium, magnesium, titanium, phosphorus, sodium, potassium.

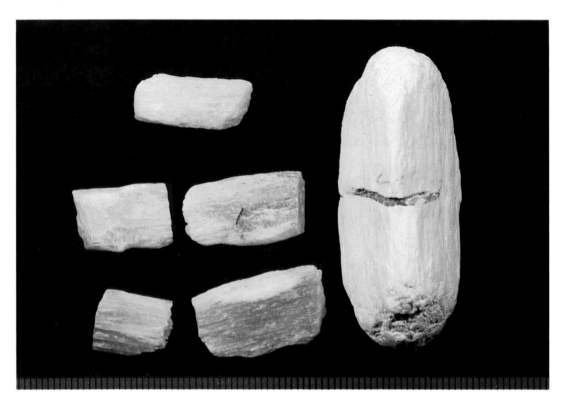

Gypsum Fibrosum: crude (left); calcined (right). (×5/3)

226 GYPSUM FIBROSUM

石膏 *shi² gao¹*. English: gypsum, fibrous gypsum. Japanese: *sekko.*

Alternate names: 軟石膏 *ruan³ shi² gao¹*, 白虎 *bai² hu³*.

Characters: This mineral, containing native calcium sulphate (CaSO₄•2H₂O), is composed of a white or gray, fibrous, crystal substance that comes in lumps of varying sizes. It is heavy and loose, breaking up easily into small lumps. The fibrous structure is visible on the cross section. If heated to 120°C, it partly looses it crystal structure, and becomes powdery. This is called calcined gypsum.

Quality: Large, clean lumps of white, highly fibrous gypsum are the best.

Production areas: China (Hubei, Anhui, Henan, Shandong, Sichuan, Hunan, Guangxi, Guangdong, Yunnan, Xinjiang).

Properties and actions: Cold; acrid and sweet; nontoxic. Enters the lung and stomach channels. Used crude, it resolves the muscles and clears heat, eliminates vexation and allays thirst. Calcined and applied topically, it engenders flesh and closes sores.

Indications: Persistent vigorous fever in heat disease; vexation and clouding of the spirit, delirious speech, and mania; lung heat with rapid dyspneic breathing; summerheat stroke with spontaneous sweating; stomach heat headache or toothache; exuberant heat toxin giving rise to maculopapular eruptions; mouth sores. Daily dosage: 15–20 g. Contraindicated in the absence of repletion heat. Used in *bai² hu³ tang¹* (White Tiger Decoction, 11), *zhu²-ye⁴ shi²-gao¹ tang¹* (Bamboo Leaf [Lophatherum] and Gypsum Decoction, 349), *ma² xing⁴ gan¹ shi² tang¹* (Ephedra, Apricot Kernel, Licorice, and Gypsum Decoction, 176), *bai² hu³ jia¹ gui⁴-zhi¹ tang¹* (White Tiger Decoction Plus Cinnamon Twig, 9), *da⁴ qing¹ long² tang¹* (Major Green-Blue Dragon Decoction, 53).

Remarks: Constituents: Hydrated calcium sulfate (CaSO₄•2H₂O) containing a small amount of calcium sulfate (CaSO₄) and minute amounts of silica, iron, magnesium, aluminum, sulfides, organic compounds.

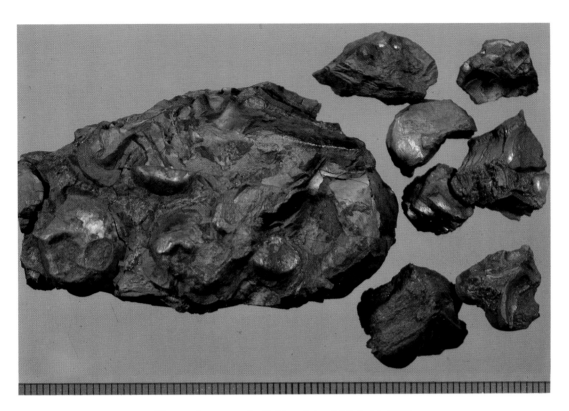

Haematitum: crude (left); calcined (right) (×5/3)

227 HAEMATITUM (OCHERUM RUBRUM)

代赭石 dai[4] zhe[3] shi[2]. English: hematite. Japanese: *taishaseki*.

Alternate names: 赤赭石 chi[4] zhe[3] shi[2], 赭石 zhe[3] shi[2]

Characters: This mineral, which has a high Fe_2O_3 content, comes in irregularly shaped lumps of varying size. It is a red-brown, and leaves a red-brown powder on the hands when handled. It has papillary protrusions on one side, and corresponding depressions on the other. It is hard in substance, and is not easily broken. The cross section reveals a structure composed of layers that bend in conformity with the protrusions visible on the exterior surface. It is crushed before use.

Quality: The best quality is red-brown, with distinct bends in the layers seen on the cross section.

Production areas: China (Shanxi, Hebei, Guangdong, Henan, Shandong, Sichuan, Hunan), and Japan.

Properties and actions: Cold; bitter and sweet; nontoxic. Enters the liver, stomach and pericardium channels. Calms the liver and settles counterflow; cools the blood and staunches bleeding. Used calcined for better counterflow-downbearing, dyspnea-calming, and blood-staunching action, and calcined with vinegar for increased astringency and power to act on the liver.

Indications: Belching; counterflow retching; esophageal constriction, stomach reflux; wheezing and dyspnea; fright epilepsy; blood ejection; spontaneous external bleeding; intestinal wind; hemorrhoids and fistulae; uterine bleeding and vaginal discharge. Daily dosage: 10–30 g. Contraindicated in pregnancy. Used in xuan[2]-fu[4] dai[4]-zhe[3] tang[1] (Inula and Hematite Decoction, 311).

Remarks: Constituents: Fe_2O_3: Fe 70%, O 30%; SiO_2, Al-salt, Mg··, Mn··, Ca··.

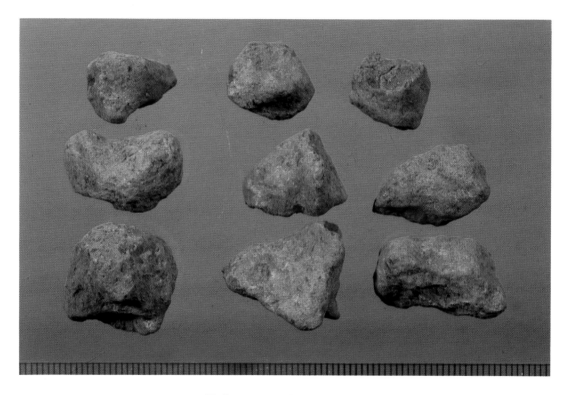

Halloysitum Rubrum. (×5/3)

228 HALLOYSITUM RUBRUM

赤石脂 *chi⁴ shi² zhi¹*. English: (red) halloysite. Japanese: *shakusekishi*.
Alternate names: 石脂 *shi² zhi¹*, 赤石土 *chi⁴ shi² tu³*.
Origin: Native brown iron oxide.
Characters: This mineral is native brown iron oxide and comes in irregularly shaped lumps of varying size. It is pinkish or purplish red in color, sometimes with pale markings. It is smooth like resin. It has a fine texture, and breaks easily and smoothly. It is highly water-absorbent and feels sticky when licked. It has the smell of earth.
Quality: Smoothness, fine texture, bright color, and stickiness when licked are signs of good quality.
Production areas: China (Fujian, Henan, Jiangsu, Shaanxi, Hubei, Shandong, Anhui, Shanxi).
Properties and actions: Warm; sweet, astringent; nontoxic. Enters the spleen, stomach, and large intestine channels. Astringes the intestines, staunches bleeding, constrains damp, and engenders flesh. Calcine for greater astringency.
Indications: Enduring diarrhea and dysentery; blood in the stool; prolapse of the rectum; uterine bleeding; vaginal discharge; persistent ulcers. Daily dosage: 10–15 g. Contraindicated in damp-heat accumulation and stagnation. Use with care in pregnancy. Used in *tao² hua¹ tang¹* (Peach Blossom Decoction, 261), *chi⁴-shi²-zhi¹ yu³-yu²-liang² tang¹* (Red Halloysite and Limonite Decoction, 41).
Remarks: Constituents; Kaorinite $Al_2O_3 \cdot 2SiO_2 \cdot 4H_2O$.
Allied drug: *bai² shi² zhi¹*, Kaolin.

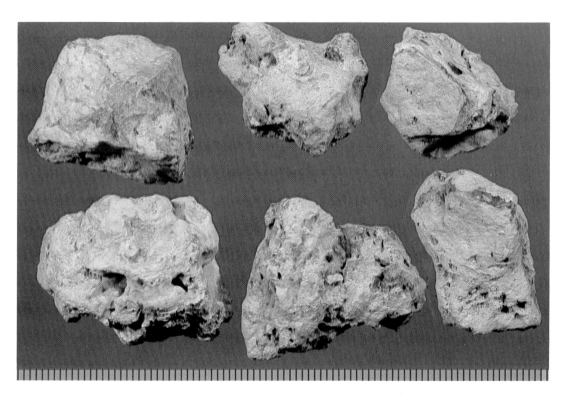

Hydrozincitum. (×5/3)

229 HYDROZINCITUM (SMITHSONITUM, CALAMINA)

爐甘石 *lu² gan¹ shi²*. English: smithsonite, hydrozincite. Japanese: *rokanseki.*

Alternate names: 盧甘石 *lu² gan¹ shi²*, 浮水甘石 *fu² shui³ gan¹ shi².*

Characters: The carbonate mineral smithsonite comes in irregular lumps of varying size. The outer surface is white or pale red, with depressions or holes. It is light and powdery in substance, and is easily broken to reveal a granular surface of the same color as the exterior. If calcined, it is white or pale yellow in non-crystal lumps, or a fine powder.

Quality: Large, light, white or pink lumps are the best.

Production areas: China (Guangxi, Sichuan, Yunnan, Hunan).

Properties and actions: Warm; sweet; nontoxic. Enters the liver, spleen, and lung channels. Eliminates eye screens and reduces eye redness; absorbs damp and contracts sores.

Indications: Used externally to treat reddening of the eyes, eye screens, wind ulceration of the eyelid rim, damp sores and persistent ulceration. Calcine to treat redness and swelling of the eyes. Used in *sheng¹ ji¹ san³* (Flesh-Engendering Powder, 236).

Remarks: Constituents: $2ZnCO_3 \cdot Zn(OH)_2$ (Calamina).

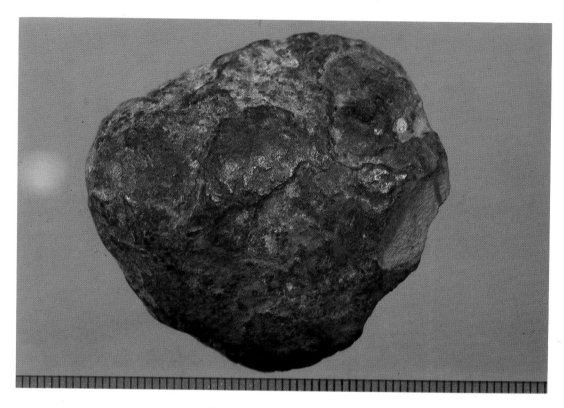

Limonitum cum Terra. (×2)

230 LIMONITUM CUM TERRA

禹餘糧 *yu³ yu² liang²*. English: limonite. Japanese: *uyoryo.*

Alternate names: 太一餘糧 *tai⁴ yi¹ yu² liang²*, 禹餘石 *yu³ yu² shi².*

Characters: Limonite mineral (Al₂O₃•2SiO₂) comes in irregular lumps about 6–10 cm long, and 1–3 cm thick. The exterior surface is yellowish or reddish brown and uneven. Sometimes it is covered with a yellow powder. The cross section is yellow brown with visible layers. Where the color is darker, it is harder in substance, but is still easily broken. Where the color is paler, it is soft enough to be scratched with the fingernail, making a powder that sticks to things easily. It has the smell of earth.

Quality: Unbroken, dark-color lumps with pronounced layers are the best.

Production areas: China (Henan, Jiangsu, Zhejiang, Sichuan).

Properties and actions: Slightly cold; sweet and astringent. Enters the spleen, stomach, and large intestine channels. Astringes the intestines and staunches bleeding. Calcination enhances the astringent quality.

Indications: Enduring diarrhea and dysentery; uterine bleeding; vaginal discharge; hemorrhoids and fistulae. Daily dosage: 10–15 g. Contraindicated in repletion patterns. Use with care in pregnancy. Used in *chi⁴-shi²-zhi¹ yu³-yu²-liang² tang¹* (Red Halloysite and Limonite Decoction, 41), *shen² xiao⁴ tai⁴ yi³ dan¹* (Wondrous Effect Tai Yi Elixir, 234).

Remarks: Constituents: Fe₂O₃•3H₂O (20–78%), Al, Mg, K, Na, PO₄.

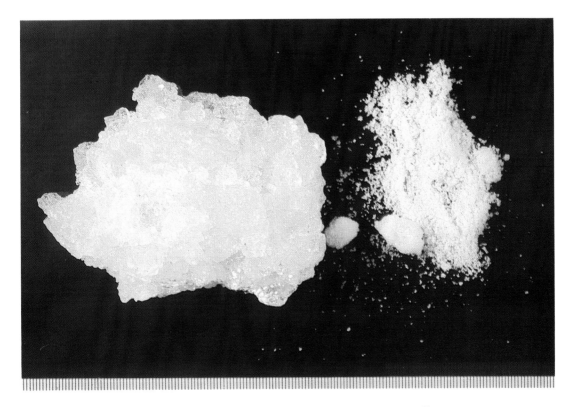

Mirabilitum (left); Mirabilitum Purum (right). (× 8/9)

231 MIRABILITUM

芒硝 *mang² xiao¹*. English: marabilite. Japanese: *bosho.*

Alternate names: 盆硝 *pen² xiao¹*.

Origin: Natural sodium sulfate.

Characters: Mirabalite, which has a high $Na_2SO_4 \cdot H_2O$ content, takes the form of prismatic or rectangular crystals, white with straight ends. It is brittle, and has no smell. Mirabalitum Purum (*xuan² ming² fen³*), which is the efflorescence of mirabilite, is a loose white powder that dissolves in water.

Quality: Colorless, transparent crystals that hold together in clumps are the best.

Production areas: China (Hebei, Henan, Jiangsu, Shanxi).

Properties and actions: Cold; acrid, bitter, salty; slightly toxic. Enters the stomach and large intestine channels. Drains heat, moistens dryness, and softens hardness.

Indications: Repletion heat stagnation and accumulation; abdominal distention; constipation; phlegm accumulation; reddening of the eyes; eye screens; cinnabar toxin; swollen yong. Marabilitum Purum is less effective for bowel conditions, and more effective as a topical dressing for sores. Daily dosage: 3–10 g. Contraindicated spleen-stomach vacuity cold and pregnancy. Used in *da⁴ cheng² qi⁴ tang¹* Major Qi-Infusing Decoction, 46), *da⁴ xian⁴ xiong¹ tang¹* (Major Chest Bind Decoction, 54), *tiao² wei⁴ cheng² qi⁴ tang¹* (Stomach-Regulating Qi-Infusing Decoction, 263).

Remarks: Constituents: Hydrated sodium sulfate ($Na_2SO_4 \cdot 10H_2O$) containing minute amounts of sodium chloride, magnesium chloride, magnesium sulfate, calcium sulfate.

Allied drugs: In former times, Epson salt, hydrated magnesium sulfate ($MgSO_4 \cdot 7H_2O$), was employed for the same purpose.

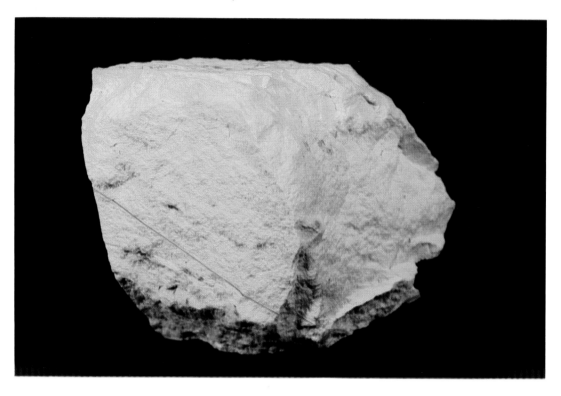

Talcum. (×5/3)

232 TALCUM

滑石 *hua² shi²*. English: talcum. Japanese: *kasseiki*.

Alternate names: 硬滑石 *ying⁴ hua² shi²*, 滑石粉 *hua² shi² fen³*.

Characters: Talcum $(3MgO \cdot 4SiO_2 \cdot H_2O)$ comes in flat, rhomboid or irregularly shaped lumps of varying sizes. It is white, sometimes with a bluish hue, or yellowish white, and has a pearly sheen. It may be opaque or semitranslucent. It is soft and fine in substance allowing a powder to be scraped off with the fingernail.

Quality: Large, clean bluish white pieces are the best.

Production areas: China (Jiangxi, Shandong, Jiangsu, Shaanxi, Shanxi, Hebei, Fujian, Zhejiang, Guangdong, Guangxi, Liaoning).

Properties and actions: Cold; sweet, bland; nontoxic. Enters the stomach and bladder channels. Clears heat, disinhibits damp and opens the portals.

Indications: Vexation and thirst in summerheat-heat; inhibited urination; water diarrhea; heat dysentery; strangury; jaundice; water swelling; spontaneous external bleeding; leg qi; damp erosion of the skin. Daily dosage: 10–15 g. Contraindicated in spleen-stomach vacuity, seminal efflux, and in febrile disease with damage to liquid. Use with care in pregnancy. Used in *liu⁴ yi¹ san³* (Six-To-One Powder, 170), *zhu¹-ling² tang¹* (Polyporus Decoction, 346), *ba¹ zheng⁴ san³* (Eight Corrections Powder, 7).

Remarks: Constituents: Hydrate magnesium silicate $(3MgO \cdot 4SiO_2 \cdot H_2O)$, usually part of magnesium is replaced by iron, sometimes contaminated by alumina.

Allied drug: Kaolinite $(Al_2O_3 \cdot 2SiO_2 \cdot 2H_2O)$ is also employed in place of talc.

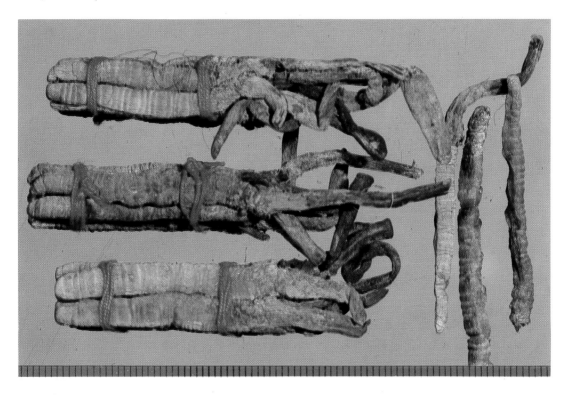

Cordyceps (×5/3)

233 CORDYCEPS

冬蟲夏草 *dong¹ chong² xia⁴ cao³*. English: cordyceps. Japanese: *tochukaso*
Alternate names: 夏草冬蟲 *xia⁴ cao³ dong¹ chong²*, 冬蟲草 *dong¹ chong² cao³*.
Origin: Clavicipitaceae family. *Cordyceps sinensis* (Berk.) Sacc. (plant), *Hepialus armoricanus* Oberthur. (insect).
Characters: This is the larva of the moth *Hepialus armoricanus,* joined to the stroma of *Cordyceps sinensis.* The larva is about 3-6 cm long, and 0.4–0.7 cm thick. It is a yellow brown, and is rough, with many transverse markings. It has eight pairs of stumpy legs on the ventral side, the four pairs in the middle section of the body being the most evident. On the transverse section it is white or slightly yellow, and deep yellow at the margins. The stroma, growing from the head of the larva, is club-shaped, swelling out in the final half and then tapering to the tip. It is brown, or blackish brown, and is 4-8 cm long, and 0.3 cm in diameter. It snaps open to reveal the white interior tissue and a hollow core.
Quality: Large, fat larvae with yellow insides and short stromata are marks of good quality.
Production areas: China (Sichuan, Qinghai, Guizhou, Yunnan, with production highest in Sichuan).
Properties and actions: Warm; sweet; slightly toxic. Enters the lung and kidney channels. Supplements vacuity and detriment; boosts essential qi; suppresses cough and transforms phlegm.
Indications: Phlegm-rheum dyspnea and cough; vacuity dyspnea; consumption cough; coughing of blood; spontaneous or night sweating; impotence and seminal emission; lumbar and knee pain; enduring vacuity preventing recovery from disease. Daily dosage: 5–10 g. Contraindicated in diseases with bleeding or exterior signs.
Method of use: Stew 15–30 g with a duck to treat vacuity dyspnea, or the same amount with pork to treat anemia, impotence, or seminal emission.
Remarks: Constituents: cordyceptic acid (ca. 7%).

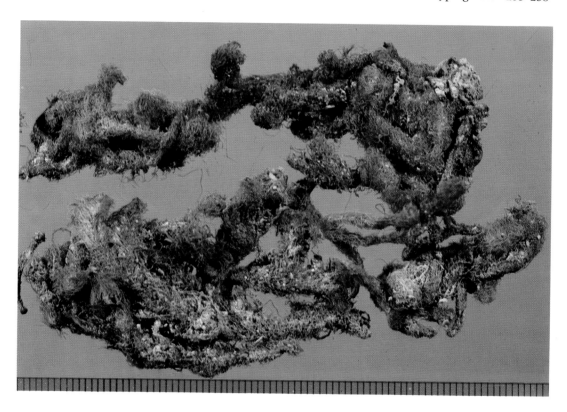

Digenea (×5/3)

234 DIGENEA

海人草 *hai³ ren² cao³*. English: digenea. Japanese: *kaininso, makuri*.

Origin: Rhodomelaceae family. *Digenea simplex* (Wulf.) C. Ag.

Characters: The dried alga is cylindrical, with many branches and forks. It is about 3–7 mm thick, and is gray-green in color, with a brown hue. It is covered with many hair-like branches, those at the bases often having been lost. It is strong and supple in texture. It is slightly slimy to the taste.

Production areas: China (Dongsha Islands, Hainan Island, Taiwan), and Japan.

Properties and actions: Balanced; salty. Kills worms.

Indications: Roundworm infestation. Daily dosage: 7–10g. Used in *qing¹ an¹ hui² tang¹* (Flesh-Clearing Roundworm-Quieting Decoction, 207).

Remarks: Constituents: Amino acids (0.15–0.2%): α-kainic acid (simply kainic acid, 0.15–0.2%), α-allokainic acid (traces); betaine. Peptides: Pro-Glu, Pro-Hypro-Lys. Acids: butyric acid, succinic acid, citric acid. Volatile oil. Saccharides: digeneaside; agarose.

Note: Kainic acid is usually used with santonin powder.

Allied drug: Dried alga of *Caloglossa leprieurii* J.Ag. (Delesseriaceae).

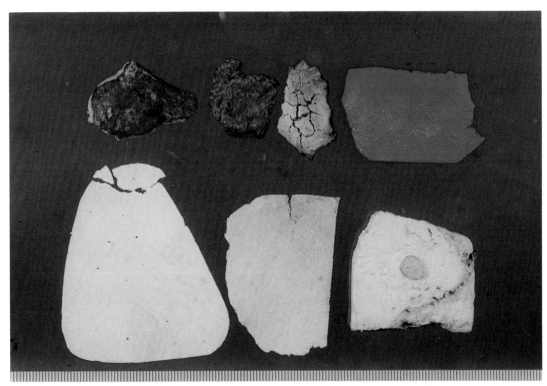

Hoelen Cortex (top left), Hoelen Album (bottom left), Hoelen Rubrum
(bottom middle), Hoelen cum Cinnabare (top right), and Hoelen cum
Radice Pini. (bottom right). (× 5/6)

235 HOELEN (PORIA) (1)

茯苓 *fu² ling²*. English: poria, hoelen, tuckahoe. Japanese: *bukuryo.*
Alternate names: 白茯苓 *bai² fu² ling²*, 雲茯苓 *yun² fu² ling²*.
Origin: Polyporaceae family. *Poria cocos* Wolf [= *Pachyma hoelen* Rumph].
Characters: The sclerotium is spherical, spheroid, or or irregular shape. It varies in size, weighing
3–5 kg. The exterior surface is a blackish brown. The outer skin is thin, rough, wrinkled, and often
has earth stuck to it. It is heavy, and breaks open with difficulty to leave a rough fracture that
is granular or farinaceous in texture. This product usually comes in the form of thin slices, with
the skin removed (this being used separately). White hoelen is white on the cut surface, while red
hoelen is peach-colored. Root hoelen comes in squared slices, with the yellow root of the pine
that grows through it clearly visible. Hoelen treatd with cinnabar is bright vermillion.
Quality: Loose, brittle sclerotia with flesh that is yellow at the margins are best.
Production areas: China (Hebei, Henan, Anhui, Zhejiang, Fujian, Guangdong, Guangxi, Hunan,
Hubei, Sichuan, Guizhou, Yunnan, Shanxi), Korea, and Japan.
Remarks: Constituents: Triterpenoids: eburicoic acid, dehydroeburicoic acid, pachymic acid
(0.10%), dehydropachymic acid, tumulosic acid (0.004–0.007%), dehydrotumulosic acid,
3β-O-acetyldehydrotumulosic acid, 3β-hydroxylanosta-7,9(11),24-trien-21-oic acid (0.008%).
Steroids: ergosterol (0.15%). Amines: lecithin, choline, adenine. Saccharides: pachyman
([$1 \rightarrow 3$]-β-D-glucan with β-[$1 \rightarrow 6$]-branchings, up to 93%).

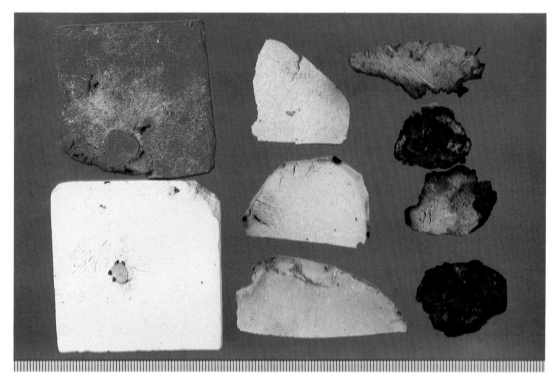

Hoelen cum Cinnabare (top left) Hoelen cum Radice Pini (bottom)
left), Hoelen Rubrum (middle), Cortex (right). (×6/7)

236 HOLELEN (PORIA) (2)

茯苓(Cont.) *fu² ling²*. English: poria, hoelen, tuckahoe. Japanese: *bukuryo.*

Origin: Polyporaceae family *Poria cocos* Wolf [= *Pachyma hoelen* Rumph].

Properties and actions: Balanced; sweet. Enters the heart, spleen, and small intestine channels. Percolates damp and disinhibits water; quiets the heart and spirit. White hoelen (Hoelen Album) is used specifically to fortify the spleen and percolate damp. Red hoelen (Hoelen Rubrum) drains damp-heat, disinhibits the portals, and moves water. The skin (Hoelen Cortex) specifically treats water swelling. Root hoelen (Hoelen cum Pini Radice) quiets the heart spirit. Cinnabar hoelen (Hoelen cum Cinnabare) has an even stronger spirit-quieting effect.

Indications: These agents treat inhibited urination; water swelling; distention and fullness; phlegm-rheum; counterflow cough; retching; diarrhea; seminal emission; turbid strangury; fright palpitation; poor memory. Daily dosage: 6–12 g. Contraindicated is seminal efflux and qi vacuity fall. Used in *wu³ ling² san³* (Poria Five Powder, 280), *xiao³ ban⁴-xia⁴ jia¹ fu²-ling² tang¹* (Minor Pinellia Decoction Plus Poria, 297), *fu²-ling² yin³* (Poria Beverage, 89), *liu⁴ jun¹ zi³ tang¹* (Six Gentlemen Decoction, 166), *gui⁴-zhi¹ fu²-ling² wan²* (Cinnamon Twig and Poria Pills, 109), *wu³ lin² san³* (Five Stranguries Powder, 279), *fu²-ling² ze²-xie⁴ tang¹* (Poria and Alisma Decoction, 90), *wu³ pi² san³* (Five Cortices Powder, 281), *shen¹ ling² bai²-zhu² san³* (Ginseng, Poria, and Atractylodes Ovata Powder, 231), *si⁴ jun¹ zi³ tang¹* (Four Gentlemen Decoction, 251), *fu²-ling² si⁴ ni⁴ tang¹* (Poria Counterflow Frigidity Decoction, 88), *zhu¹ ling²-tang¹* (Polyporus Decoction, 346).

Remarks: Although pachyman has no antitumor acitivity, on cleavage of the side chains, it affords β-$(1\rightarrow3)$-glucan, pachymaran, which exhibits antitumor activity against sarcoma-180.

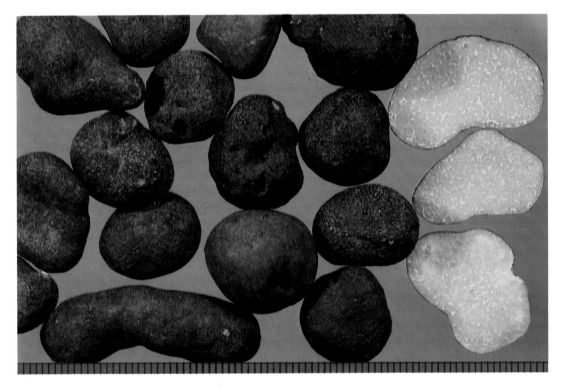

Omphalia (×5/3)

237 OMPHALIA

雷丸 *lei² wan²*. English: omphalia. Japanese: *raigan*.

Alternate name: 白雷丸 *bai² lei² wan²*.

Origin: Polyporaceae family. *Omphalia lapidescens* Schroeter [= *Polyporus mylittae* Cook. et Mass.].

Characters: This dried sclerotium is a hard mass, roughly spherical or oval in shape, with a diameter usually of 0.8–2.5 cm, and rarely as much as 4 cm. The exterior surface is brown-black with fine, dense creases. The interior is dense and fibrous, wax-white in color, semitranslucent, and slightly sticky. It produces a new fructification after the winter.

Quality: Large, full, hard sclerotia with gray skins and white interiors are the best.

Production areas: China (Sichuan, Guizhou, Hubei, Guangxi, Shaanxi).

Properties and actions: Cold; bitter; slightly toxic. Enters the stomach and large intestine channels. Disperses accumulation and kills worms.

Indications: Abdominal pain due to worm accumulation; gan disease; wind epilepsy. Daily dosage: 3–10 g. Use with caution in worm accumulations and in spleen stomach vacuity cold. Used in *lei²-wan² san³* (Omphalia Powder, 162).

Remarks: Constituents: Proteolytic enzyme, β-glucan.

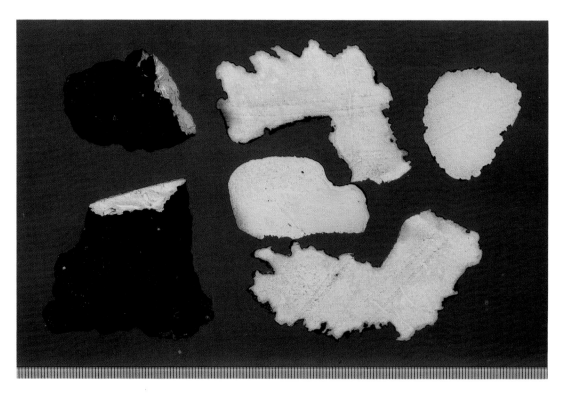

Polyporus: crude and sliced. (×7/8)

238 POLYPORUS

豬苓 *zhu¹ ling²*. English: polyporus. Japanese: *chorei*.
Alternate names: 稀苓 *xi¹ ling²*, 豬屎苓 *zhu¹ shi³ ling²*.
Origin: Polyporaceae family. *Polyporus umbellatus* (Pers.) Fr.
Characters: The dried sclerotium is a mass about 5–10 cm long and 3–8 cm in diameter, sometimes with branches. In some cases it is roughly spherical, with a diameter of 3–7 cm. The exterior skin is gray of brown black, with tumorous protuberances. It is hard, solid, and light like cork. It cuts smoothly to reveal a white, or light brown interior flesh that is granular in texture.
Quality: Large, relatively heavy sclerotia with shiny gray-black skins and white interiors are the best.
Production areas: China (Shaanxi, Henan, Hebei, Sichuan, Yunnan, and less importantly in Gansu, Zinghai, Liaoning, Jilin, Heilongjiang, Inner Mongolia, and Hubei), Japan, and Korea.
Properties and actions: Balanced; sweet, bland. Enters the spleen, kidney, and bladder channels. Disinhibits urine and percolates damp.
Indications: Inhibited urination; distention and fullness; water swelling; leg qi; diarrhea; turbid strangury; vaginal discharge. Daily dosage: 6–12 g. Contraindicated in the absence of damp. Used in *zhu¹-ling² tang¹* (Polyporus Decoction, 346), *wu³ ling² san³* (Poria Five Powder, 280), *wei⁴ ling² tang¹* (Stomach-Calming Poria Five Decoction, 267), *fen¹ xiao¹ tang¹* (Separating and Dispersing Decoction, 87).
Remarks: Constituents: Steroids: ergosterol, ergosta-4,6,8(14), 22-tetraen-3-one(0.00 2%), 5,8-epidioxy-3 β-hydroxy-5α-ergosta-6,22-diene. Acids: α-hyroxytetracosanoic acid (0.04–0.05%) Saccharides.

Appendix I   Drug Function Comparisons

1. Abducting dispersion agents 消導藥 xiao¹ dao³ yao⁴

Name	Functions	Indications	Contraindications	Daily Dosage
Crataegi Fructus shan¹ zha¹ 山楂 (131)	Disperses food accumulations; dissipates static blood; expels tapeworm. When charred, its astringent quality is enhanced, making it more effective for blood dysentery.	Concretions and conglomerations; phlegm-rheum; lump glomus; acid regurgitation; diarrhea; intestinal wind; lumbar pain; shan qi afterpain; persistent flow of the lochia; stagnation of milk in suckling infants.	Spleen-stomach vacuity.	5–10 g
Hordei Fructus Germinatus mai⁴ ya² 麥芽 (137)	Disperses food, harmonizes center, and precipitates qi. Used crude, it promotes lactation and disperses food, while stir-fried it fortifies the spleen and disperses stagnation.	Food accumulation: distention and fullness in the venter and abdomen; loss of appetite; vomiting and diarrhea: persistent distention of the breasts.		10–12 g
Asafoetida e¹ wei⁴ 阿魏 (196)	Disperses accumulation and kills worms. It is usually stir-fried to moderate the effect.	Concretions and conglomerations; lump glomus; worm and meat-type food accumulations; frigid pain in the abdomen and region of heart; malarial disease; dysenteric disease.	Pregnancy and Spleen-stomach vacuity.	0.5–1.5 g
Massa Medicata Fermentata shen² qu¹ 神麴 (201)	Fortifies the spleen and the stomach; disperses food and harmonizes the center. Used scorch-fried or stir-fried in bran to enhance its effects.	Food stagnation: thoracic glomus and abdominal distention; vomiting and diarrhea; postpartum stasis and abdominal pain; abdominal distention in children.	Use with care in excessive stomach acidity and in pregnancy.	6–12 g

2. Aromatic dampness-transforming agents 芳香化濕藥 fang¹ xiang¹ hua⁴ shi¹ yao⁴

Name	Functions	Indications	Contraindications	Daily Dosage
Magnoliae Cortex hou⁴ po⁴ 厚朴 (7)	Warms the center, precipitates qi, and dissipates fullness; dries damp; disperses stasis and breaks accumulations.	Painful distention and fullness in the chest, vomiting and diarrhea, and dyspnea and cough.	Pregnancy.	3–8 g
Atractylodis Rhizoma cang¹ zhu² 蒼朮 (77)	Fortifies the spleen, dries damp, resolves depression and repels foulness. Stir-frying with rice water, earth, or bran removes oil and reduces the dry quality. Scorch-frying warms the spleen, dispels damp, and checks diarrhea.	Exuberant damp encumbering spleen: lassitude; somnolence; glomus in the venter; abdominal distention; loss of appetite; vomiting; diarrhea; dysenteric and malarial disease; phlegm-rheum; water swelling; seasonal qi colds and flu: atony; night blindness.	Yin vacuity heat and conditions of dry bound stool and copious perspiration.	3–10 g
Amomi Cardamomi Fructus bai² dou⁴ kou⁴ 白豆蔻 (120)	Moves qi; warms the stomach; disperses food; loosens the center.	Stomach pain: abdominal distention; oppression in the venter and belching; stomach reflux; alcohol poisoning.	Retching, vomiting, stomach reflux, and abdominal pain attributable to depressed fire.	1.5–3 g

Drug	Function	Indications	Cautions	Dosage
Amomi Semen *sha¹ ren²* 砂仁 (160)	Moves qi and harmonizes the center, harmonizes stomach, and arouses the spleen. Stir-fry with brine to treat yin vacuity. Steam with the juice of Rehmanniae Radix Conquita (*shou² di⁴ huang²*) to rectify kidney qi.	Abdominal pain; glomus and distention; torpid stomach; food stagnation; esophageal constriction; vomiting; cold diarrhea and frigid dysentery; pregnancy fetus. Stir-fry with ginger juice for glomus and distention, and for vomiting.	Yin vacuity with heat.	1.5–3 g
Pogostemi Herba *huo⁴ xiang¹* 藿香 (193)	Normalizes qi, harmonizes the center, repels foulness and dispels damp. The stems regulate qi and loosen the chest.	Summerheat-damp colds and flu; fever and chills; headache; glomus and oppression in the chest and venter; vomiting and diarrhea; malarial disease; dysenteric disease; bad breath.	Effulgent yin vacuity fire, and stomach vacuity with desire to vomit.	5–10 g

3. Aromatic portal-opening agents 芳香開竅藥 *fang¹ xiang¹ kai¹ qiao¹ yao⁴*

Drug	Function	Indications	Cautions	Dosage
Benzoinum *an¹ xi² xiang¹* 安息香 (197)	Opens the portals; repels foulness; moves qi and the blood.	Sudden stroke and fulminant inversion; pain in the abdomen and region of the heart; postpartum dizziness; child fright epilepsy; wind bi lumbar pain.	Effulgent yin vacuity fire.	0.3–1 g

4. Astringing agents 收斂藥 *shou¹ lian⁴ yao⁴*

Drug	Function	Indications	Cautions	Dosage
Chebulae Fructus (Terminaliae Fructus) *he² zi³* 訶子 (127)	Contracts the lung, astringes the intestines and precipitates qi. Roasting, stir-frying with bran, and scorch-frying strengthen the intestine-astringing action.	Enduring cough and loss of voice; enduring diarrhea and dysentery; prolapse of the rectum; blood in the stool; uterine bleeding; vaginal discharge; seminal emission; frequent urination.	Initial stages of cough and dysenteric disease.	3–5 g
Mume Fructus (Pruni Mume Fructus) *wu¹ mei²* 烏梅 (144)	Promotes contraction and engenders liquid; kills worms. Used char-fried, it checks diarrhea.	Vacuity heat, vexation, and thirst; enduring diarrhea and dysentery; blood in the stool and urine; profuse uterine bleeding; roundworm with abdominal pain and vomiting; hookworm infestation; oxhide xian; outcrop.	Pathogen repletion.	3–5 g
Rubi Fructus *fu⁴ pen² zi³* 覆盆子 (150)	Supplements the liver and kidney, assists yang, secures essence and brightens the eyes.	Impotence; seminal emission; urinary frequency; enuresis; vacuity taxation; dark vision.	Exuberance of yang with difficult urination.	5–10 g

Name	Functions	Indications	Contraindications	Daily Dosage
Schisandrae Fructus wu³ wei⁴ zi³ 五味子 (151)	Constrains the lung; enriches the kidney; engenders liquid; constrains sweating; astringes essence. Use crude to clear vacuity fire and suppress cough. Treat with wine to enrich the kidney, or with vinegar to constrain the lung. Mix-fry with honey to moisten the lung.	Lung vacuity dyspnea and cough; thirst and dry mouth; spontaneous sweating; taxation emaciation; dream emissions; enduring dysentery or diarrhea.	Exterior pathogens and internal repletion heat.	1.5–3 g
Euryales Semen qian⁴ shi² zi³ 芡實 (169)	Secures the kidney and astringes essence; supplements the spleen and checks diarrhea. Stir-frying without additives enhances the sweet and astringent properties. Stir-frying in bran gives it a distinct spleen-fortifying effect.	Seminal emission; turbid strangury; vaginal discharge; incontinent urination; diarrhea.	Inhibited stool and urine.	5–10 g
Myristicae Semen rou⁴ dou⁴ kou⁴ 肉豆蔻 (176)	Warms the center; precipitates qi; disperses food; secures the intestines (especially when roasted).	Pain and distention in the abdomen and region of the heart; cold and vacuity diarrhea; retching and vomiting; retention of food.	Hot diarrhea or dysentery.	3–5 g
Galla Halepensis mo⁴ shi² zi³ 沒食子 (198)	Secures qi and astringes essence; constrains the lung and staunches bleeding.	Large intestinal vacuity efflux; persistent diarrhea; blood in the stool; seminal emission; genital sweating; cough; expectoration of blood; toothache; bleeding due to injury; persistent sores.	The initial stages of diarrhea; damp-heat or accumulation and stagnation.	3–5 g
Galla Rhois (Rhois Galla) wu³ bei⁴ zi³ 五倍子 (199)	Constrains the lung; astringes the intestine; staunches bleeding; resolves toxin.	Enduring lung vacuity cough; enduring dysentery or diarrhea; prolapse of the anus; spontaneous or night sweating; seminal emission; blood in the stool; spontaneous external or uterine bleeding; bleeding from external injury; sores and boils; ingrown eyelashes.	Cough due to exogenous wind-cold or lung repletion heat; diarrhea in which accumulation and stagnation has not been cleared.	1.5–6 g
Alumen bai² fan² 白礬 (223)	Disperses phlegm; dries damp; checks diarrhea; staunches bleeding; resolves toxin; kills worms. Alumen can be taken internally to dispel phlegm and resolve toxin (crude), and to engender flesh (calcined), and can be applied topically to astringe and to dry damp. Alumen Praeparatum is used topically as an astringent.	Epilepsy; throat yi; phlegm-drool; hepatitis; jaundice; yellow swelling; stomach and duodenal ulcers; prolapse of the uterus; white vaginal discharge; diarrhea; spontaneous external bleeding; mouth and tongue sores; hemorrhoids, jie and xian; scalds and burns.	Yin vacuity.	0.5–3 g

Halloysitum Rubrum *chi⁴ shi² zhi¹* 赤石脂 (228)	Astringes the intestines, staunches bleeding, constrains damp, and engenders flesh. Calcine for greater astringency.	Enduring diarrhea and dysentery; blood in the stool; prolapse of the rectum; uterine bleeding; vaginal discharge; persistent ulcers.	Damp-heat accumulation and stagnation. Use with care in pregnancy.	10–15 g
Limonitum cum Terra *yu³ yu² liang²* 禹餘糧 (230)	Astringes the intestines and staunches bleeding. Calcination enhances the astringent quality.	Enduring diarrhea and dysentery; uterine bleeding; vaginal discharge; hemorrhoids and fistulae.	Repletion patterns. Use with care in pregnancy.	10–15 g

5. Blood-nourishing agents 養血藥 *yang³ xue⁴ yao⁴*

Angelicae Sinensis Radix *dang¹ gui¹* 當歸 (25)	Supplements and harmonizes the blood, regulates menstruation, relieves pain, moistens dryness and lubricates the intestines. The head staunches bleeding; the body nourishes the blood, and the "tails" (branch roots) move the blood. The whole root is used to harmonize the blood. Angelica Sinensis supplements the blood and moistens the intestines when used crude, frees the channels and quickens the blood when treated with wine, and has a greater intestine-moistening power when mix-fried with honey.	Menstrual irregularities, menstrual pain, uterine bleeding, bi, impact injury, yong and ju, and blood vacuity constipation.	Spleen dampness.	5–10 g
Paeoniae Radix Alba *bai² shao² yao⁴* 白芍藥 (51)	Nourishes the blood and emolliates the liver; moderates the center and relieves pain; constrains yin and sweat. Use crude to calm the liver. Use stir-fried to nourish the blood and harmonize the liver, free the blood vessels and relieve pain. Roast to moderate the cold nature, direct the effect toward the upper body, and enhance the blood-quickening action. Stir-fry in earth to enhance pain-relieving and spleen-fortifying qualities.	Thoracic, lateral costal, and abdominal pain: diarrhea with abdominal pain; spontaneous or night sweating; yin vacuity fever; menstrual irregularities; vaginal discharge.	Thoracic fullness.	5–10 g

Name	Functions	Indications	Contraindications	Daily Dosage
Longanae Arillus (Euphoriae Longanae Arillus) long² yan³ rou⁴ 龍眼肉 (141)	Boosts the heart and spleen, supplements qi and quiets the spirit.	Vacuity taxation; marked emaciation; insomnia; impaired memory; fright palpitations and racing of the heart.	Phlegm-fire patterns and vomiting.	6-15 g
Asini Corii Gelatinum e¹ jiao¹ 阿膠 (208)	Enriches yin and supplements the blood; quiets the fetus. Stir-fry with clam-shell powder to moisten the lung and transform phlegm, suppress cough and staunch bleeding. Stir-fry with Pollen Typhae (pu² huang²) to quicken the blood, staunch bleeding, transform stasis.	Blood vacuity; vacuity taxation cough; blood ejection; spontaneous external bleeding; blood in the stool; menstrual irregularities; uterine bleeding in or outside pregnancy (stir-fry with Pollen Typhae).	Spleen-stomach vacuity.	5-10 g

6. Blood-quickening and stasis-dispelling agents 活血・祛瘀藥 huo² xue⁴, qu¹ yu¹ yao⁴

Name	Functions	Indications	Contraindications	Daily Dosage
Sappan Lignum su¹ mu⁴ 蘇木 (19)	Moves the blood, breaks stasis, disperses swelling, and relieves pain.	Postpartum stasis obstruction, menstrual block with qi congestion, swollen yong, and stasis and stagnation due to injury.	Blood vacuity.	3–5 g
Curcumae Tuber yu⁴ jin¹ 鬱金 (34)	Moves qi and resolves depression; cools the blood and breaks stasis. Use crude to move qi and resolve depression, to cool the blood and break stasis. Stir-fry to reduce the cold, bitter properties. Stir-fry with vinegar to treat upward surge of qi and blood. Stir-fry with wine to enhance the qi-moving action.	Pain in the chest, abdomen, and lateral costal region; mania and withdrawal; clouding of the spirit in febrile disease; blood ejection; spontaneous external bleeding; blood in the urine; blood strangury; vicarious menstruation; jaundice.	Yin vacuity without stasis and stagnation; pregnancy.	5-10 g
Salviae Radix dan¹ shen¹ 丹參 (60)	Quickens the blood and dispels stasis; quiets the heart and spirit; expels pus and relieves pain. Use crude to quicken and cool the blood, and dispel stasis. Char-fry to staunch bleeding. Stir-fry with rice to harmonize the stomach. Stir-fry with wine to enhance the effects. Mix with turtle's blood to enter the liver. Stir-fry with pig's blood to enter the heart and calm the spirit.	Menstrual irregularities; concretions and gatherings; swollen yong; cinnabar toxin (erysipelas); malign sores; heat vexation; wind bi.	Absence of blood stasis.	5-10 g

Drug	Actions	Indications	Contraindications	Dosage
Corydalis Tuber *yan² hu² suo³* 延胡索 (81)	Quickens the blood and dissipates stasis; rectifies qi and relieves pain.	Pain in the chest and abdomen; menstrual irregularities; concretions and conglomerations; profuse uterine bleeding; postpartum blood dizziness; lochiorrhea; impact injury.	Heat stasis and blood vacuity and pregnancy.	5–10 g
Curcumae Longae Rhizoma *jiang¹ huang²* 薑黃 (82)	Breaks blood, moves qi, promotes menstruation and relieves pain.	Painful glomus and fullness in the abdomen and region of the heart; pain in the kidney; concretions and conglomerations; menstrual block due to stasis; postpartum abdominal stasis pain; impact injuries; swollen yong.	Absence of stasis and stagnation.	3–5 g
Ligustici Rhizoma *chuan¹ xiong¹* 川芎 (88)	Moves qi and relieves depression; expels wind and dries damp; quickens the blood and relieves pain. Stir-frying in wine enhances the blood-quickening and channel-freeing action.	Wind-cold headache and dizziness; abdominal and lateral costal pain; hypertonicity of the sinews in cold bi; dizziness; menstrual block; postpartum stasis obstruction; yong, ju, and sores.	Effulgent yin vacuity fire.	3–5 g
Sparganii Rhizoma *san¹ leng²* 三稜 (96)	Moves qi and breaks blood; disperses accumulations and relieves pain; promotes menstruation. Stir-frying with vinegar to promote contraction or to disperse accumulations and relieve pain. Stir-fry with bran to disinhibit water. Stir-fry with bran and wine to move qi and break blood.	Menstrual block; concretions and conglomerations; pain in the abdomen and region of the heart; postpartum stasis and stagnation. Stir-frying with vinegar increases the accumulation-dispersing and pain-relieving effect.	Qi vacuity without stasis accumulation and pregnancy.	5–10 g
Zedoariae Rhizoma (Curcumae Zedoariae Rhizoma) *e² zhu²* 莪朮 (97)	Dispels wind and clears heat; breaks blood and disperses accumulation; disperses swelling and resolves toxin. Used crude to break blood and disperse accumulation. Used mix-fried with vinegar to harmonize the liver, resolve toxin, and relieve pain.	Distention and pain in the abdomen and region of the heart; concretions and gatherings; food stagnation; menstrual block due to blood stasis; impact injuries pain.	Dual vacuity of qi and blood; spleen-stomach vacuity without stagnation.	5–10 g
Carthami Flos *hong² hua¹* 紅花 (106)	Quickens the blood and promotes menstruation; eliminates stasis and relieves pain. Use crude to quicken the blood and dispel stasis. Boil with wine to break blood. Boil in water to nourish the blood. Triturate for topical application.	Menstrual block; concretions and conglomerations; difficult delivery; dead fetus; retention of the lochia; stasis pain; swollen yong; impact injuries.	Absence stasis and stagnation and pregnancy.	3–5 g

Name	Functions	Indications	Contraindications	Daily Dosage
Croci Stigma (Crocus) *zang⁴ hong² hua¹* 藏紅花 (110)	Quickens the blood and transforms stasis; dissipates depression and frees binds.	Binding depression due to excessive sorrow or thought; glomus and oppression in the chest and diaphragm; blood ejection; cold damage mania; fright and shock; abstraction; menstrual block; postpartum abdominal pain due to blood stasis; impact injury.	Pregnancy.	1.5–3 g
Leonuri Fructus *chong¹ wei⁴ zi³* 茺蔚子 (139)	Quickens the blood and promotes menstruation; courses wind and clears heat.	Menstrual irregularities; profuse uterine bleeding; postpartum static blood with pain; liver heat headache; reddening, soreness, and swelling of the eyes; eye screens.	Insufficiency of liver blood with dilated pupils, and in pregnancy.	5–10 g
Persicae Semen *tao² ren²* 桃仁 (177)	Breaks the blood and moves stasis; moistens dryness and lubricates the intestines.	Menstrual block; concretions and conglomerations; blood amassment in febrile disease; wind bi; malarial disease; bruises due to impact injury (static blood); constipation due to dryness blood.	Pregnancy; absence of stasis and stagnation.	5–10 g
Strychnotis Nux-Vomicae Semen *ma³ qian² zi³* 馬錢子 (186)	Dissipates blood heat, disperses swelling and relieves pain.	Throat bi; swelling and toxin of yong and ju; wind bi pain; bone fractures; facial paralysis; myasthenia gravis.	Pregnancy and vacuity.	0.3–0.6 g
Myrrha *mo⁴ yao⁴* 沒藥 (202)	Dissipates the blood and eliminates stasis; disperses swellings and settles pain.	Impact injury; incised wounds; sinew and bone pain; pain in the abdomen and region of the heart; concretions and conglomerations; menstrual block; painful, swollen yong and ju; hemorrhoids; eye screens.	Pregnancy.	3–5 g
Olibanum (Gummi Olibanum) *ru³ xiang¹* 乳香 (203)	Regulates qi and quickens the blood; relieves pain, expels toxin. Stir-fry and remove oil, or stir-fry in vinegar for strong blood-quickening and pain-relieving action.	Qi and blood stagnation; pain in the abdomen and region of the heart; swelling toxin of yong and sores; impact injury; painful menstruation; postpartum blood stasis with stabbing pain.	Pregnancy.	3–7 g
Tabanus *meng² chong²* 虻蟲 (220)	Expels stasis, breaks accumulation, and promotes menstruation.	Concretions and gatherings; blood amassment in the lower abdomen; blood stagnation and menstrual block; stasis swelling due to impact injury.	Pregnancy.	1.5–3 g

7. Blood-quickening, stasis-dispelling, and blood-staunching agents 活血祛瘀・止血藥 *huo² xue⁴ qu¹ yu¹*, *zhi³ xue⁴ yao⁴*

Typhae Pollen *pu² huang²* 蒲黃 (118)	Cools the blood and staunches bleeding; quickens the blood and disperses stasis. Use crude to quicken the blood and dispel stasis, to disinhibit urine, and to disperse swelling. Use stir-fried to staunch bleeding and supplement the blood. Char-fry (or stir-fry with vinegar) to staunch bleeding. Treat with wine to move the blood.	Use crude for treating abdominal pain due to menstrual block; postpartum stasis pain; impact injury; swelling and toxin of sores and boils. Char-fry for treating blood ejection, spontaneous external and uterine bleeding, blood in the urine, blood dysentery, and vaginal discharge. Apply topically to purulent ear, mouth sores, and genital damp itch.	Yin vacuity and pregnancy.	5–10 g

8. Blood-quickening, stasis-dispelling, and yin-supplementing agents 活血祛瘀・補陰藥 *huo² xue⁴ qu¹ yu¹*, *bu³ yin¹ yao⁴*

Achyranthis Bidentatae Radix *niu² xi¹* 牛膝 (21)	Used crude, it dissipates stasis and disperses yong swelling. With wine, its channel-freeing and blood-quickening action is enhanced. Roasted or stir-fried, it supplements the liver and kidney, and strengthens the sinews and bones. Treated with brine, its bone and sinew strengthening action is enhanced. Similar products: Achyranthis Radix (*tu³ niu² xi¹*) has the same function as Achyranthis Bidentatae Radix, while Cyathulae Radix (*chuan¹ niu² xi¹*) has an especially strong stasis-dispelling effect.	Used crude it treats menstrual block, strangury, hematuria, swollen yong, difficult delivery. When roasted, stir-fried, and treated with brine, it treats pain and weakness in the knee and lumbus.	Spleen vacuity diarrhea, and in pregnancy.	5–10 g

9. Blood-staunching agents 止血藥 *zhi³ xue⁴ yao⁴*

San-Chi Ginseng Radix (Notoginseng Radix) *san¹ qi¹* 三七 (61)	Staunches bleeding, dissipates stasis, disperses swellings, and relieves pain.	Blood ejection; coughing of blood; spontaneous external bleeding; blood in the stool; blood dysentery; uterine bleeding; concretions and conglomerations; postpartum blood dizziness; retention of the lochia; impact injury and stasis; bleeding due to trauma.	Blood vacuity without blood stasis.	5–10 g

Name	Functions	Indications	Contraindications	Daily Dosage
Sanguisorbae Radix *di⁴ yu²* 地榆 (62)	Cools the blood and staunches bleeding; clears heat and resolves toxin.	Blood ejection; spontaneous external bleeding; blood dysentery; uterine bleeding; intestinal wind; hemorrhoids and fistulae; incised wounds; burns. Use crude for all blood patterns and burns. Char-fry to cool the blood and staunch bleeding. Stir-fry with vinegar to treat uterine bleeding and blood dysentery.	Profuse uterine bleeding due to qi vacuity fall; dysentery with dark colored pus and blood in the stool.	5–10 g
Bletillae Tuber *bai² ji²* 白及 (78)	Supplements the lung; staunches bleeding; disperses swellings; engenders muscle; closes sores.	Blood ejection; spontaneous external bleeding. Topically applied for incised wounds and swollen yong.	Lung or stomach repletion heat.	3–5 g
Nelumbinis Rhizomatis Nodus *ou³ jie²* 藕節 (90)	Staunches bleeding and dissipates stasis. Use crude to clear blood heat, allay thirst, and transform stasis. Char-fry to staunch bleeding.	Blood ejection: spontaneous external bleeding; blood in the urine; blood in the stool; blood dysentery; profuse uterine bleeding.		5–10 g
Biotae Folium et Ramulus *ce⁴ bo² ye⁴* 側柏葉 (100)	Cools the blood, staunches bleeding, dispels wind-damp, dissipates swelling toxin. Use crude to cool the blood and staunches bleeding. Char for better blood-staunching effect.	Blood ejection; spontaneous external bleeding; blood in the urine; blood dysentery; intestinal wind; profuse uterine bleeding; wind-damp bi pain; bacillary dysentery; hypertension; cough; cinnabar toxin; mumps; burns and scalds.	Absence of damp-heat.	5–10 g
Celosiae Cristatae Flos *ji¹ guan¹ hua¹* 雞冠花 (108)	Staunches bleeding and cools the blood. Char-fry to staunch bleeding.	Bleeding from hemorrhoids; red and white dysentery; blood ejection; coughing of blood; blood strangury; profuse uterine bleeding; red and white vaginal discharge.	Accumulation and stagnation.	5–10 g
Sophorae Flos Immaturus *hua² hua¹* 槐花 (117)	Clears heat, cools the blood and staunches bleeding. Mix-fry with honey to moisten the lung. Char-fry to staunch bleeding.	Intestinal wind hemafecia; bleeding hemorrhoids; blood in the urine; blood strangury; uterine bleeding; spontaneous external bleeding; red and white dysentery; wind-heat reddening of the eyes; yong, ju and sores toxin. The crude drug treats hypertension. The stir-fried drug treats throat bi, blood ejection, nosebleed, and uterine bleeding. The char-fried drug is effective for red and white dysentery.	Vacuity cold diarrhea and qi vacuity uterine bleeding.	5–10 g

Drug	Function	Indications	Cautions	Dosage
Sophorae Fructus *huai² jiao³* 槐角 (152)	Clears heat, moistens the liver, cools the blood, and staunches bleeding. Charring enhances the blood-staunching effect and ability to treat hemorrhoids. Mix-frying gives it an intestine-moistening action.	Intestinal wind bleeding; hemorrhoidal bleeding; uterine bleeding; blood strangury and dysentery; vexation and oppression in the chest and heart; wind dizziness with difficulty in remaining standing; itching genital sores.	Spleen-stomach vacuity cold and pregnancy.	6–15 g

10. Blood-supplementing and blood-cooling agents 補血・涼血藥 *bu³ xue⁴, liang² xue⁴ yao⁴*

Drug	Function	Indications	Cautions	Dosage
Rehmanniae Radix *di⁴ huang²* 地黃 (59)	Enriches yin and nourishes the blood. Carbonize to supplement the spleen and stomach. Stir-fry with wine to move the blood and check bleeding.	The dry form treats blood vacuity with fever, menstrual irregularities, stirring fetus, frenetic blood heat, blood ejection, spontaneous external bleeding, precipitation of blood, uterine bleeding. The cooked form treats uterine bleeding, wasting thirst, yin vacuity cough, dyspnea, and blood vacuity.	Spleen-stomach vacuity cold.	5–10 g

11. Cough-suppressing agents 止咳藥 *zhi³ ke² yao⁴*

Drug	Function	Indications	Cautions	Dosage
Lilii Bulbus *bai³ he²* 百合 (89)	Moistens the lung and suppresses cough; clears the heart and quiets the spirit; disinhibits water. Mix-frying with honey enhances the lung-moistening action.	Taxation cough; blood ejection; vacuity vexation; fright palpitation; water swelling; hysteria.	Wind-cold or phlegm cough.	5–10 g

12. Cough-suppressing and dyspnea-calming agents 止咳・平喘藥 *zhi³ ke², ping² chuan³ yao⁴*

Drug	Function	Indications	Cautions	Dosage
Mori Cortex Radicis *sang¹ bai² pi²* 桑白皮 (8)	Drains the lung and calms dyspnea; moves water and disperses swelling.	Lung heat cough, and blood ejection, water swelling, and abdominal distention. Mix-frying with honey adds a lung-moistening action suited to patients suffering from lung vacuity cough.	Lung vacuity without fire; cold cough.	5–10 g
Asteris Radix et Rhizoma *zi³ wan³* 紫菀 (28)	Warms the lung, precipitates qi, disperses phlegm, and suppresses cough. Use crude to diffuse the lung and disperse phlegm. Stir-fry for stronger lung-warming action. Mix-fry with honey for greater lung-moistening action.	Wind-cold cough and dyspnea: coughing of blood and pus in vacuity taxation; throat bi; inhibited urination.	Yin vacuity lung heat.	5–10 g

Name	Functions	Indications	Contraindications	Daily Dosage
Peucedani Radix *qian² hu²* 前胡 (54)	Diffuses wind-heat, precipitates qi, and disperses phlegm. Use crude to diffuse wind-heat, or mix-fried with honey to moisten the lung, downbear qi, and transform phlegm.	Wind-heat cough and headache; phlegm dyspnea and fullness; counterflow retching; fullness and oppression in the chest and diaphragm.	Absence of repletion heat.	5–10 g
Stemonae Radix *bai³ bu⁴* 百部 (68)	Warms and moistens lung qi; suppresses cough; kills worms. Use crude for roundworm and pinworm. Mix-fry with honey to moisten the lung and suppress cough.	Cold cough; hookworm or pinworm infestation; jie and xian; pulmonary consumption; fulminant cough.	Spleen-stomach vacuity with diarrhea.	3–10 g
Eriobotryae Folium *pi² pa² ye⁴* 枇杷葉 (101)	Clears the lung and harmonizes the stomach; downbears qi and transforms phlegm. Has a strong lung-moistening effect when mix-fried with honey. It is usually stir-fried with ginger juice when used to treat stomach disorders.	Heat cough; copious phlegm; thirst; coughing of blood; spontaneous external bleeding; vomiting due to stomach heat.	Vacuity vexation and vomiting, and cold cough.	5–10 g
Farfarae Flos (Tussilaginis Flos) *kuan³ dong¹ hua¹* 款冬花 (112)	Moistens the lung and precipitates qi; transforms phlegm and suppresses cough. Use crude to warm the lung. Stir-fry with honey to moisten the lung and suppress cough.	Counterflow cough; dyspnea; throat bi.	Yin vacuity lung heat.	5–10 g
Aristolochiae Fructus *ma³ dou¹ ling²* 馬兜鈴 (124)	Clears the lung and downbears qi; transforms phlegm and suppresses cough. Mix-fried with honey, it has a stronger lung-moistening function.	Lung heat dyspnea and cough; expectoration of blood; loss of voice; hemorrhoids and fistulae with pain and swelling.	Vacuity cold cough and dyspnea; spleen vacuity diarrhea.	3–5 g
Perillae Fructus *zi³ su¹ zi³* 紫蘇子 (146)	Precipitates qi, disperses phlegm, moistens the lung, and loosens the intestines. Used stir-fried, it has a milder effect, and a strong qi-moving effect. Mix-fry with honey for a strong lung-moistening effect.	Counterflow cough; phlegm dyspnea; qi stagnation; constipation.	Diarrhea due to intestinal qi vacuity.	5–10 g

Armeniacae Semen (Pruni Armeniacae Semen) xing⁴ ren² 杏仁 (162)	Dispels phlegm and suppresses cough; calms dyspnea and lubricates the intestines. Steaming or stir-frying reduces toxicity. Apricot kernel frost (Armeniacae Seminis Pulvis, [xing⁴ ren² shuang¹]), i.e., the kernels crushed with the oil removed, moves the connecting vessels, diffuses the lung, dispels phlegm, and settles dyspnea.	External contraction cough; dyspnea and fullness; throat bi; constipation due to dryness intestines.	Yin vacuity cough.	5–10 g

13. Cough-suppressing and phlegm-transforming agents 止咳・化痰藥 zhi³ ke², hua⁴ tan² yao⁴

Bambusae Caulis in Taeniam zhu² ru² 竹茹 (12)	Clears heat; cools the blood; transforms phlegm; checks vomiting. Used crude to clear heat and transform phlegm. Used stir-fried to moderate the cold nature. Used treated with ginger to reduce the cold nature and enhance the power to check vomiting.	Stomach heat with counterflow retching, heat vexation in the upper burner, blood ejection, nosebleed, profuse uterine bleeding, and stirring fetus.	Spleen-stomach vacuity cold.	5–10 g
Platycodonis Radix jie² geng³ 桔梗 (55)	Opens and diffuses lung qi, eliminates phlegm, and expels pus. Use crude to diffuse the lung and dispel phlegm, to expel pus and disperse swelling, and to disinhibit the throat and relieve pain. Mix-fry with honey to moisten the lung.	External contraction cough; throat bi; pulmonary yong; blood ejection: coughing of blood and pus; fullness in the chest; pain in the lateral costal region; dysenteric disease; abdominal pain.	Yin vacuity cough.	3–5 g
Arisaematis Rhizoma tian¹ nan² xing¹ 天南星 (75)	Dries damp and transforms phlegm; dispels wind and calms fright; disperses swelling and binds. Use the processed forms for reduced toxicity. Use stir-fried with ginger to warm and dissipate, and to dispel phlegm, or processed in bile to reduce its dryness and harshness.	Wind stroke hemiplegia and deviation of the eyes and mouth; epilepsy; child fright wind; lockjaw; wind-phlegm dizziness; throat bi; scrofulous lumps; swollen yong; impact injury and bone fractures; snake and insect bites. Arisaematis Rhizoma cum Felle Bovis (with bovine bile) treats fright, epilepsy, and dizziness.	Yin vacuity and dryness phlegm.	3–5 g
Fritillariae Bulbus bei⁴ mu³ 貝母 (85)	Suppresses cough and dispels phlegm; clear heat and dissipates binds.	Cough; blood ejection; thirst; throat bi; scrofulous lumps; mammary yong; dorsal effusions; painful, swollen sores.	Spleen-stomach vacuity cold.	5–10 g

Name	Functions	Indications	Contraindications	Daily Dosage
Pinelliae Tuber *ban⁴ xia⁴* 半夏 (92)	Dries damp and transforms phlegm; downbears counterflow and suppresses vomiting; disperses glomus and dissipates binds. Use crude for topical application only. Use the ginger-treated kind, which is warm and dry in nature, to check vomiting. Use the other processed forms to dry damp and transform phlegm.	Phlegm-damp and water rheum; cough and dyspnea; dizziness. Pro formula pinellia dries damp and transforms phlegm, while ginger pinellia checks vomiting. Crude pinellia is toxic and is for external use only.	All blood patterns, pregnancy, yin vacuity, and damage to fluids.	5–10 g
Inulae Flos *xuan² fu⁴ hua¹* 旋覆花 (113)	Disperses phlegm, precipitates qi, softens hardness, and moves water. Mix-fry with honey to moisten the lung and suppress cough.	Phlegm bind in the chest; distention and fullness in the lateral costal region; cough and dyspnea; hiccough; sticky spittle; hard thoracic glomus; persistent belching; water swelling; of the upper abdomen.	Diarrhea.	5–10 g
Gleditsiae Fructus *zao⁴ jia²* 皂荚 (136)	Dispels wind-phlegm (especially when roasted or stir-fried), eliminates damp toxin, and kills worms. Boil and remove the yellow skin to treat constipation.	Deviation of eyes and mouth in wind stroke; head wind headache; phlegm-dyspnea and cough; intestinal wind hematecia; dysentery; trismus; swollen yong; inguinal lumps: sores; xian, jie, and lai.	Vacuity and pregnancy.	1–3 g
Trichosanthis Fructus *gua¹ lou²* 栝楼 (154)	Fruit: moistens the lung, transforms phlegm, and dissipates binds. Pericarp: clears heat, transforms phlegm, and disinhibits qi. Stir-fried it suppresses cold and transforms phlegm, while mix-fried with honey it loosens the center, clears heat, and moistens the intestines. Seed: moistens the lung, transforms phlegm, and moistens the intestines. Used stir-fried it treats cough and fever.	Fruit: phlegm-heat cough; thoracic bi; chest bind; pulmonary atony; coughing of blood; wasting thirst. Pericarp: phlegm-heat cough, sore throat, and blood ejection. Seed: phlegm-heat cough; constipation, and yong and ju.	Spleen-stomach vacuity cold with diarrhea; cold phlegm or damp phlegm.	10–12 g
Benincasae Semen *dong¹ gua¹ zi³* 冬瓜子 (163)	Moistens the lung; transforms phlegm; disperses yong, and disinhibits water. Stir-fry with bran to harmonize the stomach.	Phlegm-heat cough; pulmonary and intestinal yong; strangury; water swelling; leg qi; hemorrhoids; drinker's nose.	Diarrhea in enduring disease.	3–12 g

Drug	Function	Indication	Contraindication	Dosage
Sinapis Semen (Brassicae Junceae Semen) jie⁴ zi³ 芥子 (184)	Warms the center and dissipates cold; disinhibits qi and sweeps phlegm; frees the channels and the connecting vessels, disperses swelling. Stir-frying enhances the phlegm-transforming action.	Vomiting of food due to stomach cold; pain in the abdomen and region of the heart; lung cold cough; painful bi; throat bi; yin ju; cold phlegm; impact injuries.	Lung vacuity cough; effulgent yin vacuity fire.	3–5 g

14. Cough-suppressing, phlegm-transforminging, and astringing agents 止咳化痰 · 收斂藥 zhi³ ke² hua⁴ tan², shou¹ lian⁴ yao⁴

Drug	Function	Indication	Contraindication	Dosage
Ginkgo Semen bai² guo³ 白果 (171)	Constrains lung qi, calms cough and dyspnea, checks vaginal discharge, and reduces urine flow. Use crude to downbear phlegm, disperse toxin, and kill worms. Use prepared to warm the lung and boost qi, suppress cough and calm dyspnea, and to reduce urination and check vaginal discharge.	Wheezing dyspnea; phlegm cough; white turbidity; vaginal discharge; seminal emission; strangury; frequent urination.	Pathogen repletion.	5–10 g

15. Exterior-resolving and wind-damp-dispelling agents 解表 · 祛風濕藥 jie³ biao³, qu¹ feng¹ shi¹ yao⁴

Drug	Function	Indication	Contraindication	Dosage
Xanthii Fructus cang¹ er³ zi³ 蒼耳子 (156)	Dissipates wind, relieves pain, dispels damp, and kills worms. The toxin is removed by stir-frying.	Wind-cold headache; deep-source nasal congestion; toothache; wind, cold, and damp bi; hypertonicity of the limbs; jie and lai.	Blood vacuity; bi disease.	5–10 g

16. Heart-nourishing and spirit-quieting agents 養心安神藥 yang³ xin¹ an¹ shen² yao⁴

Drug	Function	Indication	Contraindication	Dosage
Polygalae Radix yuan³ zhi⁴ 遠志 (56)	Quiets the spirit and sharpens the wits; dispels wind and resolves depression.	Fright palpitations; poor memory; wet dreams; insomnia; coughing with copious phlegm; swollen yong, ju and sores. Stir-fry with honey to increase the moistening and spirit-quieting effect. Coat in cinnabar for a powerful spirit-quieting effect.	Repletion fire.	3–5 g
Zizyphi Spinosi Semen suan¹ zao³ ren² 酸棗仁 (188)	Nourishes the liver, quiets the heart, calms the spirit and contracts sweating. Use crude to drain the liver and gallbladder and to quiet the spirit. Use stir-fried to nourish liver blood and quiet the spirit.	Vacuity vexation and sleeplessness; fright palpitation; racing of the heart; vexation and thirst; vacuity sweating.	Pathogen repletion and depressed fire.	5–10 g

17. Heat-clearing and astringing agents 清熱・收斂藥 *qing¹ re⁴, shou¹ lian⁴ yao⁴*

Name	Functions	Indications	Contraindications	Daily Dosage
Nelumbinis Fructus *shí² lian² zi³* 石蓮子 (145)	Whole fruit: cold; bitter; nontoxic. Clears the heart and eliminates vexation. Seed: balanced; astringent and sweet; nontoxic. Astringes the intestines; nourishes the stomach; secures essence. Plumule: cold; bitter. Resolves heat and quiets the heart.	The whole fruit treats chronic dysentery. The seed treats spleen diarrhea and enduring diarrhea, uterine bleeding, vaginal discharge, and seminal emission. The plumule treats vexation, thirst, and blood ejection.		5–10 g (plumule 1.5–3 g)

18. Heat-clearing and blood-cooling agents 清熱・涼血藥 *qing¹ re⁴, liang² xue⁴ yao⁴*

Name	Functions	Indications	Contraindications	Daily Dosage
Lycii Cortex Radicis *di⁴ gu³ pi²* 地骨皮 (6)	Clears heat; cools the blood.	Cough, blood ejection; heat vexation; wasting thirst; taxation fever with perspiration; steaming bone tidal fever; swollen yong and malign sores.	Absence of construction heat or presence of spleen-stomach vacuity cold.	6–10 g
Moutan Cortex Radicis *mu³ dan¹ pi²* 牡丹皮 (9)	Clears heat, cools the blood, harmonizes the blood, and disperses stasis. Stir-frying enhances the stasis-dissipating action, and carbonizing adds a blood-staunching effect.	Intestinal yong, and sores; heat entering nutrition level, macules, fright epilepsy, ejection of blood, nosebleed, and hemafecia, steaming bone tidal fever, menstrual block, shan-jia, yong, and impact injury.	Spleen-stomach vacuity cold and diarrhea.	6–10 g
Cynanchi Radix *bai² wei²* 白薇 (35)	Use crude to clear heat and cool the blood. Use mix-fried with honey for external contraction with fever, cough, and dyspnea.	Yin vacuity heat; wind warmth with high fever and tendency to sleep; lung heat and coughing of blood; warm malaria; postpartum vacuity vexation and blood inversion; heat and blood strangury; rheumatic pain; scrofulous lumps.	Absence of heat in the blood aspect and center cold with diarrhea.	5–10 g
Lithospermi Radix *zi³ cao³* 紫草 (48)	Cools the blood, quickens the blood, clears heat, and resolves toxin.	Maculopapular eruptions in warm heat disease; damp-heat jaundice; purple patches; blood ejection; spontaneous external bleeding; blood in the urine; turbid strangury; blood dysentery; heat bind constipation; burns; eczema; cinnabar toxin; yong.	Gastrointestinal vacuity with diarrhea.	5–10 g
Paeoniae Radix Rubra *chi⁴ shao² yao⁴* 赤芍藥 (52)	Moves stasis, relieves pain, cools the blood, and disperses swelling. Use crude to clear heat and cool the blood. Stir-fry without additives to moderate the cool nature, or stir-fry with wine to enhance the blood-quickening and stasis-dispelling action.	Menstrual block due to blood stagnation; concretions and gatherings; pain in the abdomen and lateral costal region; spontaneous external bleeding; blood dysentery; intestinal wind bleeding; reddening of the eyes; yong swelling.	Blood vacuity.	5–10 g

				150–400 mg
Bezoar Bovis niu² pi² 牛黃 (209)	Clears the heart; transforms phlegm; disinhibits the gallbladder; and settles fright.	Clouding of the spirit and delirious speech in heat diseases; epilepsy and mania; child fright wind; gan of the teeth and gums; swollen throat; mouth sores; yong and ju; clove sores.	Pregnancy.	
Rhinocerotis Cornu xi¹ jiao³ 犀角 (219)	Clears heat, cools the blood, settles fright and resolves toxin.	Heat entering the blood aspect; fright mania; vexation and agitation; delirious frenzy; maculopapular eruptions; yellowing of the skin; blood ejection; spontaneous external bleeding; precipitation of blood; swelling and toxin of yong and ju.	Pregnancy.	1–3 g

19. Heat-clearing and damp-drying agents 清熱・燥濕藥 *qing¹ re⁴, zao⁴ shi¹ yao⁴*

				5–10 g
Fraxini Cortex qin² pi² 秦皮 (5)	Clears heat and dries damp; calms dyspnea and suppresses cough; brightens the eyes.	Bacterial dysentery; enteritis; vaginal discharge; chronic bronchitis; sore, red, swollen eyes and tearing on exposure to wind; oxhide xian.	Stomach vacuity with low food intake.	
Phellodendri Cortex huang² bo² 黃柏 (10)	Clears heat, dries damp, drains the fire and resolves toxin. Use crude to clear heat and drain fire. Use stir-fried with brine to clear vacuity heat, especially in kidney vacuity. Use stir-fried with wine to treat the upper burner or for better blood-quickening action. Use mix-fried with honey for middle burner patterns, and carbonized to staunch bleeding.	Heat dysentery and diarrhea, jaundice, steaming bones, hemorrhoids, hematecia, turbid strangury, vaginal discharge, and sores.	Spleen vacuity diarrhea or a weak stomach.	5–10 g
Gentianae Scabrae Radix (Gentianae Radix) long² dan³ 龍膽 (39)	Drains liver-gallbladder repletion fire; eliminates lower burner damp-heat. Use crude to make it act on the lower body, and stir-fry with wine to make it act on the upper body. Stir-fry with honey to make it act on the middle burner. Stir-fry with pig's bile to enhance the fire-downbearing action.	Exuberant heat in the liver channel; fright epilepsy; manic agitation; encephalitis B; headache; reddening of the eyes; sore throat; jaundice; heat dysentery; swollen yong and sores; painful swelling of the scrotum; genital damp itch.	Spleen-stomach vacuity diarrhea, and repletion fire patterns without cold-damp.	3–5 g

Name	Functions	Indications	Contraindications	Daily Dosage
Scutellariae Radix *huang² qin²* 黃芩 (65)	Drains the fire, eliminates damp-heat, staunches bleeding and quiets the fetus. Use crude to clear heat and drain fire. Stir-fry to moderate its cold nature and quiet the fetus. Stir-fry with wine to clear upper-burner damp-heat and lung heat, with ginger juice to clear heat and dispel phlegm, or with bran to reduce the agent's cold nature and minimize damage to the stomach. Carbonize to clear heat and staunch bleeding.	Vigorous fever, vexation, and thirst; lung heat cough; damp-heat diarrhea; jaundice; heat strangury; blood ejection; uterine and spontaneous external bleeding; red, sore, swollen eyes; yong and ju; stirring fetus; swollen yong and clove sores.	Spleen-stomach vacuity cold, and repletion fire patterns without damp-heat.	3–6 g
Sophorae Radix (Sophorae Flavescentis Radix) *ku³ shen¹* 苦參 (66)	Clears heat, dries damp, and kills worms.	Heat toxin and blood strangury; intestinal wind bleeding; jaundice; red and white vaginal discharge; itchy skin; jie and lai; malign sores; scrofulous lumps; scalds. Soak in wine to treat malign sores. Stir-fry without additives to treat intestinal wind. Stir-fry with wine to treat heat bind, or with vinegar to treat lower abdominal heat pain. Char-fry to staunch bleeding.	Stomach cold.	5–10 g
Coptidis Rhizoma *huang² lian²* 黃連 (80)	Drains fire, dries damp, resolves toxin and kills worms. Use crude to break blood and qi. Stir-fry without additives to regulate the blood. Stir-fry with wine to move the blood and dispel stasis. Stir-fry in vinegar to calm the liver, staunch bleeding, and relieve pain. Boil with vinegar to nourish the liver. Stir-fry with wine and vinegar to relieve pain.	Seasonal heat toxin; cold damage: exuberant heat vexation; glomus and fullness; counterflow retching; bacillary dysentery; abdominal pain due to heat diarrhea; pulmonary tuberculosis; blood ejection: spontaneous external bleeding; precipitation of blood; wasting thirst; gan accumulation: roundworm; diphtheria; sore, swollen throat; fire eye: mouth sores; toxin of yong, ju, and sores; eczema; burns and scalds.	Spleen vacuity diarrhea; vexation and fever due to either yin vacuity or postpartum blood vacuity.	1–3 g

20. Heat-clearing and fire-draining agents 清熱 · 瀉火藥 *qing¹ re⁴, xie⁴ huo³ yao⁴*

Name	Functions	Indications	Contraindications	Daily Dosage
Trichosanthis Radix *tian¹ hua¹ fen³* 天花粉 (69)	Engenders liquid and allays thirst; downbears fire; moistens dryness; expels pus; disperses swelling.	Thirst in febrile disease; wasting thirst; jaundice; lung dryness; coughing of blood; swollen yong; hemorrhoids.	Spleen-stomach vacuity cold with diarrhea; patterns without repletion heat.	10–12 g

Drug	Functions	Indications	Contraindications	Dosage
Anemarrhenae Rhizoma zhi¹ mu³ 知母 (74)	Enriches yin and downbears fire; moistens dryness and lubricates the intestines. Use crude to drain heat. Stir-fry to moderate the cold effect. Stir-fry with wine to make it act on the upper body. Stir-fry with brine to make it enter the kidney, moisten dryness, and enrich yin.	Vexation and thirst; steaming bone and taxation heat; lung heat cough; dry, bound stool; inhibited urination.	Spleen-stomach vacuity with indigestion and thin-stool diarrhea.	5–10 g
Lophatheri Folium dan⁴ zhu² ye⁴ 淡竹葉 (102)	Clears heart fire, eliminates vexation heat, and disinhibits urine.	Thirst in febrile disease; vexation: inhibited voidings of dark-colored urine; turbid stranguary; oral putrescence; tongue sores; sore, swollen gums.	Pregnancy.	6–12 g
Prunellae Spica xia⁴ ku¹ cao³ 夏枯草 (116)	Clears the liver, and dissipates binds.	Scrofulous lumps; goiter; mammary yong; nocturnal eyeball pain; tearing and aversion to light; dizziness of the head and eyes; deviated mouth and eyes; sinew and bone pain; pulmonary tuberculosis; acute icteric infectious hepatitis; uterine bleeding.	Spleen-stomach vacuity.	3–10 g
Gardeniae Fructus zhi¹ zi³ 梔子 (135)	Clears heat, drains fire, and cools the blood. Use crude to clear heat and drain fire. Stir-fry or scorch-fry for an additional blood-cooling action. Char to treat blood ejection, nosebleed, and blood dysentery. Stir-fry with ginger juice to check vexation and vomiting. Stir-fry with brine to clear vacuity fire. Remove the skin to drain heart fire, but leave it on to drain lung fire. Gardeniae Jasminoidis Grandiflorae Fructus has a strong precipitating (purgative) action.	Vacuity vexation and sleeplessness in febrile disease; jaundice and strangury; wasting thirst; reddening of the eyes; sore throat and blood ejection; spontaneous external bleeding and blood dysentery; blood in the urine; heat toxin sores; sprains.	Spleen-stomach vacuity cold.	3–10 g
Gypsum Fibrosum shi² gao¹ 石膏 (226)	Used crude, it resolves the muscles and clears heat, eliminates vexation and allays thirst. Calcined and applied topically, it engenders muscle and closes sores.	Persistent vigorous fever in heat disease; vexation and clouding of the spirit, delirious speech, and mania; lung heat with rapid dyspneic breathing; summerheat stroke with spontaneous sweating; stomach heat headache or toothache; exuberant heat toxin giving rise to maculopapular eruptions; mouth sores.	Absence of repletion heat.	15–20 g

21. Heat-clearing and toxin-resolving agents 清熱・解毒藥 *qing¹ re⁴, jie³ du² yao⁴*

Name	Functions	Indications	Contraindications	Daily Dosage
Dictamni Radicis Cortex *bai² xian¹ pi²* 白鮮皮 (3)	Dispels wind; dries damp; clears heat; and resolves toxin.	Wind bi; damp sores, jaundice, jie and xian.	Lower burner vacuity cold.	6–10 g
Sophorae Subprostratae Radix *shan¹ dou⁴ gen¹* 山豆根 (67)	Clears fire, resolves toxin, disperses swelling, and relieves pain.	Throat yong; throat wind; throat bi; sore, swollen gums; heat cough with dyspnea and fullness; jaundice; dyspnea; hemorrhoids; heat swelling; bald scalp sores; jie and xian; snake, insect and dog bites.	Spleen-stomach vacuity cold with thin stool.	3–10 g
Lonicerae Flos *jin¹ yin² hua¹* 金銀花 (114)	Clears heat and resolves toxin. Distillate of Lonicerae Flos resolves summerheat and clears heat.	Initial-stage warm disease with heat in the upper burner; swelling and toxin of sores. Char-fry to treat blood dysentery and blood in the stool. Stir-fry to treat diarrhea.	Spleen-stomach vacuity cold.	10–15 g
Forsythiae Fructus *lian² qiao²* 連翹 (134)	Clears heat, resolves toxin, dissipates binds, and disperses swelling. Use crude to clear heat and resolve toxin. Blend with cinnabar to clear the heart and quiet the spirit in febrile diseases.	Warm heat; cinnabar toxin; maculopapular eruption; swelling and toxin of yong; scrofulous lumps; dribbling urinary block. Can be applied topically to jie and xian.	Yin vacuity blood heat, gastric vacuity diarrhea, and burst yong exuding light green pus.	5–10 g
Fel Ursi *xiong² dan³* 熊膽 (214)	Clears heat, settles tetany, brightens the eyes and kills worms.	Heat jaundice; summerheat diarrhea; child fright epilepsy; gan disease; hookworm infestation; eye screens; throat bi; clove and malign sores; hemorrhoids.	Hemorrhoids.	0.15–0.3 g

22. Heat-clearing, blood-cooling, and blood-staunching agents 清熱涼血・止血藥 *qing¹ re⁴ liang² xue³, zhi³ xue⁴ yao⁴*

| Imperatae Rhizoma *bai² mao² gen¹* 白茅根 (87) | Cools the blood and staunches bleeding; clears heat; disinhibits urine. | Internal heat; vexation: inhibited urination: heat strangury; blood in the urine; blood ejection; spontaneous external bleeding. | Vacuity cold; absence of repletion heat. | 10–15 g |

23. Heavy settling and spirit-quieting agents 重鎮・安神藥 zhong⁴ zheng⁴, an¹ shen² yao⁴

Cinnabaris zhu³ sha¹ 朱砂 (224)	Quiets the spirit; calms fright; brightens the eyes; resolves toxin.	Mania and withdrawal; fright palpitations; vexation; insomnia; dizziness; clouded vision; toxin swellings; jie, xian, sores.	Absence of repletion heat.	20-35 mg.
Draconis Os (Mastodi Ossis Fossilia) long² gu³ 龍骨 (225)	Settles fright and quiets the spirit; constrains sweating and secures essence; astringes the intestines; engenders flesh and contracts sores. Use crude to subdue yang and quiet the spirit, calcined to astringe, and coated in cinnabar to quiet the heart spirit.	Diarrhea and prolapse of the anus; open sores that will not heal. fright epilepsy; mania and withdrawal; racing of the heart; poor memory; insomnia; profuse dreaming; spontaneous and night sweating; seminal emission; turbid strangury; blood ejection; spontaneous external and uterine bleeding; blood in the stool.	Damp-heat and other pathogen repletion patterns.	10-15 g

24. Heavy settling, spirit-quieting, and astringing agents 重鎮安神・收斂藥 zhong⁴ zhen⁴ an¹ shen², shou¹ lian⁴ yao⁴

Ostreae Concha mu³ li⁴ 牡蠣 (218)	Constrains yin, subdues yang, checks sweating, astringes essence, transforms phlegm, and softens hardness. Used crude, it quiets the spirit and calms the liver. Calcined, it contracts and astringes, and softens hardness.	Fright epilepsy; dizziness; spontaneous sweating; night sweating; seminal emission; turbid strangury; uterine bleeding; vaginal discharge; scrofulous lumps; goiters and tumors of the neck.	Kidney vacuity without heat, and spontaneous loss of cold semen.	10-20 g

25. Interior-warming agents 溫裡藥 wen¹ li³ yao⁴

Cinnamomi Cortex rou⁴ gui⁴ 肉桂 (2)	Supplements original yang; warms the spleen and stomach; eliminates accumulated frigidity; frees the blood vessels.	Inversion cold in the limbs, upper body heat with lower body cold, lumbar and knee pain, vacuity cold with aversion to food, clear-food diarrhea, menstrual block, abdominal pain, shan-jia, and inhibited urination.	Effulgent yin vacuity fire and pregnancy.	1-5 g
Alpiniae Officinarum Rhizoma gao¹ liang² jiang¹ 高良薑 (73)	Warms the stomach; dispels wind; dissipates cold; moves qi; relieves pain.	Spleen-stomach cold; frigid pain in the venter and abdomen; vomiting and diarrhea; esophageal constriction; food stagnation; cold pi.	Vomiting due to stomach heat, summerheat damage or choleraic disease; diarrhea due to heat or fire; heart vacuity.	3-5 g

Name	Functions	Indications	Contraindications	Daily Dosage
Zingiberis Rhizoma Exsiccatum *gan¹ jiang¹* 乾薑 (98)	Crude dried ginger warms the center. Blast-fried dried ginger warms the center and staunches bleeding.	Retching and vomiting; phlegm-rheum; cough and dyspnea; fullness and dyspnea; diarrhea; resolves toxin of Pinelliae Tuber.	Yin vacuity heat.	3–10 g
Caryophylli Flos *ding¹ xiang¹* 丁香 (107)	Warms the center, warms the kidney, and downbears counterflow.	Hiccough; vomiting; stomach reflux; diarrhea; cold pain in the abdomen and region of the heart; elusive and bowstring masses; shan qi.	Yin vacuity heat and other heat patterns; hyperchlorhydria; acute gastroenteritis; gastric hemorrhage.	1–3 g
Anisi Stellati Fructus (Illicii Veri Fructus) *ba¹ jiao³ hui² xiang¹* 八角茴香 (121)	Warms yang, dissipates cold, and rectifies qi.	Cold strike; counterflow retching; cold shan; abdominal pain; kidney vacuity; lumbar pain; dry and damp leg qi. Stir-fry lightly for lumbar pain and leg qi (beri-beri).	Effulgent yin vacuity fire.	3–5 g
Evodiae Fructus *wu² zhu¹ yu²* 吳茱萸 (132)	Warms the center and relieves pain; rectifies qi and dries damp. Treat with licorice water to reduce its harsh, pungent quality. Stir-fry with wine to quicken the blood, with vinegar to calm the liver, and with brine to enter the kidney and treat shan pain. Stir-fry with Coptidis Rhizoma (*huang² lian²*) to treat vomiting, and with ginger juice to expel cold and relieve pain. Stir-fry without additives to precipitate qi and downbear counterflow.	Counterflow retching; acid vomiting; jue yin headache; vomiting and diarrhea due to visceral cold; distention pain in the venter and abdomen; leg qi; shan qi; mouth sores and ulcers; toothache; eczema; yellow water sores.	Yin vacuity and absence of cold-damp.	1.5–3 g
Foeniculi Fructus *hui² xiang¹* 茴香 (133)	Warms the kidney and dissipates cold; harmonizes the stomach and rectifies qi.	Cold shan; frigid pain in the lower abdomen; kidney vacuity lumbar pain; stomach pain; vomiting; dry and damp leg qi. Use stir-fried for pain in the bladder, and stir-fried in brine to treat kidney vacuity lumbar pain.	Yin vacuity fire.	3–10 g
Piperis Longi Fructus *bi⁴ ba²* 蓽茇 (147)	Warms the center, dissipates cold, precipitates qi and relieves pain. Soaking in vinegar can prevent it from damaging the lung.	Frigid pain in the abdomen and region of the heart; vomiting and acid regurgitation; rumbling intestines and diarrhea; frigid dysentery; yin shan; headache; deep-source nasal congestion; toothache.	Lung-spleen repletion heat or depressed heat.	1.5–3 g

| Piperis (Nigri) Fructus hu² jiao¹ 胡椒 (148) | Warms the center, precipitates qi, disperses phlegm, and resolves toxin. | Cold phlegm; food accumulation; frigid pain in the venter and abdomen; stomach reflux; vomiting of clear fluid; diarrhea; frigid dysentery. | Upflaming yin vacuity fire. | 1.5–3 g |
| Zanthoxyli Fructus hua¹ jiao¹ 花椒 (157) | Warms the center and dissipates cold; eliminates damp, relieves pain, kills worms, and resolves fish toxin. | Food accumulation; frigid pain in the abdomen and heart; vomiting; belching and hiccough; cough and qi counterflow; wind, cold, and damp bi; diarrhea; dysenteric disease; shan pain; toothache; roundworm and pinworm infestation; genital itch; jie. | Effulgent yin vacuity fire; pregnancy. | 1.5–5 g |

26. Interior-warming and blood-staunching agents 溫裡 · 止血藥 wen¹ li³, zhi³ xue⁴ yao⁴

| Artemisiae Argyi Folium ai⁴ ye⁴ 艾葉 (99) | Rectifies qi and the blood; expels cold-damp; warms the channels; staunches bleeding; quiets the fetus. Use crude to dissipate cold and relieve pain, and stir-fried with vinegar to relieve abdominal pain and staunch bleeding. Char for enhanced blood-staunching action. | Abdominal cold pain; frigid dysentery; menstrual block; uterine bleeding in pregnancy; blood ejection or nosebleed; vaginal discharge; stirring fetus; yong, jie, and xian. | Yin vacuity and blood heat. | 3–5 g |

27. Liver-calming and wind-extinguishing agents 平肝 · 熄風藥 ping² gan¹, xi² feng¹ yao⁴

Uncariae Ramulus et Uncus gou¹ teng² 鉤藤 (20)	Clears heat and calms the liver; extinguishes wind and settles fright.	Dizziness and infantile fright epilepsy.	Absence of wind-heat or repletion heat.	5–10 g
Gastrodiae Rhizoma tian¹ ma² 天麻 (86)	Extinguishes wind and calms fright. Treats dizziness, head wind and headache, numbness of the limbs, hemiplegia, impeded speech, child fright epilepsy.	Dizziness and blackouts; head wind and headache; wind stroke with hemiplegia and speech difficulty; child fright epilepsy; wind, cold, and damp bi.	Yin vacuity.	3–5 g
Tribuli Fructus ci⁴ ji² li² 刺蒺藜 (153)	Dissipates wind, brightens the eyes, precipitates qi, moves the blood. Stir-fry in brine for extra kidney-supplementing action.	Headache (use crude form); generalized itch; red swollen eyes; thoracic fullness; counterflow cough; concretions and conglomerations; mammary yong; yong and ju: scrofulous lumps. For eye diseases stir-fry till yellow.	Blood and qi vacuity; pregnancy.	10–12 g

Name	Functions	Indications	Contraindications	Daily Dosage
Antelopis Cornu *ling² yang² jiao³* 羚羊角 (207)	Calms the liver and extinguishes wind; clears heat and settles fright; resolves toxin.	Tetany and clouding of the spirit in febrile disease; delirious mania; headache and dizziness; fright epilepsy and spasm; reddening of the eyes; eye screens.	Absence heat in the liver channel.	1.5-3 g
Bombyx Batryticatus *bai² jiang¹ can²* 白僵蠶 (210)	Dispels wind and resolves tetany; transforms phlegm and dissipates binds. Stir-frying enhances the power to "combat toxin with toxin." Mix-frying with honey reduces irritation to the stomach.	Wind stroke loss of voice; fright epilepsy; head wind; throat wind; itchy throat; scrofulous lumps; wind sores; dormant papules (urticaria); cinnabar toxin (erysipelas); mastitis.	External contractions; uterine bleeding.	5-10 g
Haliotidis Concha *shi² jue² ming²* 石决明 (215)	Calms the liver and subdues yang; eliminates heat; brightens the eyes. Calcined, it helps the active agents to dissolve during decoction, and has an enhanced liver-supplementing action.	Headache, dizziness, and fright convulsions due to welling up of wind yang; steaming bone tidal fever; clear-eye blindness and internal obstructions of the eye.	Spleen-stomach vacuity cold.	10-15 g
Haematitum *dai⁴ zhe³ shi²* 代赭石 (227)	Calms the liver and settle counterflow; cools the blood and staunches bleeding. Used calcined for better counterflow-downbearing, dyspnea-calming, and blood-staunching action, and calcined with vinegar for increased astringency and power to act on the liver.	Belching; counterflow retching; esophageal constriction, stomach reflux; wheezing and dyspnea; fright epilepsy; blood ejection; spontaneous external bleeding; intestinal wind; hemorrhoids and fistulae; uterine bleeding and vaginal discharge.	Pregnancy.	10-30 g

28. Liver-clearing and eye-brightening agents 清肝・明目藥 *qing¹ gan¹ · ming² mu⁴ yao⁴*

Name	Functions	Indications	Contraindications	Daily Dosage
Buddleiae Flos *mi⁴ meng² hua¹* 密蒙花 (105)	Dispels wind, cools the blood, moistens the liver, and brightens the eyes.	Red, sore, and swollen eyes; copious tears; aversion to light; clear-eye blindness; eye screens; wind ulceration of the eyes.		3-5 g
Cassiae Torae Semen *jue² ming² zi³* 决明子 (165)	Clears liver fire, brightens the eyes, disinhibits water, and frees the stool. Stir-fry to disinhibit urine and dispel summerheat.	Wind-heat reddening of the eyes; clear-eye blindness; night blindness; hypertension; hepatitis; ascites due to cirrhosis; habitual constipation.	Diarrhea.	5-10 g

29. Moist precipitating agents 潤下藥 run⁴ xia⁴ yao⁴

Cannabis Semen huo³ ma² ren² 火麻仁 (164)	Moistens dryness; lubricates the intestine; frees strangury; quickens the blood.	Constipation due to intestinal dryness; wasting thirst; heat strangury; wind bi; dysenteric disease; menstrual irregularities; jie and xian.	Diarrhea.	10-15 g
Lini Semen ya³ ma² ren² 亞麻仁 (174)	Frees the stool and kills worms.	Leprosy; itchy skin; alopecia; dry stool.	Vomiting due to a weak stomach.	5-10 g
Pini Semen hai³ song¹ zi³ 海松子 (179)	Nourishes humor, extinguishes wind, moistens the lung, and lubricates the intestines.	Wind bi; dizziness; dryness cough; blood ejection; constipation.	Loose bowels or in damp phlegm disorders.	5-10 g

30. Portal-opening agents 開竅藥 kai¹ qiao⁴ yao⁴

Acori Graminei Rhizoma shi² chang¹¹ pu² 石菖蒲 (71)	Opens the portals; sweeps phlegm; rectifies qi; quickens the blood; dissipates wind; eliminates damp. Stir-fry with ginger juice to open the chest and relieve pain, warm the stomach and open the portals. Mix-fry with bran and honey to open the portals and fortify the spleen. Coat in cinnabar for a stronger spirit-quieting action.	Mania and withdrawal; phlegm inversion; clouding inversion in febrile disease; poor memory; qi block deafness; vexation and oppression in the chest; stomach pain; abdominal pain; wind, cold, and damp bi; swelling and toxin of yong and ju; impact injury.	Yang exuberance due to yin vacuity with cough and expectoration of blood.	3-6 g
Ambra Grisea long² xian² xiang¹ 龍涎香 (205)	Transforms phlegm and opens the portals; moves qi and quickens the blood; dissipates binds and relieves pain; disinhibits water and frees strangury. Has an antispasmodic effect similar to that of Moschus (she⁴ xiang¹).	Cough and dyspnea; qi counterflow; qi bind; concretions and gatherings; pain in the abdomen and region of the heart; strangury.	Wind-cold dyspnea.	0.3-1 g

Name	Functions	Indications	Contraindications	Daily Dosage
Moschus *she⁴ xiang²* 麝香 (216)	Opens the portals, exorcises foulness, frees the connecting vessels and dissipates stasis.	Wind stroke; phlegm inversion; fright epilepsy; malignity sores; vexation and oppression; fulminant pain in the abdomen and region of the heart; concretions and conglomerations; elusive masses; impact injuries; swelling and toxin of yong and ju.	Pregnancy.	5–10 mg

31. Precipitating agents 瀉下藥 *xie⁴ xia⁴ yao⁴*

Name	Functions	Indications	Contraindications	Daily Dosage
Rhei Rhizoma *da⁴ huang²* 大黃 (95)	Drains heat toxin; breaks accumulation and stagnation; moves static blood. It has a milder precipitating effect when cooked, and bears upward when treated with wine (head and eye disorders).	Repletion heat constipation; delirious mania; food accumulation glomus and fullness; initial stage of dysentery; abdominal urgency and rectal heaviness; menstrual block; concretions and gatherings; seasonal heat toxin; blood ejection; spontaneous external bleeding; fulminant reddening and swelling of the eyes; yang jaundice; water swelling; turbid strangury; dark-colored urine; yong, ju, sores, burns, scalds.	Absence of depressed heat in the blood aspect or absence of food stagnation.	3–10 g
Aloe *lu² hui⁴* 蘆薈 (195)	Clears heat, frees the stools and kills worms. Usually used calcined to moderate the effect.	Heat bind constipation; menstrual block; child fright epilepsy; gan heat; worm accumulation; hemorrhoids and fistulae; atrophic rhinitis; scrofulous lumps.	Spleen-stomach vacuity.	0.5–1.5 g
Mirabilitum *mang² xiao¹* 芒硝 (231)	Drains heat, moistens dryness, and softens hardness.	Repletion heat stagnation and accumulation; abdominal distention; constipation; phlegm accumulation; reddening of the eyes; eye screens; cinnabar toxin; yong swelling. Marabilitum Purum is less effective for bowel conditions, and more effective as a topical dressing for sores.	Spleen-stomach vacuity cold and pregnancy.	3–10 g

32. Qi-boosting agents 益氣藥 yi⁴ qi⁴ yao⁴

			5–10 g
Astragali Radix *huang² qí²* 黃耆 (29, 30)	Boosts defense qi and secures exterior; disinhibits water and disperses swelling; expels sore toxin and engenders flesh; supplements the center and boosts qi. Use crude both to promote and check sweating according to need. Use mix-fried with honey to supplement the center, boost original qi, warm the triple burner, and strengthen the stomach and spleen.	Spontaneous external bleeding; night sweating; blood bi; water swelling; persistent young and ju.	Repletion patterns and yang exuberance due to yin vacuity.

33. Qi-rectifying agents 理氣藥 li³ qi⁴ yao⁴

Aquilariae Lignum *chen² xiang¹* 沉香 (11)	Downbears qi and warms the center; warms the kidney and promotes qi absorption.	Vomiting, hiccough, pain in the abdomen and region of the heart, toxin dysentery with inability to eat, large intestinal vacuity constipation, vacuity cold of the lumbus and knees, counterflow qi dyspnea.	Effulgent yin vacuity fire; qi vacuity fall.	1.5–3 g
Santali Albi Lignum *tan² xiang¹* 檀香 (18)	Rectifies qi and harmonizes the stomach.	Pain in the venter and abdomen, esophageal constriction, and retching and vomiting.	Exuberant yin vacuity heat.	1.5–3 g
Linderae Radix *wu¹ yao⁴* 烏藥 (47)	Normalizes qi, opens depression, dissipates cold, and relieves pain. Stir-fry with brine to warm the kidney and contain urine, or with bran to disinhibit qi.	Wind stroke; pain in the abdomen and region of the heart; thoracic glomus; perduring food; stomach reflux; vomiting; frequent urination; cold shan; qi counterflow.	Qi vacuity with internal heat.	5–10 g
Saussureae Radix *mu⁴ xiang¹* 木香 (63)	Moves qi and relieves pain; warms the center and harmonizes the stomach. Use crude to rectify qi and relieve pain. Stir-fry with Coptidis Rhizoma (*huang² lian²*) to check dysentery. Roast to check diarrhea and allay thirst.	Fullness pain in the chest and abdomen; dysenteric disease with tenesmus; cold shan.	Blood vacuity and damage to liquid.	1.5–5 g

Name	Functions	Indications	Contraindications	Daily Dosage
Cyperi Rhizoma *xiang¹ fu⁴ zi³* 香附子 (83)	Rectifies qi and resolves depression; relieves pain and regulates menstruation. Use crude to resolve depression. Stir-fry with vinegar to enter the liver, rectify qi and blood, and relieve pain. Treat with wine to move channel and vessel flow. Stir-fry with brine to enter the blood aspect and moisten dryness. Stir-fry with ginger juice to transform phlegm and rheum. Char-fry to staunch bleeding.	Menstrual irregularities; qi depression; distention and pain in the chest and abdomen; liver-stomach disharmony; phlegm-rheum; glomus and fullness; uterine bleeding and vaginal discharge; yong and ju.	Yin vacuity blood heat.	5–10 g
Aurantii Fructus Immaturus (Citri Aurantii Fructus Immaturus) *zhi³ shi²* 枳實 (125)	Breaks qi, dissipates glomus, drains phlegm, and disperses accumulation. Use crude to break qi and disperse accumulations, stir-fried with bran to produce a milder effect and strengthen the spleen, and scorch-fried to staunch bleeding and to loosen the center. The mature fruit, Aurantii Fructus, is milder in action, and is therefore more suitable for weaker patients.	Distention and fullness in the chest and abdomen; thoracic bi; glomus pain; phlegm pi; water swelling; food accumulation; constipation; gastroptosis (downward displacement of the stomach); prolapse of the uterus and rectum.	Spleen-stomach vacuity.	3–5 g
Citri Exocarpium *chen² pi²* 陳皮 (128)	Rectifies qi; regulates the center; dries damp; transforms phlegm; resolves fish and crab toxin. The red part of the peel, Citri Exocarpium Rubrum, is stronger in its drying, warming, and qi-rectifying effect. The white part, Citri Exocarpium Album, is milder in its effect. The seeds of the fruit, Citri Semen, rectifies qi and relieves pain, while the vascular bundles of the fruit, Citri Fasciculus Vascularis, free the connecting vessels.	Distention and fullness in the chest and abdomen; no thought of food or drink; retching, vomiting, and hiccough; cough with copious phlegm.	Yin vacuity with thirst.	3–10 g
Kaki Calyx (Diospyroris Kaki Calyx) *shi⁴ di⁴* 柿蒂 (138)	Downbears counterflow qi. Used char-fried to staunch bleeding.	Counterflow cough; lower esophageal qi constriction; stomach reflux.		5–10 g

34. Qi-rectifying and water-disinhibiting agents 理氣・利水藥 li³ qi⁴, li⁴ shui³ yao⁴

Drug	Action	Indication	Contraindication	Dosage
Arecae Pericarpium da⁴ fu⁴ pi² 大腹皮 (123)	Precipitates qi and loosens the center; moves water. Wash in wine or licorice water to reduce toxicity.	Abdominal glomus and distention; leg qi; water swelling.	Qi vacuity.	5–10 g

35. Qi-rectifying and worm-expelling agents 理氣・驅蟲藥 li³ qi⁴, qu¹ chong² yao⁴

Drug	Action	Indication	Contraindication	Dosage
Meliae Toosendan Fructus chuan¹ lian⁴ zi³ 川楝子 (143)	Eliminates damp-heat; clears liver fire; relieves pain; and kills worms. Used crude to clear liver fire.	Heat inversion; heart pain; lateral costal pain; shan pain; abdominal pain due to worm accumulation. Stir-fry to treat shan pain.	Spleen-stomach vacuity cold.	5–10 g

36. Qi-supplementing agents 補氣藥 bu³ qi⁴ yao⁴

Drug	Action	Indication	Contraindication	Dosage
Codonopsitis Radix dang³ shen¹ 黨參 (33)	Supplements the center, boosts qi and engenders liquid. Mix-fry with honey to increase the center-supplementing action. Stir-fry with rice for better stomach-harmonizing and spleen-fortifying action. Treat with Halloysitum Rubrum (chi⁴ shi² zhi¹) to enhance the spleen-supplementing action.	Spleen-stomach vacuity; dual depletion of qi and blood; fatigue and lack of strength; low food intake; thirst; enduring diarrhea; prolapse of the rectum.	Pathogen repletion patterns.	5–10 g
Ginseng Radix ren² shen¹ 人參 (40) (White ginseng)	Greatly supplements original qi, stems desertion and engenders liquids, and quiets the spirit.	Taxation damage with low food intake and lassitude; stomach reflux; efflux diarrhea; vacuity cough with rapid, distressed, dyspneic breathing; spontaneous sweating; fulminant desertion; fright palpitation; dizziness; impotence; frequent urination; uterine bleeding; chronic fright wind; enduring vacuity; insufficiency of qi, blood, and fluids.	Pathogen repletion patterns.	1.5–10 g
Gingseng Radix Rubra hong² shen¹ 紅參 (41) (Red ginseng)	Red ginseng has the same nature and sapor as white ginseng, but has a stronger supplementing action. It is especially suitable for yang vacuity patterns with inversion cold in the limbs.	See Ginseng Radix (ren² shen¹) above.	Pathogen repletion patterns.	1.5–10 g

Name	Functions	Indications	Contraindications	Daily Dosage
Glycyrrhizae Radix *gan¹ cao³* 甘草 (42)	Harmonizes the center and relieves tension; moistens the lung; resolves toxin. Harmonizes all drugs. Use crude to drain fire and resolve toxin, relieve pain and tension, stir-fried to fortify the stomach and spleen, and boost original qi, and mix-fried with honey to supplement the center and boost qi, as well as to eliminate unpleasant odors or flavors of decoctions. Use the fine roots in formulae designed to disinhibit water.	Used crude for sore throat, yong, ju, digestive tract ulcers and food poisoning. Used mix-fried for spleen-stomach vacuity, low food intake, abdominal pain and thin stool, fatigue and fever, pulmonary atony with cough, and for palpitations and epilepsy.	Spleen-stomach damp and center fullness with nausea and retching.	1.5–10 g
Atractylodis Ovatae Rhizoma *bai² zhu²* 白朮 (76)	Supplements the spleen and boosts the stomach; dries damp; harmonizes the center. Use crude to dry damp and disinhibit water. Use stir-fried for greater spleen-fortifying action. Use stir-fried with earth to fortify the spleen and check diarrhea. Use stir-fried with bran to disperse fullness and distention and to supplement the spleen.	Spleen vacuity with fullness and distention; vexation and oppression in the chest and diaphragm; diarrhea; water swelling; phlegm-rheum; spontaneous sweating.	Yin vacuity with thirst.	5–10 g
Dioscoreae Rhizoma *shan¹ yao⁴* 山藥 (84)	Fortifies the spleen, supplements the lung, secures the kidney and boosts essence. Use crude to enrich yin. Stir-fry (with or without bran or earth) to harmonize the stomach and spleen.	Spleen vacuity diarrhea; enduring dysentery; cough due to vacuity taxation; wasting thirst; seminal emission; frequent urination.	Damp-heat repletion patterns.	10–15 g
Polygonati Rhizoma *huang² jing¹* 黃精 (93)	Supplements the center and boosts qi; moistens the lung; strengthens the sinews and bones. The commercial processing enhances the supplementing action.	Fever and chills in vacuity detriment; pulmonary consumption; coughing of blood; weak constitution after disease; weak sinews and bones; wind lai and xian.	Spleen vacuity with exuberant damp and food accumulations; unsuitable for patients with thin stool diarrhea.	10–15 g
Zizyphi Fructus *da⁴ zao³* 大棗 (158)	Supplements the spleen and harmonizes the stomach; reinforces qi and engenders liquids; regulates construction-defense; resolves drug toxins.	Stomach vacuity; low food intake; thin stool due to spleen vacuity; insufficiency of qi, blood and fluids; construction-defense disharmony; palpitations and racing of the heart; visceral agitation in women.	Phlegm-heat.	10–15 g

Drug	Functions	Indications	Contraindications	Dosage
Lablab (Vulgaris) Semen *bian³ dou⁴* 扁豆 (173)	Fortifies qi and harmonizes the center; dispels summerheat and transforms damp. Use crude to dispel summerheat. Stir-fry without additives to fortify the spleen and check diarrhea. Stir-fry with earth to check diarrhea. Stir-fry with vinegar to treat vomiting with diarrhea.	Summerheat-damp vomiting and diarrhea; Spleen vacuity counterflow retching; low food intake; enduring diarrhea; wasting thirst; red and white vaginal discharge; child gan accumulation.	Disease cold-heat complexes.	5–12 g

37. Potent precipitating and water-expelling agents 峻下・逐水藥 *jun⁴ xia⁴*, *zhu² shui³ yao⁴*

Drug	Functions	Indications	Contraindications	Dosage
Euphorbiae Kansui Radix *gan¹ sui⁴* 甘遂 (37)	Drains water-yin, breaks accumulations and gatherings, frees the urine and stool. Stir-frying with vinegar, roasting, and boiling with beancurd (tofu) reduces toxicity. Boiling with Glycyrrhizae Radix (*gan¹ cao³*) and Platycodonis Radix (*jie² geng³*) reduces the side-effect of vomiting.	Water swelling; phlegm-rheum; chest bind; mania and withdrawal; esophageal constriction; concretions, conglomerations, accumulations, and gatherings; urinary and fecal stoppage.	Pregnancy and general debilitation.	1.5–3 g
Knoxiae Radix *hong² da⁴ ji³* 紅大戟 (43)	Expels water and phlegm-drool; disperses swelling and fullness. Use roasted to reduce toxicity and enhance water-moving effects.	Pain in the chest, back, lumbus and the lateral costal region; dry retching.	Yin water due to vacuity cold. pregnancy.	1.5–3 g
Daphnes Genkwa Flos *yuan² hua¹* 芫花 (111)	Expels water and flushes phlegm. Stir-fry with vinegar for milder action.	Phlegm-rheum; elusive masses; dyspnea and cough; water swelling; lateral costal pain; distention and fullness in the abdomen and heart; food poisoning; mother of malaria; swollen yong.	Original qi vacuity and pregnancy.	1.5–3 g
Euphorbiae Lathyridis Semen *qian¹ jin¹ zi³* 千金子 (168)	Expels water and disperses swelling; breaks concretions and kills worms. Remove oil for milder action.	Water swelling and distention; phlegm-rheum; perduring stagnation; stomach pain; concretions and gatherings; menstrual block; jie, xian, and sores; insect bites; warts.	Insufficiency of center qi; spleen vacuity diarrhea; pregnancy.	0.3–1.5 g
Pharbitidis Semen *qian¹ niu² zi³* 牽牛子 (178)	Drains water, precipitates qi, and kills worms.	Water swelling; dyspnea and fullness; phlegm-rheum; leg qi; worm accumulation; food stagnation; bound stool.	Pregnancy and stomach qi vacuity.	3–6 g

Name	Functions	Indications	Contraindications	Daily Dosage
Tiglii Semen (Crotonis Semen) *ba¹ dou⁴* 巴豆 (187)	Drains cold accumulations; free the jaw and portals; expels phlegm; moves water; kills worms. Use frost (Tiglii Seminis Pulvis, [*ba¹ dou⁴ shuang¹*]) for milder precipitating action.	Frigid accumulations; distention and acute pain in the chest and abdomen; blood conglomerations; phlegm pi; diarrhea; water swelling; Applied externally to throat wind, throat bi, malign sores, jie and xian.	Pregnancy; general weakness; absence of repletion cold accumulation and stagnation.	0.15–0.3 g

38. Topically applied agents 外用藥 *wai⁴ yong⁴ yao⁴*

Name	Functions	Indications	Contraindications	Daily Dosage
Hydnocarpi Semen *da⁴ feng¹ zi³* 大風子 (172)	Dispels wind and dries damp; attacks toxin and kills worms.	Leprosy; jie and xian; red bayberry (syphilitic) sores.	Yin vacuity blood heat.	1.5–3 g
Momordicae Semen *mu⁴ bie¹ zi³* 木鱉子 (175)	Disperses swelling and bind; dispels toxin.	Bake or stir-fry to treat gan accumulation and diarrhea. Swollen yong; clove sores; scrofulous lumps; hemorrhoids; innominate swollen toxin sores; xian; wind-damp bi pain; hypertonicity of the sinews. Use crude for topical treatment of sores. Make into a frost to moderate the effect.	Pregnancy and debilitation.	0.5–1 g
Ricini Semen *bi⁴ ma² zi³* 蓖麻子 (182)	Disperses swelling and draws out pus; lubricates the intestines and frees stagnation.	Swelling and toxin of yong and ju; scrofulous lumps; throat bi; jie, lai, and xian; water swelling; and abdominal fullness; dry, bound stool.	Pregnancy.	4–16 cc at a time taken orally.
Gambir Catechu (Catechu) *hai² er² cha²* 孩兒茶 (200)	Clears heat, transforms phlegm, staunches bleeding, disperses food, engenders flesh, and settles pain.	Phlegm-heat cough; wasting thirst; blood ejection; spontaneous external bleeding; blood in the urine; blood dysentery; profuse uterine bleeding; child indigestion; gan of the teeth and gums; mouth sores; throat bi.	Cold-damp patterns.	1–3 g
Pini Resina *song¹ xiang¹* 松香 (204)	Dispels wind, dries damp, expels pus, draws out toxin, engenders flesh, and relieves pain.	Yong and ju; clove sores; hemorrhoids and fistulae; malign sores; jie and xian; bald white sores; incised wounds; sprains; wind-damp bi pain; itching due to pestilential wind.		Apply topically in powder form.

Drug	Functions	Indications	Cautions	Dosage
Bufonis Venenum chan² su¹ 蟾酥 (211)	Resolves toxin, disperses swelling, strengthens the heart and relieves pain. Its harshness is moderated by stir-frying with vinegar.	Clove sores; yong and ju; dorsal effusions; scrofulous lumps; chronic osteomyelitis; sore, swollen throat; child gan accumulation; heart failure; toothache due to caries or wind.	Oral administration contraindicated in vacuity and pregnancy.	1.5–3 mg
Mylabris (Cantharis) ban¹ mao² 斑蝥 (217)	Attacks toxin and expels stasis.	Applied topically for malign sores; stubborn xian: deviated mouth and eyes; throat moth. To be taken internally for scrofulous lumps; rabid dog bites. Grind to a powder for external use, and stir-fry before grinding for oral administration.	Vacuity and in pregnancy. Use with care when administering orally in view of its toxicity.	0.03–0.05g
Hydrozincitum (Smithsonitum, Calamina) lu² gan¹ shi² 爐甘石 (229)	Eliminates eye screens and reduces redness of the eyes; absorbs damp and closes sores.	Used externally to treat reddening of the eyes, eye screens, wind ulceration of the eyelid rim, damp sores and persistent ulceration. Calcine to treat redness and swelling of the eyes.		

39. Water-disinhibiting and damp-percolating agents 利水・渗湿藥 li⁴ shui³, shen⁴ shi¹ yao⁴

Drug	Functions	Indications	Cautions	Dosage
Hocquartiae Caulis (Mutong Caulis) mu⁴ tong¹ 木通 (16)	Drains fire and moves water; frees the blood vessels.	Damp-heat strangury, inhibited urination, water swelling, menstrual block and absence of breast milk.	The absence of damp-heat.	3–5 g
Junci Medulla deng¹ xin¹ cao³ 燈心草 (17)	Clears the heart and downbears fire; disinhibits urine and frees strangury. Coated in cinnabar, it quiets the spirit. Charred, it cools the blood and staunches bleeding, clears heat and resolves toxin.	Strangury; water swelling; inhibited urination; damp-heat jaundice; vexation and insomnia; night crying in infants; throat bi; and wounds.	Vacuity cold.	1.5–3 g
Kwang-Fang-Chi Radix (Fangji Radix) guang³ fang² ji³ 廣防己 (44)	Resolves heat; disinhibits urine; relieves pain. Use crude for damp-heat and roasted or stir-fried for wind-damp.	Water swelling, leg qi, bi pain in the flesh, rheumatic arthritis, and inhibited urination.	Absence of damp-heat.	5–10 g

Name	Functions	Indications	Contraindications	Daily Dosage
Alismatis Rhizoma *ze² xie⁴* 澤瀉 (72)	Disinhibits water, percolates damp, and drains heat. Use crude to fortify the spleen and disinhibit water. Stir-fry with brine to make it act on the kidney and have an even stronger water-disinhibiting effect. Stir-fry with wine and brine for use in supplementing formulae.	Inhibited urination; water swelling; distention and fullness; diarrhea; phlegm-rheum; leg qi; strangury; blood in the urine.	Liver or kidney vacuity in the absence of damp-heat.	6–12 g
Coicis Semen *yi⁴ yi³ ren²* 薏苡仁 (166)	Fortifies the spleen and supplements the lung; clears heat and disinhibits damp. Use crude to disinhibit water-damp, and stir-fried with earth for better spleen-fortifying and diarrhea-checking action.	Diarrhea; damp bi; hypertonicity of the limbs; water swelling; leg qi; pulmonary atony and yong; intestinal yong; turbid strangury; vaginal discharge.	Pregnancy.	10–30 g
Plantaginis Semen *che¹ qian² zi³* 車前子 (180)	Clears heat (especially when used crude); disinhibits water (especially when stir-fried in brine); brightens the eyes; dispels phlegm.	Urinary stoppage; turbid strangury; vaginal discharge; blood in the urine; jaundice; water swelling; heat dysentery; diarrhea; nosebleed; reddening, soreness, and swelling of the eyes; throat bi; throat moth; cough; ulcers.	Profuse urination with constipation, and in the absence of damp-heat.	5–10 g
Artemisiae Capillaris Herba *yin¹ chen² hao¹* 茵陳蒿 (189)	Clears heat and disinhibits damp.	Damp and heat jaundice; inhibited urination; itchy wind sores and jie.	Jaundice not caused by damp-heat.	10–15 g
Talcum *hua² shi²* 滑石 (232)	Clears heat, disinhibits damp and opens the portals.	Vexation and thirst in summerheat-heat; inhibited urination; water diarrhea; heat dysentery; strangury; jaundice; water swelling; spontaneous external bleeding; leg qi; damp erosion of the skin.	Spleen-stomach vacuity, seminal efflux, and in febrile disease with damage to liquid. Use with care in pregnancy.	10–15 g
Hoelen (Poria) *fu² ling²* 茯苓 (235, 236)	Percolates damp and disinhibits water; quiets the heart and spirit. White hoelen is used specifically to fortify the spleen and percolate damp. Red hoelen drains damp-heat, disinhibits the portals, and moves water. The skin specifically treats water swelling. Root hoelen quiets the heart spirit. Cinnabar hoelen has an even stronger spirit-quieting effect.	Inhibited urination; water swelling; distention and fullness; phlegm-rheum; counterflow cough; retching; diarrhea; seminal emission; turbid strangury; fright palpitation; poor memory.	Seminal efflux and qi vacuity fall.	6–12 g

			Absence of damp.	6-12 g
Polyporus zhu1 ling2 豬苓 (238)	Disinhibits urine and percolates damp.	Inhibited urination; distention and fullness; water swelling; leg qi; diarrhea; turbid strangury; vaginal discharge.	Absence of damp.	6-12 g

40. Wind-cold-effusing agents 發散風寒藥 fa1 san4 feng1 han2 yao4

Cinnamomi Ramulus gui4 zhi1 桂枝 (2)	Promote sweating, and warm and free the channels.	Wind-cold exterior patterns, with cold in the joins, as well as thoracic bi with phlegm and rheum, and menstrual block with concretions and conglomerations.	Pregnancy or warm heat disease manifesting in yang exuberance and yin vacuity, or blood patterns.	1.5-5 g
Angelicae Dahuricae Radix bai2 zhi3 白芷 (23)	Dispels wind; dries damp; disperses swelling; relieves pain. Char-fry for vaginal discharge.	All diseases of the head and face including headache and toothache; red and white vaginal discharge; dry itchy skin.	Yin vacuity and depressed fire.	3-7 g
Asiasari Radix (Asari Radix) xi4 xin1 細辛 (26)	Dispels wind, dissipates cold, moves water, and opens the portals.	Wind-cold headache; deep-source nasal congestion; toothache; phlegm-rheum; counterflow cough; wind-damp bi pain.	Qi vacuity sweating; blood vacuity headache; yin vacuity cough.	1-3 g
Ledebouriellae Radix (Saposhnikoviae Divaricatae Radix) fang2 feng1 防風 (45)	Effuses the exterior, dispels wind, percolates damp, relieves pain. Use crude to resolve the exterior, dispel wind-damp, and relieve tetany. Use stir-fried to check diarrhea and dispel wind. Stir-fry with wine to check perspiration, and char to staunch bleeding.	Headache, dizziness, and stiffness of the neck in external wind-cold patterns; wind, cold, and damp bi; aching pain in the joints; hypertonicity of the limbs; lockjaw.	Effulgent yin vacuity fire; pathogen patterns without wind.	5-10 g
Ligustici Sinensis Rhizoma et Radix gao3 ben3 藁本 (46)	Dissipates wind, cold and damp pathogens.	Wind-cold headache; vertex headache; cold-damp abdominal pain; diarrhea; concretions and conglomerations; jie and xian.	Internal yin vacuity heat.	3-5 g
Zingiberis Rhizoma Recens sheng1 jiang1 生薑 (98)	Diffuses cold and resolves the exterior.	Wind-cold colds and flu; resolves toxin of Pinelliae Tuber, Arisaematis Rhizoma, fish crabs, animals, birds.	Yin vacuity heat.	3-10 g

Name	Functions	Indications	Contraindications	Daily Dosage
Perillae Folium *zi³ su¹ ye⁴* 紫蘇葉 (104)	Effuses exterior, dissipates cold, rectifies qi, and harmonizes nutrition. Char-fry to staunch bleeding.	External wind-cold; aversion to cold and fever; cough and dyspnea; distention and fullness in the chest and abdomen; stirring fetus.	Qi vacuity and exterior vacuity.	5–10 g
Magnoliae Flos *xin¹ yi²* 辛夷 (115)	Dispels wind and frees the portals.	Headache; deep-source nasal congestion; nasal obstruction; toothache.	Effulgent yin vacuity fire.	3–5 g
Ephedrae Herba *ma² huang²* 麻黃 (190)	Promotes sweating, calms dyspnea, and disinhibits water. Honey mix-frying reduces the diaphoretic action, making it suitable for debilitated patients with qi vacuity.	Exterior repletion cold damage patterns with aversion to cold, adiaphoretic fever, headache and nasal congestion, generalized joint pain; cough and dyspnea; wind water swelling; inhibited urination; stubborn wind bi; wind numbness; wind papules.	General weakness with spontaneous or night sweats and dyspnea.	1.5–6 g
Schizonepetae Herba seu Flos *jing¹ jie⁴* 荊芥 (194)	Effuses the exterior, dispels wind, and rectifies the blood; staunches bleeding when used char-fried.	Colds and fever; headache; sore, swollen throat; wind stroke with clenched jaws; spontaneous external bleeding; blood in the stool; uterine bleeding; postpartum blood dizziness; yong, jie, and sores; scrofulous lumps.	Exterior vacuity with spontaneous sweating; yin vacuity headache.	5–10 g

41. Wind-damp-dispelling agents 祛風濕藥 *qu¹ feng¹ shi¹ yao⁴*

Name	Functions	Indications	Contraindications	Daily Dosage
Acanthopanacis Radicis Cortex *wu³ jia¹ pi²* 五加皮 (1)	Dispels wind-damp; strengthens sinew and bone; quickens the blood and eliminates stasis.	Wind-cold-damp bi, leg qi, wind-damp in the skin, impotence, and scrotal damp.	Effulgent yin vacuity fire.	5–10 g
Angelicae Laxiflorae Radix *chuan¹ du² huo²* 川獨活 (24)	Dispels wind, percolates damp, dissipates cold and relieves pain.	Wind-cold-damp bi, especially damp bi of the lower limbs; painful, swollen knees; hypertonicity of the limbs.	Effulgent yin vacuity fire; high fever without aversion to cold.	3–5 g
Clematidis Radix *wei¹ ling² xian¹* 威靈仙 (32)	Dispels wind-damp, frees the channels, disperses phlegm, and dissipates elusive masses. Prepare with wine to dispel wind and free the channels.	Cold pain in the lumbus and knees; leg qi; stubborn xian; gout; malarial disease; concretions and gatherings; tetanus; tonsillitis; bones stuck in the throat.	Hypertonicity of the sinews due to blood vacuity; pathogen repletion patterns without wind-damp.	3–10 g

Gentianae Macrophyllae Radix *qin² jiao¹* 秦艽 (38)	Dispels wind and eliminates damp; harmonizes the blood and soothes the sinews; clears heat and disinhibits urine.	Wind-damp bi pain; hypertonicity of the sinews and bones; jaundice; blood in the stool; steaming bone tidal fever; child gan heat; inhibited urination.	Persistent pain in the limbs due to inability of qi and blood to provide adequate nourishment.	5–10 g
Tsao-Wu-Tou Tuber *cao³ wu¹ tou²* 草烏頭 (70)	Tracks down wind and percolates damp; dissipates cold and relieves pain; sweeps phlegm, and disperses swelling.	Wind, cold, and damp bi; wind stroke paralysis; lockjaw; head wind; frigid pain in the venter and abdomen; phlegm pi; qi lumps; cold dysentery; throat bi; yong and ju: clove sores; scrofulous lumps.	Severe vacuity; pregnancy; effulgent yin vacuity fire; heat patterns with pain.	1–3 g
Chaenomelis Fructus *mu⁴ gua¹* 木瓜 (126)	Calms the liver and harmonizes the stomach: eliminates damp and soothes the sinews.	Choleraic cramp; leg qi; damp bi.	Gastrointestinal stagnation.	5–10 g
Tigris Os *hu³ gu³* 虎骨 (222)	Chases wind and settles pain; fortifies the bones, and settles fright. Stir-fry with vinegar or wine, or without additives to dissipate wind-cold and fortify the sinews and bones.	Articular wind pain, hypertonicity of the limbs, stiff lumbus (use the limb bones); fright palpitation and epilepsy (use the skull); hemorrhoids and fistulae: prolapse of the rectum.	Exuberant fire due to blood vacuity.	10–15 g

42. Wind-damp-dispelling and interior-warming agents 祛風濕 · 溫裡藥 *qu¹ feng¹ shi¹* , *wen¹ li³ yao⁴*

Aconiti Tuber Laterale *fu⁴ zi³* 附子 (22)	Returns yang and supplements the fire; dissipates cold and eliminates damp.	Exuberant yin repelling yang; profuse sweating in yang collapse; blood conglomerations; cold-damp atony; hypertonicity; pain in the knees with difficulty in walking.	Yang exuberance due to yin vacuity; true heat and false cold; pregnancy.	2–5 g

43. Wind-dispelling, exterior-resolving, and wind-damp-dispelling agents 祛風解表 · 祛風濕藥 *qu¹ feng¹ jie³ biao³* , *qu¹ feng¹ shi¹ yao¹*

Notopterygii Rhizoma *qiang¹ huo²* 羌活 (91)	Dissipates exterior cold, dispels wind-damp, and disinhibits the joints.	Contraction of wind-cold with headache and absence of sweating; wind, cold, and damp bi; stiffness of the neck; wind water swelling: yong, ju, and sores.	Blood vacuity.	3–10 g

44. Wind-heat-effusing agents 發散風熱藥 fa¹ san⁴ feng¹ re⁴ yao⁴

Name	Functions	Indications	Contraindications	Daily Dosage
Bupleuri Radix chai² hu² 柴胡 (31)	Harmonizes exterior and interior, courses the liver, and upbears yang. Use crude to resolve the exterior. Stir-fry to moderate the effusing and dissipating action. Mix-fry with honey for greater center-supplementing, lung-moistening, and cough-suppressing action. Prepare with wine to move the blood and free the channels. Prepare with vinegar to soothe the liver, quicken the blood, and relieve pain. Stir-fry in turtle's blood for greater yin-supplementing action.	Alternating fever and chills; thoracic fullness; pain in the lateral costal region; bitter taste in the mouth; deafness; headache and dizziness; malarial and dysenteric disease; menstrual irregularities; prolapse of the uterus.	Intense yin vacuity fire.	3–5 g
Puerariae Radix ge² gen¹ 葛根 (58)	Raises yang and resolves the muscles; outthursts papules and checks diarrhea; eliminates vexation and allays thirst. Use crude to resolve the exterior, outthrust macules, and engender liquid. Roast to moderate the diaphoretic action and help supplement stomach qi.	Headache and stiffness of the neck in cold damage or warm heat; heat vexation; wasting thirst; diarrhea; dysenteric disease; non-eruption of measles; hypertension; angina pectoris; deafness.	Flaming yin vacuity fire; upper body exuberance with lower body vacuity.	3–7 g
Cimicifugae Rhizoma sheng¹ ma² 升麻 (79)	Upbears yang, promotes exterior effusion, outthrusts papules and resolves toxin. Use crude to outthrust papules, clear heat, resolve toxin, and effuse wind-heat. Use mix-fried with honey for stronger lung-moistening and cough-suppressing action.	Seasonal and epidemic pestilential qi; yang ming headache; sore throat; maculopapular eruption; wind heat sores; center qi fall; enduring diarrhea; prolapse of the rectum; uterine bleeding and vaginal discharge.	Upper body exuberance and lower body vacuity and effulgent yin vacuity fire.	3–5 g
Mori Folium sang¹ ye⁴ 桑葉 (103)	Dispels wind and clears heat; cools the blood and brightens the eyes. It is mix-fried with honey to moisten the lung, and steamed to brighten the eyes. The fruit, Mori Fructus (sang¹ shen⁴), supplements the liver and boost the kidney, extinguishes wind and enriches humor.	Wind warmth fever; headache; reddening of eyes; thirst; lung heat cough; wind bi; dormant papules; elephantiasis of the lower limbs. The fruit treats liver-kidney depletion, wasting thirst, dim vision, tinnitus, scrofulous lumps, and inhibited movement of the joints.		5–10 g

Chrysanthemi Flos ju2 hua1 菊花 (109)	Courses wind-heat, calms the liver and brightens the eyes. Use crude to course wind-heat. Char-fry to clear heat and resolve toxin.	Headache; dizziness; reddening of the eyes; heat vexation in the heart and chest; clove sores; toxin swelling.		3–10 g
Arctii Fructus niu2 bang4 zi3 牛蒡子 (122)	Courses wind and dissipates heat; diffuses the lung and outthrusts papules; disperses swelling and resolves toxin.	Wind-heat cough; sore, swollen throat; non-outthrust macules and papules; itchy wind papules; swollen yong and toxin of sores.	Spleen-stomach vacuity with diarrhea.	5–10 g
Viticis Fructus man4 jing1 zi3 蔓荆子 (155)	Courses wind-heat; clears the head and eyes. Stir-frying reduces the pungent, dissipating quality and helps it to ascend to clear the head and eyes.	Wind-heat colds; ambilateral and hemilateral headache; toothache; reddening of the eyes; inner eyes pain; clouded vision; tearing; damp bi and hypertonicity.	Headache or dizziness in patterns of blood vacuity with heat; stomach vacuity.	5–10 g
Sojae Semen Praeparatum dan4 dou4 chi3 淡豆豉 (185)	Resolves the exterior, eliminates vexation, diffuses depression, and resolves toxin.	Cold damage febrile disease; fever and chills; headache; vexation and agitation; thoracic oppression.	Absence of external contraction of wind-cold.	10–12 g
Menthae Herba bo4 he2 薄荷 (192)	Courses wind, dissipates heat, exorcises foulness and resolves toxin. Used crude to dissipate wind-heat, and mix-fried with honey to produce a stronger cough-suppressing action.	External wind-heat; headache; reddening of the eyes; sore, swollen throat; food stagnation and qi distention; mouth sores; toothache; sores; dormant papules.	Yin vacuity and blood dryness; exterior vacuity with copious sweating.	1.5–5 g

45. Worm-expelling agents 驅蟲藥 qu1 chong2 yao4

Quisqualis Fructus shi3 jun1 zi3 使君子 (149)	Kills worms, disperses stagnation, fortifies the spleen.	Abdominal pain due to roundworm; child gan accumulations; stagnation of milk and food in infants; abdominal distention; diarrhea.	Tea is contraindicated when taking this drug.	5–10 g
Arecae Semen bin1 lang2 檳榔 (161)	Kills worms, breaks accumulation, precipitates qi, and moves water. Use crude to kill worms. Scorch-fry for a stronger dispersing and abducting action.	Worm accumulation; food stagnation; distention pain in the venter and abdomen; diarrhea with rectal heaviness; malarial disease; water swelling; leg qi; phlegm pi; concretions and conglomerations. Char-fry to treat malarial disease.	Qi vacuity fall and the absence of food stagnation.	5–10 g

Name	Functions	Indications	Contraindications	Daily Dosage
Digenea hai³ ren² cao³ 海人草 (234)	Kills worms.	Roundworm infestation.		7–10 g
Omphalia lei² wan² 雷丸 (237)	Disperses accumulation and kills worms.	Abdominal pain due to worm accumulation; gan disease; wind epilepsy.	Worm accumulations and spleen-stomach vacuity cold.	3–10 g

46. Yang-assisting agents 助陽藥 zhu⁴ yang² yao⁴

Name	Functions	Indications	Contraindications	Daily Dosage
Eucommiae Cortex du⁴ zhong⁴ 杜仲 (4)	Supplements the liver and kidney; strengthens sinew and bone; quiets the fetus.	Lumbar and knee pain.	Yin vacuity fire.	6–10 g
Cistanches Caulis rou⁴ cong¹ rong² 肉從容 (13)	Supplements the kidney and boosts essence; moistens dryness and lubricates the intestines. Treated with black beans, it has a great supplementing and moistening action.	Impotence, cold pain in the lumbus and knees, dribble after urinary voiding, infertility, uterine bleeding, vaginal discharge, and constipation due to blood dryness.	Constipation, heat in the kidney, impotence, and seminal emission.	7–10 g
Cynomorii Caulis suo³ yang² 鎖陽 (14)	Supplements the kidney and boosts essences; moistens the intestines.	Impotence, seminal emission, and weak lumbus and knees.	Yin vacuity fire and diarrhea.	5–10 g
Dipsaci Radix xu⁴ duan⁴ 續斷 (36)	Supplements the liver and kidney, joins sinew and bones and regulates the blood vessels.	Aching pain in the lumbus and back; lack of strength in the knees and foot; uterine bleeding in pregnancy; profuse uterine bleeding and vaginal discharge; seminal emission; impact injuries; incised wounds; hemorrhoids and fistulae; yong, ju, and sores. Stir-fry to treat uterine bleeding. Mix-fry with brine for lower burner patterns (stirring fetus, and precipitation of blood).	Intense yin vacuity fire.	5–10 g

Drug	Functions	Indications	Contraindications	Dosage
Morindae Radix ba¹ ji³ tian¹ 巴戟天 (49)	Supplements kidney yang; strengthens the sinews and bone; dispels wind-damp.	Impotence; wind-damp leg qi; weak, aching sinews and bones; pain in the lumbus and knees. Stir-fry with brine to supplement the kidney. Boil in licorice water to reduce toxicity. Stir-fry with wine to dissipate wind-damp.	Exuberant yin vacuity fire patterns with dry, bound stool.	5-10 g
Alpiniae Oxyphyllae Fructus yi⁴ zhi⁴ ren² 益智仁 (119)	Warms the spleen and kidney, secures qi, astringes essence. Stir-fry to reduce dryness and prevent damage to the kidney. Stir-fry with brine to warm the spleen and check diarrhea.	Frigid qi pain in the abdomen; vomiting and diarrhea due to cold stroke; profuse sleeping; seminal emission; dribbling urination; nocturia.	Dryness and heat patterns.	3-10 g
Allii Tuberosi Semen jiu³ zi³ 韭子 (159)	Supplements the liver and kidney, warms lumbus and knees, strengthens yang and secures essence. Has a more moderate effect when scorch-fried.	Impotence; dream emissions; frequent urination; enuresis; frigid pain and limp, aching lumbus and knees; diarrhea; vaginal discharge; turbid strangury.	Effulgent yin vacuity fire.	5-10 g
Cuscutae Semen tu⁴ si¹ zi³ 菟絲子 (167)	Supplements the kidney and liver, boosts essence and brightens the eyes. Stir-fry with brine to supplement the kidney, with wine to warm the flesh, and with wine and rice to treat diarrhea.	Aching pain in the lumbus and knees; seminal emission; wasting thirst; dribble after voiding; dark vision.	Pregnancy, uterine bleeding; prolonged erection; bound stool, fire in the kidney, and fire stirring from to yin vacuity.	10-12 g
Foeni-Graeci Semen (Trigonellae Foeni-Graeci Semen) hu² lu² ba¹ 胡蘆巴 (170)	Supplements kidney yang, and dispels cold-damp. Soak in wine to warm the kidney. Steam to increase the enriching effect. Stir-fry to invigorate original yang.	Cold shan; distention and fullness in the abdomen and lateral costal region; cold-damp leg qi; aching lumbus due to kidney vacuity; impotence.	Effulgent yin vacuity fire.	3-5 g
Psoraleae Semen bu³ gu³ zhi¹ 補骨脂 (181)	Supplements the kidney and assists yang. Stir-frying in brine enhances the kidney-supplementing effect.	Frigid diarrhea due to kidney vacuity; enuresis; seminal efflux; frequent urination; impotence; frigid pain in the lumbus and knees; cough and dyspnea due to vacuity cold. Applied topically to white patch wind.	Effulgent yin vacuity fire, blood in the urine, and constipation.	5-10 g
Epimedii Herba yin² yang² huo⁴ 淫羊藿 (191)	Supplements the kidney and fortifies yang; dispels wind and eliminates damp. Used mix-fried in sheep fat to enhance the yang-invigorating action.	Impotence; dribbling urination; hypertonicity of the sinews and bones; hemiplegia; lack of strength in lumbus and knees; wind-damp bi pain; insensitivity of the extremities.	Yin vacuity and stirring ministerial fire.	3-10 g

Name	Functions	Indications	Contraindications	Daily Dosage
Callorhini Testis et Penis ha^3 gou^3 $shen^4$ 海狗腎 (212)	Warms the kidney and strengthens yang; boosts the essence and supplements marrow.	Vacuity taxation; impotence; atony of the lumbus and knees.	Effulgent yin vacuity fire and steaming bone tidal fever with cough.	3-10 g
Cervi Cornu Parvum lu^4 $rong^2$ 鹿茸 (213)	Invigorates original yang, supplements qi and blood, boosts essence and marrow, strengthens sinew and bone.	Vacuity taxation and marked emaciation; exhaustion of essence-spirit; dizziness; deafness; dark vision; aching pain in the lumbus and knees; impotence; seminal efflux; vacuity cold of the uterus; uterine bleeding; vaginal discharge.	Exuberance of yang due to yin vacuity.	1-3 g
Cordyceps $dong^1$ $chong^2$ xia^4 cao^3 冬蟲夏草 (233)	Supplements vacuity and detriment; boosts essential qi; suppresses cough and transforms phlegm.	Phlegm-rheum dyspnea and cough; vacuity dyspnea; consumption cough; coughing of blood; spontaneous or night sweating; impotence and seminal emission; lumbar and knee pain; enduring vacuity preventing recovery from disease.	Diseases with bleeding or exterior signs.	5-10 g

47. Yang-assisting and worm-expelling agents 助陽・驅蟲藥 zhu^4 $yang^2$, qu^1 $chong^2$ yao^4

Name	Functions	Indications	Contraindications	Daily Dosage
Cnidii Monnieri Fructus she^2 $chuang^2$ zi^3 蛇床子 (129)	Warms the kidney and assists yang; dispels wind, dries damp, and kills worms.	Impotence; infertility due to uterine cold; wind-damp bi. Apply topically to damp scrotal itch; genital itch (e.g., trichomonas vaginitis), jie, xian, and damp sores.	Lower burner damp-heat; insufficiency of kidney yin.	3-10 g

48. Yin-supplementing agents 補陰藥 bu^3 yin^1 yao^4

Name	Functions	Indications	Contraindications	Daily Dosage
Dendrobii Caulis shi^2 hu^2 石斛 (15)	Engenders liquid and boosts the stomach; clears heat and nourishes yin. Stir-frying with brine enhances the power to supplement the kidney, and clear kidney and stomach fire.	Damage to liquid in heat diseases, dry mouth, thirst, vexation, and vacuity heat after illness.	Damp warmth and warm heat before transformation into dryness.	5-10 g
Asparagi Tuber $tian^1$ men^2 $dong^1$ 天門冬 (27)	Enriches yin and moistens dryness; clears the lung and downbears fire. Mix-frying with honey enhances the lung-moistening and cough-suppressing action. Coating in cinnabar adds a spirit-quieting action.	Yin vacuity fever; cough; blood ejection; pulmonary atony; pulmonary yong; sore, swollen throat; wasting thirst; constipation.	Spleen-stomach vacuity cold with diarrhea.	1.5-10 g

Drug	Actions	Indications	Cautions	Dosage
Ophiopogonis Tuber *mai⁴ men² dong¹* 麥門冬 (50)	Nourishes yin and moistens lung, clears the heart and eliminates vexation, boosts stomach and engenders liquid. Remove the heart to treat vexation. Stir-fry with rice to moderate the cool nature. Cover with cinnabar to quiet the heart-spirit.	Dryness pulmonary; dry cough; blood ejection; expectoration of blood; pulmonary yong and atony; vacuity taxation; heat vexation: wasting thirst; damage to liquid in febrile disease; dry mouth and throat; constipation.	Spleen-stomach vacuity cold with diarrhea.	5–10 g
Panacis Quinquefolii Radix *xi¹ yang² shen¹* 西洋參 (53)	Boosts lung yin and clears vacuity fire; engenders liquid and allays thirst.	Enduring cough; pulmonary atony; vacuity vexation; thirst with scant liquid; toothache due to stomach fire.	Spleen-stomach cold-damp.	3–5 g
Polygonati Officinalis Rhizoma *yu⁴ zhu²* 玉竹 (94)	Nourishes yin; moistens dryness; eliminates vexation; allays thirst. Use crude to clear heat and nourish yin. Use processed forms to supplement the center and boost qi, and to enrich yin and moisten dryness.	Damage to yin in febrile disease; cough, vexation, and thirst; vacuity taxation with fever; swift digestion with rapid hungering; frequent urination.	Debilitation of yang and exuberance of yin, in spleen vacuity with thoracic oppression, and stagnant phlegm-damp.	5–10 g
Ligustri Fructus *nü³ zhen¹ zi³* 女貞子 (140)	Supplements the liver and kidney, strengthens the lumbus and knees. Steaming with vinegar or brine eliminates the side effect of diarrhea.	Internal heat due to yin vacuity; dizziness; flowery vision; tinnitus; limp, aching lumbus and knees; premature graying.	Spleen-stomach vacuity diarrhea; yang vacuity.	5–10 g
Lycii Fructus *gou³ qi³ zi³* 枸杞子 (142)	Enriches the kidney, moistens the lung, supplements the liver, and brightens the eyes.	Liver-kidney yin depletion; limp, aching knees and lumbus; dizziness; copious tears; vacuity taxation cough; wasting thirst; seminal emission.	Repletion heat due to external contraction; spleen vacuity with damp.	5–10 g
Sesami Semen Atrum *hei¹ zhi¹ ma²* 黑脂麻 (183)	Supplements the liver and kidney and moistens the five viscera. Stir-fried to bring out the aroma, it promotes lactation. Steamed with wine, it expels wind and supplements.	Insufficiency of the liver and kidney; vacuity wind dizziness; wind bi; paralysis; vacuity marked emaciation after disease; premature graying; scant breast milk.	Spleen vacuity with thin stool.	5–10 g

Name	Functions	Indications	Contraindications	Daily Dosage
Amydae Sinensis Carapax *bie¹ jia³* 鱉甲 (206)	Nourishes yin and clears heat; calms the liver and extinguishes wind; softens hardness and dissipates binds. Used crude to enrich yin and subdue yang, stir-fried for steaming bone fever, and mix-fried with vinegar to soften hardness and dissipate binds.	Steaming bone taxation fever; stirring wind due to yin vacuity; mother of taxation malaria; concretions and conglomerations; elusive and bowstring masses; menstrual block; scant uterine bleeding; child fright epilepsy.	Pregnancy; Spleen-stomach yang debilitation with reduced food intake and thin stool.	10-12 g
Testudinis Plastrum *gui¹ ban³* 龜板 (221)	Enriches yin, subdues yang, supplements the kidney and fortifies the bones. Stir-frying with vinegar improves the yang-subduing action.	Insufficiency of kidney yin; steaming bone taxation fever; blood ejection; spontaneous external bleeding; enduring cough; seminal emission; uterine bleeding; vaginal discharge; lumbar pain; bone atony; yin vacuity wind; enduring dysentery and malaria; hemorrhoids; non-closure of the fontanels.	Vacuity patterns without heat signs.	10-20 g

49. Yin-supplementing and astringing agents 補陰・收斂藥 *bu³ yin¹, shou¹ lian⁴ yao⁴*

Name	Functions	Indications	Contraindications	Daily Dosage
Corni Fructus *shan¹ zhu¹ yu²* 山茱萸 (130)	Supplements the liver and kidney; astringes essential qi and checks vacuity desertion.	Lumbar and knee pain; dizziness; tinnitus; impotence; seminal emission; frequent urination; fever and chills due to liver vacuity; incessant vacuity sweating; weak heart with scattered pulse.	Intense life gate fire usually due to insufficiency of kidney yin, with signs such as inhibited urination, insomnia, and profuse dreaming.	5-10 g

50. Yin-supplementing and blood-nourishing agents 補陰・養血藥 *bu³ yin¹, yang³ xue⁴ yao⁴*

Name	Functions	Indications	Contraindications	Daily Dosage
Polygoni Multiflori Radix *he² shou³ wu¹* 何首烏 (57)	Supplements the liver and boosts the kidney; nourishes the blood and dispels wind. It is used crude to moisten the intestines and free the stool, steamed in wine to increase humor, and treated with black beans to enhance the channel-freeing action.	Liver-kidney yin depletion with signs such as premature graying of the hair, limp lumbus and knees, and seminal emission; blood vacuity dizziness; uterine bleeding; vaginal discharge; enduring malaria; swollen yong; intestinal wind; hemorrhoids.	Damp-phlegm and watery diarrhea.	10-15 g

51. Yin-supplementing, heat-clearing, and blood cooling agents 補陰 · 清熱 · 涼血藥 bu^3 yin^1, $qing^1$ re^4, $liang^2$ xue^4 yao^4

Scrophulariae Radix $xuan^2$ $shen^1$ 玄參 (64)	Enriches yin; downbears fire; eliminates vexation; resolves toxin. Use crude to drain fire, resolve toxin, and disinhibit the throat. Stir-fry with brine to enhance the yin-enriching action.	Vexation and thirst in febrile disease; swelling of yong; macular eruption; sore, swollen throat; scrofulous lumps; constipation.	Spleen vacuity diarrhea.	5-10 g

Appendix II Drug Processing

Chinese medicinal agents are "natural" in the sense that they are simply prepared animal, vegetable, and mineral products. Most items on sale in a Chinese pharmacy are readily recognizable as leaves, flowers, seeds, insects, etc. Nevertheless, most require minimum washing, cutting, and drying which is carried out according to established methods. Some agents require more complicated methods of processing before they can be administered. The finished materials are called decocting pieces (*yin³ pian⁴*), i.e., materials ready for boiling into a decoction. The preparation of decocting pieces is a necessity in as far as it facilitates extraction of active ingredients and ensures that the properties of agents are properly adjusted to the needs of the patient before decoction. At the same time, it is an art: the Chinese pharmacist goes to great pains to present his drugs in an attractive form.

The Aims of Processing

Elimination or reduction of toxicity: For example, Pinelliae Tuber Crudum (*sheng¹ ban⁴ xia⁴*) is treated with Zingiberis Succus (*jiang¹ zhi¹*), Alumen (*ming² fan²*), or Glycyrrhizae Radix (*gan¹ cao³*) to prevent poisoning and sore throat. The toxicity of Euphorbiae Kansui Radix (*gan¹ sui⁴*) is reduced by boiling in vinegar. The precipitating (purgative) action of Tiglii Semen (*ba¹ dou⁴*) is moderated be removing its oil content. Dichroae Radix (*chang² shan¹*) is treated stir-fried with wine to eliminate is emetic side-effects.

Enhancing action: Processing can enhance the effectiveness of some agents. For example, Corydalis Tuber (*yan² hu² suo³*) after being treated with vinegar has a strong pain-relieving effect. When Farfarae Flos (*kuan³ dong¹ hua¹*) is mix-fried with honey, it has a greater lung-moistening and cough-suppressing action. Atractylodis Ovatae Rhizoma (*bai² zhu²*) stir-fried with earth supplements the spleen and checks diarrhea more effectively. Bupleuri Radix (*chai² hu²*) mix-fried with vinegar has a greater liver-coursing and depression-resolving action.

Changing properties: Some agents have different actions depending on whether or not they are processed. For example, Rehmanniae Glutinosae Radix (*di⁴ huang²*) is cold in nature and has a blood-cooling action when raw, but is warm in nature and supplements the blood when steamed with wine (Chinese rice wine). Typhae Pollen (*pu² huang²*) moves the blood and resolves stasis when raw, and can check bleeding when char-fried. The effect of a drug can be changed by adjuvants. Processing with wine, for example, tends to check an agent's cold nature and make it bear upward. Below is a list of commonly used additives and the way in which the affect the nature and action of drugs according to traditional theory.

Additive	*Aim*
Wine	Checks cold and uplifts
Ginger	Warms, dissipates and sweeps phlegm
Honey	Sweetens, moistens dryness, and boosts the origin
Salt	Penetrates the kidney, moves downward, softens hardness
Vinegar	Penetrates the liver, induces contraction, and relieves pain
Earth (oven earth, Terra Flava Usta)	Fortifies the spleen and stomach and harmonizes the center
Rice	Eiminates dryness and nourishes the stomach
Bran	Eliminates harshness and prevents damage to stomach

Soaking in black bean and licorice decoction	Resolves toxin, and enhances supplementing action
Sheep's or goat's fat and pork lard	Penetrates bone products and helps calcination; used to stir-fry materials, it enters the spleen; used to char-fry materials, it checks bleeding

Methods of Processing

Older Chinese books discuss drug processing under three headings, water treatment (e.g., washing), fire treatment (e.g., baking), and fire and water treatment (e.g., boiling). Many, if not most, materials require fire, water, or fire and water treatment, yet a few need only basic preparation such as cutting or grinding. These basic methods are discussed first.

BASIC METHODS

Pounding (搗 *dao³*): Some small fruits and seeds are pounded just before use with a heavy-duty steel pestle and mortar. Gardeniae Fructus (*shan¹ zhi¹*), Amomi Semen (*sha¹ ren²*), and Alpiniae Katsumadae Semen (*cau⁴ kou⁴*) are pounded in small quantities prior to decoction to ensure that all the active constituents are extracted. Agents should not be stored for long periods after pounding since they may lose their oil content and other constituents, thus becoming less effective.

Grinding to a fine powder (研末, *yan² mo⁴*) (or trituration) with a pestle and mortar, is the method used to prepare formula that are administered or applied in powder form, but it is also used to ensure extraction of active constituents of hard materials such as minerals and shells in decoction. Cinnabaris (*zhu¹ sha¹*) and Margarita (*zhen¹ zhu¹*) are treated in this way.

Grating (鑢,剉 *cuo⁴*): Some hard bony materials such as Antelopis Cornu (*ling² yang² jiao³*) and Rhinocerotis Cornu (*xi¹ jiao³*) are grated in small particles using a steel rasp to facilitate decoction.

Cutting (切, *qie¹*): Cutting helps materials to dry, and to disintegrate during preparation. It enables the dispenser to achieve greater accuracy of quantities, and ensures that the active constituents are extracted during decoction. It is often facilitated by soaking or steeping (see *water treatment* ahead). Kitchen knives, herbal knives, guillotines, and nowadays cutting machines are used to cut materials into lumps, slices of various sizes. Many agents are cut with an herbal knife or cutting machines. Herb cutters save labor time, but cut less cleanly than an experienced hand cutter. The correct length or thickness and shape of slices depends on the material. There is transverse cutting, oblique cutting and longitudinal cutting; transverse shredding and longitudinal shredding. Roots, rhizomes, stems, vines, and woody materials that are hard in substance are cut Into thin slices, i.e., about 0.15 cm, while softer, less dense materials are cut in slices 0.3 cm or more thick. Materials that are long and thin, such as Imperatae Rhizoma (*mao² gen¹*) can be cut into lengths of 1–1.5 cm. Skins and barks, such as Phellodendri Cortex (*huang² bo²*), that are hard and thick can be cut into shreds of 0.6 cm. Thinner, less dense barks, such as Eucommiae Radicis Cortex (*du⁴ zhong⁴*) are cut into 1–1.5 cm broad strips. Brittle, fragile materials like Lycii Cortex Radicis (*di⁴ gu³ pi²*) need not be cut. Leaves that are thick and flexible, such as Pyrrosiae Folium (*shi² wei²*) are cut into strips 1–1.5 cm. Thick ones that are brittle after drying, such as Mori Folium (*su¹ ye⁴*) are either not cut or are simply rubbed between the hands. Whole plants with thin stems are cut into lengths of 1.5 cm; ones with thicker stems are cut into shorter lengths. Flowers and small fruits and seeds are generally not cut. Large fruits or ones that do not dry easily, such as Crataegi Fructus (*shan¹ zha¹*) are cut into three of four slices. Some pericarps such as Trichosanthis Pericarpium (*gua¹ lou² pi²*), are roughly shredded.

Frosting (制霜 *zhi⁴ shuang¹*): The production of a fine crisp powder by methods other than simple grinding is known as frosting. This is not one, but three distinct methods:

a) One method involves the defatting and trituration of seeds. The seeds are first sun-dried or stir-fried, the husks are removed, and the kernels is rolled pounded to an almost paste-like consistency. The materials are sandwiched between layers of paper, and then sun-dried, baked, or pressed, so that the paper absorbs the oil. The paper is repeatedly changed until the materials are light, loose and no longer stick together. Tiglii Pulvis Seminis (*ba¹ dou⁴ shuang¹*) and (*gua¹ ren² shuang¹*) are produced in this way.

b) Another method, used to treat certain gourds, is efflorescence. For example, Citrulli Fructus (*xi¹ gua¹*), or watermelon, is frosted by gouging out a small lump to form a hole in which a small amount of Mirabilitum (*mang² xiao¹*) is placed. The lump is then replaced, and the water melon is hung up to air. The Mirabilitum (*mang² xiao¹*) comes out and effloresces, and a fine, white frost forms on the surface of the watermelon, which it brushed off ready for use.

c) The production of Kaki Pulvis (*shi⁴ shuang¹*) represents a third method of frosting. Kaki Fructus Praeparatio (*shi⁴ bing³*) is exposed to the sun in the day and to the dew at night and then is covered to allow the skin to saccharify and form a frost.

WATER TREATMENT

Water treatment includes various ways of treating medicinal materials with clean water. The aim is to remove impurities, foreign bodies, and unwanted elements (such as sand, earth, salt, unpleasant odors), to increase suppleness to facilitate cutting, to purify and refine minerals, and to reduce toxicity. Methods must be carefully chosen to prevent loss of active constituents. Below are the commonest water processing methods.

Washing (洗, *xi³*) is the method used to remove earth and in some cases unwanted parts. With the exception of flowers, whose active constituents are easily lost in water, most materials are washed before use. Materials should not be left in water too long otherwise they lose their active constituents. Light, soft materials in particular should be washed as quickly as possibly.

Maceration (漂,水漂, *piao³, shui³ piao³*) is the process whereby materials are steeped in clean water that is continually or continuously replaced, to eliminate toxic constituents, salts, or bad odor, or remove foreign matter.

Soaking (浸泡 *jin⁴ pao⁴*) is allowing materials stand in water for a short time until the water has been absorbed. Its aim is to soften materials to facilitate cutting.

Water-grinding (水飛 *shui³ fei¹*) is the trituration of materials in water. The materials are first roughly crushed. They are then placed in a porcelain mortar, covered with water, and ground until the grating sound of rough lumps ceases. At this point, more water is mixed in, and the water containing suspended particles is then poured off and reserved. More water and materials are added, and the process is repeated. The reserved suspension is allowed to stand until the particles have settled, and the excess clear water is poured off. The remaining sludge is sun-dried, after which it is ready for use. This method is used for minerals and shells. Its advantage over dry trituration is that fine particles are not blown away and lost, and that impurities dissolved in the water are (at least partially) removed. The much finer powder it produces makes for greater assimilation of orally taken agents and reduces irritation by topically applied agents. Cinnabaris (*zhu¹ sha¹*), Talcum (*hua² shi²*), Smithsonitum (*lu² gan¹ shi²*), Realgar (*xiong² huang²*) are treated in this way for laryngeal insufflation, eye dab, or for coating pills.

FIRE TREATMENT

Fire treatment methods involve either direct or indirect contact of materials with a heat source, sometimes with additives. Care is required in controlling time and temperature, and the quantity of any additive used. Excessively high temperatures can cause undesirable changes in drug characteristics. The most common forms of fire treatment are as follows:

I.   **Stir-Frying** (炒 , *chao³*) is the most common form of fire treatment. Its aims are threefold:

   a) To eliminate unwanted constituents, change the nature of agents, and reduce irritation or other side-effects, and reduce extreme cold or dryness. For example, the fierce draining precipitant (downward draining or purgative) action of Rhei Rhizoma (*da⁴ huang²*) in its raw form is moderated by stir-frying, and even more markedly reduced by char-frying.

b) To increase aromatic and spleen-fortifying qualities. For example, Atractylodis Ovatae Rhizoma (*bai² zhu²*) and Hordei Fructus Germinatus (*mai⁴ ya²*) are stir-fried until yellow, while Crataegi Fructus (*shan¹ zha¹*) and Massa Medicata Fermentata (*shen² qu¹*) are scorch-fried.

c) To facilitate crushing, storage, and extraction of active constituents through decoction. For example, some seeds when lightly fried crispen and crack open facilitating decoction. Some materials become looser after stir-frying, so that they are more easily crushed, and their active constituents are more easily extracted. Also, stir-frying reduces moisture content and destroys ferments, thus preventing the breakdown of active constituents during storage. Stir-frying includes plain stir-frying and stir-frying with adjuvants.

1) **Plain Stir-Frying** (清炒 *qing¹ chao³*, 單炒 *dan¹ chao³*), i.e., stir-frying without any adjuvants, includes the following forms:

Light stir-frying (微炒 *wei² chao³*) is of short duration, and its aim is to remove the moisture content so that the material is left dry, at least on the outer surface, but without producing any change in form or characteristics of the agent.

Scorch-frying (炒焦 *chao³ jiao¹*): Materials are turned in the wok over a high flame until they become a burnt brown on the outside and emit a burnt smell. Abducting dispersers such as Massa Medicata Fermentata (*shen² qu¹*) and Crataegi Fructus (*shan¹ zha¹*) are treated in this way to strengthen their spleen-fortifying and food-dispersing action.

Blast-frying (炮 *pao¹*): Materials are turned quickly and vigorously over a very high flame until their surface becomes scorched, swollen, and cracked. Zingiberis Rhizoma (*gan¹ jiang¹*), Aconiti Tuber Laterale (*fu⁴ zi³*), and Aconiti Tuber Laterale Tianxiong (*tian¹ xiong²*) are treated in this way to reduce their harshness.

Char-frying (炒炭 *chao³ tan⁴*) is similar to scorch-frying, but uses a yet higher flame. The aim is to make the materials charred and black on the outside, brown on the inside, and brittle. Although a large proportion of the materials is carbonized, the original properties are still present. This is what is known as ''nature-preservative burning.'' To ensure that the nature is partially preserved in this way it is important that the materials should not be completely carbonized. Because of the high temperature used in char-frying materials easily catch fire. In this event, water should be sprinkled on until no sparks are seen. Some materials, such as Typhae Pollen (*pu² huang²*) require particularly vigorous stirring to clear the smoke they produce. Char-frying moderates the properties of drugs, and increases its capacity to promote contraction and check bleeding. Some modern experiments show that blood-staunching properties may be destroyed through the process. Further research is necessary.

2) **Stir-Frying with Adjuvants** (副料炒 *fu³ liao⁴ chao³*) means stir-frying materials together with a secondary solid material that is sifted off when frying is completed.

Earth-frying (土炒 *tu³ chao³*) is stir-frying materials together with Terra Flava Usta (*zao⁴ xin¹ tu³*), which, being pungent and warm, gives them the power supplement the spleen and staunch bleeding, and harmonize the stomach and check vomiting. Terra Flava Usta (*zao⁴ xin¹ tu³*), through its long exposure to high temperatures, contains zinc oxide and little water or organic matter, and being slightly alkaline it reduces stomach acidity. Atractylodis Ovatae Rhizoma (*bai² zhu²*) and Dioscoreae Rhizoma (*shan¹ yao⁴*) may be treated in this way.

Bran-frying (麩炒 *fu¹ chao³*): The materials and bran are placed in the wok together, and fried until a thick yellow-black smoke is given off. This process, increases a drug's capacity to fortify the spleen and stomach, and absorbs oils that would cause side effects. In addition, it removes unpleasant odors. Atractylodis Ovatae Rhizoma (*bai² zhu²*) and Aurantii Fructus (*zhi³ ke²*) may be treated in this way.

Rice-frying (米炒 *mi³ chao³*) reduces the dryness of agents, and increases their capacity to supplement the center and boost qi. It can also reduce the toxicity of a small number of agents. Codonopsitis Radix (*dang³ shen¹*) and Mylabris (*ban¹ mao²*) are treated in this way.

Stir-frying with clam shell powder (蛤粉炒*ge² fen³ chao³*): Clam shell powder is fine, and conducts heat slowly, and hence poses little danger of burning. For this reason, is often used to treat animal gelatinous products, which are allow to turn yellow or bubble up at the surface before removal. Ass hide glue pellets, Asini Corii Gelatini Pilula (*e¹ jiao¹ zhu¹*), are made in this way. Talcum (*hua² shi²*) is used in exactly the same way as clam shell.

3) **Mix-frying** (炙*zhi⁴*) is stir-frying with liquid adjuvants, which soak into the materials. The aim of mix-frying is to make the adjuvant gradually soak into the materials. The aim of mix-frying is to change drug characteristics, enhance effectiveness, improve flavor and smell, resolve toxicity, and prevent rotting. Usually, the adjuvant and materials are first blended, covered, and left to stand for a short time before frying.

Honey mix-frying (蜜炙*mi⁴ zhi⁴*): Honey is sweet in flavor and balanced in nature. It relieves pain and tension, boosts the origin, moistens the lung and calms cough, resolves toxin, and improves the flavor. It can moderate the qualities of other drugs and harmonize the various drugs in a formula, as well as improving the effectiveness of other drugs. Mix-frying with honey is usually used to moisten the lung and suppress cough, to boost and nourish, and to moderate the powerful nature of agents such as Asteris Radix et Rhizoma (*zi³ wan³*) and Astragali Radix (*huang² qi²*).

Wine mix-frying (酒炙*jiu³ zhi⁴*): Usually, "yellow wine" (rice or millet wine, such as Shaoxing) is used, but "white wine," colorless spirits such as sorghum liquor, are also used on occasions. Wine is pungent, sweet, and very hot. It can conduct agents upwards, reduce the cold nature of agents, and can quicken the blood and free the connecting channels. Also, wine is also an excellent organic solvent: alkaloids and volatile oils all easily dissolve in it. Mix-frying in wine thus helps to release active constituents, thereby increasing the effectiveness of medication. It also serves to improve the flavor and smell, and remove fishy or putrid smells. Scutellariae Radix (*huang² qin²*), Rhei Rhizoma (*da⁴ huang²*), and Paeoniae Radix, Alba (*bai² shao²*) can all be treated in this way. One method is to sprinkle yellow wine over the materials, which are then covered and left to stand for a while to allow the wine to soak in. They are then transferred to the wok, where they are continuously stirred over a low flame until they turn pale yellow and the aroma of the materials can be smelled. Another way is to sprinkle the wine over the materials after they have been heated over a low flame, and continue stir-frying until the aroma of the materials can be smelled. Whichever method is used, the duration of frying and the size of flame should not be excessive. Smell and color are good guides. Frying should cease before any burnt smell arises and before any change of color occurs inside the materials. The amount of wine used depends on the material. Generally it is 60–90 g for 500g of materials.

Vinegar mix-frying (醋炙*cu⁴ zhi⁴*): Vinegar is sour, bitter, and slightly warm, hence it can enter the liver channel, promote contraction, and relieve pain. Mix-frying with vinegar gives agents increased power to enter the blood and promote contraction, emolliate the liver and relieve pain. It also improves the flavor and removes unpleasant odors, such as in the case of Trogopteri seu Pteromydis Excrementum (*wu³ ling² zhi¹*). Containing acetic acid, vinegar is also a good solvent: it can combine with free alkaloids to form soluble salts, allowing active constituents to be easily extracted through decoction and increasing the speed with which the agent takes effect, as in the case of Corydalis Tuber (*yan² hu² suo³*). Agents most commonly vinegar mix-fried are liver-calming and qi-rectifying agents such as Citri Pericarpium Immaturum (*qing¹ pi²*), Cyperi Rhizoma (*xiang¹ fu⁴*), Bupleuri Radix (*chai² hu²*), and Corydalis Tuber (*yan² hu² suo³*). One method of mix-frying with vinegar, which is usually used for herbs, is to first blend the vinegar (rice vinegar) with the agent and leave it to soak in. The agent is then stir-fried over a low flame until it gives off its own smell and turns slightly golden. It is then taken out of the wok and left to cool ready for use. Another method, used mainly for animal products and shells, is to put the materials in the wok and heat them over a low flame, turning them constantly while sprinkling the vinegar over them. Stir-frying continues until the materials completely absorb the vinegar, give off their own smell, and turn slightly golden. One or more parts of vinegar to five parts of materials represents the usual proportion, i.e., roughly 60 g of vinegar for every 500 g of materials.

Brine mix-frying (鹽炙 *yan² zhi⁴*): Stir-frying with a salt solution is known as brine mix-frying. Being salty and cold, salt clears clears heat and cools the blood, enter the kidney, and softens hardness. It can also improve the flavor and act as preservative. Brine stir-frying is a common method of processing agents that supplement the kidney, secure essence, treat shan qi, and drain kidney fire such as Psoraleae Semen (*bu³ gu³ zhi¹*), Foeniculi Fructus (*xiao³ hui² xiang¹*), Anemarrhenae Rhizoma (*zhi¹ mu³*), Phellodendri Cortex (*huang² bo²*), and Alismatis Rhizoma (*ze² xie⁴*).

Ginger juice mix-frying (薑炙 *jiang¹ zhi⁴*): Fresh ginger, Zingiberis Rhizoma Recens (*sheng¹ jiang¹*), is pungent and warm. It warms the stomach, checks vomiting, sweeps phlegm and opens the portals. Stir-frying agents with its juice gives them better able to fortify the stomach, settle vomiting, and dispel phlegm. At the same time, it can counteract the cold and cool nature of some agents, reduce toxicity, and eliminate such side effects as vomiting.

Fat-frying (油炙 *you² zhi⁴*) is stir-frying agents in oil, or mixing them with fat or oil before stir-frying. Usually, sesame seed or sheep fat is used. Fat-frying makes materials crisp and easier to crush, and can eliminate toxicity, such as in the case of Tigris Os (*hu³ gu³*), and Strychnotis Nux-Vomicae Semen (*ma³ qian² zi³*).

II. **Calcination** (煆 *duan⁴*) is a process whereby materials are heated until red hot (over 760°C by a charcoal or coal to make them crisp, soft, and easily crushed, and to facilitate the extraction of their active constituents in decoction. Some materials are calcined by placing them directly in the fire, some in containers, some in a wok. Especially hard materials need to be dipped in water or vinegar after heating. This is called dip-calcination.

III. **Roasting** (煨 *wei¹*) is a method of drawing out unwanted oils or irritants from materials and reducing their toxicity by exposure to heat. Materials are usually wrapped in wet paper or coated in flour and water paste, and placed in hot embers until the wrapping becomes burnt and black. They may also be put at the side of the fire, in an oven, or tossed in a wok. Myristicae Semen (*rou⁴ dou⁴ kou⁴*) and Euphorbiae Kansui Radix (*gan¹ sui⁴*) may be treated in this way.

IV. **Stone-baking** (焙 *bei⁴*) is heating agents gently on a stone slab or tile without allowing them to change color. This process is similar to light stir-frying.

FIRE AND WATER TREATMENT

Fire and water treatment involves treatment with both fire and water, sometimes with the use of adjuvants. The main forms are steaming, boiling, distillation, and soaking in boiling water.

Steaming (蒸 *zheng¹*): Steaming involves placing materials in pots or baskets, with or without adjuvants, over boiling water. The aim is to change the nature of the drug, improve its effectiveness, and facilitate slicing and storage.

Boiling (煮 *zhu³*): The main purpose of boiling is to eliminate toxicity, irritants or prevent side-effects, or increase effectiveness. Boiling in some cases facilitates storage.

Distillation (蒸露 *zheng¹ lu⁴*): Agents that have a high volatile oil content can be distilled.

Lonicerae Flos (*jin¹ yin² hua¹*), Pogostemi seu Agastaches Herba (*huo⁴ xiang¹*), and Menthae Herba (*bo⁴ he²*) can all be made into distillates.

Dip calination (淬 *cui⁴*): Described under the heading *fire treatment.*

Appendix III Formulas

1 *an¹ gong¹ niu²-huang² wan²* 安宮牛黃丸
Peaceful Palace Bovine Bezoar Pills
Source: 溫病條辨 (*wen¹ bing⁴ tiao² bian⁴*)
Bezoar Bovis *niu² huang²* 3 g
Rhinocerotis Cornu *xi¹ jiao³* 30 g
Curcumae Tuber *yu⁴ jin¹* 30 g
Coptidis Rhizoma *huang² lian²* 30 g
Scutellariae Radix *huang² qin²* 30 g
Gardeniae Fructus *shan¹ zhi¹ zi³* 30 g
Cinnabaris *zhu¹ sha¹* 30 g
Realgar *xiong² huang²* 30 g
Margarita *zhen¹ zhu¹* 15 g
Moschus *she⁴ xiang¹* 7.5 g
Borneolum *bing¹ pian⁴* 7.5 g
Preparation method: Form into 3 g pills.
Actions and Indications: Clears the heart and opens the portals; drains fire and resolves toxin. Treats: 1) Warm heat disease with high fever, clouding of the spirit and, in severe cases, tetanic inversion. 2) Acute child fright wind. 3) Wind stroke loss of consciousness due to phlegm-heat clouding the portals of the heart.
Dosage: 1 pill 3 times a day.

2 *an¹-xi²-xiang¹ wan²* 安息香丸
Benzoin Pills
Source: 金幼心鑑 (*jin¹ you⁴ xin¹ jian⁴*)
Benzoinum *an¹ xi² xiang¹* (steamed in wine to form a paste) 1.5 g
Aquilariae Lignum *chen² xiang¹* 3 g
Saussureae Radix *mu⁴ xiang¹* 3 g
Caryophylli Flos *ding¹ xiang¹* 3 g
Agastaches seu Pogostemi Herba *huo⁴ xiang¹* 3 g
Anisi Stellati Fructus *ba¹ jiao³ hui² xiang¹* 3 g
Cyperi Rhizoma *xiang¹ fu⁴ zi³* 5 g
Amomi Semen *sha¹ ren²* 5 g
Glycyrrhizae Radix *gan¹ cao³* (mix-fried) 5 g
Preparation method: Grind to a powder, blend with honey, and form into 1 g pills.
Actions and Indications: Treats child epilepsy; abdominal pain; lumbar pain.
Dosage: 3 pills 3 times a day.

3 *an¹ zhong¹ san³* 安中散
Center-Quieting Powder
Source: 和劑局方 (*he³ ji⁴ ju² fang¹*)
Corydalis Tuber *yan² hu² suo³* 3 g
Alpiniae Officinarum Rhizoma *gao¹ liang² jiang¹* 0.5 g
Amomi Semen *sha¹ ren²* 1 g
Foeniculi Fructus *hui² xiang¹* 1.5 g
Cinnamomi Ramulus *gui⁴ zhi¹* 4 g
Ostreae Concha *mu³ li⁴* 3 g
Glycyrrhizae Radix *gan¹ cao³* 1 g
Actions and Indications: Treats nervous gastric pain; stomach or duodenal ulcers; chronic gastritis; menstrual pain; vomiting in pregnancy.

4 *ba¹ li² san³* 八厘散
Eight Pinches Powder
Source: 醫宗金鑑 (*yi¹ zong¹ jin¹ jian⁴*)
Sappan Lignum *su¹ mu⁴* 5 g
Strychnotis Nux-Vomicae Semen *ma³ qian² zi³* 0.5 g
Pyritum *zi⁴ ran² tong²* 3 g
Olibanum *ru³ xiang¹* 3 g
Myrrha *mo⁴ yao⁴* 3 g
Draconis Sanguis *xue⁴ jie²* 3 g
Moschus *she⁴ xiang¹* 0.1 g
Carthami Flos *hong² hua¹* 2 g
Caryophylli Flos *ding¹ xiang¹* 0.5 g
Preparation method: Grind to a fine powder.
Actions and Indications: Dissipates stasis. Treats impact injury.
Dosage: 0.3 g 3 times a day.

5 *ba¹ wei⁴ dai⁴ xia⁴ fang¹* 八味帶下方
Eight-Ingredient Discharge Formula
Source: 名家方選 (*ming² jia¹ fang¹ xuan³*)
Angelicae Sinensis Radix *dang¹ gui¹* 5 g
Ligustici Rhizoma *chuan¹ xiong¹* 3 g
Poria *fu² ling²* 3 g
Mutong Caulis *mu⁴ tong¹* 4 g
Smilacis Glabrae Rhizoma *tu³ fu² ling²* 4 g
Citri Exocarpium *chen² pi²* 2 g
Lonicerae Flos *jin¹ yin² hua¹* 1 g
Rhei Rhizoma *da⁴ huang²* 1 g
Actions and Indications: Treats vaginal discharge with foul smell.

6 *ba¹ wei⁴ di⁴-huang² wan²* 八味地黃丸
Eight-Ingredient Rehmannia Pills
Source: 金匱要略 (*jin¹ gui⁴ yao⁴ lue⁴*)
Rehmanniae Radix Exsiccata *gan¹ di⁴ huang²* 5 g
Poriae *fu² ling²* 3 g
Cinnamomi Ramulus *gui⁴ zhi¹* 1 g
Alismatis Rhizoma *ze² xie⁴* 3 g

Aconiti Tuber Laterale *fu⁴ zi³* 1 g
Moutan Radicis Cortex *mu³ dan¹ pi²* 3 g
Corni Fructus *shan¹ zhu¹ yu²* 3 g
Dioscoreae Rhizoma *shan yao* 3g
Actions and Indications: Treats disorders of the kidney and bladder, diabetes, hypertension, neurasthenia, lumbar pain, cataracts, impotence, and paralysis of the lower limbs.

7 *ba¹ zheng⁴ san³* 八正散
Eight Corrections Powder
Source:和劑局方 (*he² ji⁴ ju² fang¹*)
Dianthi Herba *qu¹ mai⁴* 6–12 g
Polygoni Avicularis Herba *bian³ xu⁴* 6–12 g
Plantaginis Semen *che¹ qian² zi³* 9–15 g
Mutong Caulis *mu⁴ tong¹* 3–6 g
Talcum *hua² shi²* 12–30 g
Glycyrrhizae Radix Tenuis *gan¹ cao³ shao¹* 3–9 g
Gardeniae Fructus *zhi¹ zi³* 3–9 g
Rhei Rhizoma *da⁴ huang²* (prepared) 6–9 g
Preparation method: The original formula included Junci Medulla (*deng¹ xin¹ cao³*), and was grind to a powder before decoction. Now it is simply prepared as a decoction.
Actions and Indications: Clears heat and drains fire; disinhibits water and frees stranguary. Treats downpour of damp-heat into the bladder giving rise to dribbling, difficult, and painful voidings of dark-colored urine, and stone stranguary or unctuous stranguary.

8 *bai² hu³ jia¹ cang¹-zhu² tang¹* 白虎加蒼朮湯
White Tiger Decoction Plus Atractylodes
Alternate name:石膏知母蒼朮湯 *shi²-gao¹ zhi¹-mu³ cang¹-zhu² tang¹* Gypsum, Anemarrhena and Atractylodes Decoction
Source:活人書 (*huo² ren² shu¹*)
Gypsum Crudum *sheng¹ shi² gao¹* 16 g
Anemarrhenae Rhizoma *zhi¹ mu³* 6 g
Glycyrrhizae Radix *gan¹ cao³* (mix-fried) 2 g
Oryzae Semen *geng¹ mi³* 8–10 g
Atractylodis Rhizoma *cang¹ zhu²* 2 g
Actions and Indications: Clears heat and dries damp. Treats: 1) Damp warmth with copious sweating, heavy body, and cold feet. 2) Damp bi transforming into heat. 3) Summer fever with signs of damp encumbrance such as bag-over-the-head sensation, oppression in the chest, thirst without desire for fluids, painful, swollen joints, and a slimy white tongue fur.

9 *bai² hu³ jia¹ gui⁴-zhi¹ tang¹* 白虎加桂枝湯
White Tiger Decoction Plus Cinnamon Twig
Alternate name:石膏知母桂枝湯 *shi²-gao¹ zhi¹-mu³*

gui⁴-zhi¹ tang¹ Gypsum, Anemarrhena and Cinnamon Twig Decoction
Source:金匱要略 (*jin¹ gui⁴ yao⁴ lue⁴*)
Gypsum Crudum *sheng¹ shi² gao¹* 15 g
Anemarrhenae Rhizoma *zhi¹ mu³* 5 g
Glycyrrhizae Radix *gan¹ cao³* 2 g
Oryzae Semen *geng¹ mi³* 8 g
Cinnamomi Ramulus *gui⁴ zhi¹* 2–4 g
Actions and Indications: Clears pathogenic heat; frees the channels. Treats warm malaria characterized by fever without chills, and pain in the joints, and periodic retching. 2) Heat bi. 3) High fever in the summer with vexation, thirst, sweating and aversion to wind.

10 *bai² hu³ jia¹ ren²-shen¹ tang¹* 白虎加人參湯
White Tiger Decoction Plus Ginseng
Source:傷寒論 (*shang¹ han² lun⁴*)
Gypsum Crudum *sheng¹ shi² gao¹* 15 g
Anemarrhenae Rhizoma *zhi¹ mu³* 5 g
Glycyrrhizae Radix *gan¹ cao³* 2 g
Oryzae Semen *geng¹ mi³* 10 g
Ginseng Radix *ren² shen¹* 3 g
Actions and Indications: Clears heat; boosts qi; engenders liquid. Treats White Tiger Decoction patterns in which excessive sweating has caused damage to both qi and liquid; summerheat stroke in the summer months, with fever, thirst, and copious sweating. Pulse: large and forceful.

11 *bai² hu³ tang¹* 白虎湯
White Tiger Decoction
Alternate name:石膏知母湯 *shi²-gao¹ zhi¹-mu³ tang¹* Gypsum and Anemarrhena Decoction
Source:傷寒論 (*shang¹ han² lun⁴*)
Gypsum Crudum *sheng¹ shi² gao¹* 15–60 g
Anemarrhenae Rhizoma *zhi¹ mu³* 10–15 g
Glycyrrhizae Radix *gan¹ cao³* 3–5 g
Oryzae Semen *geng¹ mi³* 15–30 g
Actions and Indications: Clears pathogen heat in the qi aspect; eliminates vexation and allays thirst. Treats yang-ming cold damage or qi aspect warm heat disease, characterized by high fever, vexation and agitation, thirst with desire for fluids, large surging or slippery rapid pulse. Also treats exuberant stomach fire manifesting as headache, toothache, or wasting thirst.

12 *bai²-ji²-li² san³* 白蒺藜散
Tribulus Powder
Source:證治準繩 (*zheng⁴ zhi⁴ zhun³ sheng²*)
Tribuli Fructus *ci⁴ ji² li²* (stir-fried)
Dictamni Radicis Cortex Radicis *bai² xian¹ pi²*

Ledebouriellae Radix *fang² feng¹*
Rhei Rhizoma *da⁴ huang²* (stir-fried),
Paeoniae Radix Rubrae *chi⁴ shao² yao⁴*
Gardeniae Fructus *shan¹ zhi¹ zi³*
Scutellariae Radix *huang² qin²*
Ophiopogonis Tuber *mai⁴ men² dong¹* (stone-baked)
Scrophulariae Radix *xuan² shen¹*
Platycodonis Radix *jie² geng³*
Glycyrrhizae Radix *gan¹ cao³* (mix-fried)
Peucedani Radix *qian² hu².*
All agents in equal proportions. Preparation method:
Grind to a powder.
Actions and Indications: Treats itchy heat toxin sores
with vexation and agitation.
Dosage: 3 g 3 times a day.

13   *bai²-ji² pi²-pa² wan²* 白及枇杷丸....78, 90, 101
Bletilla and Loquat Pills
Source: 證治準繩 (*zheng⁴ zhi⁴ zhun³ sheng²*)
Bletillae Tuber *bai² ji²* 3 g
Eriobotryae Folium *pi² pa² ye⁴* 1.5 g
Nelumbinis Rhizomatis Nodus *ou³ jie²* 1.5 g
Rehmanniae Radix Cruda *sheng¹ di⁴ huang²* 1.5 g
Asini Corii Gelatinum *e¹ jiao¹* (stir-fried with
    clamshell powder)
Preparation method: Form into 1-2 g pills.
Actions and Indications: Clears the lung and sup-
presses cough. Treats cough with expectoration of
blood.
Dosage: 1 g a day.

14   *bai²-jiang¹-can² san³* 白僵蠶散..................210
Silkworm Powder
Source: 楊氏方 (*yang² shi⁴ fang¹*)
Bombyx Batryticatus *bai² jiang¹ can²* 3 g
Arisaematis Rhizoma *tian¹ nan² xing¹* (blast-fried)
    3 g
Preparation method: Grind to a powder.
Actions and Indications: Treats throat bi and swollen
throat. Grind to a powder.
Dosage: 3 g 3 times a day.

15   *bai² jin¹ wan²* 白金丸 34, 223
Alum and Curcuma Pills
Source: 醫方考 (*yi¹ fang¹ kao³*)
Curcumae Tuber *yu⁴ jin¹* 210 g
Alumen *bai² fan²* 90 g
Actions and Indications: Dispels phlegm and opens
the portals. Treats epilepsy with copious phlegm, sud-
den clouding collapse and foaming at the mouth.
Dosage: 3-6 g. twice daily.

16   *bai²-tou²-weng¹ tang¹* 白頭翁湯 5, 10
Pulsatilla Decoction
Source: 傷寒論 (*shang¹ han² lun⁴*)

Pulsatillae Radix *bai² tou² weng¹* 15-30 g
Fraxini Cortex *qin² pi²* 9-15 g
Coptidis Rhizoma *huang² lian²* 6-9 g
Phellodendri Cortex *huang² bo²* 9-12 g
Preparation method: Decoct with water.
Actions and Indications: Clears heat and resolves tox-
in; cools the blood and checks dysentery. Treats heat
dysentery with pus and blood in the stool, tenesmus,
burning sensation in the anus, and sometimes fever
and bitter taste in the mouth.

17   *bai²-wei² tang¹* 白薇湯 35
Baiwei Decoction
Source: 普濟和事方 (*pu³ ji⁴ he² shi⁴ fang¹*)
Cynanchi Radix *bai² wei²* 3 g
Angelicae Sinensis Radix *dang¹ gui¹* 3 g
Ginseng Radix *ren² shen¹* 1.5 g
Glycyrrhizae Radix *gan¹ cao³* 1.5 g
Actions and Indications: Treats cold damage that fails
to resolve.

18   *bai²-xian¹-pi² san³* 白鮮皮散........................3
Dictamnus Powder
Source: 聖濟總錄 (*sheng⁴ ji⁴ zong³ lu⁴*)
Dictamni Radicis Cortex *bai² xian¹ pi²* 3 g
Ledebouriellae Radix *fang² feng¹* 3 g
Ginseng Radix *ren² shen¹* 3 g
Anemarrhenae Rhizoma *zhi¹ mu³* 3 g
Adenophorae seu Glehniae Radix *sha¹ shen¹* 3. g
Scutellariae Radix *huang² qin²* 1.5 g
Actions and Indications: Treats lung wind-heat; tox-
ic qi causing itchy skin; inhibited sensation in the chest
and diaphragm with vexation and agitation.

19   *bai³-bu⁴ san³* 百部散................................68
Stemona Powder
Source: 聖惠方 (*sheng⁴ hui⁴ fang¹*)
Stemonae Radix *bai³ bu⁴* 5 g
Fritillariae Bulbus *bei² mu³* (roasted until yellow) 5 g
Asteris Radix et Rhizoma *zi³ wan³* 5 g
Puerariae Radix *ge² gen¹* 5 g
Gypsum *shi² gao¹* 10 g
Preparation method: Grind to a powder.
Actions and Indications: Treats cough, vexation and
fever in children.
Dosage: 3 g 2-3 times a day.

20   *bai³-he² gu⁴ jin¹ tang¹* 百合固金湯 85, 89
Lily Bulb Metal-Securing Decoction
New name: 百合固肺湯 *bai³-he² gu⁴ fei⁴ tang¹* Lily
Bulb Lung-Securing Decoction
Source: 醫方集解 (*yi¹ fang¹ ji² jie³*)
Lilii Bulbus *bai³ he²* 6-9 g
Rehmanniae Radix Cruda *sheng¹ di⁴* 6-9 g
Rehmanniae Radix Conquita *shou² di⁴ huang²* 6-9 g

Ophiopogonis Tuber *mai⁴ dong¹* 6–9 g
Scrophulariae Radix *xuan² shen¹* 6–9 g
Fritillariae Bulbus bei mu   3–6 g
Platycodonis Radix *jie² geng³* 3–5 g
Angelicae Sinensis Radix *dang¹ gui¹* 3–6 g
Paeoniae Radix *shao² yao⁴* 3–6 g
Glycyrrhizae Radix Cruda *sheng¹ gan¹ cao³* 3–5 g
Actions and Indications: Nourishes yin and clears
heat; moistens the lung and transforms phlegm. Treats
lung-kidney yin vacuity with upflaming vacuity fire,
characterized by signs such as sore throat, cough,
dyspnea, phlegm containing blood, dry mouth, heat
in the heart of the soles and palms, a red tongue with
scant fur, and a fine, rapid pulse.

**21 *bai³-he² zhi¹-mu³ tang¹* 百合知母湯 74, 89
Lily Bulb and Anemarrhena Decoction**
Source: 金匱要略 (*jin¹ gui⁴ yao⁴ lue⁴*)
Lilii Bulbus *bai³ he²* 3 g
Anemarrhenae Rhizoma *zhi¹ mu³* 3 g
Actions and Indications: Treats heart-lung vacuity pat-
terns known as "lily disease" (*bai³ he² bing⁴*).

**22 *bai³ hua¹ gao¹* 百花膏 89, 112
Lily Bulb and Tussilago Paste**
Source: 濟生方 (*ji⁴ sheng¹ fang¹*)
Lilii Bulbus *bai³ he²*
Tussilaginis Flos *kuan³ dong¹ hua¹*
Both agents in equal proportions.
Preparation method: Grind to a powder, blend with
honey, and form into 2–3 g pills.
Actions and Indications: Moistens the lung and sup-
presses cough. Treats cough and rapid, dyspneic
breathing, dry mouth, and hoarse voice, and phlegm
streaked with blood.
Dosage: 1 pill after meals.

**23 *ban¹-mao² tong¹ jing¹ wan²* 斑蝥通經丸 217
Mylabris Channel-Freeing Pills**
Source: 濟陰綱目 (*ji⁴ yin¹ gang¹ mu⁴*)
Mylabris *ban¹ mao²* (stir-fried with glutinous rice)
   10 pieces
Persicae Semen *tao² ren²* (stir-fried) 50 pieces
Rhei Rhizoma *da⁴ huang²* 15 g
Preparation method: Grind to a fine powder, blend
with honey, and form into 300 mg pills.
Actions and Indications: Itchy heat toxin sores with
vexation and agitation.
Dosage: Take 3 g at a time.

**24 *ban⁴-xia⁴ bai²-zhu² tian¹-ma² tang¹* 半夏白朮天
      麻湯 76, 86, 92, 137
Pinellia, Atractylodes Ovata, and Gastrodia Decoction**

Source: 醫學心悟 (*yi¹ xue² xin¹ wu⁴*)
Pinelliae Tuber *ban⁴ xia⁴* (prepared) 6–9 g
Hordei Fructus Germinatus *mai⁴ ya²* 2–3 g
Gastrodiae Rhizoma *tian¹ ma²* 6–9 g
Atractylodis Ovatae Rhizoma *bai² zhu²* 9–12 g
Citri Exocarpium Rubrum *ju² hong²*
   6–9 g
Poria *fu² ling²* 6–9 g
Glycyrrhizae Radix *gan¹ cao³* 1.5–3 g
Zingiberis Rhizoma Recens *sheng¹ jiang¹*
   2–3 slices
Zizyphi Fructus *da⁴ zao³* 3–5 pieces
Preparation method: Decoct with water.
Actions and Indications: Transforms phlegm and ex-
tinguishes wind; fortifies the spleen and dries damp.
Treats dizziness and headache, copious phlegm, and
oppression in the chest. Tongue fur: white and slimy.

**25 *ban⁴-xia⁴ hou⁴-po⁴ tang¹* 半夏厚朴湯 7, 92
Pinellia and Magnolia Bark Decoction**
Source: 金匱要略 (*jin¹ gui⁴ yao⁴ lue⁴*)
Pinelliae Tuber *ban⁴ xia⁴* 6–9 g
Magnoliae Cortex *hou⁴ po⁴* 3–6 g
Poria *fu² ling²* 9–12 g
Perillae Caulis et Calyx *zi³ su¹* 6–9 g
Zingiberis Rhizoma Recens *sheng¹ jiang¹* 4–5 slices.
Preparation method: Decoct with water.
Actions and Indications: Rectifies qi and resolves
depression; downbears counterflow and transforms
phlegm. Treats emotional depression with congealing
phlegm-drool and "plum pit qi" (globus hystericus);
congesting phlegm-damp causing fullness in the chest
and rapid breathing; painful glomus in the middle
venter with vomiting.

**26 *ban⁴-xia⁴ xie⁴ xin¹ tang¹* 半夏瀉心湯 92
Pinellia Heart-Draining Decoction**
Source: 傷寒論 (*shang¹ han¹ lun⁴*)
Pinelliae Tuber *ban⁴ xia⁴* 6–9 g
Scutellariae Radix *huang² qin²* 6–9 g
Zingiberis Rhizoma *gan¹ jiang¹* 3–6 g
Coptidis Rhizoma *huang² lian²* 3–6 g
Ginseng Radix *ren² shen¹*
Glycyrrhizae Radix *gan¹ cao³* 3–6 g
Zizyphi Fructus *da⁴ zao³* 4 pieces
Actions and Indications: Harmonizes the stomach and
downbears counterflow; frees binds and eliminates
glomus.
Treats impaired gastrointestinal function with the
presence of both cold and heat, characterized by
fullness and glomus below the heart, no desire for food
or drink, nausea and vomiting, rumbling intestines,
and diarrhea. Tongue fur: thin, yellow and slimy.

27 bei⁴-mu³ tang¹ 貝母湯.............................85
Fritillaria Decoction
Source: 本事方 (ben³ shi⁴ fang¹)
Fritillariae Bulbus bei mu 2 g
Scutellariae Radix huang² qin² 2.5 g
Schisandrae Fructus wu³ wei⁴ zi³ 2.5 g
Zingiberis Rhizoma gan¹ jiang¹ 0.5 g
Citri Exocarpium chen² pi² 2.5 g
Mori Radicis Cortex sang¹ bai² pi² 2.5 g
Bupleuri Radix chai² hu² 3 g
Pinelliae Tuber ban⁴ xia⁴ 1 g
Cinnamomi Ramulus gui⁴ zhi¹ 2 g
Saussureae Radix mu⁴ xiang¹ 1 g
Glycyrrhizae Radix gan¹ cao³ 1 g
Armeniacae Semen xing⁴ ren² 2 g
Actions and Indications: Treats all persistent coughs.

28 bo²-ye⁴ tang¹ 柏葉湯.............................100
Biota Leaf Decoction
Source: 金匱要略 (jin¹ gui⁴ yao⁴ lue⁴)
Biotae Folium et Ramulus ce⁴ bo² ye⁴ 9–15 g
Zingiberis Rhizoma gan¹ jiang¹ 3–6 g
Artemisiae Argyi Folium ai⁴ ye⁴ 3–6 g
Actions and Indications: Warms the center and staunches bleeding. Treats persistent blood ejection with withered yellow complexion. Tongue: pale. Pulse: vacuous and forceless.

29 bu² huan⁴ jin¹ zheng⁴ qi⁴ san³ 不換金正氣散
....193
Satisfaction Guaranteed Qi-Correcting Powder
Source: 和劑局方 (he² ji⁴ ju² fang¹)
Agastaches seu Pogostemi Herba huo⁴ xiang¹ 1 g
Pinelliae Tuber ban⁴ xia⁴ 6 g
Atractylodis Rhizoma cang¹ zhu² 4 g
Magnoliae Cortex hou² po⁴ 3 g
Citri Exocarpium chen² pi² 3 g
Glycyrrhizae Radix gan¹ cao³ 1.5 g
Zizyphi Fructus da⁴ zao³ 1–3 g
Zingiberis Rhizoma Recens sheng¹ jiang¹ 2–3 g
Actions and Indications: Transforms damp and resolves the exterior; harmonizes the center and stops vomiting. Treats damp-heat collecting internally with external contraction, manifesting as vomiting, abdominal distention, aversion to cold and fever.

30 bu³ fei⁴ tang¹ 補肺湯.............................112
Lung-Supplementing Decoction
Source: 千金方 (qian¹ jin¹ fang¹)
Ophiopogonis Tuber mai⁴ men² dong¹ 4 g
Schisandrae Fructus wu³ wei⁴ zi³ 3 g
Cinnamomi Ramulus gui⁴ zhi¹ 3 g
Zizyphi Fructus da⁴ zao³ 3 g
Oryzae Semen geng¹ mi³ 3 g

Mori Radicis Cortex sang¹ bai² pi² 3 g
Tussilaginis Flos kuan³ dong¹ hua¹ 2 g
Zingiberis Rhizoma Recens sheng¹ jiang¹ 2 g
Preparation method: Decoct with water.
Actions and Indications: Treats hoarse voice and cough.

31 bu³ gan¹ san³ 補肝散.............................116
Liver-Supplementing Powder
Source: 沈氏尊書方 (shen³ shi⁴ zun¹ shu¹ fang¹)
Prunellae Spica xia⁴ ku¹ cao³ 5 g
Cyperi Rhizoma xiang¹ fu⁴ zi³ 10 g
Preparation method: Grind to a fine powder.
Actions and Indications: enriches yin and supplements the blood. Treats insufficiency of liver blood.
Dosage: 3 g at a time.

32 bu³-gu³-zhi¹ wan² 補骨脂丸......181, 202, 203
Psoralea Pills
Source: 和劑局方 (he² ji⁴ ju² fang¹)
Psoraleae Semen bu³ gu³ zhi¹ (stir-fried till aroma comes out) 120 g
Cuscutae Semen tu⁴ si¹ zi³ (steamed in wine) 12 g
Juglandis Semen hu² tao² ren² (with skin removed) 30 g
Olibanum ru³ xiang¹ 10 g
Aquilariae Lignum chen² xiang¹ 10 g
Myrrha mo⁴ yao⁴ 10 g
Preparation method: Form into 300 mg pills.
Actions and Indications: Strengthens the sinews and bone; boosts the lower origin. Treats vacuity of the lower origin, with heavy arms and legs, and frequent night sweating.
Dosage: 10-15 pills a day.

33 bu³ zhong¹ yi⁴ qi⁴ tang¹ 補中益氣湯.....76, 79
Center-Supplementing Qi-Boosting Decoction
Source: 脾胃論 (pi² wei⁴ lun⁴)
Astragali Radix huang² qi² 9–15 g
Ginseng Radix ren² shen¹ 9–12 g
  (or Codonopsitis Radix dang³ shen¹)
Atractylodis Ovatae Rhizoma bai² zhu² 9–12 g
Glycyrrhizae Radix gan¹ cao³ (mix-fried) 3–6 g
Angelicae Sinensis Radix dang¹ gui¹ 6–9 g
Citri Exocarpium chen² pi² 6–9 g
Cimicifugae Rhizoma sheng¹ ma² 3–6 g
Bupleuri Radix chai² hu² 3–9 g
Actions and Indications: Boosts qi and upbears yang; regulates and supplements the stomach and spleen. Treats insufficiency of spleen, stomach and center qi with low food intake, fatigue, spontaneous sweating sometimes with fever, and a forceless large, vacuous pulse. Specific forms include: dizziness due to failure of clear yang to bear upward; displacement of the in-

ternal organs; enduring diarrhea with prolapse of the rectum; prolapse of the uterus; enuresis; unctuous strangury; uterine bleeding due to qi failing to contain the blood.

34 *cang¹-er³ san³* 蒼耳散 23, 115, 156
Xanthium Powder
Alternate name: 蒼耳子散 *cang¹-er³-zi³ san³*
Source: 濟生方 (*ji⁴ sheng¹ fang¹*)
Xanthii Fructus *cang¹ er³ zi³* 6–9 g
Angelicae Dahuricae Radix *bai² zhi³* 3–6 g
Magnoliae Flos *xin¹ yi²* 3–6 g
Menthae Herba *bo⁴ he²* 3–6 g
Actions and Indications: Courses wind and frees the portals. Treats deep-source nasal congestion due to wind-heat attacking the upper body. Signs: nasal congestion, inability to smell, turbid nasal mucus, pain and feeling of distention in the forehead.

35 *cao³-wu¹-tou² san³* 草烏頭散 70
Wild Aconite Powder
Source: 聖濟總錄 (*sheng⁴ ji⁴ zong³ lu⁴*)
Aconiti Tsao-wu-tou Tuber *cao³ wu¹ tou²*
Preparation method: Grind to a powder.
Actions and Indications: Disperses swelling and resolves toxin. Treats swelling and toxin of yong and ju.

36 *chai²-hu² gui⁴-zhi¹ gan¹-jiang¹ tang¹*
柴胡桂枝乾薑湯 2, 31, 98, 218
Bupleurum, Cinnamon Twig, and Dried Ginger Decoction
Alternate name: 柴胡桂薑湯   *chai²-hu² gui⁴ jiang¹ tang¹* Bupleurum, Cinnamon Twig and Ginger Decoction
Source: 金匱要略 (*jin¹ gui⁴ yao⁴ lue⁴*)
Bupleuri Radix *chai² hu²* 5–6 g
Cinnamomi Ramulus *gui⁴ zhi¹* 3 g
Zingiberis Rhizoma *gan¹ jiang¹* 2 g
Trichosanthis Radix *tian¹ hua¹ fen³* 3–4 g
Scutellariae Radix *huang² qin²* 3 g
Ostreae Concha *mu³ li⁴* 3 g
Glycyrrhizae Radix *gan¹ cao³* 2 g
Actions and Indications: Harmonizes and resolves the shao yang; dissipates cold and terminates malaria. Treats malarial disease with pronounced chills and mild fever, or complete absence of fever.

37 *chai²-hu² gui⁴-zhi¹ tang¹* 柴胡桂枝湯......2, 31
Bupleurum and Cinnamon Twig Decoction
Source: 傷寒論 (*shang¹ han² lun⁴*)
Bupleuri Radix *chai² hu²* 5 g
Scutellariae Radix *huang² qin²* 2 g
Pinelliae Tuber *ban⁴ xia⁴* 4 g

Zingiberis Rhizoma Recens *sheng¹ jiang¹* 2–3 g
Glycyrrhizae Radix *gan¹ cao³* 1.5–2 g
Ginseng Radix *ren² shen¹* 2 g
Cinnamomi Ramulus *gui⁴ zhi¹* 2–3 g
Paeoniae Radix *shao² yao⁴* 2–3 g
Zizyphi Fructus *da⁴ zao³* 2 g
Actions and Indications: Harmonizes and resolves the shao yang; resolves the muscles and effuses the exterior. Treats tai yang and shao yang combination disease, with fever, slight aversion to cold, pain in the joints, mild retching, and oppressive distention below the heart.

38 *chai²-hu² jia¹ long²-gu³ mu³-li⁴ tang¹*
柴胡加龍骨牡蠣湯 31, 218, 225
Bupleurum Decoction Plus Dragon Bone and Oyster Shell
Source: 傷寒論 (*shang¹ han² lun⁴*)
Bupleuri Radix *chai² hu²* 4–5 g
Scutellariae Radix *huang² qin²* 2.5 g
Pinelliae Tuber *ban⁴ xia⁴* 4 g
Ginseng Radix *ren² shen¹* 2–2.5 g
Cinnamomi Ramulus *gui⁴ zhi¹* 4 g
Draconis Os (Mastodi Ossis Fossilia) *long² gu³* 2–2.5 g
Ostreae Concha *mu³ li⁴* 2–2.5 g
Rhei Rhizoma *da⁴ huang²* 1 g
Poria *fu² ling²* 2–3 g
Zingiberis Rhizoma Recens *sheng¹ jiang¹* 2–3 g
Zizyphi Fructus *da⁴ zao³* 2–2.5 g
Actions and Indications: Harmonizes the shao yang; settles fright and quiets the spirit. Treats inappropriate precipitation in cold damage giving rise to fullness in the chest, vexation and fright, delirious speech, general heaviness preventing the patient from turning, and, in some cases, inhibited urine.

39 *chen²-xiang¹ jiang⁴ qi⁴ tang¹* 沉香降氣湯.....11
Aquilaria Qi-Downbearing Decoction
Source: 和劑局方 (*he² ji⁴ ju² fang¹*)
Aquilariae Lignum *chen² xiang¹* 3 g
Cyperi Rhizoma *xiang¹ fu⁴ zi³* 6 g
Glycyrrhizae Radix *gan¹ cao³* (mix-fried) 5 g
Amomi Semen *sha¹ ren²* 4 g
Actions and Indications: Fortifies the stomach and relieves pain. Treats qi stagnation with glomus and oppression in the chest and lateral costal region, shortness of breath, and acid regurgitation.

40 *chen²-xiang¹ tian¹-ma² tang¹* 沉香天麻湯11, 86
Aquilaria and Gastrodia Decoction
Source: 證治準繩 (*zheng⁴ zhi⁴ zhun³ sheng²*)
Aquilariae Lignum *chen² xiang¹* 2 g
Gastrodiae Rhizoma *tian¹ ma²* 3 g

Alpiniae Oxyphyllae Fructus *yi⁴ zhi⁴ ren²* 2 g
Aconiti Tuber *chuan¹ wu¹ tou²*
  (blast-fried) 2 g
Ledebouriellae Radix *fang² feng¹* 3 g
Pinelliae Tuber *ban⁴ xia⁴* 3 g
Notopterygii Rhizoma *qiang¹ huo²* 2.5 g
Glycyrrhizae Radix *gan¹ cao³* (mix-fried) 1.5 g
Angelicae Sinensis Radix *dang¹ gui¹* 1.5 g
Zingiberis Rhizoma Recens *sheng¹ jiang¹* 1.5 g
Angelicae Duhuo Radix *du² huo²* 2 g
Preparation method: Decoct with water.
Actions and Indications: Treats child fright epilepsy.

41 *chi⁴-shi²-zhi¹ yu³-yu²-liang² tang¹* 赤石脂禹餘糧
  湯 228, 230
Red Halloysite and Limonite Decoction
Source: 傷寒論 (*shang¹ han² lun⁴*)
Halloysitum Rubrum *chi⁴ shi² zhi¹* 6 g
Limonitum cum Terra *yu³ yu² liang²* 6 g
Actions and Indications: Astringes the intestines and
checks diarrhea (used for enduring cases). Treats per-
sistent diarrhea efflux desertion.

42 *chuan¹-xiong¹ cha² tiao² san³* 川芎茶調散
  ....88, 91, 192
Tea-Blended Ligusticum (Cnidium) Powder
Source: 和劑局方 (*he² ji⁴ ju² fang¹*)
Ligustici Rhizoma *chuan¹ xiong¹* 120 g
Theae Folium *cha² ye⁴* 60 g
Angelicae Dahuricae Radix *bai² zhi³* 360 g
Notopterygii Rhizoma *qiang¹ huo²* 60 g
Glycyrrhizae Radix *gan¹ cao³* 60 g
 Schizonepetae Herba seu Flos *jing¹ jie⁴* 120 g
Ledebouriellae Radix *fang² feng¹* 45 g
Menthae Herba *bo⁴ he²* 240 g
Actions and Indications: Dissipates the wind
pathogen; relieves headache. Treats general,
hemilateral, or vertex headache due to external wind
or wind-cold, with aversion to cold, fever, dizziness
and clear, runny nasal mucus.

43 *da⁴ ban⁴-xia⁴ tang¹* 大牛夏湯 92
Major Pinellia Decoction
Source: 金匱要略 (*jin¹ gui⁴ yao⁴ lue⁴*)
Pinelliae Tuber *ban⁴ xia⁴* 4–7 g
Ginseng Radix *ren² shen¹* (or Codonopsitis Radix
  dang³ shen¹) 3 g
Mel *feng¹ mi⁴* 20 g
Actions and Indications: Supplements qi; downbears
counterflow and relieves retching. Treats stomach qi
vacuity with stomach reflux vomiting, fatigued
essence-spirit, and constipation.

44 *da⁴ bu³ yin¹ wan²* 大補陰丸 10, 74, 221
Major Yin Supplementation Pills

Alternate name: 大補丸 *da⁴ bu³ wan²* Major Supplementation Pills
Source: 丹溪心法 (*dan¹ xi¹ xin¹ fa³*)
Phellodendri Cortex *huang² bo²* 120 g
Anemarrhenae Rhizoma *zhi¹ mu³*   120 g
Rehmanniae Radix Conquita
  shou² di⁴ huang² 180 g
Testudinis Plastrum *gui¹ ban³* 180 g
Actions and Indications: Enriches yin and downbears
fire. Treats effulgent yin vacuity fire, upbearing fire
flush, steaming bone tidal fever, night sweats, aching
lumbus and limp legs, dizziness and tinnitus, cough
and expectoration of blood, vexation and irascibility, reduced sleep and profuse dreaming, and seminal
emission.

45 *da⁴ chai²-hu² tang¹* 大柴胡湯 31
Major Bupleurum Decoction
Source: 傷寒論 (*shang¹ han² lun⁴*)
Bupleuri Radix *chai² hu²* 6–12 g
Scutellariae Radix *huang² qin²* 6–9 g
Pinelliae Tuber *ban⁴ xia⁴* 6–9 g
Aurantii Fructus Immaturus *zhi³ shi²* 6–9 g
Rhei Rhizoma *da⁴ huang²* 6–9 g
Paeoniae Radix Alba *bai² shao² yao⁴* 6–9 g
Zingiberis Rhizoma Recens *sheng¹ jiang¹* 3–5 g
Zizyphi Fructus *da⁴ zao³* 5–7 g
Preparation method: Decoct with water.
Actions and Indications: Harmonizes the shao yang;
precipitates heat binds. Treats alternating fever and
chills, thoracic oppression and lateral costal pain, pain
and distention in the venter and abdomen, failure to
defecate or inhibited diarrhea, bitter taste in the
mouth. Tongue fur: yellow. Pulse: wiry and forceful.

46 *da⁴ cheng² qi⁴ tang¹* 大承氣湯 95, 231
Major Qi-Infusing Decoction
Source: 傷寒論 (*shang¹ han² lun⁴*)
Rhei Rhizoma *da⁴ huang²* (add near end) 6–12 g
Mirabilitum *mang² xiao¹* (infused) 9–15 g
Magnoliae Cortex *hou⁴ po⁴* 6–12 g
Aurantii Fructus Immaturus *zhi³ shi²* 6–12 g
Preparation method: Decoct with water, and take
warm.
Actions and Indications: Precipitates heat binds;
drains fire and resolves toxin. Treats yang ming bowel
repletion patterns with constipation, abdominal
fullness and distention with pain exacerbated by
pressure, vexation, agitation and delirious speech.
Tongue: prickly with burnt yellow fur. Pulse: deep,
replete and forceful. Also specifically indicated for heat
bind with circumfluence (*re⁴ jie² pang² liu²*), and
tetanic inversion.

47 *da⁴-huang² fu⁴-zi³ tang¹* 大黃附子湯 22, 95
Rhubarb and Aconite Decoction
Source: 金匱要略 (*jin¹ gui⁴ yao⁴ lue⁴*)
Rhei Rhizoma *da⁴ huang²* 6–9 g
Aconiti Tuber Laterale *fu⁴ zi³* 6–9 g
Asiasari Radix *xi⁴ xin¹* 3–6 g
Actions and Indications: Warms yang and dispels cold;
frees urine and relieves pain. Treats interior cold ac-
cumulation with abdominal pain, constipation, frigid
limbs, and fear of cold. Tongue fur: white. Pulse: deep,
tight and wiry.

48 *da⁴-huang² gan¹-cao³ tang¹* 大黃甘草湯 ..42, 95
Rhubarb and Licorice Decoction
Source: 金匱要略 (*jin¹ gui⁴ yao⁴ lue⁴*)
Rhei Rhizoma *da⁴ huang²* 4 g
Glycyrrhizae Radix *gan¹ cao³* 2 g
Actions and Indications: Treats constipation.

49 *da⁴-huang² gan¹-sui⁴ tang¹* 大黃甘遂湯 37
Rhubarb and Kansui Decoction
Source: 金匱要略 (*jin¹ gui⁴ yao⁴ lue⁴*)
Rhei Rhizoma *da⁴ huang²* 4 g
Euphorbiae Kansui Radix *gan¹ sui⁴* 2 g
Asini Corii Gelatinum *e¹ jiao¹* 2 g
Actions and Indications: Treats lower abdominal
distention and difficult urination.

50 *da⁴-huang² mu³-dan¹ tang¹* 大黃牡丹湯
....9, 95, 163, 177
Rhubarb and Moutan Decoction
Alternate name: 大黃牡丹皮湯方 (*da⁴ -huang² mu³-
dan¹- pi² tang¹ fang¹*, Rhubarb and Moutan
Decoction Formula
Source: 金匱要略 (*jin¹ gui⁴ yao⁴ lue⁴*)
Rhei Rhizoma *da⁴ huang²* 9–12 g
Moutan Radicis Cortex *mu³ dan¹ pi²* 9–12 g
Persicae Semen *tao² ren²* 9–15 g
Benincasae Semen *dong¹ gua¹ zi³* 15–30 g
Mirabilitum *mang² xiao¹* (infused) 9–12 g
Actions and Indications: Drains heat and expels stasis;
dissipates binds and disperses yong. Treats intestinal
yong, with pain on the right side of the lower abdomen
that is exacerbated by pressure, inability to stretch out
the right leg, fever and fear of cold, a wiry pulse that
is tight or rapid, and a yellow tongue fur that is either
slimy or dry.

51 *da⁴ jian⁴ zhong¹ tang¹* 大建中湯 33, 98, 157
Major Center-Fortifying Decoction
Source: 金匱要略 (*jin¹ gui⁴ yao⁴ lue⁴*)
Zanthoxyli Fructus *hua¹ jiao¹* 3–6 g
Zingiberis Rhizoma *gan¹ jiang¹* 6–9 g

Ginseng Radix *ren² shen¹* (or Codonopsitis Radix
dang³ shen¹) 6–9 g
Granorum Saccharon *yi² tang²* 30–60 g
Actions and Indications: Warms the center and supplements vacuity; downbears counterflow and relieves
pain. Treats middle burner vacuity cold with acute
pain in the venter and abdomen, aggravated at the
slightest touch, retching and inability to take food or
drink, and, in some cases, gurgling in the abdomen.
Tongue: pale with slimy fur. Pulse: wiry and slow or
deep and fine.

52 *da⁴ qin²-jiao¹ tang¹* 大秦芃湯 38
Macrophylla Decoction
Source: 素問病機 (*su⁴ wen⁴ bing⁴ ji¹*)
Gentianae Macrophyllae Radix *qin² jiao¹* 5 g
Notopterygii Rhizoma *qiang¹ huo²* 2.5 g
Angelicae Duhuo Radix *du² huo²* 2.5 g
Ledebouriellae Radix *fang² feng¹* 2.5 g
Asiasari Radix *xi⁴ xin¹* 1.5 g
Angelicae Dahuricae Radix *bai² zhi³* 2.5 g
Angelicae Sinensis Radix *dang¹ gui¹* 2.5 g
Ligustici Rhizoma *chuan¹ xiong¹* 2.5 g
Paeoniae Radix Alba *bai² shao² yao⁴* 2.5 g
Rehmanniae Radix Conquita *shou² di⁴ huang²* 2.5 g
Poria *fu² ling²* 2.5 g
Atractylodis Ovatae Rhizoma *bai² zhu²* 2.5 g
Glycyrrhizae Radix *gan¹ cao³* 2.5 g
Rehmanniae Radix Cruda *sheng¹ di⁴* 2.5 g
Gypsum *shi² gao¹* 5 g
Scutellariae Radix *huang² qin²* 2.5 g
Actions and Indications: Dispels wind and clears heat;
regulates qi and the blood. Treats initial-stage chan-
nel or connecting-vessel wind stroke with bitter taste
in the mouth, vexation and fever, inability to move
the limbs, and stiff tongue preventing speech.

53 *da⁴ qing¹ long² tang¹* 大青龍湯 2, 162, 190, 226
Major Green-Blue Dragon Decoction
New name: 麻桂石膏湯 *ma² gui⁴ shi²-gao¹ tang¹*
Ephedra, Cinnamon Twig and Gypsum Decoction
Source: 傷寒論 (*shang¹ han¹ lun⁴*)
Ephedrae Herba *ma² huang²* 6 g
Armeniacae Semen *xing⁴ ren²* 5 g
Cinnamomi Ramulus *gui⁴ zhi¹* 3 g
Glycyrrhizae Radix *gan¹ cao³* (mix-fried) 2 g
Gypsum *shi² gao¹* 10 g
Zingiberis Rhizoma Recens *sheng¹ jiang¹* 3 g
Zizyphi Fructus *da⁴ zao³* 3 g
Actions and Indications: Induces sweating and resolves
the exterior; clears heat and eliminates vexation.
Treats Ephedra Decoction patterns with interior heat
causing vexation and agitation, as well as wind water
swelling.

54 *da⁴ xian⁴ xiong¹ tang¹* 大陷胸湯 .. *37, 95, 231*
Major Chest Bind Decoction
Source: 傷寒論 (*shang¹ han² lun⁴*)
Rhei Rhizoma *da⁴ huang²* 9 g
Mirabilitum *mang² xiao¹* 15 g
Euphorbiae Kansui Radix *gan¹ sui⁴* 1.5 g
Actions and Indications: Drains heat and expels water. Treats hard fullness below the heart with pain exacerbated by the slightest pressure, constipation, shortness of breath, vexation and agitation, postmeridian tidal fever, dry mouth and tongue. Pulse: deep, tight and forceful.

55 *da⁴ zao⁴ wan²* 大造丸 *4, 21, 27*
Greatly Supplementing Pills
Alternate name: 河車大造丸 *he²-che¹ da⁴ zao⁴ wan²*
Greatly Supplementing Placenta Pills
Source: 醫方集解 (*yi¹ fang¹ ji² jie³*)
Hominis Placenta *zi³ he² che¹* 10 g
Rehmanniae Radix *di⁴ huang²* 4 g
Testudinis Plastrum *gui¹ ban³* 6 g
Phellodendri Cortex *huang² bo²* 3 g
Eucommiae Cortex *du⁴ zhong⁴* 3 g
Ginseng Radix *ren² shen¹* 2 g
Asparagi Tuber *tian¹ men² dong¹* 3 g
Ophiopogonis Tuber *mai⁴ dong¹* 3 g
Achyranthis Bidentatae Radix *niu² xi¹* 3 g
Amomi Semen *sha¹ ren²* (optional) 3 g
Poria *fu² ling²* (optional) 3 g
Actions and Indications: Enriches yin and downbears fire; boosts essence-blood; supplements the lung and kidney. Treats vacuity taxation and depletion with cough, tidal fever, dry mouth and throat, emaciation, and seminal emission, taxation damage with cough and tidal fever.

56 *dan¹-shen¹ yin³* 丹參飲 *18, 60*
Salvia Beverage
Source: 時方歌括 (*shi² fang¹ ge¹ kuo⁴*)
Salviae Radix *dan¹ shen¹* 9–15 g
Santali Albi Lignum *tan² xiang¹* 3–6 g
Amomi Semen *sha¹ ren²* 3–6 g
Actions and Indications: Quickens the blood and transforms stasis; rectifies qi and relieves pain. Treats blood stasis and qi stagnation with pain in the abdomen and region of the heart. Modern clinical analysis shows that it is effective for coronary disease causing thoracic oppression and shortness of breath.

57 *dang¹-gui¹ jian⁴ zhong¹ tang¹* 當歸建中湯 ... *25*
Tangkuei Center-Fortifying Decoction
Source: 千金翼方 (*qian¹ jin¹ yi⁴ fang¹*)
Variant of 小建中湯 *xiao³ jian⁴ zhong¹ tang¹* Minor

Center-Fortifying Decoction
Cinnamomi Ramulus *gui⁴ zhi¹* 4 g
Paeoniae Radix Alba *bai² shao² yao⁴* 5-6 g
Glycyrrhizae Radix *gan¹ cao³* 2 g
Zingiberis Rhizoma Recens *sheng¹ jiang¹* 4 g
Zizyphi Fructus *da⁴ zao³* 4 g
Angelicae Sinensis Radix *dang¹ gui¹* 4 g
Granorum Saccharon *yi² tang²* 20 g
Actions and Indications: Warms the center and supplements vacuity; nourishes and harmonizes the blood. Treats: 1) Postpartum construction-blood vacuity with gripping pain in the lower abdomen relieved by warmth and pressure. 2) Middle burner vacuity cold with insufficiency of construction-blood.

58 *dang¹-gui¹ long² hui⁴ wan²* 當歸龍薈丸
.... *25, 39, 195*
Tangkuei, Gentian, and Aloe Pills
Source: 錢氏方 (*qian² shi⁴ fang¹*)
Gentianae Scabrae Radix *long² dan³* 10 g
Angelicae Sinensis Radix *dang¹ gui¹* 10 g
Gardeniae Fructus *zhi¹ zi³* 10 g
Coptidis Rhizoma *huang² lian²* 10 g
Scutellariae Radix *huang² qin²* 10 g
Phellodendri Cortex *huang² bo²* 10 g
Rhei Rhizoma *da⁴ huang²* 5 g
Aloe *lu² hui⁴* 1.5 g
Indigo Pulverata Levis *qing¹ dai⁴* (water-ground) 5 g
Saussureae Radix *mu⁴ xiang¹* 2.5 g
Moschus *she⁴ xiang¹* 0.5 g
Preparation method: Grind to a fine powder, blend with honey, and form into 100 mg pills.
Actions and Indications: Drains liver fire and frees the stool. Treats liver-gallbladder repletion fire manifesting in dizziness, fright palpitations, clonic spasm, mania, constipation, dark-colored urine, and high blood pressure.
Dosage: 20 pills 1–2 times a day.

59 *dang¹-gui¹ san³* 當歸散 *25, 76*
Tangkuei Powder
Source: 金匱要略 (*jing¹ gui⁴ yao⁴ lue⁴*)
Angelicae Sinensis Radix *dang¹ gui¹* 3 g
Paeoniae Radix *shao² yao⁴* 3 g
Ligustici Rhizoma *chuan¹ xiong¹* 3 g
Atractylodis Ovatae Rhizoma *bai² zhu²* 1.5 g
Scutellariae Radix *huang² qin²* 3 g
Actions and Indications: Nourishes the blood and quiets the fetus. Treats blood vacuity with heat stirring the fetus.

60 *dang¹-gui¹ shao²-yao⁴ san³* 當歸芍藥散 .. *25, 51*
Tangkuei and Peony Powder

Source: 金匱要略 (*jin¹ gui⁴ yao⁴ lue⁴*)
Angelicae Sinensis Radix *dang¹ gui¹* 3 g
Paeoniae Radix *shao² yao⁴* 4–6 g
Poria *fu² ling²* 4 g
Atractylodis Ovatae Rhizoma *bai² zhu²* 4 g
Alismatis Rhizoma *ze² xie⁴* 4–5 g
Ligustici Rhizoma *chuan¹ xiong¹* 3 g
Actions and Indications: Nourishes the blood and quiets the fetus; fortifies the stomach and spleen, and disinhibits urine. Treats mild abdominal pain in pregnancy, especially where there are gastrointestinal signs.

61 *dang¹-gui¹ si⁴ ni⁴ jia¹ wu²-zhu¹-yu² sheng¹-jiang¹ tang¹* 當歸四逆加吳茱萸生薑湯 25, 98, 132
Tangkuei Counterflow Frigidity Decoction Plus Evodia and Fresh Ginger
Source: 傷寒論 (*shang¹ han² lun⁴*)
Angelicae Sinensis Radix *dang¹ gui¹* 3 g
Cinnamomi Ramulus *gui⁴ zhi¹* 3 g
Paeoniae Radix *shao² yao⁴* 3 g
Glycyrrhizae Radix *gan¹ cao³* 2 g
Asiasari Radix *xi⁴ xin¹* 3 g
Mutong Caulis *mu⁴-tong¹* 3g
Zizyphi Fructus *da⁴ zao³* 5 g
Evodiae Fructus *wu² zhu¹ yu²* 2 g
Zingiberis Rhizoma Recens *sheng¹ jiang¹* 4 g
Actions and Indications: Warms the channels and dissipates cold. Treats inversion frigidity in the extremities, faint pulse verging on expiry in patients suffering from enduring cold.

62 *dang¹-gui¹ si⁴ ni⁴ tang¹* 當歸四逆湯 16, 25, 26
Tangkuei Counterflow Frigidity Decoction
Source: 傷寒論 (*shang¹ han² lun⁴*)
Angelicae Sinensis Radix *dang¹ gui¹* 6–9 g
Cinnamomi Ramulus *gui⁴ zhi¹* 3–9 g
Paeoniae Radix *shao² yao⁴* 6–9 g
Asiasari Radix *xi⁴ xin¹* 3–6 g
Glycyrrhizae Radix *gan¹ cao³* (mix-fried) 3–6 g
Mutong Caulis *mu⁴-tung¹* 3–6 g
Zizyphi Fructus *da⁴ zao³* 5–12 pieces.
Actions and Indications: Warms the channels and dissipates cold; nourishes the blood and frees the vessels. Treats: 1) Contraction of cold in blood vacuity patients, characterized by counterflow frigidity in the limbs, and a fine pulse verging on expiry. 2) Wind-damp bi patterns. 3) Delayed menses and cold-type menstrual pain.

63 *dang¹-gui¹ yin³ zi³* 當歸飲子 25, 57, 153
Tangkuei Drink
Source: 證治準繩 (*zheng⁴ zhi⁴ zhun³ sheng²*)
Angelicae Sinensis Radix *dang¹ gui¹* 5 g

Paeoniae Radix *shao² yao⁴* 3 g
Ligustici Rhizoma *chuan¹ xiong¹* 3 g
Rehmanniae Radix Cruda *sheng¹ di⁴* 4 g
Tribuli Fructus *ci⁴ ji² li²* 3 g
Schizonepetae Herba seu Flos *jing¹ jie⁴* 1.5 g
Ledebouriellae Radix *fang² feng¹* 3 g
Polygoni Multiflori Radix *he² shou³ wu¹* 2 g
Astragali Radix *huang² qi²* 1.5 g
Glycyrrhizae Radix *gan¹ cao³* 1 g
Actions and Indications: Quickens the blood and transforms stasis; expels wind and clears heat. Treats chronic itchy eczema in yin vacuity patients with scant secretions.

64 *dao³ chi⁴ san³* 導赤散 16, 102
Red-Abducting Powder
Source: 小兒藥證直訣 (*xiao³ er² yao⁴ zheng⁴ zhi⁴ jue²*)
Rehmanniae Radix Cruda *sheng¹ di⁴ zhi¹* 15 g
Mutong Caulis *mu⁴ tong¹* 3 g
Lophatheri Folium *dan⁴ zhu² ye⁴* 3 g
Glycyrrhizae Radix Tenuis *gan¹ cao³ shao¹* 3 g
Actions and Indications: Clears heart fire; disinhibits urine. Treats acute cystitis or urethritis with inhibited urination.

65 *dao³ qi⁴ tang¹* 導氣湯 133, 143
Qi-Abducting Decoction
Source: 沈氏尊書方 (*shen³ shi⁴ zun¹ shu¹ fang¹*)
Meliae Toosendan Fructus *chuan¹ lian⁴ zi³* 9–12 g
Saussureae Radix *mu⁴ xiang¹* 6–9 g
Foeniculi Fructus *hui² xiang¹* 6–9 g
Evodiae Fructus *wu² zhu¹ yu²* 5–6 g
Preparation method: Decoct with water.
Actions and Indications: Moves qi, dissipates cold, and relieves pain. Treats small intestinal hernia with lower abdominal pain.

66 *dao³ shui³ fu²-ling² tang¹* 導水茯苓湯 . 17, 123
Water-Abducting Poria Decoction
Source: 奇效良方 (*qi² xiao⁴ liang² fang¹*)
Poria *fu² ling²* 3 g
Alismatis Rhizoma *ze² xie⁴* 3 g
Atractylodis Ovatae Rhizoma *bai² zhu²* 3 g
Ophiopogonis Tuber *mai⁴ men² dong¹* 5 g
Mori Radicis Cortex *sang¹ bai² pi²* 1 g
Perillae Caulis et Calyx *zi³ su¹* 1 g
Arecae Pericarpium *da⁴ fu⁴ pi²* 1 g
Amomi Semen *sha¹ ren²* 1 g
Saussureae Radix *mu⁴ xiang¹* 1 g
Junci Medulla *deng¹ xin¹ cao³* 1 g
Arecae Semen *bin¹ lang²* 2 g
Chaenomelis Fructus *mu⁴ gua¹* 2 g
Citri Exocarpium *chen² pi²* 1.5 g
Actions and Indications: Treats water swelling,

dyspnea and fullness, and extremely small, painful urinary voidings.

67 *di³ dang¹ tang¹* 抵當湯 220
Dead-On Decoction
Source: 傷寒論 (*shang¹ han² lun⁴*)
Hirudo seu Whitmania *shui³ zhi⁴*   1–3 g
Tabanus *meng² chong²* 0.3–1 g
Rhei Rhizoma *da⁴ huang²* (washed in wine) 6–12 g
Persicae Semen *tao² ren²* 6–9 g
Preparation method: Decoct with water.
Actions and Indications: Breaks blood and expels stasis. Treats blood amassment in the lower burner and stasis heat in the interior, with mania and uninhibited urination; or inhibited menstruation with painful fullness or hardness in the lateral lower abdomen.

68 *di⁴-huang² yin³ zi³* 地黃飲子.................27, 59
Rehmannia Drink
Source: 易簡方 (*yi⁴ jian³ fang¹*)
Rehmanniae Radix Cruda *sheng¹ di⁴ huang²* 9–12 g
Rehmanniae Radix Conquita *shou² di⁴ huang²* 9–12 g
Asparagi Tuber *tian¹ men² dong¹* 6–12 g
Ophiopogonis Tuber *mai⁴ men² dong¹*   6–12 g
Dendrobii Caulis *shi² hu²* 9–15 g
Ginseng Radix *ren² shen¹* 9–12 g
Astragali Radix *huang² qi²* (mix-fried) 6–9 g
Glycyrrhizae Radix *gan¹ cao³* 3–6 g
Eriobotryae Folium *pi² pa² ye⁴* 6–9 g
Alismatis Rhizoma *ze² xie⁴* 6–9 g
Aurantii Fructus *zhi³ ke²* 6–9 g
Actions and Indications: Enriches yin and boosts qi; engenders liquid and allays thirst. Treats wasting thirst characterized by thirst with desire for fluid, emaciation, and lack of strength.

69 *di⁴-yu² wan²* 地榆丸.................................62
Sanguisorba Pills
Source: 證治準繩 (*zheng⁴ zhi⁴ zhun³ sheng²*)
Sanguisorbae Radix *di⁴ yu²* (stir-fried) 5 g
Angelicae Sinensis Radix *dang¹ gui¹* (stir-fried)   5 g
Asini Corii Gelatinum *e¹ jiao¹* (stir-fried with glutinous rice) 5 g
Coptidis Rhizoma *huang² lian²* 5 g
Chebulae Fructus *he¹ zi³* (stir-fried) 5 g
Saussureae Radix *mu⁴ xiang¹* 5 g
Mume Fructus *wu¹ mei²* 5 g
Preparation method: Grind to a find powder, blend with honey, and form into 300 mg. pills.
Actions and Indications: Treats diarrhea and blood dysentery.
Dosage: 10 pills on an empty stomach.

70 *ding¹-xiang¹ shi⁴-di⁴ tang¹* 丁香柿蒂湯
....107, 138, 203
Clove and Persimmon Decoction
Source: 萬病回春 (*wan⁴ bing⁴ hui² chun¹*)
Caryophylli Flos *ding¹ xiang¹* 1 g
Alpiniae Officinarum Rhizoma *gao¹ liang² jiang¹* 1 g
Saussureae Radix *mu⁴ xiang¹* 1 g
Aquilariae Lignum *chen² xiang¹* 1 g
Foeniculi Fructus *hui² xiang¹* 1 g
Agastaches seu Pogostemi Herba *huo⁴ xiang¹* 1 g
Magnoliae Cortex *hou⁴ po⁴* 1 g
Amomi Semen *sha¹ ren²* 1 g
Glycyrrhizae Radix *gan¹ cao³* 1 g
Olibanum *ru³ xiang¹* 1 g
Kaki Calyx *shi⁴ di⁴* 3 g
Cinnamomi Ramulus *gui⁴ zhi¹* 3 g
Pinelliae Tuber *ban⁴ xia⁴* 3 g
Citri Exocarpium *chen² pi²* 3 g
Actions and Indications: Treats cold-type hiccough.

71 *ding⁴ chuan³ tang¹* 定喘湯.........112, 146, 171
Dyspnea- Stabilizing Decoction
Source: 攝生眾妙方 (*she⁴ shen¹ zhong⁴ miao⁴ fang¹*)
Ginkgo Semen *bai² guo³* (with shell removed) 5-7 pieces
Ephedrae Herba *ma² huang²* 6–9 g
Armeniacae Semen *xing⁴ ren²* 6–9 g
Glycyrrhizae Radix *gan¹ cao³* 3–4.5 g
Perillae Fructus *zi³ su¹ zi³* 6–9 g
Mori Radicis Cortex *sang¹ bai² pi²* 6–9 g
Scutellariae Radix *huang² qin²* 6–9 g
Pinelliae Tuber *ban⁴ xia⁴* 6–9 g
Tussilaginis Flos *kuan³ dong¹ hua¹* 6–9 g
Preparation method: Decoct with water.
Actions and Indications: Diffuses the lung and calms dyspnea; clears heat and transforms phlegm. Treats phlegm-heat wheezing and dyspnea, cough, with rapid breathing, copious yellow phlegm.

72 *ding⁴ zhi⁴ wan²* 定志丸 56, 71
Orientation-Stabilizing Pills
Alternate name: 定志小丸 *ding⁴ zhi⁴ xiao³ wan²*
Small Orientation-Stabilizing Pills
Source: 千金方 (*qian¹ jin¹ fang¹*)
Ginseng Radix *ren² shen¹*
(or Codonopsitis Radix *dang³ shen¹*) 30 g
Poria *fu² ling²* 30 g
Acori Graminei Rhizoma *shi² chang¹ pu² ye⁴* (stir-fried) 20 g
Polygalae Radix *yuan³ zhi⁴* 20 g
Actions and Indications: Boosts qi and nourishes the heart; opens the portals and quiets the spirit. Treats fright palpitations and poor memory.

73 *du²-huo² ji⁴-sheng¹ tang¹* 獨活寄生湯 4, 24, 52
Duhuo and Mistletoe Decoction
Source: 千金方 (*qian¹ jin¹ fang¹*)
Angelicae Duhuo Radix *du² huo²* 6–9 g
Ledebouriellae Radix *fang² feng¹* 6–9 g
Gentianae Macrophyllae Radix *qin² jiao¹* 6–9 g
Angelicae Sinensis Radix *dang¹ gui¹* 6–9 g
Paeoniae Radix Rubra *chi⁴ shao² yao⁴* 6–9 g
Ligustici Rhizoma *chuan¹ xiong¹* 6–9 g
Ginseng Radix *ren² shen¹* 6–9 g
Poria *fu² ling²* 6–9 g
Eucommiae Cortex *du⁴ zhong⁴* 6–9 g
Achyranthis Bidentatae Radix *niu² xi¹* 6–9 g
Asiasari Radix *xi⁴ xin¹* 3–6 g
Rehmanniae Radix *di⁴ huang²* 12–20 g
Glycyrrhizae Radix *gan¹ cao³* (mix-fried) 3–9 g
Loranthi seu Visci Ramus *sang¹ ji⁴ sheng¹*
     15–30 g
Cinnamomi Cortex Rasus *gui⁴ xin¹* 3–5 g
Preparation method: Decoct with water.
Actions and Indications: Dispels wind-damp; supplements qi and blood; boosts the liver and kidney. Treats wind-cold-damp bi, depletion of both liver and kidney, weak, aching lumbus and knees, and pain in the joints.

74 *du⁴-zhong⁴ san³* 杜仲散 4
Eucommia Powder
Source: 聖惠方 (*sheng⁴ hui⁴ fang¹*)
Eucommiae Cortex *du⁴ zhong⁴* 6 g
Salviae Radix *dan¹ shen¹* 6 g
Ligustici Rhizoma *chuan¹ xiong¹* 4.5 g
Cinnamomi Cassiae Guixin *gui⁴ xin¹* 3 g
Asiasari Radix *xi⁴ xin¹* 1 g
Actions and Indications: Treats sudden excruciating lumbar pain.

75 *e¹-jiao¹ san³* 阿膠散 208
Ass Hide Glue Powder
Alternate name: 補肺阿膠湯 *bu³ fei⁴ e¹-jiao¹ tang¹*
Lung-Supplementing Ass Hide Glue Decoction
Source: 小兒藥證直訣 (*xiao³ er² yao⁴ zheng⁴ zhi² jue²*)
Asini Corii Gelatinum *e¹ jiao¹* (dissolved) 9–12 g
Aristolochiae Fructus *ma³ dou¹ ling²* 6–9 g
Arctii Fructus *niu² bang⁴ zi³* 6–9 g
Armeniacae Semen *xing⁴ ren²* 6–9 g
Oryzae Semen *nuo⁴ mi³* 10 g
Glycyrrhizae Radix *gan¹ cao³* (mix-fried) 15–30 g
Actions and Indications: Nourishes yin and supplements the lung; suppresses cough and staunches bleeding. Treats bronchial asthma in children forming lung vacuity patterns.

76 *e¹-jiao¹ shao²-yao⁴ tang¹* 阿膠芍藥湯 52, 208
Ass Hide Glue and Peony Decoction
Source: 聖濟總錄 (*sheng⁴ ji⁴ zong³ lu⁴*)
Asini Corii Gelatinum *e¹ jiao¹* (mix-fried) 10 g
Paeoniae Radix Rubra *chi⁴ shao² yao⁴* 10 g
Angelicae Sinensis Radix *dang¹ gui¹* 10 g
Glycyrrhizae Radix *gan¹ cao³* (mix-fried) 5 g
Actions and Indications: Treats blood in the stool.

77 *e¹-wei⁴ hua⁴ pi³ gao¹* 阿魏化痞膏 97, 182, 196
Asafoetida Glomus-Transforming Paste
Source: 經驗方 (empirical formula)
Asafoetida *e¹ wei⁴* 60 g
Sparganii Rhizoma *san¹ leng²* 60g
Zedoariae Rhizoma *e² zhu²* 60 g
Manitis Squama *chuan¹ shan¹ jia³* 60 g
Rhei Rhizoma *da⁴ huang²* 60 g
Cyperi Rhizoma *xiang¹ fu⁴ zi³* 60 g
Angelicae Sinensis Radix *dang¹ gui¹* 60 g
Aconiti Tuber *chuan¹ wu¹ tou²* 60 g
Allii Sativi Bulbus *da⁴ suan⁴* 60 g
Angelicae Dahuricae Radix *bai² zhi³* 60 g
Quisqualis Fructus *shi³ jun¹ zi³* 60 g
Ricini Semen *bi⁴ ma² zi³* 60 g
Magnoliae Cortex *hou⁴ po⁴* 60 g
Momordicae Semen *mu⁴ bie¹ zi³* 60 g
Tsao-wu-tou Tuber *cao³ wu¹ tou²* 60 g
Catharsius *qiang¹ lang²* 60 g
Picrorhizae Rhizoma *hu² huang² lian²* 60 g
Cinnamomi Cortex *rou⁴ gui⁴* 60 g
Realgar *xiong² huang²* 45 g
Camphora *zhang¹ nao³* 45 g
Olibanum *ru³ xiang¹* 10 g
Myrrha *mo⁴ yao⁴* 10 g
Draconis Sanguis *xue⁴ jie²* 10 g
Aloe *lu² hui⁴* 10 g
Actions and Indications: Disperses accumulations and transforms glomus. Treats accumulations and gatherings with distention in the chest and lateral costal region, and women's concretions and conglomerations.

78 *e¹-wei⁴ hua⁴ pi³ san³* 阿魏化痞散 196
Asafoetida Glomus-Transforming Powder
Source: 張氏醫通 (*zhang¹ shi⁴ yi¹ tong⁴*)
Ligustici Rhizoma *chuan¹ xiong¹* 1 g
Angelicae Sinensis Radix *dang¹ gui¹* 1 g
Atractylodis Ovatae Rhizoma *bai² zhu²* 1 g
Poria *fu² ling²* 1 g
Carthami Flos *hong² hua¹* 1 g
Asafoetida *e¹ wei⁴* 1 g
Fagopyri Farina *qiao² mai⁴ mian⁴* 10 g
Rhei Rhizoma *da⁴ huang²* (stir-fried in wine) 8 g
Amydae Carapax *bie¹ jia³* 3 g

Preparation method: Grind to a powder.

Actions and Indications: Treats malarial disease with fever and chills, and accumulations and gatherings with abdominal pain.

Dosage: 4 g 3 times a day.

79   e¹-wei⁴ wan² 阿魏丸 196
Asafoetida Pills
Source: 衛生寶鑑 (wei⁴ sheng¹ bao³ jian⁴)
Asafoetida e¹ wei⁴ (steeped in wine)   2.5 g
Crataegi Fructus shan¹ zha¹   10 g
Arisaematis Rhizoma tian¹ nan² xing¹ (steeped in Gleditsia water)   10 g
Coptidis Rhizoma huang² lian²   10 g
Pinelliae Tuber ban⁴ xia⁴ (steeped in Gleditsiae Sinensis Spina water)   10 g
Hordei Fructus Germinatus mai² ya²   10 g
Massa Medicata Fermentata shen² qu¹   10 g
Raphani Semen lai² fu² zi¹ (steamed)   10 g
Forsythiae Fructus lian² qiao²   5 g
Fritillariae Bulbus bei⁴ mu³ lan²   5 g
Trichosanthis Fructus gua¹ lou²   5 g
Mirabilitum Purum xuan² ming² fen³   2.5 g
Picrorhizae Rhizoma hu² huang² lian²   2.5 g
Sinapis Semen bai² jie⁴ zi³   2.5 g
Preparation method: form into 250 mg pills.
Actions and Indications: Treats concretions, conglomerations, accumulations and gatherings.
Dosage: 8 pills 3 times a day.

80   er⁴ chen² tang¹ 二陳湯 92, 128
Double Vintage Decoction
Source: 和劑局方 (he² ji⁴ ju² fang¹)
Pinelliae Tuber ban⁴ xia⁴   5 g
Citri Exocarpium chen² pi²   4 g
Poria fu² ling²   5 g
Glycyrrhizae Radix gan¹ cao³   1 g
Zingiberis Rhizoma Recens sheng¹ jiang¹   3 g

The last two ingredients are now commonly omitted.
Actions and Indications: Dries damp and transforms phlegm; rectifies qi and harmonizes the center. Treats damp phlegm manifesting as cough with copious phlegm, distention and fullness in the chest and diaphragm, nausea and vomiting. Tongue fur: white, slimy, and glossy.

81   er⁴ shen² wan² 二神丸 118, 147
Two Spirits Pills
Source: 陳氏方 (chen³ shi⁴ fang¹)
Typhae Pollen pu² huang² (soaked)
Piperis Longi Fructus bi⁴ ba²
In equal proportions.
Preparation method: Grind to a fine powder, cook

with honey, and form into 300 mg pills.
Actions and Indications: Treats qi pain, hemorrhage, and menstrual irregularities in women.
Dosage: 10 pills 2 times a day.

82   er⁴ xian¹ tang¹ 二仙湯 49, 191
Two Immortals Decoction
Source: 中醫方劑臨床手冊 (zhong¹ yi¹ fang¹ ji⁴ lin² chuang² shou³ ce⁴)
Curculiginis Rhizoma xian¹ mao²   6–15 g
Epimedii Herba yin² yang² huo⁴   9–15 g
Angelicae Sinensis Radix dang¹ gui¹   9 g
Morindae Radix ba¹ ji³ tian¹   9 g
Phellodendri Cortex huang² bo²   6–9 g
Anemarrhenae Rhizoma zhi¹ mu³   6–9 g
Actions and Indications: Supplements the kidney and drains fire; regulates the penetrating and conception vessels. Treats menopausal syndrome, dizziness, hypertension, and other diseases affecting the penetrating and conception vessels.

83   fang²-feng¹ tong¹ sheng⁴ san³ 防風通聖散
....45, 134
Ledebouriella Sage-Inspired Powder
Source: 宣明論 (xuan¹ ming² lun⁴)
Ledebouriellae Radix fang² feng   1.2 g
Schizonepetae Herba seu Flos jing¹ jie⁴   1.2 g
Ephedrae Herba ma² huang²   1.2 g
Forsythiae Fructus lian² qiao²   1.2 g
Menthae Herba bo⁴ he²   1.2 g
Ligustici Rhizoma chuan¹ xiong¹   1.2 g
Angelicae Sinensis Radix dang¹ gui¹   1.2 g
Paeoniae Radix Alba bai² shao² yao⁴   1.2 g
Atractylodis Ovatae Rhizoma bai² zhu²   2 g
Gardeniae Fructus shan¹ zhi¹ zi³   1.2 g
Rhei Rhizoma da⁴ huang²   1.5 g
Mirabilitum mang² xiao¹   1.5 g
Gypsum shi² gao¹   2–3 g
Scutellariae Radix huang² qin²   2 g
Platycodonis Radix jie² geng³   2 g
Glycyrrhizae Radix gan¹ cao³   2 g
Talcum hua² shi²   3–5 g
Zingiberis Rhizoma Recens sheng¹ jiang¹   1.2 g
Actions and Indications: Resolves the exterior and frees the interior; courses wind and clears heat. Treats exuberant wind-heat forming a pattern of interior and exterior repletion. Signs: generalized fever, aversion to cold, headache, dry throat, constipation and dark-colored urine, itchy skin and eczema.
Dosage: 3 g 2–3 times a day.

84   fang²-ji³ fu²-ling² tang¹ 防己茯苓湯.....44, 236
Fangji and Poria Decoction
Source: 金匱要略 (jin¹ gui⁴ yao⁴ lue⁴)

Fangji Radix *fang² ji³* 3 g
Astragali Radix *huang² qi²* 3 g
Glycyrrhizae Radix *gan¹ cao³* 2 g
Poria *fu² ling²* 6 g
Cinnamomi Ramulus *gui⁴ zhi¹* 3 g
Actions and Indications: Boosts qi, frees yang, and disinhibits water. Treats skin water patterns with generalized swelling, and swollen distended limbs.

85 *fang²-ji³ huang²-qi² tang¹* 防己黃耆湯 .. 30, 44
Fangji and Astragalus Decoction
Source: 金匱要略(*jin¹ gui⁴ yao⁴ lue⁴*)
Fangji Radix *fang² ji³* 6–12 g
Astragali Radix *huang² qi²* 9–30 g
Atractylodis Ovatae Rhizoma *bai² zhu²* 6–9 g
Glycyrrhizae Radix *gan¹ cao³* 3–6 g
Zingiberis Rhizoma Recens *sheng¹ jiang¹* 2–3 g
Zizyphi Fructus *da⁴ zao³* 3 pieces
Preparation method: Decoct with water.
Actions and Indications: Boosts qi and fortifies the spleen; disinhibits water and disperses swelling. Treats generalized wind swelling with sweating, aversion to wind, inhibited urination, and wind-damp bi with heaviness and numbness of the limbs.

86 *fei² er² wan²* 肥兒丸 161
Chubby Child Pills
Source: 和劑局方(*he² ji⁴ ju² fang¹*)
Quisqualis Fructus *shi³ jun¹ zi³* 150 g
Myristicae Semen *rou⁴ dou⁴ kou⁴* 150 g
Hordei Fructus Germinatus *mai⁴ ya²* 150 g
Massa Medicata Fermentata *shen² qu¹* 300 g
Coptidis Rhizoma *huang² lian²* 300 g
Arecae Semen *bin¹ lang²* 20 g
Saussureae Radix *mu⁴ xiang¹* 60 g
Suis Bilis *zhu¹ dan³ zhi¹*
Actions and Indications: Kills worms and disperses accumulations. Treats worm accumulations with indigestion and diarrhea.

87 *fen¹ xiao¹ tang¹* 分消湯 123, 238
Separating and Dispersing Decoction
Source: 萬病回春(*wan⁴ bing⁴ hui² chun¹*)
Atractylodis Rhizoma *cang¹ zhu²* 2.5 g
Atractylodis Ovatae Rhizoma *bai² zhu²* 2.5 g
Poria *fu² ling²* 2.5 g
Citri Exocarpium *chen² pi²* 2 g
Magnoliae Cortex *hou⁴ po⁴* 2 g
Cyperi Rhizoma *xiang¹ fu⁴ zi³* 2 g
Polyporus *zhu¹ ling²* 2 g
Alismatis Rhizoma *ze² xie⁴* 2 g
Aurantii Fructus Immaturus *zhi³ shi²* 1 g
Arecae Pericarpium *da⁴ fu⁴ pi²* 1 g
Amomi Semen *sha¹ ren²* 1 g

Saussureae Radix *mu⁴ xiang¹* 1 g
Junci Medulla *deng¹ xin¹ cao³* 1 g
Astragali Radix Cruda *sheng¹ huang² qi²* 1 g
Actions and Indications: Treats exudative peritonitis, nephritis, and drum distention, and cirrhosis of the liver.

88 *fu²-ling² si⁴ ni⁴ tang¹* 茯苓四逆湯 236
Poria Counterflow Frigidity Decoction
Source: 傷寒論(*shang¹ han² lun⁴*)
Aconiti Tuber Laterale *fu⁴ zi³* 1 g
Zingiberis Rhizoma *gan¹ jiang¹* 2 g
Glycyrrhizae Radix *gan¹ cao³* (mix-fried) 2 g
Ginseng Radix *ren² shen¹* 2 g
Poria *fu² ling²* 4 g
Actions and Indications: Returns yang and stems counterflow; quiets the heart and eliminates vexation. Treats shao yang disease with vexation and agitation.

89 *fu²-ling² yin³* 茯苓飲 235, 236
Poria Beverage
Source: 金匱要略(*jin¹ gui⁴ yao⁴ lue⁴*)
Poria *fu² ling²* 4 g
Ginseng Radix *ren² shen¹* 3 g
Atractylodis Ovatae Rhizoma *bai² zhu²* 4 g
Aurantii Fructus Immaturus *zhi³ shi²* 1–2 g
Citri Exocarpium *chen² pi²* 3 g
Zingiberis Rhizoma Recens *sheng¹ jiang¹* 3 g
Actions and Indications: Treats water collecting in the area of the stomach, giving rise to fullness, vomiting, palpitations, and loss of appetite.

90 *fu²-ling² ze²-xie⁴ tang¹* 茯苓澤瀉湯 72, 236
Poria and Alisma Decoction
Source: 金匱要略(*jin¹ gui⁴ yao⁴ lue⁴*)
Poria *fu² ling²* 4 g
Alismatis Rhizoma *ze² xie⁴* 4 g
Cinnamomi Ramulus *gui⁴ zhi¹* 2 g
Atractylodis Ovatae Rhizoma *bai² zhu²* 3 g
Zingiberis Rhizoma Recens *sheng¹ jiang¹* 3–5 g
Glycyrrhizae Radix *gan¹ cao³* 1.5 g
Actions and Indications: Disinhibits urine.

91 *fu² tu⁴ dan¹* 茯菟丸 167, 236
Poria and Cuscuta Pills
Source: 和劑局方(*he² ji⁴ ju² fang¹*)
Cuscutae Semen *tu⁴ si¹ zi³* 10 g
Poria *fu² ling²* 3 g
Nelumbinis Semen *shi² lian² zi³* 3 g
Schisandrae Fructus *wu³ wei⁴ zi³* 8 g
Dioscoreae Rhizoma *shan¹ yao⁴* 6 g
Actions and Indications: Boosts the kidney and astringes essence; fortifies the spleen and percolates damp.

Treats kidney vacuity with seminal emission, white turbid urine, and wasting thirst.
Dosage: 3–6 g twice a day.

92 *gan¹-cao³ fu⁴-zi³ tang¹* 甘草附子湯 22, 42
Licorice and Aconite Decoction
Source: 金匱要略 (*jin¹ gui⁴ yao⁴ lue⁴*)
Glycyrrhizae Radix *gan¹ cao³* 2 g
Aconiti Tuber Laterale *fu⁴ zi³* 1 g
Atractylodis Ovatae Rhizoma *bai² zhu²* 4 g
Cinnamomi Ramulus *gui⁴ zhi¹* 3.5 g
Actions and Indications: Warms the yang of the heart and kidney to eliminate wind-damp. Treats contention of wind and damp with vexing pain in the joints that is exacerbated by pressure and that prevents bending and stretching. Other signs include sweating, shortness of breath, inhibited urination, aversion and to cold deterring the patient from removing his clothing, and in some cases slight generalized swelling.

93 *gan¹-cao³ gan¹-jiang¹ tang¹* 甘草乾薑湯 ..42, 98
Licorice and Dried Ginger Decoction
Source: 金匱要略 (*jin¹ gui⁴ yao⁴ lue⁴*)
Glycyrrhizae Radix *gan¹ cao³* 4 g
Zingiberis Rhizoma *gan¹ jiang¹* 2 g
Actions and Indications: Warms the center and boosts qi; restores yang and stems inversion. Treats frigid legs, dry throat, vexation and agitation, vomiting; pulmonary atony, bronchial asthma, and enuresis.

94 *gan¹-cao³ xie⁴ xin¹ tang¹* 甘草瀉心湯 42
Licorice Heart-Draining Decoction
Source: 傷寒論 (*shang¹ han² lun⁴*)
Pinellia Heart-Draining Decoction (*ban⁴-xia⁴ xie⁴ xin¹ tang¹*, 26) plus extra Glycyrrhizae Radix *gan¹ cao³*
Actions and Indications: Boosts qi and supplements vacuity. Indications as for Pinellia Heart-Draining Decoction, i.e., glomus below the heart, dry retching, diarrhea, and vexation, but with extra licorice to boost qi and supplement vacuity.

95 *gan¹-jiang¹ ren²-shen¹ ban⁴-xia⁴ wan²*
乾薑人參半夏丸 40, 92, 98
Dried Ginger, Ginseng, and Pinellia Pills
Source: 金匱要略 (*jin¹ gui⁴ yao⁴ lue⁴*)
Zingiberis Rhizoma *gan¹ jiang¹* 1–3 g
Ginseng Radix *ren² shen¹* 1–3 g
Pinelliae Tuber *ban⁴ xia⁴* 2–6 g
Actions and Indications: Treats morning sickness.

96 *gan¹ lu⁴ yin³* 甘露飲 15, 27
Sweet Dew Beverage
Source: 和劑局方 (*he² ji⁴ ju² fang¹*)
Rehmanniae Radix Exsiccata *gan¹ di⁴* 2.5 g

Rehmanniae Radix Conquita *shou² di⁴ huang²* 2.5 g
Asparagi Tuber *tian¹ men² dong¹* 2.5 g
Ophiopogonis Tuber *mai⁴ dong¹* 2.5 g
Dendrobii Caulis *shi² hu²* 2.5 g
Artemisiae Capillaris Herba *yin¹ chen² hao¹* 2.5 g
Scutellariae Radix *huang² qin²* 2.5 g
Aurantii Fructus *zhi³ ke²* 2.5 g
Eriobotryae Folium *pi² pa² ye⁴* 2.5 g
Glycyrrhizae Radix *gan¹ cao³* 2.5 g
Actions and Indications: Nourishes yin, clears heat, and engenders liquid. Treats damage to yin by pathogen heat with signs such as heat vexation, thirst, bad breath, mouth and tongue sores, sore, swollen throat, erosion of the gums; yin vacuity constitution, with a dry, red or crimson tongue, jaundice, and wasting thirst.

97 *gan¹ mai⁴ da⁴-zao³ tang¹* 甘麥大棗湯 42, 158
Licorice, Wheat, and Jujube Decoction
Source: 金匱要略 (*jin¹ gui⁴ yao⁴ lue⁴*)
Glycyrrhizae Radix *gan¹ cao³* 3–9 g
Tritici Semen Leve *fu² xiao³ mai⁴* 15–30 g
Zizyphi Fructus *da⁴ zao³* 6 g
Actions and Indications: Nourishes the heart and quiets the spirit. Treats visceral agitation with abstraction, sorrowfulness, weepiness, lack of emotional control, vexation and agitation. Tongue red with little fur. Pulse: fine and rapid.

98 *gao¹-liang²-jiang¹ tang¹* 高良薑湯 73
Lesser Galangal Decoction
Source: 千金方 (*qian¹ jin¹ fang¹*)
Alpiniae Officinarum Rhizoma *gao¹ liang² jiang¹* 5 g
Magnoliae Cortex *hou⁴ po⁴* 2 g
Angelicae Sinensis Radix *dang¹ gui¹* 3 g
Cinnamomi Cortex Rasus *gui⁴ xin¹* 3 g
Actions and Indications: Treats sudden gripping heart pain, propping fullness in both lateral costal regions, and oppression.

99 *ge²-gen¹ hong²-hua¹ tang¹* 葛根紅花湯 ..58, 106
Pueraria and Carthamus Decoction
Source: 本朝經驗 (*ben³ chao² jing¹ yan⁴*)
Puerariae Radix *ge² gen¹* 3 g
Paeoniae Radix *shao² yao⁴* 3 g
Rehmanniae Radix *di⁴ huang²* 3 g
Coptidis Rhizoma *huang² lian²* 1.5 g
Gardeniae Fructus *shan¹ zhi¹ zi³* 1.5 g
Carthami Flos *hong² hua¹* 1 g
Rhei Rhizoma *da⁴ huang²* 0.5–1 g
Glycyrrhizae Radix *gan¹ cao³* 1 g
Actions and Indications: Treats chloasma hepaticum (skin discoloration due to liver disease) and drinker's nose.

100 *ge²-gen¹ huang²-qin² huang²-lian² tang¹*
葛根黃芩黃連湯 58, 65, 80
Pueraria, Scutellaria, and Coptis Decoction
Source: 傷寒論 (*shang¹ han² lun⁴*)
Puerariae Radix *ge² gen¹*9–15 g
Scutellariae Radix *huang² qin²* 6–9 g
Coptidis Rhizoma *huang² lian²* 3–6 g
Glycyrrhizae Radix *gan¹ cao³* 3–6 g
Actions and Indications: Resolves the exterior and clears the interior. Treats early-stage febrile disease patterns such as: a) heat in the exterior and interior giving rise to vexation and thirst, and a red tongue with yellow fur; b) non-resolution of the exterior with pathogen heat entering the interior, causing diarrhea; and c) inappropriate precipitation leaving the patient with fever, skipping pulse, dyspnea, and sweating.

101 *ge²-gen¹ tang¹* 葛根湯 58
Pueraria Decoction
Source: 傷寒論 (*shang¹ han² lun⁴*)
Puerariae Radix *ge² gen¹* 9–12 g
Ephedrae Herba *ma² huang²* 2–5 g
Cinnamomi Ramulus *gui⁴ zhi¹* 2–6 g
Paeoniae Radix *shao² yao⁴* 6–9 g
Glycyrrhizae Radix *gan¹ cao³* 2–5 g
Zingiberis Rhizoma Recens *sheng¹ jiang¹* 2–4 g
Zizyphi Fructus *da⁴ zao³* 3–5 g
Preparation method: Decoct with water.
Actions and Indications: Promotes sweating and resolves the exterior. Treats contraction of external wind-cold with fever, absence of sweating, aversion to cold, stiff neck and back. Pulse: floating. Tongue fur: thin and white.

102 *ge²-gen¹ tang¹ jia¹ chuan¹-xiong¹ xin¹-yi²*
葛根湯加川芎辛夷 58, 88, 115
Pueraria Decoction Plus Ligusticum (Cnidium) and Magnolia Flower
Source: 本朝經驗 (*ben³ chao² jing¹ yan⁴*)
Puerariae Radix *ge² gen¹* 8 g
Ephedrae Herba *ma² huang²* 4 g
Zizyphi Fructus *da⁴ zao³* 4 g
Cinnamomi Ramulus *gui⁴ zhi¹* 3 g
Paeoniae Radix *shao² yao⁴* 3 g
Ligustici Rhizoma *chuan¹ xiong¹* 2–3 g
Magnoliae Flos *xin¹ yi²* 2–6 g
Actions and Indications: Treats chronic rhinitis.

103 *gou¹-teng² tang¹* 鉤藤湯 20
Uncaria Decoction
Source: 婦人良方 (*fu⁴ ren² liang² fang¹*)
Uncariae Ramulus et Uncus *gou¹ teng²* 3 g
Angelicae Sinensis Radix *dang¹ gui¹* 3 g
Poria cum Pini Radice *fu² shen²* 3 g

Ginseng Radix *ren² shen¹* 3 g
Loranthi seu Visci Ramus *sang¹ ji⁴ sheng¹* 3 g
Platycodonis Radix *jie² geng³* 4.5 g
Actions and Indications: Extinguishes wind and quiets the fetus. Treats epilepsy in pregnancy with jerking of the limbs, stirring of the fetus, and abdominal pain.

104 *gua¹-lou² gui⁴-zhi¹ tang¹* 栝樓桂枝湯 2, 69
Trichosanthes and Cinnamon Twig Decoction
Source: 金匱要略 (*jin¹ gui⁴ yao⁴ lue⁴*)
Trichosanthis Radix *gua¹ lou² gen¹* 2 g
Cinnamomi Ramulus *gui⁴ zhi¹* 3 g
Paeoniae Radix *shao² yao⁴* 3 g
Glycyrrhizae Radix *gan¹ cao³* 2 g
Zingiberis Rhizoma *gan¹ jiang¹* 1 g
Zizyphi Fructus *da⁴ zao³* 3 g
Actions and Indications: Treats tetanic disease; spastic paralysis.

105 *gua¹-lou² zhi³-shi² tang¹* 栝樓枳實湯 125, 154
Trichosanthes and Unripe Bitter Orange Decoction
Source: 萬病回春 (*wan⁴ bing⁴ hui² chun¹*)
Angelicae Sinensis Radix *dang¹ gui¹* 3 g
Platycodonis Radix *jie² geng³* 2 g
Glycyrrhizae Radix *gan¹ cao³* 1 g
Poria *fu² ling²* 3 g
Citri Exocarpium *chen² pi²* 2 g
Gardeniae Fructus *zhi¹ zi³* 1 g
Fritillariae Bulbus *bei⁴ mu³* 3 g
Scutellariae Radix *huang² qin²* 2 g
Aurantii Fructus Immaturus *zhi³ shi²* 1 g
Trichosanthis Semen *gua¹ lou² ren²* 2 g
Amomi Semen *sha¹ ren²* 1 g
Bambusae Succus Exsiccatus *zhu² li⁴* 1 g
Saussureae Radix *mu⁴ xiang¹* 1 g
Zingiberis Rhizoma Recens *sheng¹ jiang¹* 2 g
Actions and Indications: Treats acute and chronic bronchitis; pneumonia; intercostal neuralgia; dyspnea; cerebral hemorrhage; pulmonary tuberculosis; hyperchlorhydria; arteriosclerosis.

106 *gui¹-ban³ tang¹* 龜板湯 221
Tortoise Plastron Decoction
Source: 本朝經驗 (*ben³ chao² jing¹ yan⁴*)
Angelicae Sinensis Radix *dang¹ gui¹* 6 g
Rehmanniae Radix Conquita *shou² di⁴ huang²* 6 g
Testudinis Plastrum *gui¹ ban³* 4 g
Paeoniae Radix *shao² yao⁴* 4 g
Ligustici Rhizoma *chuan¹ xiong¹* 4 g
Haliotidis Concha *shi² jue² ming²* 4 g
Actions and Indications: Treats numbness in the lumbus and lower limbs; infantile paralysis; diseases of the spine.

107 *gui¹ bo² jiang¹ zhi¹ wan²* 龜柏薑梔丸 221
Tortoise Plastron, Phellodendron, Ginger, and Gardenia Pills
Source: 醫學入門 (*yi¹ xue² ru⁴ men²*)
Testudinis Plastrum *gui¹ ban³*   30 g
Phellodendri Cortex *huang² bo²*   10 g
Zingiberis Rhizoma Exsiccatum *gan¹ jiang¹*   1 g
Gardeniae Fructus *zhi ¹ zi³*   2.5 g
Preparation method: 10 pills (each weighing 300 mg) 2–3 times a day.
Actions and Indications: Treats red and white vaginal discharge and abdominal pain.

108 *gui¹ pi² tang¹* 歸脾湯 56, 141, 188
Spleen-Returning Decoction
Source: 濟生方 (*ji⁴ sheng¹ fang¹*)
Atractylodis Ovatae Rhizoma *bai² zhu²*   2–3 g
Poria *fu² ling²*   2–3 g
Astragali Radix *huang² qi²*   2–3 g
Ginseng Radix *ren² shen¹*   2–3 g
Glycyrrhizae Radix *gan¹ cao³*   1 g
Saussureae Radix *mu⁴ xiang¹*   1 g
Angelicae Sinensis Radix *dang¹ gui¹*   2 g
Polygalae Radix *yuan³ zhi⁴*   1–2 g
Longanae Arillus *long² yan³ rou⁴*   2–3 g
Zizyphi Spinosi Semen *suan¹ zao³ ren²*   2–3 g
Actions and Indications: Fortifies the spleen and boosts qi; supplements the blood and nourishes the heart. Treats a) vacuity of the both heart and spleen, and insufficiency of qi and blood, with signs such as fatigue of spirit and body, palpitations or racing of the heart, insomnia, and poor memory; b) spleen failing to manage the blood with blood in the stool or urine or uterine bleeding.

109 *gui⁴-zhi¹ fu²-ling² wan²* 桂枝茯苓丸
....2, 9, 177, 236
Cinnamon Twig and Poria Pills
Source: 金匱要略 (*jin¹ gui⁴ yao⁴ lue⁴*)
Cinnamomi Ramulus *gui⁴ zhi¹*   4 g
Poria *fu² ling²*   4 g
Moutan Radicis Cortex *mu³ dan¹ pi²*   4 g
Persicae Semen *tao² ren²*   4 g
Paeoniae Radix *shao² yao⁴*   4 g
Actions and Indications: Transforms stasis and disperses concretions. Treats tender lesser abdominal concretion lumps in women with inhibited menstruation, menstrual pain, or persistent flow of lochia.

110 *gui⁴-zhi¹ jia¹ hou⁴-po⁴ xing⁴-ren² tang¹*
桂枝加厚朴杏仁湯 2, 7, 162
Cinnamon Twig Decoction Plus Magnolia Bark and Apricot Kernel
Source: 傷寒論 (*shang¹ han² lun⁴*)

Cinnamomi Ramulus *gui⁴ zhi¹*   3–4 g
Paeoniae Radix *shao² yao⁴*   3–4 g
Glycyrrhizae Radix *gan¹ cao³*   3–4 g
Zingiberis Rhizoma Recens *sheng¹ jiang¹*   3–4 g
Zizyphi Fructus *da⁴ zao³*   3–4 g
Magnoliae Cortex *hou⁴ po⁴*   1–4 g
Armeniacae Semen *xing⁴ ren²*   3–4 g
Actions and Indications: Regulates construction and defense; downbears counterflow and calms dyspnea. Treats attacks of dyspnea presenting with Cinnamon Twig Decoction signs, or tai yang disease with mild dyspnea.

111 *gui⁴-zhi¹ jia¹ huang²-qi² tang¹* 桂枝加黃耆湯
....29, 30
Cinnamon Twig Decoction Plus Astragalus
Source: 金匱要略 (*jin¹ gui⁴ yao⁴ lue⁴*)
Cinnamomi Ramulus *gui⁴ zhi¹*   3–4 g
Paeoniae Radix *shao² yao⁴*   3–4 g
Glycyrrhizae Radix *gan¹ cao³*   2 g
Zingiberis Rhizoma Recens *sheng¹ jiang¹*   4 g
Zizyphi Fructus *da⁴ zao³*   3–4 g
Astragali Radix *huang² qi²*   3–4 g
Actions and Indications: Boosts qi and secures the exterior; regulates construction and defense. Treats yellow perspiration; general vacuity with susceptibility to colds and flu; exterior vacuity spontaneous sweating.

112 *gui⁴-zhi¹ jia¹ long²-gu³ mu³-li⁴ tang¹*
桂枝加龍骨牡蠣湯 218, 225
Cinnamon Twig Decoction Plus Dragon Bone and Oyster Shell
Source: 金匱要略 (*jin¹ gui⁴ yao⁴ lue⁴*)
Cinnamomi Ramulus *gui⁴ zhi¹*   3–4 g
Paeoniae Radix *shao² yao⁴*   3–4 g
Glycyrrhizae Radix *gan¹ cao³*   2 g
Zingiberis Rhizoma Recens *sheng¹ jiang¹*   3–4 g
Zizyphi Fructus *da⁴ zao³*   3–4 g
Draconis Os (Mastodi Ossis Fossilia) *long² gu³*   2 g
Ostreae Concha *mu³ li⁴*   3 g
Actions and Indications: Warms yang and dissipates cold; promotes contraction. Treats vacuity cold in the lower burner with tense abdomen, seminal emission, or impotence; insomnia with profuse dreaming; child enuresis.

113 *gui⁴-zhi¹ jia¹ shao²-yao⁴ tang¹* 桂枝加芍藥湯
....51
Cinnamon Twig Decoction Plus Peony
Source: 傷寒論 (*shang¹ han² lun⁴*)
Cinnamomi Ramulus *gui⁴ zhi¹*   4 g
Paeoniae Radix *shao² yao⁴*   6 g
Glycyrrhizae Radix *gan¹ cao³* (mix-fried)   2 g

Zingiberis Rhizoma Recens *sheng¹ jiang¹* 4 g
Zizyphi Fructus *da⁴ zao³* 4 g
Actions and Indications: Resolves the exterior and relaxes tension. Treats abdominal fullness and periodic pain in tai yang disease patients wrongly given precipitating treatment.

114 *gui⁴-zhi¹ tang¹* 桂枝湯 2
Cinnamon Twig Decoction
Source: 傷寒論 (*shang¹ han² lun⁴*)
Cinnamomi Ramulus *gui⁴ zhi¹* 5–9 g
Paeoniae Radix *shao² yao⁴* 6–9 g
Glycyrrhizae Radix *gan¹ cao³* (mix-fried) 3–6 g
Zingiberis Rhizoma Recens *sheng¹ jiang¹* 2–4 g
Zizyphi Fructus *da⁴ zao³* 4–6 g
Usually white peony (Peoniae Radix Alba) is used.
Actions and Indications: Resolves the muscles and effuses the exterior; harmonizes construction and defense. Treats contraction of external wind cold. Signs: Headache, fever, sweating, aversion to wind, nasal congestion with clear nasal mucous, dry retching, absence of thirst. Tongue fur: thin, white, moist and glossy. Pulse: floating and moderate, or floating and weak.

115 *hao¹ qin² qing¹ dan³ tang¹* 蒿芩清膽湯 12
Sweet Wormwood and Scutellaria Glallbladder-Clearing Decoction
Source: 重訂通俗傷寒論 (*chong² ding⁴ tong¹ su²
shang¹ han² lun⁴*)
Artemisiae Apiaceae seu Annuae Herba *qing¹ hao¹*
9–12 g
Scutellariae Radix *huang² qin²* 9–12 g
Pinelliae Tuber *ban⁴ xia⁴* 6–9 g
Aurantii Fructus *zhi³ ke²* 6–9 g
Bambusae Caulis in Taeniam *zhu² ru²* 6–9 g
Poria *fu² ling²* 9–12 g
Jasper Jade Powder *bi⁴ yu⁴ san³* 9–12 g
Citri Exocarpium *chen² pi²* 4–6 g
Actions and Indications: Clears the gallbladder and discharges heat; harmonizes the stomach and transforms damp. Treats pathogen heat depressed in the gallbladder channel and phlegm-damp obstructing the middle burner, characterized by mild aversion to cold and fever, heavy head and fatigued limbs, oppressive glomus in the chest and venter, retching and nausea, bitter taste in the mouth, dry mouth or thirst without desire for fluids, dark-colored urine, and sometimes diarrhea. Tongue fur: white or yellow slimy. Pulse: soggy and rapid. Also treats malaria.

116 *he¹-zi³ yin³* 訶子飲 127
Chebule Beverage
Source: 濟生方 (*ji⁴ sheng¹ fang¹*)

Chebulae Fructus *he¹ zi³* (with kernel removed) 10 g
Armeniacae Semen *xing⁴ ren²* 10 g
Mutong Caulis *mu⁴ tong¹* 2.5 g
Preparation method: Take with warm after meals.
Actions and Indications: Treats loss of voice from enduring cough.

117 *he² ren² yin³* 何人飲 57
Flowery Knotweed and Ginseng Beverage
Source: 景岳全書 (*jing³ yue⁴ quan² shu¹*)
Polygoni Multiflori Radix *he² shou³ wu¹* 9–30 g
Angelicae Sinensis Radix *dang¹ gui¹* 6–9 g
Codonopsitis Radix *dang³ shen¹* 9–15 g
Citri Exocarpium *chen² pi²* 6 g
Zingiberis Rhizoma *jiang¹* (roasted) 3 slices
Preparation method: Decoct with water.
Actions and Indications: Supplements qi and the blood; treats vacuity malaria. Treats persistent malaria with dual vacuity of qi and blood. Signs: Withered yellow complexion, attacks that are brought on by taxation. Tongue: pale tongue. Pulse: large, vacuous and forceless. Take three hours before an expected attack.

118 *hei¹ hu³ dan¹* 黑虎丹 107
Black Tiger Elixir
Source: 經驗方 (empirical formula)
Bombyx Batryticatus *bai² jiang¹ can²* 2 g
Buthus *quan² xie¹* 4.5 g
Scolopendra *wu² gong¹* 6 g
Moschus *she⁴ xiang¹* 0.5 g
Bovis Calculus *niu² huang²* 0.3 g
Magnetitum *ci² shi²* 4.5 g
Manitis Squama *chuan¹ shan¹ jia³* 3 g
Caryophylli Flos *ding¹ xiang¹* 3 g
Caryophylli Fructus *mu³ ding¹ xiang¹* 3 g
Borneolum *bing¹ pian⁴* 3 g
Aranea *zhi¹ zhu¹* 7 pieces.
Actions and Indications: Draws out pus and poison; disperses swelling and softens hardness. Treats yong and ju, effusions of the back, mouth-level nape sores (*dui⁴ kou³ chuang¹*), clove sores, and innominate swollen toxin sores.

119 *hong²-hua¹ san³* 紅花散 106
Carthamus Powder
Source: 保命集 (*bao³ ming⁴ ji²*)
Carthami Flos *hong² hua¹*
Nelumbinis Folium Exsiccatum *gan¹ he² ye⁴*
Moutan Radicis Cortex *mu³ dan¹ pi²*
Angelicae Sinensis Radix *dang¹ gui¹*
Typhae Pollen *pu² huang²* (stir-fried)
All agents in equal proportions.
Preparation method: Grind to a fine powder.

Actions and Indications: Treats postpartum dizziness; blood dizziness; profuse uterine bleeding.
Dosage: 5 g twice a day.

120 *hou⁴-po⁴ san¹ wu⁴ tang¹* 厚朴三物湯............7
Magnolia Bark Three Agents Decoction
Source: 金匱要略(*jin¹ gui⁴ yao⁴ lue⁴*)
Magnoliae Cortex *hou⁴ po⁴*   5 g
Rhei Rhizoma *da⁴ huang²*   2.5 g
Aurantii Fructus Immaturus *zhi³ shi²*   2.5 g
Actions and Indications: Treats abdominal pain; abdominal fullness; constipation.

121 *hu²-lu²-ba¹ san³* 胡蘆巴散......................170
Fenugreek Powder
Source: 濟生方(*ji⁴ sheng¹ fang¹*)
Foeni-Graeci Semen *hu² lu² ba¹* (stir-fried) 5 g
Sparganii Rhizoma *san¹ leng²* (steeped in wine and stone-baked) 5 g
Zingiberis Rhizoma *gan¹ jiang¹* (blast-fried) 2.5 g
Preparation method: Grind to a powder.
Actions and Indications: Treats headache cold-damp leg qi.
Dosage: 3 g at a time.

122 *hu³-gu³ mu⁴-gua¹ jiu³* 虎骨木瓜酒.....126, 222
Tiger Bone and Chaenomeles Wine
Source: 經驗方 (empirical formula)
Tigris Os *hu³ gu³*   10 g
Chaenomelis Fructus *mu⁴ gua¹*   30 g
Ligustici Rhizoma *chuan¹ xiong¹*   10 g
Cyathulae Radix *chuan¹ niu² xi¹*   10 g
Angelicae Sinensis Radix *dang¹ gui¹*   10 g
Gastrodiae Rhizoma *tian¹ ma²*   10 g
Acanthopanacis Radicis Cortex *wu³ jia¹ pi²*   10 g
Carthami Flos *hong² hua¹*   10 g
Dipsaci Radix *xu⁴ duan⁴*   10 g
Solani Melongenae Radix *qie² gen¹*   10 g
Polygonati Officinalis Rhizoma *yu⁴ zhu²*   20 g
Gentianae Macrophyllae Radix *qin² jiao¹*   5 g
Ledebouriellae Radix *fang² feng¹*   5 g
Mori Ramulus *sang¹ zhi¹*   40 g
Sorghi Spiritus *gao¹ liang² jiu³*   3,000 cc.
Saccharon Granulatum *sha¹ tang²*   300 g
Actions and Indications: Expels wind and relieves pain; eliminates cold and damp; strengthens the sinews and bone.

123 *hu³ qian² wan²* 虎潛丸.....................14, 222
Hidden Tiger Pills
Alternate name:健步虎潛丸*jian⁴ bu⁴ hu³ qian² wan²*
Steady Gait Hidden Tiger Pills
Source:丹溪心法 (*dan¹ xi¹ xin¹ fa³*)

Rehmanniae Radix Conquita *shou² di⁴ huang²*   20 g
Testudinis Plastrum *gui¹ ban³*   40 g
Anemarrhenae Rhizoma *zhi¹ mu³*   20 g
Phellodendri Cortex *huang² bo²*   30 g
Paeoniae Radix Alba *bai² shao² yao⁴*   20 g
Citri Exocarpium *chen² pi²*   10 g
Cynomorii Caulis *suo³ yang²*   20 g
Tigris Os *hu³ gu³*   15 g
Zingiberis Rhizoma *gan¹ jiang¹*   5 g
Actions and Indications: Enriches yin and downbears fire; boosts essence blood; strengthens the sinews and bones. Treats liver-kidney yin vacuity and insufficiency of qi and blood, with weak, aching lumbus and knees, emaciation of the legs, and feeble gait.

124 *hua⁴ shi² yang³ pi² tang¹* 化食養脾湯........201
Food-Transforming Spleen-Nourishing Decoction
Source:證治大還 (*zheng⁴ zhi⁴ da⁴ huan²*)
Ginseng Radix *ren² shen¹*   4 g
Atractylodis Ovatae Rhizoma *bai² zhu²*   4 g
Poria *fu² ling²*   4 g
Pinelliae Tuber *ban⁴ xia⁴*   4 g
Citri Exocarpium *chen² pi²*   2 g
Zizyphi Fructus *da⁴ zao³*   2 g
Massa Medicata Fermentata *shen² qu¹*   2 g
Hordei Fructus Germinatus *mai⁴ ya²*   2 g
Crataegi Fruitus *shan¹ zha¹*   2 g
Amomi Semen *sha¹ ren²*   1.5 g
Zingiberis Rhizoma *gan¹ jiang¹*   1 g
Glycyrrhizae Radix *gan¹ cao³*   1 g
Actions and Indications: Treats indigestion, stomach pain, and vomiting.

125 *huai²-hua¹ san³* 槐花散...................100, 117
Sophora Flower Powder
Source:本事方 (*ben³ shi⁴ fang¹*)
Sophorae Flos *huai² hua¹* (stir-fried) 9–15 g
Biotae Folium et Ramulus *ce⁴ bo² ye⁴* (stir-fried) 9–12 g
Schizonepetae Herba Carbonisata *hei¹ jing¹ jie⁴* (stir-fried) 6–9 g
Aurantii Fructus *zhi³ ke²* (stir-fried) 6–9 g
Preparation method: Originally a powder; now prepared as a decoction.
Actions and Indications: Clears yang and staunches bleeding. Treats damp-heat brewing internally with blood in the stool; or bleeding hemorrhoids with bright colored blood.

126 *huai²-jiao³ wan²* 槐角丸.........................152
Sophora Fruit Pills
Source:和劑局方 (*he² ji⁴ ju² fang¹*)
Sophorae Fructus *huai² jiao³*   40 g
Ledebouriellae Radix *fang² feng¹*   20 g

Aurantii Fructus *zhi³ ke²* (stir-fried with bran)　20 g
Sanguisorbae Radix *di⁴ yu²* 20 g
Angelicae Sinensis Radix *dang¹ gui¹* (steeped in wine and stone-baked)　20 g
Scutellariae Radix *huang² qin²* 20 g
Preparation method: Form into 300 mg pills.
Actions and Indications: Cools the blood and staunches bleeding. Treats blood in the stool, and bleeding hemorrhoids.
Dosage: 10 pills twice a day.

127 *huai² xiang¹ san³* 槐香散 117
Sophora Flower and Musk Powder
Source: 聖濟總錄 (*sheng⁴ ji⁴ zong³ lu⁴*)
Sophorae Flos *huai² hua¹*
Preparation method: Grind to a fine powder and add a pinch of musk.
Actions and Indications: Treats vomiting of blood.

128 *huan² shao⁴ dan¹* 還少丹 13, 49
Rejuvenation Elixir
Source: 洪氏集驗方 (*hong² shi⁴ ji⁴ yan⁴ fang¹*)
Rehmanniae Radix Conquita *shou² di⁴ huang²* 5 g
Dioscoreae Rhizoma *shan¹ yao⁴* 15 g
Achyranthis Bidentatae Radix *niu² xi¹* (steeped in wine and stone-baked)　15 g
Lycii Fructus *gou³ qi³ zi³* (steeped in wine) 5 g
Corni Fructus *shan¹ zhu¹ yu²* 10 g
Poria *fu² ling²* 10 g
Eucommiae Cortex *du⁴ zhong⁴* 10 g
Polygalae *yuan³ zhi⁴* 10 g
Schisandrae Fructus *wu³ wei⁴ zi³* (stir-fried) 10 g
Broussonetiae Fructus *chu³ shi²* (steamed in wine) 10 g
Foeniculi Fructus *hui² xiang¹* (stir-fried with brine) 10 g
Morindae Radix *ba¹ ji³ tian¹* 10 g
Cistanches Caulis *rou⁴ cong¹ rong²* 10 g
Acori Grarminei Rhizoma *shi² chang¹ pu²* 5 g
Zizyphi Pericarpium *zao³ rou⁴*
Preparation method: From into 300 mg pills.
Actions and Indications: Nourishes the heart and kidney. Treats vacuity taxation and heart-kidney insufficiency with weak, aching lumbus and kdnees, insomnia, poor memory, dizziness, turbid urine, seminal emission, premature senility, fatigue and lack of strength.
Dosage: 10 pills 3 times a day.

129 *huang²-lian² e¹-jiao¹ tang¹* 黃連阿膠湯 .80, 208
Coptis and Ass Hide Glue Decoction
Source: 傷寒論 (*shang¹ han² lun⁴*)
Coptidis Rhizoma *huang² lian²* 1.5–3 g
Scutellariae Radix *huang² qin²* 6–9 g

Asini Corii Gelatinum *e¹ jiao¹* 6–9 g
Paeoniae Radix Alba *bai² shao² yao⁴* 6–9 g
Galli Vitellus *ji¹ zi³ huang²* 2 g
Preparation method: Decoct and strain, add Asini Corii Gelatinum, Allow to cool off before stirring in the egg yolks. Split into two doses.
Actions and Indications: Enriches yin and downbears fire; eliminates vexation and quiets the spirit. Treats: 1) Effulgent yin vacuity fire with heat vexation in the heart and insomnia. Tongue: red with dry fur. Pulse: fine and rapid. 2) Latter stages of febrile diseases with residual heat and depletion of yin humor giving rise to vacuity vexation and insomnia.

130 *huang²-lian² jie³ du² tang¹* 黃連解毒湯
....10, 65, 80
Coptis Toxin-Resolving Decoction
Source: 外臺秘要 (*wai⁴ tai² mi² yao⁴*)
Coptidis Rhizoma *huang² lian²* 3–9 g
Phellodendri Cortex *huang² bo²* 6–12 g
Gardeniae Fructus *shan¹ zhi¹ zi³* 6–12 g
Scutellariae Radix *huang² qin²* 6–12 g
Actions and Indications: Drains fire and resolves toxin; clears heat and transforms damp. Treats all types of pathogen fire and heat toxin giving rise to vigorous fever, vexation, agitation, and in some cases clouding of the spirit, and delirious speech. Tongue: red with yellow fur. Pulse: rapid and forceful. Also treats exuberant heat giving rise to vomiting of blood and macular eruption, damp-heat heat jaundice, dysentery, and clove and other sores.

131 *huang²-lian² tang¹* 黃連湯 80
Coptis Decoction
Source: 傷寒論 (*shang¹ han² lun⁴*)
Variant of 半夏瀉心湯 *ban⁴-xia⁴ xie⁴ xin¹ tang¹*
Pinellia Heart-Draining Decoction
Pinelliae Tuber *ban⁴ xia⁴* 5–6 g
Zingiberis Rhizoma *gan¹ jiang¹* 3 g
Coptidis Rhizoma *huang² lian²* 3 g
Ginseng Radix *ren² shen¹* (or Codonopsitis Radix *dang³ shen¹*) 2–3 g
Glycyrrhizae Radix *gan¹ cao²* 3 g
Zizyphi Fructus *da⁴ zao³* 3 g
Cinnamomi Ramulus *gui⁴ zhi¹* 3 g
Actions and Indications: Downbears counterflow and eliminates glomus; warms the center and harmonizes the stomach. Treats impaired gastrointestinal function, with heat vexation in the chest, glomus and oppression, qi counterflow with desire to vomit, abdominal pain, sometimes with rumbling of the intestines and diarrhea. Tongue fur: glossy and white. Pulse: wiry. Such patterns sometimes include fever and chills. For sever abdominal pain due to interior cold, Cinnamomi

Ramulus may be replaced by Cinnamomi Cortex (rou⁴ gui⁴) to increase the interior-warming, cold-dispelling, and pain-relieving action.

132 huang²-qi² bie¹-jia³ san³ 黃耆鱉甲散
Astragalus and Turtle Shell Powder
Source:衛生寶鑑 (wei⁴ sheng¹ bao³ jian⁴)
Astragali Radix huang² qi² 2 g
Amydae Carapax bie¹ jia³ 2 g
Gentianae Macrophyllae Radix qin² jiao¹ 1 g
Bupleuri Radix chai² hu² 2 g
Lycii Radicis Cortex di⁴ gu³ pi² 2 g
Asparagi Tuber tian¹ men² dong¹ 2.5 g
Rehmanniae Radix di⁴ huang² 2 g
Ginseng Radix ren² shen¹ 1 g
Anemarrhenae Rhizoma zhi¹ mu³ 1 g
Mori Radicis Cortex sang¹ bai² pi² 1 g
Asteris Radix et Rhizoma zi³ wan³ 1 g
Pinelliae Tuber ban⁴ xia⁴ 1 g
Paeoniae Radix Rubra chi⁴ shao² yao⁴ 2 g
Poria fu² ling² 2.5 g
Platycodonis Radix jie² geng³ 1 g
Cinnamomi Ramulus gui⁴ zhi¹ 1 g
Glycyrrhizae Radix gan¹ cao³ 1 g
Actions and Indications: Boosts qi and nourishes yin; clears vacuity heat; transforms phlegm and suppresses cough. Treats dual vacuity of qi and yin with steaming bone tidal fever, emaciation, spontaneous sweating, and cough. Tongue: red. Pulse: vacuous.

133 huang²-qi² gui⁴-zhi¹ wu³ wu⁴ tang¹
黃耆桂枝五物湯
Astragalus and Cinnamon Twig Five Agents Decoction
Source:金匱要略 (jin¹ gui⁴ yao⁴ lue⁴)
Astragali Radix huang² qi² 3 g
Paeoniae Radix shao² yao⁴ 3 g
Cinnamomi Ramulus gui⁴ zhi¹ 3 g
Zingiberis Rhizoma Recens sheng¹ jiang¹ 6 g
Zizyphi Fructus da⁴ zao³ 3 g
Actions and Indications: Boosts qi and warms the channels; quickens the blood and frees bi. Treats blood bi with numbness of the skin. Pulse: faint and rough pulse.

134 huang²-qi² jian⁴ zhong¹ tang¹ 黃耆建中湯…30
Astragalus Center-Fortifying Decoction
Source:金匱要略 (jin¹ gui⁴ yao⁴ lue⁴)
Variant of 小建中湯 xiao³ jian⁴ zhong¹ tang¹ Minor Center-Fortifying Decoction
Cinnamomi Ramulus gui⁴ zhi¹ 3–4 g
Paeoniae Radix Alba bai² shao² yao⁴ 6 g

Glycyrrhizae Radix gan¹ cao³ 2–3 g
Zingiberis Rhizoma Recens sheng¹ jiang¹ 3–4 g
Zizyphi Fructus da⁴ zao³ 3–4 g
Granorum Saccharon yi² tang² 20 g
Astragali Radix huang² qi² 3–4 g
Actions and Indications: Warms the center and supplements vacuity; boosts qi and secures the exterior. Treats: 1) Abdominal pain due to middle burner vacuity cold with spontaneous sweating due to exterior vacuity. 2) Minor Center-Fortifying Decoction patterns with pronounced qi vacuity.

135 huang²-qin² tang¹ 黃芩湯
Scutellaria Decoction
Source:傷寒論 (shang¹ han² lun⁴)
Scutellariae Radix huang² qin² 4 g
Paeoniae Radix shao² yao⁴ 3 g
Glycyrrhizae Radix gan¹ cao³ 3 g
Zizyphi Fructus da⁴ zao³ 4 g
Actions and Indications: Clears heat and checks diarrhea; relaxes tension and relieves pain. Treats generalized fever with bitter taste in the mouth, and abdominal pain, diarrhea or or dysentery. Tongue: red with yellow fur. Pulse: wiry and rapid.

136 hui²-xiang¹ wan² 茴香丸
Star Anise Pills
Source:脚氣治法總錄 (jiao³ qi⁴ zhi⁴ fa³ zong³ lu⁴)
Anisi Stellati Fructus ba¹ jiao³ hui² xiang¹ (stir-fried) 10 g
Lumbricus di⁴ long² (stir-fried) 10 g
Aconiti Tuber chuan¹ wu¹ tou² (blast-fried) 10 g
Linderae Radix wu¹ yao⁴ (grated) 10 g
Pharbitidis Semen qian¹ niu² zi³ (stir-fried) 10 g
Preparation method: Grind to a powder, boil in wine, and form into 300 mg pills. Take 15 pills twice a day before meals.
Actions and Indications: Treats wind toxin and damp qi; cold shan abdominal pain.

137 huo⁴-xiang¹ zheng⁴ qi⁴ san³ 藿香正氣散…193
Agastache/Patchouli Qi-Correcting Powder
Source:和劑局方 (he² ji⁴ ju² fang¹)
Agastaches seu Pogostemi Herba huo⁴ xiang¹ 9–15 g
Perillae Caulis et Calyx zi³ su¹ 6–9 g
Angelicae Dahuricae Radix bai² zhi³ 3–6 g
Platycodonis Radix jie² geng³ 3–6 g
Atractylodis Ovatae Rhizoma bai² zhu² 6–9 g
Magnoliae Cortex hou⁴ po⁴ 3–6 g
Pinelliae Massa Fermentata ban⁴ xia⁴ qu¹ 9 g
Arecae Pericarpium da⁴ fu⁴ pi² 6–9 g
Poria fu² ling² 9–12 g
Citri Exocarpium chen² pi² 5–9 g
Glycyrrhizae Radix gan¹ cao³ 3 g

Zingiberis Rhizoma Recens *sheng¹ jiang¹* 3 slices
Zizyphi Fructus *da⁴ zao³* 1 piece
Last two ingredients are added for decoction form.
Preparation method: Usually prepared as a decoction,
but also available in pill and tablet form.
Actions and Indications: Transforms damp and
resolves the exterior; rectifies qi and harmonizes the
center. Contraction of external wind-cold with internal damp stagnation, manifesting as aversion to cold,
fever, headache, cough, oppression in the chest,
nausea and vomiting, rumbling intestines, diarrhea,
and bland taste in the mouth. Tongue fur: white and
slimy.
Dosage: 3–6 g 2–3 times a day, with water.

138 *ji¹-guan¹ san³* 雞冠散............................108
Cockscomb Powder
Source:太平聖惠方(*tai⁴ ping² sheng⁴ hui⁴ fang¹*)
Celosiae Cristatae Flos *ji¹ guan⁴ hua¹*
Preparation method: Stir-fry with seeds and grind to
a powder.
Actions and Indications: Treats precipitation of blood
after defecation.

139 *ji¹ ming² san³* 雞鳴散........................126, 132
Cockcrow Powder
Source:證治準繩(*zheng⁴ zhi⁴ zhun³ sheng²*)
Arecae Semen *bin¹ lang²* 6–9 g
Citri Exocarpium *chen² pi²* 3–6 g
Chaenomelis Fructus *mu⁴ gua¹* 6–9 g
Evodiae Fructus *wu² zhu¹ yu²* 2–4 g
Platycodonis Radix *jie² geng³* 3–6 g
Perillae Caulis et Calyx *zi³ su¹* 3–9 g
Zingiberis Rhizoma Recens *sheng¹ jiang¹* 3–5 slices
Preparation method: Now prepared in decoction form.
Actions and Indications: Dissipates damp, downbears
qi and turbidity. Treats damp-type leg qi characteriz-
ed by swelling and numbness of the legs and feet, and
difficulty in walking, or downpour of wind-damp with
feet so painful that they cannot even be put on the
ground. Take on an empty stomach.

140 *jia¹ wei⁴ gui¹ pi² tang¹* 加味歸脾湯......31, 135
Supplemented Spleen-Returning Decoction
Source:濟生方(*ji⁴ sheng¹ fang¹*)
Bupleuri Radix *chai² hu²* 3 g
Gardeniae Fructus *shan¹ zhi¹ zi³* 2 g
Atractylodis Ovatae Rhizoma *bai² zhu²* 3 g
Ginseng Radix *ren² shen¹* 3 g
Astragali Radix *huang² qi²* 3 g
Angelicae Sinensis Radix *dang¹ gui¹* 2 g
Glycyrrhizae Radix *gan¹ cao³* 1 g
Poria *fu² ling²* 3 g
Polygalae Radix *yuan³ zhi⁴* 1.5–2 g

Zizyphi Spinosi Semen *suan¹ zao³ ren²* 2 g
Saussureae Radix *mu⁴ xiang¹* 1 g
Longanae Arillus *long² yan³ rou⁴* 2 g
Zingiberis Rhizoma Recens *sheng¹ jiang¹* 1.5 g
Zizyphi Fructus *da⁴ zao³* 1 g
Actions and Indications: Blood vacuity and anemia,
palpitations, poor memory, insomnia, and bleeding.

141 *jia¹ wei⁴ jie³ du² tang¹* 加味解毒湯.............17
Supplemented Toxin-Resolving Decoction
Source:壽世保元(*shou⁴ shi⁴ bao³ yuan²*)
Scutellariae Radix *huang² qin²* 2 g
Coptidis Rhizoma *huang² lian²* 2 g
Phellodendri Cortex *huang² bo²* 2 g
Gardeniae Fructus *zhi¹ zi³* 2 g
Bupleuri Radix *chai² hu²* 2 g
Artemisiae Capillaris Herba *yin¹ chen² hao¹* 2 g
Gentianae Scabrae Radix *long² dan³* 2 g
Mutong Caulis *mu⁴ tong¹* 2 g
Talcum *hua² shi²* 3 g
Cimicifugae Rhizoma *sheng¹ ma²* 1.5 g
Glycyrrhizae Radix *gan¹ cao³* 1.5 g
Rhei Rhizoma *da⁴ huang²* 1.5 kgr.
Junci Medulla *deng¹ xin¹ cao³* 1.5 g
Actions and Indications: Treats triple burner repletion
heat.

142 *jia¹ wei⁴ ping² wei⁴ san³* 加味平胃散 131
Supplemented Stomach-Calming Powder
Source: 醫方考 (*yi¹ fang¹ kao³*)
Atractylodis Ovatae Rhizoma *bai² zhu²* 4–6 g
Magnoliae Cortex *hou⁴ po⁴* 3–4.5 g
Citri Exocarpium *chen² pi²* 3–4.5 g
Glycyrrhizae Radix *gan¹ cao³* 1–1.5 g
Zingiberis Rhizoma Recens *sheng¹ jiang¹* 2–3 g
Zizyphi Fructus *da⁴ zao³* 2–3 g
Massa Medicata Fermentata *shen² qu¹* 2–3 g
Hordei Fructus Germinatus *mai⁴ ya²* 2–3 g
Crataegi Fructus *shan¹ zha¹* 2–3 g
Actions and Indications: Treats glomus in the venter,
watery diarrhea, and poor appetite.

143 *jia¹ wei⁴ xiao¹ yao² san³* 加味逍遙散...........9
Supplemented Free Wanderer Powder
Source:和劑局方(*he² ji⁴ ju² fang¹*)
Moutan Radicis Cortex *mu³ dan¹ pi²* 2 g
Paeoniae Radix Rubrae *chi¹ shao² yao⁴* 3 g
Bupleuri Radix *chai² hu²* 3 g
Angelicae Sinensis Radix *dang¹ gui¹* 3 g
Atractylodis Ovatae Rhizoma *bai² zhu²* 3 g
Poria *fu² ling²* 3 g
Glycyrrhizae Radix *gan¹ cao³* 1–5.2 g
Zingiberis Rhizoma Recens *sheng¹ jiang¹* 1 g
Menthae Herba *bo⁴ he²* 1 g

Actions and Indications: Treats menstrual disorders, psychasthenia, and sensations of cold.

144 *jiang¹-huang² san³* 薑黃散 82
Turmeric Powder
Source: 聖濟總錄 (*sheng⁴ ji⁴ zong³ lu⁴*)
Curcumae Longae Rhizoma *jiang¹ huang²* (lightly stir-fried) 10 g
Angelicae Sinensis Radix *dang¹ gui¹* (stone-baked) 10 g
Linderae Radix *wu¹ yao⁴* (stir-fried) 5 g
Saussureae Radix *mu⁴ xiang¹* 5 g
Preparation method: Grind to a fine powder.
Actions and Indications: Treats heart pain.
Dosage: 2 g 2–3 times a day.

145 *jiao¹ mei² tang¹* 椒梅湯 144, 157
Zanthoxylum and Mume Decoction
Source: 萬病回春 (*wan⁴ bing⁴ hui² chun¹*)
Mume Fructus *wu¹ mei²* 2 g
Zanthoxyli Fructus *hua¹ jiao¹* 2 g
Arecae Semen *bin¹ lang²* 2 g
Aurantii Fructus Immaturus *zhi³ shi²* 2 g
Saussureae Radix *mu⁴ xiang¹* 2 g
Cyperi Rhizoma *xiang¹ fu⁴ zi³* 2 g
Amomi Semen *sha¹ ren²* 2 g
Cinnamomi Cortex *rou⁴ gui⁴* 2 g
Magnoliae Cortex *hou⁴ po⁴* 2 g
Zingiberis Rhizoma *gan¹ jiang¹* 2 g
Glycyrrhizae Radix *gan¹ cao³* 2 g
Meliae Toosendan Fructus *chuan¹ lian⁴ zi³* 2 g
Actions and Indications: Treats hookworm.

146 *jie²-geng³ bai² san³* 桔梗白散 55, 85
Platycodon White Powder
Source: 傷寒論 (*shang¹ han² lun⁴*)
Platycodonis Radix *jie² geng³* 1 g
Fritillariae Bulbus *bei⁴ mu³* 1 g
Crotonis Semen *ba¹ dou⁴* 0.3 g
Preparation method: Grind to a powder.
Actions and Indications: Treats dyspnea; acute pneumonia; diphtheria; wind stroke. Dosage: Take in small frequent doses.

147 *jie² nue⁴ qi¹ bao³ yin³* 截瘧七寶飲 161
Malaria-Terminating Seven-Jewel Beverage
Source: 楊氏家藏方 (*yang² shi⁴ jia¹ cang² fang¹*)
Dichroae Radix *chang² shan¹* 6–9 g
Arecae Semen *bin¹ lang²* 6–9 g
Amomi Tsao-Ko Fructus *cao³ guo³* 6–9 g
Magnoliae Cortex *hou⁴ po⁴* 6–9 g
Citri Exocarpium Immaturum *quing¹ pi²* 4–6 g
Citri Exocarpium *chen² pi²* 4–6 g
Glycyrrhizae Radix *gan¹ cao³* (mix-fried) 3 g

Preparation method: Add one spoonful of yellow rice wine after boiling.
Actions and Indications: Dries damp and dispels phlegm; terminates malaria. Treats recurrent malarial attacks in strong patients with pronounced phlegm-damp signs. Pulse: large, slippery, wiry and forceful. Take three hours before an expected attack.

148 *jin¹-fei⁴-cao³ san³* 金沸草散 113
Inula Powder
Source: 類證活人書 (*lei⁴ zheng⁴ huo² ren² shu¹*)
Inulae Flos *jin¹ fei⁴ hua¹* 6–9 g
Peucedani Radix *qian² hu²* 6–9 g
Schizonepetae Herba seu Flos *jing¹ jie⁴* 6–9 g
Asiasari Radix *xi⁴ xin¹* 3–5 g
Pinelliae Tuber cum Zingibere Praeparatum *jiang¹ ban⁴ xia⁴* 6–9 g
Paeoniae Radix Rubra *chi⁴ shao² yao⁴* 6–9 g
Glycyrrhizae Radix *gan¹ cao³* 2–3 g
Zingiberis Rhizoma Recens *sheng¹ jiang¹* 2–3 slices
Zizyphi Fructus *da⁴ zao³* 2–3 pieces
Actions and Indications: Dissipates wind-cold; downbears qi, transforms phlegm and suppresses cough. Treats external contraction of wind-cold with cough and expectoration of copious amounts of thin drool-like phlegm, rapid breathing and oppression in the chest.

149 *jin¹ suo³ gu⁴ jing¹ wan²* 金鎖固精丸 169, 218, 225
Golden Lock Essence-Securing Pills
Source: 醫方集解 (*yi¹ fang¹ ji² jie³*)
Astragali Complanati Semen *sha¹ yuan⁴ zi³* 100 g
Euryales Semen *qian⁴ shi²* 100 g
Nelumbinis Stamen *lian² xu¹* 100 g
Fossilia Ossis Mastodi (Draconis Os) *long² gu³* (calcined) 50 g
Ostreae Concha *mu³ li⁴* (calcined) 50 g
Nelumbinis Semen *lian² rou⁴* 200 g
Preparation method: Form into 300 mg pills.
Actions and Indications: Secures the kidney and astringes essence. Treats seminal emission due to spleen vacuity.
Dosage: 10 Pills 3 times a day.

150 *jing¹ fang² bai⁴ du² san³* 荊防敗毒散 54, 134, 194
Schizonepeta and Ledebouriella Toxin-Vanquishing Powder
Source: 攝生眾妙方 (*she⁴ sheng¹ zhong⁴ miao⁴ fang¹*)
Schizonepetae Herba seu Flos *jing¹ jie⁴* 6–9 g
Ledebouriellae Radix *fang² feng¹* 6–9 g
Forsythiae Fructus *lian² qiao²* 2–3 g

Notopterygii Rhizoma *qiang¹ huo²* 6–9 g
Angelicae Duhuo Radix *du² huo²* 6–9 g
Ligustici Rhizoma *chuan¹ xiong¹* 5–6 g
Menthae Herba *bo⁴ he²* 2–3 g
Bupleuri Radix *chai² hu²* 6–9 g
Peucedani Radix *qian² hu²* 6–9 g
Platycodonis Radix *jie² geng³* 3–6 g
Aurantii Fructus *zhi³ ke²* 5–6 g
Poria *fu² ling²* 6–9 g
Glycyrrhizae Radix *gan¹ cao³* 2–5 g
Zingiberis Rhizoma Recens *sheng¹ jiang¹* 3 slices
Preparation method: Decoct with water.
Actions and Indications: Induces sweating and resolves the exterior; dispels wind and relieves pain. Treats external contraction of wind, cold and damp pathogens. Signs: aversion to cold, fever, headache and stiffness of the nape, aching limbs, absence of sweating. Tongue fur: thin and white. Pulse: rapid and floating pulse. Also used for initial-stage reddening of the eyes, mumps and sores when exterior signs are present.

151 *jing¹-jie⁴ lian²-qiao² tang¹* 荊芥連翹湯 134, 194
Schizonepeta and Forsythia Decoction
Source: 一貫堂 (*yi² guan⁴ tang²*)
Schizonepetae Herba seu Flos *jing¹ jie⁴* 1.5 g
Forsythiae Fructus *lian² qiao²* 1.5 g
Ledebouriellae Radix *fang² feng¹* 1.5 g
Angelicae Sinensis Radix *dang¹ gui¹* 1.5 g
Ligustici Rhizoma *chuan¹ xiong¹* 1.5 g
Paeoniae Radix *shao² yao⁴* 1.5 g
Bupleuri Radix *chai² hu²* 1.5–2.5 g
Aurantii Fructus Immaturus *zhi³ shi²* 1.5 g
Scutellariae Radix *huang² qin²* 1.5 g
Coptidis Rhizoma *huang² lian²* 1.5 g
Phellodendri Cortex *huang² bo²* 1.5 g
Menthae Folium *bo⁴ he² ye⁴* 1.5 g
Platycodonis Radix *jie² geng³* 1.5–2.5 g
Glycyrrhizae Radix *gan¹ cao³* 1–1.5
Angelicae Dahuricae Radix *bai² zhi³* 1.5–2.5 g
Gardeniae Fructus 1.5 g
Rehmanniae Radix *di⁴ huang²* 1.5 g
Actions and Indications: Treats chronic rhinitis and chronic tonsillitis.

152 *jiu³ wei⁴ qiang¹-huo² tang¹* 九味羌活湯 91
Nine-Ingredient Notopterygium Decoction
Source: 此事難知 (*ci³ shi⁴ nan² zhi¹*)
Notopterygii Rhizoma *qiang¹ huo²* 4.5 g
Ledebouriellae Radix *fang² feng¹* 3 g
Asiasari Radix *xi⁴ xin¹* 1.5 g
Angelicae Dahuricae Radix *bai² zhi³* 2.5 g
Ligustici Rhizoma *chuan¹ xiong¹* 2.5 g
Atractylodis Rhizoma *cang¹ zhu²* 3 g

Rehmanniae Radix Cruda *sheng¹ di⁴ huang²* 2.5 g
Scutellariae Radix *huang² qin²* 2.5 g
Glycyrrhizae Radix *gan¹ cao³* 2 g
Actions and Indications: Resolves the exterior and dispels damp; clears interior heat. Treats contraction of external wind, cold and damp pathogens. Signs: aversion to cold, fever, absence of sweating, headache and stiff neck, pain in the limbs, thirst and bitter taste in the mouth. Tongue: red. Pulse: rapid and floating.

153 *ju²-pi² tang¹* 橘皮湯 98, 128
Tangerine Peel Decoction
Source: 金匱要略 (*jin¹ gui⁴ yao⁴ lue⁴*)
Citri Exocarpium *ju² pi²* 6 g
Zingiberis Rhizoma Recens *sheng¹ jiang¹* 6 g
Actions and Indications: Treats dry retching and inversion frigidity of the limbs.

154 *ju²-pi² zhi³-shi² sheng¹-jiang¹ tang¹*
橘皮枳實薑湯 98, 125, 128
Tangerine Peel, Unripe Bitter Orange, and Fresh Ginger Decoction
Source: 金匱要略 (*jin¹ gui⁴ yao⁴ lue⁴*)
Citri Exocarpium *ju² pi²* 6 g
Citri Aurantii Fructus Immaturus *zhi³ shi²* 3 g
Zingiberis Rhizoma Recens *sheng¹ jiang¹* 8 g
Preparation method: Decoct in water.
Actions and Indications: Treats chest pain; intercostal neuralgia; dyspnea; pulmonary emphysema.

155 *ju²-pi² zhu²-ru² tang¹* 橘皮竹茹湯 12, 128
Tangerine Peel and Bamboo Shavings Decoction
Source: 金匱要略 (*jin¹ gui⁴ yao⁴ lue⁴*)
Citri Exocarpium *ju² pi²* 6–9 g
Bambusae Caulis in Taeniam *zhu² ru²* 3–6 g
Ginseng Radix *ren² shen¹* (or Codonopsitis Radix *dang³ shen¹*) 6–9 g
Glycyrrhizae Radix *gan¹ cao³* (mix-fried) 3–6 g
Zingiberis Rhizoma Recens *sheng¹ jiang¹* 3–5 slices
Zizyphi Fructus *da⁴ zao³* 3 pieces.
Preparation method: Decoct with water.
Actions and Indications: Harmonizes the stomach and downbears counterflow; boosts qi and clears heat. Treats vacuity due to enduring sickness with stomach vacuity heat, counterflow qi, hiccoughing, nausea and vomiting.

156 *juan¹ bi⁴ tang¹* 蠲痺湯 203
Bi-Alleviating Decoction
Source: 醫學心悟 (*yi¹ xue² xin¹ wu²*)
Notopterygii Rhizoma *qiang¹ huo²* 6–10 g
Angelicae Duhuo Radix *du² huo²* 6–10 g
Gentianae Macrophyllae Radix *qin² jiao¹* 6–10 g
Angelicae Sinensis Radix *dang¹ gui¹* 6–10 g

Ligustici Rhizoma *chuan¹ xiong¹* 6–10 g
Cinnamomi Ramulus *gui⁴ zhi¹* 6–10 g
Saussureae Radix *mu⁴ xiang¹* 3–6 g
Olibanum *ru³ xiang¹* 3–6 g
Glycyrrhizae Radix *gan¹ cao³* (mix-fried) 3–6 g
Mori Ramulus *sang¹ zhi¹* 15–30 g
Piperis Kadsurae Caulis *hai³ feng¹ teng²* 15–30 g
Preparation method: Decoct with water.
Actions and Indications: Dispels wind-damp and relieves bi pain. Treats wind-cold-damp bi, with pain in the limb joints relieved by warmth and exacerbated by cold, and sometimes associated with heaviness and numbness.

157 *jue²-ming²-zi³ san³* 决明子散 165
Fetid Cassia Powder
Source: 聖惠方(*sheng⁴ hui⁴ fang¹*)
Cassiae Torae Semen *jue² ming² zi³* 10 g
Viticis Fructus *man⁴ jing¹ zi³* 10 g
Preparation method: Grind to a powder.
Actions and Indications: Brightens the eyes. Treats dim vision.
Dosage: 3 g 3 times a day after meals.

158 *kai¹ jin⁴ san³* 開噤散 145
Food Denial Powder
Source: 百一選方(*bai³ yi¹ xuan³ fang¹*)
Nelumbinis Semen *shi² lian² zi³*
Preparation method: Grind to a powder.
Actions and Indications: Treats food denial dysentery (dysentery characterized by complete loss of appetite and vomiting of anything ingested).

159 *kong⁴ xian² dan¹* 控涎丹 37, 43, 184
Drool-Controlling Elixir
Alternate name: 子龍丸*zi³ long² wan²* Young Dragon Pills
Source: 三因方 (*san¹ yin¹ fang¹*)
Euphorbiae Kansui Radix *gan¹ sui⁴*
Knoxiae Radix *da⁴ ji³*
Sinapis Semen *bai² jie⁴ zi³*
All agents in equal proportions.
Actions and Indications: Dispels phlegm and rheum. Treats water-rheum collecting in the chest and diaphragm with dull pain in the chest and lateral costal region, cough; phlegm-drool congestion with wood saw rasping sound in the throat. Dosage: 1–2 g taken with water twice a day after meals.

160 *ku³-shen¹ tang¹* 苦參湯 66
Bitter Ginseng Decoction
Source:金匱要略 (*jin¹ gui⁴ yao⁴ lue⁴*)
Sophorae Flavescentis Radix *ku³ shen¹* 6–10 g
Actions and Indications: Treats Hongkong foot with

severe itching.

161 *kuan³-dong¹-hua¹ tang¹* 款多花湯 112
Tussilago Decoction
Source:聖濟總錄(*sheng⁴ ji⁴ zong³ lu⁴*)
Tussilaginis Farfarae Flos *kuan³ dong¹ hua¹* 20 g
Fritillariae Bulbus *bei⁴ mu³* 5 g
Glycyrrhizae Radix *gan¹ cao³* (mix-fried) 5 g
Mori Radicis Cortex *sang¹ bai² pi²* 5 g
Anemarrhenae Rhizoma *zhi¹ mu³* 1 g
Armeniacae Semen *xing⁴ ren²* 3 g
Schisandrae Fructus *wu³ wei⁴ zi³* 5 g
Actions and Indications: Treats fulminant cough.

162 *lei²-wan² san³* 雷丸散 237
Omphalia Powder
Source:聖濟總錄(*sheng⁴ ji⁴ zong³ lu⁴*)
Omphaliae *lei² wan²*
Ligustici Rhizoma *chuan¹ xiong¹*
Both agents in equal proportions.
Actions and Indications: Expels worms.

163 *ling² gan¹ jiang¹ wei⁴ xin¹ xia⁴ ren² tang¹* 苓甘薑味辛夏仁湯 151
Poria, Licorice, Ginger, Schisandra, Pinellia, and Apricot Kernel Decoction
Source: 金匱要略 (*jin¹ gui⁴ yao⁴ lue⁴*)
Poria *fu² ling²* 4 g
Pinelliae Tuber *ban⁴ xia⁴* 4 g
Armeniacae Semen *xing⁴ ren²* 4 g
Glycyrrhizae Radix *gan¹ cao³* 2 g
Zingiberis Rhizoma *gan¹ jiang¹* 2 g
Asiasari Radix *xi⁴ xin¹* 2 g
Schisandrae Fructus *wu³ wei⁴ zi³* 3 g
Actions and Indications: Treats acute and chronic bronchitis and bronchial asthma; pulmonary emphysema; edema; ascites; chronic nephritis; leg qi; pulmonary edema.

164 *ling²-jiao³ gou¹-teng² tang¹* 羚角鉤藤湯 12, 20, 207
Antelope Horn and Uncaria Decoction
Source:通俗傷寒論(*tong¹ su² shang¹ han² lun⁴*)
Antelopis Cornu *ling² yang² jiao³* (grated) 0.3–0.6 g
Uncariae Ramulus et Uncus *gou¹ teng²* (add near end) 9–15 g
Chrysanthemi Chuzhouensis Flos *chu² ju²* 9–15 g
Mori Folium Praeustum *jing¹ shuang¹ sang¹ ye⁴* 9–12 g
Rehmanniae Succus Radicis *xian¹ sheng¹ di⁴ zhi¹* 15–30 g
Paeoniae Radix Alba Cruda *sheng¹ bai² shao²* 9–12 g
Glycyrrhizae Radix *gan¹ cao³* 3 g
Fritillaria Cirrhosae Bulbus *chuan¹ bei⁴ mu³* 6–9 g
Bambusae Caulis in Taeniam *zhu² ru²* 6–12 g

Poria cum Pini Radice *fu² shen²*   9–12 g

Preparation method: Decoct with water.

Actions and Indications: Clears the liver and extinguishes wind; calms and downbears liver yang. Treats: 1) Warm heat disease with pathogen heat damaging the liver channel giving rise to high fever and clouded spirit, vexation, agitation and oppression, and convulsive spasm of the limbs developing into tetanic inversion. Tongue: crimson and dry. Pulse: fine, wiry and rapid. 2) Ascendant liver yang with headache, dizziness, and tremor.

165 *ling²-yang²-jiao³ wan²* 羚羊角丸 207
Antelope Horn Pills

Source: 聖濟總錄 (*sheng⁴ ji⁴ zong³ lu⁴*)

Antelopis Cornu *ling² yang² jiao³*   3 g

Rhinocerotis Cornu *xi¹ jiao³*   1 g

Notopterygii Rhizoma *qiang¹ huo²*   4.5 g

Ledebouriellae Radix *fang² feng¹*   4.5 g

Coicis Semen *yi⁴ yi³ ren²* (stir-fried)   6 g

Gentianae Macrophyllae Radix *qin² jiao¹*   6gr

Preparation method: Grind to a fine powder, blend with honey, and form into pills the size of firmiana seeds (*wu² tong² zi³*).

Actions and Indications: Treats shaky hands in wind stroke.

Dosage: 20 pills at a time.

166 *liu⁴ jun¹ zi³ tang¹* 六君子湯 40, 236
Six Gentlemen Decoction

New name: 健脾化痰湯 *jian⁴ pi² hua⁴ tan² tang¹* spleen-Fortifying Phlegm-Transforming Decoction

Source: 醫學正傳 (*yi¹ xue² zheng⁴ chuan²*)

Ginseng Radix *ren² shen¹*   4 g

Atractylodis Ovatae Rhizoma *bai² zhu²*   4 g

Poria *fu² ling²*   4 g

Glycyrrhizae Radix *gan¹ cao³*   1 g

Citri Exocarpium *chen² pi²*   2 g

Pinelliae Tuber *ban⁴ xia⁴*   4 g

Actions and Indications: Boosts qi and fortifies the spleen; harmonizes the stomach and transforms phlegm. Treats spleen-stomach qi vacuity with no thought of food and drink, qi distention in the venter and abdomen, vomiting, acid regurgitation, thin stool, dizziness, palpitations, or cough with copious phlegm.

167 *liu⁴ shen² wan²* 六神丸 211, 216
Six Spirits Pills

Source: 中國醫學大辭典 (*zhong¹ guo² yi¹ xue² da⁴ ci² dian³*)

Moschus *she⁴ xiang¹*   0.3 g

Bovis Calculus *niu² huang²*   0.5 g

Borneolum *bing¹ pian⁴*   3 g

Margarita *zhen¹ zhu¹*   5 g

Bufonis Venenum *chan² su¹*   3 g

Realgar *xiong² huang²*   3 g

Actions and Indications: Resolves toxin; disperses swelling. Treats throat moth, sore throat, diphtheria, putrefying throat sha, yong, ju, clove sores, and innominate swollen toxin sores.

168 *liu⁴ wei⁴ di⁴-huang² wan²* 六味地黃丸 59, 130
Six-Ingredient Rehmannia Pills

Original name: 地黃丸 *di⁴-huang² wan²* Rehmannia Pills

Source: 小兒藥證直訣 (*xiao³ er² yao⁴ zheng⁴ zhi² jue²*)

Rehmanniae Radix Conquita *shou² di⁴ huang²* 240 g

Corni Fructus *shan¹ zhu¹ yu²* 120 g

Dioscoreae Rhizoma *shan¹ yao⁴* 120 g

Alismatis Rhizoma *ze² xie⁴* 90 g

Moutan Radicis Cortex *mu³ dan¹ pi²* 90 g

Poria *fu² ling²* 90 g

Actions and Indications: Enriches yin and supplements the kidney. Treats insufficiency of kidney yin with weak, aching lumbus and knees, dizziness, deafness, tinnitus, spontaneous or night sweating, seminal emission or dream emissions, wasting thirst, sore throat and oss of voice, loosening fo the teeth, pain in the heel, red tongue, dry mouth. In children, the signs are poor development and non-closure of the fontanels.

169 *liu⁴ wei⁴ xiang¹-ru² yin³* 六味香薷飲 173
Six Ingredient Elsholtzia Beverage

Source: 醫方集解 (*yi¹ fang¹ ji² jie³*)

This is Elsholtzia Powder (*xiang¹-ru² san³*) with plus Poria (*fu² ling²*) and Glycyrrhizae Radix (*gan¹ cao³*).

Actions and indications: Dispels summerheat in the exterior; transforms damp and harmonizes the center; relieves leg cramp. Treats Elsholtzia Powder patterns with cramp in the legs.

170 *liu⁴ yi¹ san³* 六一散 232
Six-To-One Powder

Source: 傷寒標本 (*shang¹ han² biao¹ ben³*)

Talcum *hua² shi²*   60 g

Glycyrrhizae Radix Cruda *sheng¹ gan¹ cao³*   10 g

Preparation method: Take mixed with warm water and a little honey or decoct in a cloth bag.

Actions and Indications: Clears summerheat and disinhibits damp. Treats downpour of damp-heat into the lower burner with difficult voidings of dark-colored urine; or contraction of summerheat-damp with fever, vexation, thirst, and short voidings of dark-colored urine.

171 *long¹-gu³ er²-cha² san³* 龍骨兒茶散 200
Dragon Bone and Cutch Powder

Source: 實用正骨學(*shi² yong⁴ zheng⁴ gu³ xue²*)
Fossilia Ossis Mastodi (Draconis Os), *long² gu³*
(calcined)
Elephantis Corium *xiang⁴ pi²*
Saxum Calcareum Vetum *chen² shi² hui¹*
Pini Resina Praeparata Veta *lao³ song¹ xiang¹*
Dalbergiae Ligni Pulvis *jiang⁴ xiang¹ mo⁴*
Draconis Sanguis *xue⁴ jie²*
Catechu Atrum *er² cha² gao¹*
Bletillae Striatae Tuber *bai² ji²*
All agents in equal proportions.
Preparation method: All agents in equal proportions.
Grind to a powder, and apply topically.
Actions and Indications: Staunches bleeding.

172 *long²-dan³ xie⁴ gan¹ tang¹* 龍膽瀉肝湯 ..16, 39
Gentian Liver-Draining Decoction
Source: 醫宗金鑑(*yi¹ zong¹ jin¹ jian⁴*)
Gentianae Scabrae Radix *long² dan³* 3-9 g
Scutellariae Radix *huang² qin²* 6-12 g
Gardeniae Fructus *shan¹ zhi¹ zi³* 6-12 g
Bupleuri Radix *chai² hu²* 3-9 g
Angelicae Sinensis Radix *dang¹ gui¹* 6-12 g
Rehmanniae Radix Cruda *sheng¹ di⁴ huang²* 9-15 g
Plantaginis Semen *che¹ qian² zi³* 9-15 g
Alismatis Rhizoma *ze² xie⁴* 6-12 g
Mutong Caulis *mu⁴ tong¹* 3-6 g
Glycyrrhizae Radix *gan¹ cao³* 3-6 g
Preparation method: Decoct with water
Actions and Indications: Drains liver and gallbladder
fire; clears heat and disinhibits damp. Treats: 1) Liver-
gallbladder repletion heat characterized by headache,
red eyes, bitter taste in the mouth, lateral costal pain,
painful swelling of the ears and deafness. 2) Downpour
of damp-heat manifesting as strangury, swelling of the
scrotum, genital itch, or vaginal discharge.

173 *lu²-hui⁴ wan²* 蘆薈丸 195
Aloe Pills
Source: 本草切要(*ben³ cao³ qie⁴ yao⁴*)
Aloe *lu² hui⁴* 1 g
Pinelliae Tuber Crudum *sheng¹ ban⁴ xia⁴* (stir-fried
   with ginger juice) 3 g
Atractylodis Ovatae Rhizoma *bai² zhu²* 3 g
Glycyrrhizae Radix *gan¹ cao³* (stir-fried) 1.4 g
Preparation method: Gind to a powder, blend with
honey, and form into 300 mg. pills.
Actions and Indications: Treats epilepsy. Dosage: 5-10
pills 1-3 times a day. Half dose for infants.

174 *ma²-huang² fu⁴-zi³ xi⁴-xin¹ tang¹*
        麻黃附子細辛湯................................26, 190
Ephedra, Aconite, and Asarum Decoction
Source: 傷寒論 (*shang¹ han² lun⁴*)

Ephedrae Herba *ma² huang²* 3-6 g
Aconiti Tuber Laterale *fu⁴ zi³* 6-10 g
Asiasari Radix *xi⁴ xin¹* 2-3 g
Actions and Indications: Reinforces yang and resolves
the exterior. Treats contraction of external wind-cold
in patients suffering from yang vacuity, with signs such
as pronounced aversion to cold, slight fever, absence
of sweating, and headache. Pulse: deep rather than
floating.

175 *ma²-huang² tang¹* 麻黃湯 162, 190
Ephedra Decoction
Source: 傷寒論(*shang¹ han² lun⁴*)
Ephedrae Herba *ma² huang²* 3-9 g
Cinnamomi Ramulus *gui⁴ zhi¹* 3-9 g
Armeniacae Semen *xing⁴ ren²* 6-12 g
Glycyrrhizae Radix *gan¹ cao³* 2-5 g
Preparation method: Decoct with water.
Actions and Indications: Induces sweating and resolves
the exterior; perfuses the lung and calms dyspnea.
Treats wind-cold contraction with fever, aversion to
cold, absence of sweating, cough and dyspnea,
headache and generalized pain. Pulse: tight and
floating. Tongue fur: thin and white.

176 *ma² xing⁴ gan¹ shi² tang¹* 麻杏甘石湯
        ....44, 162, 190, 226
**Ephedra, Apricot Kernel, Licorice, and Gypsum
Decoction**
Source: 傷寒論 (*shang¹ han² lun⁴*)
Ephedrae Herba *ma² huang²* 4 g
Armeniacae Semen *xing⁴ ren²* 3 g
Gypsum *shi² gao¹* 10 g
Glycyrrhizae Radix *gan¹ cao³* 2 g
Actions and Indications: Clears heat; diffuses the lung;
calms dyspnea. Treats pathogen heat congesting the
lung with cough, dyspnea, vexation, agitation, and
thirst.

177 *ma² xing⁴ yi⁴ gan¹ tang¹* 麻杏薏甘湯 166
**Ephedra, Apricot Kernel Coix, and Licorice
Decoction**
Source: 金匱要略 (*jin¹ gui⁴ yao⁴ lue⁴*)
Ephedrae Herba *ma² huang²* 4 g
Armeniacae Semen *xing⁴ ren²* 3 g
Coicis Semen *yi⁴ yi³ ren²* 10 g
Glycyrrhizae Radix *gan¹ cao³* 2 g
Actions and Indications: Treats myalgia, neuralgia,
and pain in the joints.

178 *ma²-zi³-ren² wan²* 麻子仁丸 164
Cannabis Seed Pills
Alternate names:脾約麻仁丸*pi² yue¹ ma²-ren² wan²*
Cannabis Splenic Jam Pills

Source: 傷寒論 (shang[1] han[2] lun[4])
Cannabis Semen huo[3] ma[2] ren[2] 125 g
Armeniacae Semen xing[4] ren[2] 125 g
Rhei Rhizoma da[4] huang[2] 125 g
Magnoliae Cortex hou[4] po[4] 125 g
Aurantii Fructus Immaturus zhi[3] shi[2] 60 g
Paeoniae Radix Alba bai[2] shao[3] yao[4] 90 g
Actions and Indications: Moistens the intestines and frees the stool. Treats dryness-heat in the stomach and intestines, with constipation, distention and fullness in the venter and abdomen, pain in the abdomen. Also used for constipation with hemorrhoids.

179 ma[3]-dou[1]-ling[2] san[3] 馬兜鈴散 124
Aristolochia Fruit Powder
Source: 證治準繩 (zheng[4] zhi[4] zhun[3] sheng[2])
Aristolochiae Fructus ma[3] dou[1] ling[2] 5 g
Platycodonis Radix jie[2] geng[3] 5 g
Ginseng Radix ren[2] shen[1] 5 g
Glycyrrhizae Radix gan[1] cao[3] 5 g
Fritillariae Bulbus bei[4] mu[3] 5 g
Perillae Folium zi[3] su[1] ye[4] 10 g
Arecae Pericarpium da[4] fu[4] pi[2] 10 g
Citri Exocarpium chen[2] pi[2] 10 g
Mori Radicis Cortex sang[1] bai[2] pi[2] 10 g
Schisandrae Fructus wu[3] wei[4] zi[3] 2.5 g
Preparation method: Grind to a powder.
Actions and Indications: Treats congestion of fetal qi in pregnant women, with cough and rapid dyspneic breathing.
Dosage: 3 g 3 times a day.

180 mai[4]-men[2]-dong[1] tang[1] 麥門冬湯 50
Ophiopogon Decoction
Source: 金匱要略 (jin[1] gui[4] yao[1] lue[4])
Ophiopogonis Tuber mai[4] men[2] dong[1] 9–18 g
Ginseng Radix ren[2] shen[1] 9–12 g
Pinelliae Tuber ban[4] xia[4] 5–6 g
Glycyrrhizae Radix gan[1] cao[3] 3–5 g
Oryzae Semen geng[1] mi[3] 12–15 g
Zizyphi Fructus da[4] zao[3] 4–5 pieces.
Actions and Indications: Enriches yin and nourishes the stomach; downbears counterflow and precipitates qi. Treats damage to lung and stomach yin with qi fire accending counterflow, characterized by coughing up of drool and foam, dry mouth and pharynx, red tongue with scant fur, a rapid, and vacuous pulse; also treats patterns involving vomiting or hiccough.

181 mai[4]-men[2]-dong[1] yin[3] zi[3] 麥門冬飲子 50, 69
Ophiopogon Drink
Source: 宣明論 (xuan[1] ming[2] lun[4])
Ophiopogonis Tuber mai[4] men[2] dong[1] 3.5 g
Ginseng Radix ren[2] shen[1] 3.5 g
Anemarrhenae Rhizoma zhi[1] mu[3] 3.5 g

Rehmanniae Radix Exsiccata gan[1] di[4] huang[2] 3 g
Poria fu[2] ling[2] 2.5 g
Schisandrae Fructus wu[3] wei[4] zi[3] 2 g
Trichosanthis Radix tian[1] hua[1] fen[3] 2 g
Puerariae Radix ge[2] gen[1] 2 g
Glycyrrhizae Radix gan[1] cao[3] 2 g
Lophatheri Folium zhu[2] ye[4] 1 g
Actions and Indications: Treats wasting thirst with vexation.

182 man[4]-jing[1]-zi[3] san[3] 蔓菁子散 93
Daikon Seed Powder
Source: 聖惠方 (sheng[4] hui[4] fang[1])
Raphani Semen man[4] jing[1] zi[3] 20 g
Polygonati Rhizoma huang[2] jing[1] 10 g
Preparation method: Grind to a powder.
Actions and Indications: Brightens the eyes; supplements liver qi.
Dosage: 1.5 g twice a day.

183 mao[2]-gen[1] tang[1] 茅根湯 87
Imperata Decoction
Source: 小品方 (xiao[3] pin[3] fang[1])
Imperatae Rhizoma bai[2] mao[2] gen[1] 5 g
Puerariae Radix ge[2] gen[1] 5 g
Preparation method: Decoct with water.
Actions and Indications: Treats sudden cold and vomiting after drinking water in warm disease with fever.

184 mi[4] jing[1] wan[2] 秘精丸 159
Essence-Containing Pills
Allii Tuberosi Semen jiu[3] zi[3]
Cuscutae Semen tu[4] si[1] zi[3]
Fossilia Ossis Mastodi (Draconis Os) long[2] gu[3]
Ostreae Concha mu[3] li[4]
Schisandrae Fructus wu[3] wei[4] zi[3]
Mantidis Ootheca sang[1] piao[1] xiao[1]
Kaolin bai[2] shi[2] zhi[1]
Poria fu[2] ling[2]
Preparation method: All agents in equal proportion. grind to a powder, cook with honey, and form into pills.
Actions and Indications: Invigorates yang and secures essence. Treats impotence and seminal emission.

185 mi[4]-meng[2]-hua[1] san[3] 密蒙花散 105
Buddleia Powder
Source: 太平惠方 (tai[4] ping[2] hui[4] fang[1])
Buddleiae Flos mi[4] meng[2] hua[1]
Notopterygii Rhizoma qiang[1] huo[2]
Chrysanthemi Flos ju[2] hua[1]
Haliotidis Concha shi[2] jue[2] ming[2]
Tribuli Fructus ci[4] ji[2] li[2]

Equiseti Herba *mu⁴ zei²*
All agents in equal proportions.
Preparation method: Grind to a fine powder.
Actions and Indications: Treats liver-gallbladder vacuity with eye screens and aversion to light. Dosage: 3 g after meals.

186 *mo⁴-shi²-zi³ wan²* 沒食子丸....................198
Aleppo Gall Pills
Source: 和劑局方 (*he² ji⁴ ju² fang¹*)
Sanguisorbae Radix *di⁴ yu²* 1.5 g
Galla Halepensis *mo⁴ shi² zi³* 1.5 g
Phellodendri Cortex *huang² bo²* (stir-fried with honey) 6 g
Coptidis Rhizoma *huang² lian²* (stir-fried) 4.5 g
Granati Pericarpium *shi² liu² pi²* 3 g
Preparation method: Grind to a powder, cook with vinegar to form into a paste, and form into 100 mg. pills. Actions and Indications: Treats diarrhea and abdominal pain in children.
Dosage: 10–20 pills before meals.

187 *mu³-li⁴ san³* 牡蠣散 218
Oyster Shell Powder
Source: 和劑局方 (*he² ji⁴ ju² fang¹*)
Ostreae Concha *mu³ li⁴* 15–30 g
Astragali Radix *huang² qi²* 9–12 g
Ephedrae Radix *ma² huang² gen¹* 3–9 g
Tritici Semen Leve *fu² xiao³ mai4* 15 g
Actions and Indications: Boosts qi and secures the exterior; constrains yin and checks perspiration. Treats night or spontaneous sweating due to vacuity.

188 *mu⁴-bie¹-zi³ wan²* 木鱉子丸 175
Momordica Pills
Source: 楊氏方 (*yang² shi⁴ fang¹*)
Aquilariae Lignum *chen² xiang¹* 2 g
Aurantii Fructus *zhi³ ke²* 8 g
Trogopteri seu Pteromi Excrementum *wu³ ling² zhi¹* 8 g
Momordicae Semen *mu⁴ bie² zi³* 8 g
Preparation method: Grind to powder and mix, boil in vinegar, and make into pills with flour dough.
Actions and Indications: Treats enduring diarrhea and prolapse of the anus in children.

189 *mu⁴- gua¹ wan²* 木瓜丸 126
Chaenomeles Pills
Source: 聖惠方 (*sheng⁴ hui⁴ fang¹*)
Chaenomelis Fructus *mu⁴ gua¹* 10 g
Citri Exocarpium *ju² pi²* 10 g
Ginseng Radix *ren² shen¹* 10 g
Cinnamomi Cortex Rasus *gui⁴ xin¹* 5 g
Caryophylli Flos *ding¹ xiang¹* 5 g

Arecae Semen *bin¹ lang²* 20 g
Preparation method: Grind to a find powder, blend with honey, and form into 300 mg pills.
Actions and Indications: Treats damp leg qi, and phlegm counterflow.
Dosage: 10 pills 3 times a day with a decoction of ginger.

190 *mu⁴-xiang¹ bin¹-lang² wan²* 木香檳榔丸
....63, 97, 161
Saussurea and Areca Pills
Source: 醫方集解 (*yi¹ fang¹ ji² jie³*)
Saussureae Radix *mu⁴ xiang¹* 30 g
Arecae Semen *bin¹ lang²* 30 g
Citri Exocarpium Immaturum *qing¹ pi²* 30 g
Citri Exocarpium *chen² pi²* 30 g
Aurantii Fructus *zhi³ ke²* 30 g
Zedoariae Rhizoma *e² zhu²* 30 g
Sparganii Rhizoma *san¹ leng²* 30 g
Rhei Rhizoma *da⁴ huang²* 90 g
Coptidis Rhizoma *huang² lian²* 90 g
Phellodendri Cortex *huang² bo²* 90 g
Cyperi Rhizoma *xiang¹ fu⁴ zi³* 90 g
Pharbitidis Semen *qian¹ niu² zi³* 120 g
Mirabilitum *mang² xiao¹* 60 g
Preparation method: Can also be prepared as a decoction.
Actions and Indications: Moves qi and abducts stagnation; drains heat and frees stool. Treats food accumulation and qi stagnation with damp and heat obstructing each other, giving rise to distention, fullness and sometimes pain in the venter and abdomen, slimy tongue fur, and constipation. Can also be used for the initial stages of dysenteric disease with tenesmus and stagnation in the digestive tract.
Dosage: 5–9 g twice daily.

191 *niu²-bang⁴-zi³ san³* 牛蒡子散 122
Arctium Powder
Source: 本事方 (*ben³ shi⁴ fang¹*)
Arctii Fructus *niu² bang⁴ zi³* 30 g
Sojae Semen Praeparatum *dan⁴ dou⁴ chi³* (stir-fried) 30 g
Notopterygii Rhizoma *qiang¹ huo²* 30 g
Rehmanniae Radix *di⁴ huang²* 15 g
Astragali Radix *huang² qi²* 15 g
Preparation method: Grind all constituents to a fine powder.
Actions and Indications: Treats hypertonicity of the limbs.
Dosage: Take 3 g 3 times a day.

192 *niu² che¹ shen⁴ qi⁴ wan²* 牛車腎氣丸...21, 180
Achyranthes and Plantago Kidney Qi Pills

Source: 濟生方 (ji⁴ sheng¹ fang¹)
Rehmanniae Radix Conquita shou² di⁴ huang²   5 g
Dioscoreae Rhizoma shan¹ yao⁴ 3 g
Corni Fructus shan¹ zhu¹ yu² 3 g
Poria fu² ling² 3 g
Moutan Radicis Cortex mu³ dan¹ pi² 3 g
Alismatis Rhizoma ze² xie⁴ 3 g
Achyranthis Bidentatae Radix niu² xi¹ 3 g
Plantaginis Semen che¹ qian² zi³ 3 g
Aconiti Tuber Laterale fu⁴ zi³ 0.5 g
Cinnamomi Ramulus gui⁴ zhi¹ 1 g
Actions and Indications: Treats nephritis; albuminuria; nocturia; arteriosclerosis; hypertension; diabetes mellitus; sciatica; amnesia; dream emissions.

193 niu²-huang² qing¹ xin¹ wan² 牛黃清心丸 ..209
Bovine Bezoar Heart-Clearing Pills
Source: 痘疹心法 (dou⁴ zhen³ xin¹ fa³)
Bezoar Bovis niu² huang² 0.25 g
Cinnabaris zhu¹ sha¹ 1.5 g
Coptidis Rhizoma huang² lian² 5 g
Scutellariae Radix huang² qin² 2.5 g
Gardeniae Fructus shan¹ zhi¹ zi³ 3 g
Curcumae Tuber yu⁴ jin¹ 1–2 g
Preparation method: Form into 500 mg pills.
Actions and Indications: Clears heat and resolves toxin; opens the portals and quiets the spirit. Treats heat entering the pericardium, clouded spirit and delirious speech, vexation and agitation, and fright inversion.
Dosage: 1–2 pills 1–2 times a day.

194 niu²-xi¹ san³ 牛膝散 21
Achyranthes Powder
Source: 婦人良方 (fu⁴ ren² liang² fang¹)
Achyranthis Bidentatae Radix niu² xi¹ 3 g
Cinnamomi Ramulus gui⁴ zhi¹ 3 g
Paeoniae Radix shao² yao⁴ 3 g
Persicae Semen tao² ren² 3 g
Angelicae Sinensis Radix dang¹ gui¹ 3 g
Moutan Radicis Cortex mu³ dan¹ pi² 3 g
Corydalis Tuber yan² hu² suo³ 3 g
Saussureae Radix mu⁴ xiang¹ 1 g
Actions and Indications: Treats dysmenorrhea and painful menstruation.

195 nü³-zhen¹ tang¹ 女貞湯 140
Ligustrum Decoction
Source: 醫醇賸义 (yi¹ chun² sheng⁴ cha¹)
Ligustri Fructus nü³ zhen¹ zi³ 2 g
Rehmanniae Radix Cruda sheng¹ di⁴ huang² 3 g
Testudinis Plastrum gui¹ ban³ 3 g
Angelicae Sinensis Radix dang¹ gui¹ 2 g
Poria fu² ling² 2 g
Dendrobii Caulis shi² hu² 2 g

Trichosanthis Radix tian¹ hua¹ fen³ 2 g
Dioscoreae Hypoglaucae Rhizoma bei¹ xie⁴ 2 g
Achyranthis Bidentatae Radix niu² xi¹ 2 g
Plantaginis Semen che¹ qian² zi³ 2 g
Preparation method: Decoct with water.
Actions and Indications: Treats turbid strangury with pain on urination and weak, aching lumbus.

196 ping² wei⁴ san³ 平胃散 7, 77, 128
Stomach-Calming Powder
Source: 和劑局方 (he² ji⁴ ju² fang¹)
Atractylodis Rhizoma cang¹ zhu¹ 6–9 g
Magnoliae Cortex hou⁴ po⁴ 3–6 g
Citri Exocarpium chen² pi² 3–6 g
Glycyrrhizae Radix gan¹ cao³ 3 g
Zingiberis Rhizoma Recens sheng¹ jiang¹ 3 g
Zizyphi Fructus da⁴ zao³ 2 pieces
Preparation method: Originally prepared as a powder, but now usually prepared in decoction form.
Actions and Indications: Dries damp and fortifies the spleen. Treats damp encumbering the stomach and spleen with distention and fullness in the venter and abdomen, bland taste in the mouth, reduced food intake, fatigued limbs, and thin stool. Tongue fur: white and slimy or thick slimy and moist.

197 qi¹ wu⁴ jiang⁴ xia⁴ tang¹ 七物降下湯 20
Seven Agents Downbearing Decoction
Source: 修琴堂 (xiu¹ qin² tang²)
Angelicae Sinensis Radix dang¹ gui¹ 3–4 g
Paeoniae Radix shao² yao⁴ 3–4 g
Ligustici Rhizoma chuan¹ xiong¹ 3–4 g
Rehmanniae Radix di⁴ huang² 3–4 g
Uncariae Ramulus et Uncus gou¹ teng² 3–4 g
Astragali Radix huang² qi² 2–3 g
Phellodendri Cortex huang² bo² 2 g
Preparation method: Decoct with water.
Actions and Indications: General vacuity with tendency to hypertension, counterflow ascent, shoulder pain, and tinnitus.

198 qi³ ju² di⁴-huang² wan² 杞菊地黃丸 109, 142
Lycium, Chrysanthemum, and Rehmannia Pills
Source: 醫級 (yi¹ ji²)
Variant of 六味地黃丸 liu⁴ wei⁴ di⁴-huang² wan²
Rehmannia Six Pills
Rehmanniae Radix Conquita shou² di⁴ huang² 40 g
Corni Fructus shan¹ zhu¹ yu² 20 g
Dioscoreae Rhizoma shan¹ yao⁴ 20 g
Alismatis Rhizoma ze² xie⁴ 15 g
Moutan Radicis Cortex mu³ dan¹ pi² 15 g
Poria fu² ling² 15 g
Lycii Fructus gou³ qi³ zi³ 15 g
Chrysanthemi Flos ju² hua¹ 10 g

Actions and Indications: Enriches yin and supplements the kidney; nourishes the liver and brightens the eyes. Treats insufficiency of liver and kidney with dizziness, poor vision, wasting thirst, and high blood pressure.

199 *qi³ pi² tang¹* 啓脾湯 131
Spleen-Arousing Decoction
Source: 萬病回春 (*wan⁴ bing⁴ hui² chun¹*)
Ginseng Radix *ren² shen¹* 3 g
Atractylodis Ovatae Rhizoma *bai² zhu²* 4 g
Poria *fu² ling²* 4 g
Nelumbinis Semen *lian² rou⁴* 3 g
Citri Exocarpium *chen² pi²* 2 g
Crataegi Fructus *shan¹ zha¹* 2 g
Glycyrrhizae Radix *gan¹ cao³* 1 g
Alismatis Rhizoma *ze² xie⁴* 2 g
Zizyphi Fructus *da⁴ zao³* 1 g
Zingiberis Rhizoma Recens *sheng¹ jiang¹* 3 g
Actions and Indications: Fortifies the spleen and disperses food; checks diarrhea and disinhibits urine. Treats spleen-stomach vacuity with fatigue and lack of strength, indigestion, and diarrhea.

200 *qian¹ jin¹ wei³ jing¹ tang¹*千金葦莖湯163, 166
Thousand Gold Pieces Phragmites Decoction
Source: 千金方 (*qian¹ jin¹ fang¹*)
Phragmititis Caulis *lu² jing¹* 3 g
Coicis Semen *yi⁴ yi³ ren²* (stir-fried) 10 g
Persicae Semen *tao² ren²* 3 g
Benincasae Semen *dong¹ gua¹ zi³* 5 g
Actions and Indications: Treats pulmonary yong characterized by vexation and fullness, cough and mild fever.

201 *qian¹-niu² wan²* 牽牛丸 178
Morning Glory Pills
Source: 楊氏方 (*yang² shi⁴ fang¹*)
Corydalis Tuber *yan² hu² suo³* 20 g
Psoraleae Semen *bu³ gu³ zhi¹* (stir-fried) 20 g
Pharbitidis Semen Atrum *hei¹ chou³* (stir-fried) 30 g
Preparation method: Grind all agents to a fine powder, mixed with crushed, baked garlic, and form into 300 mg pills.
Actions and Indications: Treats lumbar pain.
Dosage: 15 pills 3 times a day before meals.

202 *qiang¹-huo² bai²-zhi³ san³* 羌活白芷散
....23, 91, 155
Notopterygium and Angelica Powder
Source: 證治準繩 (*zheng⁴ zhi⁴ zhun³ sheng²*)
Notopterygii Rhizoma *qiang¹ huo²* 3 g
Angelicae Dahuricae Radix *bai² zhi³* 3 g
Bupleuri Radix *chai² hu²* 3 g
Schizonepetae Herba seu Flos *jing¹ jie⁴* 3 g

Viticis Fructus *man⁴ jing¹ zi³* 3 g
Ledebouriellae Radix *fang² feng¹* 3 g
Gleditsiae Spina *zao⁴ jiao³ ci⁴* 3 g
Glycyrrhizae Radix *gan¹ cao³* 3 g
Coptidis Rhizoma *huang² lian²* (stir-fried) 3 g
Preparation method: Decoct with water.
Actions and Indications: Treats wind-heat and blood dryness with sores on the head and face.

203 *qiang¹-huo² fang²-feng¹ tang¹* 羌活防風湯
....45, 46, 91
Notopterygium and Ledebouriella Decoction
Source: 病機氣宜 (*bing⁴ ji¹ qi⁴ yi²*)
Notopterygii Rhizoma *qiang¹ huo²* 2 g
Ledebouriellae Radix *fang² feng¹* 2 g
Angelicae Sinensis Radix *dang¹ gui¹* 2 g
Paeoniae Radix *shao² yao⁴* 2 g
Ligustici Sinensis Radix et Rhizoma *gao³ ben³* 2 g
Glycyrrhizae Radix *gan¹ cao³* 2 g
Ligustici Rhizoma *chuan¹ xiong¹* 2 g
Sanguisorbae Radix *di⁴ yu²* 1.5 g
Asiasari Radix *xi⁴ xin¹* 1.5 g
Actions and Indications: Treats lockjaw.

204 *qiang¹-huo² sheng⁴ shi¹ tang¹* 羌活勝濕湯
....46, 91
Notopterygium Dampness-Overcoming Decoction
Source: 內外傷辨惑論 (*nei⁴ wai⁴ shang¹ bian⁴ huo⁴ lun⁴*)
Notopterygii Rhizoma *qiang¹ huo²* 3–10 g
Angelicae Duhuo Radix *du² huo²* 3–10 g
Ligustici Sinensis Radix et Rhizoma *gao³ ben³* 9–12 g
Ledebouriellae Radix *fang² feng¹* 3–10 g
Ligustici Rhizoma *chuan¹ xiong¹* 3–6 g
Viticis Fructus *man⁴ jing¹ zi³* 6–12 g
Glycyrrhizae Radix *gan¹ cao³* 3 g
Actions and Indications: Dispels wind and resolves the exterior; relieves pain. Treats wind-damp in the exterior with headache and heavy-headedness, or generalized pain, aversion to cold with mild fever. Tongue fur: white. Pulse: floating.

205 *qin²-jiao¹ bie¹-jia³ san³* 秦艽鱉甲散......38, 206
Macrophylla and Turtle Shell Powder
Source: 衛生寶鑑 (*wei⁴ sheng¹ bao³ jian⁴*)
Gentianae Macrophyllae Radix *qin² jiao¹* 2 g
Amydae Carapax *bie¹ jia³* 3 g
Lycii Radicis Cortex *di⁴ gu³ pi²* 3 g
Bupleuri Radix *chai² hu²* 3 g
Anemarrhenae Rhizoma *zhi¹ mu³* 2 g
Angelicae Sinensis Radix *dang¹ gui¹* 3 g
Mume Fructus *wu¹ mei²* 2 g
Artemiseae Apiaceae Seu Annuae Folium *qing¹ hao¹ ye⁴* 2 g

Actions and Indications: Enriches yin and nourishes the blood; clears heat and eliminates steam. Treats steaming bone tidal fever, emaciation, night sweating, and red cheeks and lips. Pulse: fine and rapid.

206 *qing¹ gong¹ tang¹* 清宮湯 145
Palace-Clearing Decoction
Source: 溫病條辨 (*wen¹ bing⁴ tiao² bian⁴*)
Rhinocerotis Cornu *xi¹ jiao³* 1.5 g
Scrophulariae Radix *xuan² shen¹* 3 g
Ophiopogonis Tuber *mai⁴ dong¹* 3 g
Forsythiae Fructus *lian² qiao²* ¹ 2 g
Lophatheri Folium *zhu² ye⁴* 2 g
Nelumbinis Plumula *lian² zi³ xin¹* 1 g
Preparation method: Decoct with water.
Actions and Indications: Clears the heart and resolves toxin; nourishes yin and engender liquid. Treats excessive sweating in warm heat disease that causes damage to fluids and allows the pathogen to enter the pericardium, giving rise to clouded spirit and delirious speech. Tongue: red or crimson.

207 *qing¹ ji¹ an¹ hui² tang¹* 清肌安蛔湯 234
Flesh-Clearing Roundworm-Quieting Decoction
Source: 蔓難錄 (*man⁴ nan² lu⁴*)
Bupleuri Radix *chai² hu²* 4–7 g
Pinelliae Tuber *ban⁴ xia⁴* 4–5 g
Zingiberis Rhizoma Recens *sheng¹ jiang¹* 4 g
Ginseng Radix *ren² shen¹* 2–3 g
Scutellariae Radix *huang² qin²* 3 g
Glycyrrhizae Radix *gan¹ cao³* 2 g
Digenea *hai³ ren² cao³* 3 g
Ophiopogonis Tuber *mai⁴ men² dong¹* 3 g
Actions and Indications: Treats roundworm infestation.

208 *qing¹ shang⁴ fang²-feng¹ tang¹* 清上防風湯
.... 45, 192
Upper-Body-Clearing Ledebouriella Decoction
Source: 萬病回春 (*wan⁴ bing⁴ hui² chun¹*)
Ledebouriellae Radix *fang² feng¹* 3.5 g
Schizonepetae Herba seu Flos *jing¹ jie⁴* 1.5 g
Gardeniae Fructus *shan¹ zhi¹ zi³* 1.5 g
Coptidis Rhizoma *huang² lian²* 1.5 g
Menthae Folium *bo⁴ he² ye⁴* 1.5 g
Aurantii Fructus *zhi³ ke²* 1.5 g
Forsythiae Fructus *lian² qiao²* 2.5 g
Angelicae Dahuricae Radix *bai² zhi³* 2.5 g
Platycodonis Radix *jie² geng³* 2.5 g
Ligustici Rhizoma *chuan¹ xiong¹* 2 g
Scutellariae Radix *huang² qin²* 2 g
Glycyrrhizae Radix *gan¹ cao³* 1 g
Actions and Indications: Treats eczema and other skin disease; hyperemia of the eye; drinker's nose; sores and boils on the head and face.

209 *qing¹ shi¹ hua⁴ tan² tang¹* 清濕化痰湯 75
Dampness-Clearing   Phlegm-Transforming Decoction
Source: 壽世保元 (*shou⁴ shi⁴ bao³ yuan²*)
Arisaematis Rhizoma *tian¹ nan² xing¹* 3 g
Pinelliae Tuber *ban⁴ xia⁴* 4 g
Citri Exocarpium *chen² pi²* 2–3 g
Poria *fu² ling²* 4 g
Atractylodis Rhizoma *cang¹ zhu²* 4 g
Notopterygii Rhizoma *qiang¹ huo²* 1.5 g
Scutellariae Radix *huang² qin²* 3 g
Angelicae Dahuricae Radix *bai² zhi³* 1.5 g
Sinapis Semen *bai² jie⁴ zi³* 1.5 g
Glycyrrhizae Radix *gan¹ cao³* 1–1.5 g
Actions and Indications: Treats generalized migratory pain; pain in the chest radiating through to the back.

210 *qing¹ shu³ yi⁴ qi⁴ tang¹* 清暑益氣湯 ... 33, 151
Summerheat-Clearing Qi-Boosting Decoction
Source: 脾胃論 (*pi² wei⁴ lun²*)
Astragali Radix *huang² qi²* 9–12 g
Ginseng Radix *ren² shen¹* (or Codonopsitis Radix *dang³ shen¹*) 9–12 g
Atractylodis Rhizoma *cang¹ zhu²* 6 g
Atractylodis Ovatae Rhizoma *bai² zhu²* 6 g
Ophiopogonis Tuber *mai⁴ dong¹* 9–12 g
Schisandrae Fructus *wu³ wei⁴ zi³* 3–6 g
Puerariae Radix *ge² gen¹* 6–9 g
Citri Exocarpium *chen² pi²* 3–6 g
Citri Exocarpium Immaturum *qing¹ pi²* 3–6 g
Massa Medicata Fermentata *shen² qu¹* 9 g
Angelicae Sinensis Radix *dang¹ gui¹* 6–9 g
Alismatis Rhizoma *ze² xie⁴* 6–9 g
Phellodendri Cortex *huang² bo²* 6–9 g
Glycyrrhizae Radix *gan¹ cao³* 3 g
Cimicifugae Rhizoma *sheng¹ ma²* 3–6 g
Actions and Indications: Clears summerheat and boosts qi; fortifies the spleen and safeguards the lung. Treats contraction of summerheat-damp in patients usually suffering from qi vacuity. Signs include general fever, headache, thirst, spontaneous sweating, fatigued cumbersome limbs, no thought of food or drink, thoracic fullness, heavy body, thin stool, short voidings of dark-colored urine, a soft, vacuous pulse, and a thin, slimy tongue fur.

211 *qing¹ xin¹ lian²-zi³ yin³* 清心蓮子飲 145
Heart-Clearing Lotus Seed Beverage
Source: 和劑局方 (*he² ji⁴ ju² fang¹*)
Nelumbinis Semen *lian² rou⁴* 4 g
Ophiopogonis Tuber *mai⁴ dong¹* 4 g
Scutellariae Radix *huang² qin²* 3 g
Lycii Radicis Cortex *di⁴ gu³ pi²* 2 g
Ginseng Radix *ren² shen¹* 3 g

Astragali Radix *huang² qi²* 2 g
Glycyrrhizae Radix *gan¹ cao³* (mix-fried) 2 g
Poria *fu² ling²* 3 g
Plantaginis Semen *che¹ qian² zi³* 3 g
Actions and Indications: Clears heart heat; boosts qi and yin; treats turbid strangury. Treats effulgent heart fire with qi and yin vacuity, with general signs such as dry mouth, vexing heat in the five hearts, and troubled sleep. Specific patterns include seminal emission, turbid strangury, wasting thirst, uterine bleeding, and vaginal discharge.

212 *qiong² yu⁴ gao¹* 瓊玉膏 33
Fine Jade Paste
Source: 洪氏集驗方 (*hong² shi⁴ ji² yan⁴ fang¹*)
Rehmanniae Radix Cruda *sheng¹ di⁴ huang²* 800 g
Codonopsitis Radix *dang³ shen¹* 72 g
Poria *fu² ling²* 150 g
Mel *feng¹ mi⁴* 320 g
Actions and Indications: Nourishes yin and moistens the lung. Treats lung vacuity with enduring cough, dry throat, expectoration of blood or dry cough without phlegm.

213 *qu¹ zhu² wan²* 麴尢丸 77, 201
Medicated Leaven and Atractylodes Pills
Source: 和劑局方 (*he² ji⁴ ju² fang¹*)
Massa Medicata Fermentata *shen² qu¹* (stir-fried)
Atractylodis Rhizoma *cang¹ zhu²* (steeped in rice water)
Both agents in equal proportions.
Actions and Indications: Treats summerheat diarrhea with glomus and oppression in the chest and diaphragm.

214 *ren²-shen¹ bai⁴ du² san³* 人參敗毒散 54, 55
Ginseng Toxin-Vanquishing Powder
Source: 醫方集解 (*yi¹ fang¹ ji² jie³*)
Ginseng Radix *ren² shen¹* 2 g
Bupleuri Radix *chai² hu²* 2 g
Peucedani Radix *qian² hu²* 2 g
Notopterygii Rhizoma *qiang¹ huo²* 2 g
Angelicae Duhuo Radix *du² huo²* 2 g
Aurantii Fructus *zhi³ ke²* 2 g
Ligustici Rhizoma *chuan¹ xiong¹* 2 g
Platycodonis Radix *jie² geng³* 2 g
Poria *fu² ling²* 2 g
Glycyrrhizae Radix *gan¹ cao³* 1 g
Zingiberis Rhizoma Recens *sheng¹ jiang¹* 1 g
Menthae Herba *bo⁴ he²* 1 g
Actions and Indications: Treats colds and coughs, nasal congestion, and initial-stage yong and sores.

215 *ren²-shen¹ ge²-jie⁴ san³* 人參蛤蚧散 40, 162
Ginseng and Gecko Powder

Source: 衛生寶鑒 (*wei⁴ sheng¹ bao³ jian⁴*)
Gecko *ge² jie⁴* 2 pieces
Armeniacae Semen *xing⁴ ren²* 150 g
Glycyrrhizae Radix *gan¹ cao³* (mix-fried) 150 g
Ginseng Radix *ren² shen¹* 60 g
Poria *fu² ling²* 60 g
Fritillariae Bulbus *bei⁴ mu³* 60 g
Mori Radicis Cortex *sang¹ bai² pi²* 60 g
Anemarrhenae Rhizoma *zhi¹ mu³* 60 g
Actions and Indications: Supplements qi and clears the lung; suppresses cough and calms dyspnea. Treats cough due to enduring sickness, qi ascent with dyspnea and fullness, coughing up of pus and blood, vexation and heat in the chest, and tabid emaciated body.

216 *ren²-shen¹ tang¹* 人參湯 40
Ginseng Decoction
Source: 傷寒論 (*shang¹ han² lun⁴*)
Ginseng Radix *ren² shen¹* 3 g
Zingiberis Rhizoma *gan¹ jiang¹* 3 g
Atractylodis Ovatae Rhizoma *bai² zhu²* 3 g
Glycyrrhizae Radix *gan¹ cao³* 3 g
Actions and Indications: Warms the center and dispels cold; boosts qi and fortifies the spleen. Treats chronic gastroenteritis, gastroptosis, vomiting in pregnancy.

217 *ren²-shen¹ yang³ rong² tang¹* 人參養榮湯 40
Ginseng Construction-Nourishing Decoction
Source: 和劑局方 (*he² ji⁴ ju² fang¹*)
Ginseng Radix *ren² shen¹* 3 g
Astragali Radix *huang² qi²* 2.5 g
Atractylodis Ovatae Rhizoma *bai² zhu²* 4 g
Poria *fu² ling²* 4 g
Glycyrrhizae Radix *gan¹ cao³* 1.5 g
Angelicae Sinensis Radix *dang¹ gui¹* 4 g
Rehmanniae Radix *di⁴ huang²* 2.5 g
Paeoniae Radix *shao² yao⁴* 4 g
Cinnamomi Ramulus *gui⁴ zhi¹* 2.5 g
Schisandrae Fructus *wu³ wei⁴ zi³* 1.5 g
Polygalae Radix *yuan³ zhi⁴* 1.5 g
Citri Exocarpium *chen² pi²* 2.5 g
Zingiberis Rhizoma Recens *sheng¹ jiang¹*
Zizyphi Fructus *da⁴ zao³*
Actions and Indications: Boosts qi and supplements the blood; nourishes the heart and quiets the spirit. Treats vacuity of qi and blood, fatigued spirit and lack of strength, fright palpitations, and insomnia.

218 *run⁴ chang² tang¹* 潤腸湯 164
Intestine-Moistening Decoction
Source: 萬病回春 (*wan⁴ bing⁴ hui² chun¹*)
Angelicae Sinensis Radix *dang¹ gui¹* 3 g
Rehmanniae Radix Conquita *shou² di⁴ huang²* 3 g

Rehmanniae Radix Exsiccata *gan¹ di⁴ huang²* 3 g
Cannabis Semen *huo³ ma² ren²* 3 g
Persicae Semen *tao² ren²* 2 g
Armeniacae Semen *xing⁴ ren²* 2 g
Aurantii Fructus Immaturus *zhi³ shi²* 0.5–2 g
Scutellariae Radix *huang² qin²* 2 g
Magnoliae Cortex *hou⁴ po⁴* 2 g
Rhei Rhizoma *da⁴ huang²* 1–3 g
Glycyrrhizae Radix *gan¹ cao³* 1–1.5 g
Actions and Indications: Nourishes the blood and moistens the intestines. Treats constipation.

219 *san¹-leng² wan²* 三稜丸 96, 97
Sparganium Pills
Source:六科準繩 (*liu⁴ ke¹ zhun³ sheng²*)
Sparganii Rhizoma *san¹ leng²* (stir-fry with vinegar) 10 g
Ligustici Rhizoma *chuan¹ xiong¹* 10 g
Achyranthis Bidentatae Radix *niu² xi¹* 10 g
Corydalis Tuber *yan² hu² suo³* 10 g
Zedoariae Rhizoma *e² zhu²* (stir-fry with vinegar) 10 g
Moutan Cortex Radicis *mu³ dan¹ pi²* 10 g
Daphnes Genkwa Flos *yuan² hua¹* (stir-fry with vinegar) 10 g
Angelicae Dahuricae Radix *bai² zhi³* 10 g
Angelicae Sinensis Radix *dang¹ gui¹* 10 g
Lumbricus *di⁴ long²* (stir-fried after soaking in wine) 10 g
Zingiberis Rhizoma *gan¹ jiang¹* (blast-fried) 10 g
Rhei Rhizoma *da⁴ huang²* 20 g
Preparation method: Grind rhubarb root (Rhei Rhizoma) into a fine powder, and cook with vinegar to form a paste. Grind other agents and blend with rhubarb paste, and form into 300 mg pills.
Actions and Indications: Treats qi pain, vaginal discharge, and blood conglomerations in women.
Dosage: 10 pills on an empty stomach.

220 *san¹ ren² tang¹* 三仁湯 120, 162, 166
Three Kernels Decoction
Source:溫病條辨 (*wen¹ bing¹ tiao² bian⁴*)
Armeniacae Semen *xing⁴ ren²* 9–15 g
Amomi Cardamomi Fructus *bai² dou⁴ kou⁴* 3–6 g
Coicis Semen Crudum *sheng¹ yi⁴ ren²* 9–18 g
Magnoliae Cortex *hou⁴ po⁴* 3–6 g
Tetrapanacis Medulla *tong¹ cao³* 3–6 g
Talcum *hua² shi²* 12–18 g
Lophatheri Herba *zhu² ye⁴* 3–6 g
Pinelliae Tuber *ban⁴ xia⁴* (prepared) 6–9 g
Preparation method: Decoct with water.
Actions and Indications: Diffuses qi; clears heat and disinhibits damp. Treats initial stages of damp warmth or summerheat warmth with damp, in which the

pathogens are in the qi aspect, and the damp is more pronounced than the heat. Signs: oppression in the chest, upflow and nausea, no desire for food, headache, generalized heaviness, postmeridian generalized fever. Tongue fur: white and slimy. Pulse: soggy.

221 *san¹ shen² wan²* 三神丸 81
Three Spirits Pills
Source:濟生方 (*ji⁴ sheng¹ fang¹*)
Corydalis Tuber *yan² hu² suo³* 10 g
Angelicae Sinensis Radix *dang¹ gui¹* 10 g
Citri Exocarpium Rubrum *ju² hong²* 20 g
Preparation method: Grind to a powder, blend with honey, and form into 300 mg. pills.
Actions and Indications: Treats contention between qi and blood in virgins with abdominal pain and menstrual irregularities.
Dosage: 10 pills on an empty stomach.

222 *san¹ sheng¹ yin³* 三生飲 75
Three Raw Agents Beverage
Source:和劑局方 (*he² ji⁴ ju² fang¹*)
Arisaematis Rhizoma Crudum *sheng¹ tian¹ nan² xing¹* 3–6 g
Aconiti Tuber Crudum *sheng¹ chuan¹ wu¹* 1.5–3 g
Aconiti Tuber Laterale Crudum *sheng¹ fu⁴ zi³* 1.5–3 g
Saussureae Radix *mu⁴ xiang¹* 3–6 g
Zingiberis Rhizoma Recens *sheng¹ jiang¹* 3–5 slices
Preparation method: Decoct with water.
Actions and Indications: Dispels wind and transforms phlegm. Treats sudden wind stroke with loss of consciousness, leaving the patient with hemiplegia, wryness of the mouth, and phlegm congesting in the throat. Tongue fur: white and glossy. Pulse: deep or hidden.

223 *san¹ wu⁴ bei⁴ ji² wan²* 三物備急丸 95, 98, 187
Three Agents Emergency Pills
Source:金匱要略 (*jin¹ gui⁴ yao⁴ lue⁴*)
Crotonis Seminis Pulvis *ba¹ dou⁴ shuang¹* 1 g
Rhei Rhizoma *da⁴ huang²* 1 g
Zingiberis Rhizoma *gan¹ jiang¹* 1 g
Actions and Indications: Expels cold accumulations. Treats cold food accumulation with pain and distention in the venter and abdomen, constipation, rapid breathing, green-blue complexion and inversion frigidity of the limbs.

224 *san¹ wu⁴ huang²-qin² tang¹* 三物黃芩湯
....59, 65, 66
Three Agents Scutellaria Decoction
Source:金匱要略 (*jin¹ gui⁴ yao⁴ lue⁴*)

Scutellariae Radix *huang² qin²*   3 g
Sophorae Flavescentis Radix *ku³ shen¹*   3 g
Rehmanniae Radix Exsiccata *gan¹ di⁴ huang²*   6 g
Preparation method: Decoct with water.
Actions and Indications: Treats vexing pain in the limbs, and blood heat.

225 *sang¹ ju² yin³* 桑菊飲 103, 109, 162
Mulberry Leaf and Chrysanthemum Beverage
Source: 溫病條辨 (*wen¹ bing⁴ tiao² bian⁴*)
Mori Folium *sang¹ ye⁴*   6–9 g
Chrysanthemi Flos *ju² hua¹*   6–9 g
Armeniacae Semen *xing⁴ ren²*   6–12 g
Forsythiae Fructus *lian² qiao²*   9–12 g
Menthae Herba *bo⁴ he²* (add near end)   3–5 g
Platycodonis Radix *jie² geng³*   3–6 g
Glycyrrhizae Radix *gan¹ cao³*   2–5 g
Phragmititis Rhizoma *lu² gen¹*   15–30 g
Preparation method: Decoction with water.
Actions and Indications: Courses wind and clears heat; diffuses the lung and suppresses cough. Treats initial-stage wind warmth with cough, unpronounced fever, and slight thirst. Tongue fur: thin. Pulse: floating.

226 *sang¹ ma² wan²* 桑麻丸 103, 183
Mulberry Leaf and Sesame Pills
Alternate name: 扶桑丸 *fu² sang¹ wan²*
Source: 中國醫學大辭典 (*zhong¹ guo² yi¹ xue² da⁴ ci² dian³*)
Mori Folium *sang¹ ye⁴*   80 g
Sesami Semen *hei¹ zhi¹ ma²* 40 g
Preparation method: Crush sesame seeds, blend with honey, add the powdered mulberry leaves, and make into 300 mg pills.
Actions and Indications: Supplements the liver and kidney; clears the head and eyes. Treats yin vacuity and blood dryness, with dizziness, clouded vision, and dry, bound stool.
Dosage: 10 pills on an empty stomach.

227 *sang¹ xing⁴ tang¹* 桑杏湯 103, 162
Mulberry Leaf and Apricot Kernel Decoction
Source: 溫病條辨 (*wen¹ bing⁴ tiao² bian⁴*)
Mori Folium *sang¹ ye⁴*   3 g
Armeniacae Semen *xing⁴ ren²*   3 g
Adenophorae seu Glehniae Radix *sha¹ shen¹*   5 g
Fritillariae Verticillatae Bulbus *zhe⁴ bei⁴ mu³*   3 g
Sojae Semen Praeparatum *dou⁴ chi³*   3 g
Gardeniae Fructus *shan¹ zhi¹ zi³*   3 g
Pyri Exocarpium *li² pi²*   3 g
Actions and Indications: Diffuses dryness heat with light agents; nourishes yin and moistens the lung. Treats external contraction of warm dryness giving rise to headache, generalized fever, dry cough without phlegm or with small amounts of sticky phlegm, and dry mouth. Tongue: red with dry, thin fur.

228 *shan¹-dou⁴-gen¹ tang¹* 山豆根湯 67
Bushy Sophora Root Decoction
Source: 直指方 (*zhi² zhi³ fang¹*)
Sophorae Subprostratae Radix *shan¹ dou⁴ gen¹*
Perillae Folium *zi³ su¹ ye⁴*
In equal proportions.
Preparation method: Decoct with water.
Actions and Indications: Scrofulous lumps.

229 *shao²-yao⁴ gan¹-cao³ tang¹* 芍藥甘草湯 ..42, 51
Peony and Licorice Decoction
Source: 傷寒論 (*shang¹ han² lun⁴*)
Paeoniae Radix *bai² shao² yao⁴*   6 g
Glycyrrhizae Radix *gan¹ cao³*   6 g
Actions and Indications: Relaxes tension and relieves pain. Treats various forms of pain in the venter and abdomen; hypertonicity of the limbs; sciatica; lumbar pain.

230 *she²-chuang²-zi³ san³* 蛇床子散 129
Cnidium Fruit Powder
Source: 婦產科學 (*fu⁴ chan³ ke¹ xue²*)
Cnidii Monnieri Fructus *she² chuang² zi³*   15 g
Sophorae Flavescentis Radix *ku³ shen¹*   15 g
Zanthoxyli Fructus *hua¹ jiao¹*   15 g
Stemonae Radix *bai³ bu⁴*   15 g
Alumen Praeparatum *ku¹ fan²*   15 g
Actions and Indications: Dries damp; kills worms; relieves itching. Treats pudendal itch.

231 *shen¹ ling² bai²-zhu² san³* 參苓白朮散173, 236
Ginseng, Poria, and Atractylodes Ovata Powder
Source: 和劑局方 (*he² ji⁴ ju² fang¹*)
Ginseng Radix *ren² shen¹* (or Codonopsitis Radix *dang³ shen¹*)   1 kg.
Atractylodis Ovatae Rhizoma *bai² zhu²*   1 kg.
Poria *fu² ling²*   1 kg.
Glycyrrhizae Radix *gan¹ cao³* (mix-fried)   1 kg.
Dioscoreae Rhizoma *shan¹ yao⁴*   1. kg.
Lablab Semen *bian³ dou⁴*   500 g
Nelumbinis Semen *lian² rou⁴*   500 g
Platycodonis Radix *jie² geng³*   500 g
Coicis Semen *yi⁴ yi³ ren²*   500 g
Amomi Semen *sha¹ ren²*   500 g
Actions and Indications: Fortifies the spleen and supplements qi; harmonizes the stomach and percolates damp. Treats spleen-stomach vacuity with poor appetite, vomiting or diarrhea, emaciation, lack of strength in the limbs, inhibited feeling in the chest and venter, and a moderate, vacuous pulse.

232 *shen¹ su¹ yin³* 參蘇飲 54, 104
Ginseng and Perilla Beverage
Source: 和劑局方 (*he² ji⁴ ju² fang¹*)
Ginseng Radix *ren² shen¹* 1.5 g
Perillae Caulis et Calyx *zi³ su¹* 1–1.5 g
Citri Exocarpium *chen² pi²* 2 g
Glycyrrhizae Radix *gan¹ cao³* 1 g
Peucedani Radix *qian² hu²* 2 g
Pinelliae Tuber *ban⁴ xia⁴* 3 g
Poria *fu² ling²* 3 g
Aurantii Fructus *zhi³ ke²* 1–1.5 g
Platycodonis Radix *jie² geng³* 2 g
Puerariae Radix *ge² gen¹* 2 g
Saussureae Radix *mu⁴ xiang¹* 1–1.5 g
Zingiberis Rhizoma Recens *sheng¹ jiang¹* 1.5 g
Zizyphi Fructus *da⁴ zao³* 1.5 g
Preparation method: Decoct with water and drink cold.
Actions and Indications: Boosts qi and resolves the exterior; harmonizes the stomach and transforms phlegm. Treats external wind-cold contraction with internal phlegm-rheum. Signs: Aversion to cold, fever, headache, nasal congestion, cough with copious phlegm, fullness and oppression in the chest and diaphragm. Tongue fur: thin and white. Pulse: weak and floating.

233 *shen²-qu¹ san³* 神麴散 201
Medicated Leaven Powder
Source: 聖惠方 (*sheng⁴ hui⁴ fang¹*)
Massa Medicata Fermentata *shen² qu¹* 30 g
Rehmanniae Radix Conquita *shou² di⁴ huang²* 10 g
Atractylodis Ovatae Rhizoma *bai² zhu²* 15 g
Preparation method: Grind to a powder.
Actions and Indications: Treats postpartum frigid diarrhea with abdominal pain.
Dosage: 4 g 3 times a day.

234 *shen² xiao⁴ tai⁴ yi³ dan¹* 神效太乙丹.........230
Wondrous Effect Tai Yi Elixir
Source: 聖惠方 (*sheng⁴ hui⁴ fang¹*)
Limonitum cum Terra *yu³ yu² liang²* 120 g
Aconiti Tuberis Extremitas *wu¹ tou² fu⁴ zi³ jian¹* 30 g
Preparation method: Grind and combine constituents, boil in vinegar, blend with flour, and form into pills the size of adzuki beans (100mg). Take five pills with warm water before meals.
Actions and Indications: Treats frigid taxation with persistent large intestinal diarrhea.

235 *sheng¹ hua⁴ tang¹* 生化湯 88
Engendering Transformation Decoction
Source: 傅青主女科 (*fu⁴ qing¹ zhu³ nü³ ke¹*)
Angelicae Sinensis Radix *dang¹ gui¹* 3–4 g
Ligustici Rhizoma *chuan¹ xiong¹* 3 g

Persicae Semen *tao² ren²* 3 g
Zingiberis Rhizoma *jiang¹* (blast-fried) 1 g
Glycyrrhizae Radix *gan¹ cao³* 1 g
Preparation method: Decoct with water (the original book says decoct in equal proportions of yellow wine and Urina Infantis, *tong² bian⁴*).
Actions and Indications: Quickens the blood and transforms stasis; warms the channels and relieves pain. Treats retention of the lochia and lower abdominal pain.

236 *sheng¹ ji¹ san³* 生肌散 229
Flesh-Engendering Powder
Source: 中醫外科手冊 (*zhong¹ yi¹ wai⁴ ke¹ shou³ ce⁴*)
Smithsonitum *lu² gan¹ shi²* (prepared) 15 g
Stalactitum Tubiforme *di¹ ru³ shi²* 9 g
Talcum *hua² shi²* 30 g
Draconis Sanguis *xue⁴ jie²* 9 g
Cinnabaris *zhu¹ sha¹* 3 g
Borneolum *bing¹ pian⁴* 0.3 g
Actions and Indications: Engenders muscle and closes wounds. Treats yong, ju and other sores that have burst, nearly finished suppurating and are starting to heal.

237 *sheng¹-jiang¹ ban⁴-xia⁴ tang¹* 生薑半夏湯 ...98
Fresh Ginger and Pinellia Decoction
Source: 金匱要略 (*jin¹ gui⁴ yao⁴ lue⁴*)
Pinelliae Tuber *ban⁴ xia⁴* 8 g
Zingiberis Succus *jiang¹ zhi¹* 20 g
Preparation method: Boil Pinelliae Tuber in 120 ml water, and reduce to 80 ml. Add ginger jiuice and reduce to 60 ml.
Actions and Indications: Frees binds and checks vomiting. Treats vexation and oppression in the chest with a semblance of dyspnea, retching, and hiccoughing. Can be used in food damage, drug poisoning, and morning sickness.

238 *sheng¹-ma² ge²-gen¹ tang¹* 升麻葛根湯 ..58, 79
Cimicifuga and Pueraria Decoction
Source: 閻氏小兒方論 (*yan² shi⁴ xiao³ er² fang¹ lun⁴*)
Cimicifugae Rhizoma *sheng¹ ma²* 3–9 g
Puerariae Radix *ge² gen¹* 9–12 g
Paeoniae Radix *shao² yao⁴* 6–9 g
Glycyrrhizae Radix *gan¹ cao³* (mix-fried) 3–5 g
Preparation method: Decoct with water.
Actions and Indications: Resolves the muscles and outthrusts papules. Treats unerupted or poorly erupting measles with generalized fever and headache.

239 *sheng¹ mai⁴ san³* 生脈散........ 33, 40, 50, 151
Pulse-Engendering Powder

Source: 內外傷辨惑論 (*nei⁴ wai⁴ shang¹ bian⁴ huo⁴*)
Ginseng Radix *ren² shen¹* (or Codonopsitis Radix *dang³ shen¹*) 9–15 g
Ophiopogonis Tuber *mai⁴ dong¹ zhi¹* 9–12 g
Schisandrae Fructus *wu³ wei⁴ zi³* 3–6 g
Actions and Indications: Nourishes yin and boosts qi; constrains sweat and engenders the pulse. Treats damage to original qi and yin liquid by heat, manifesting in signs such as copious perspiration, thirst, rapid dyspneic breathing verging on desertion, forceless vacuous pulse, and a dry, red tongue. Also treats heart-lung vacuity arising in enduring disease with insufficiency of both qi and yin, characterized by signs such as cough with little phlegm, shortness of breath and spontaneous sweating, dry mouth and tongue, and a soft vacuous pulse.

240 *shi¹ xiao⁴ san³* 失笑散 118
Sudden Smile Dowder
Source: 和劑局方 (*he² ji⁴ ju² fang¹*)
Trogopteri seu Pteromi Excrementum *wu³ ling² zhi¹* 3 g
Typhae Pollen *pu² huang²* 3 g
Actions and Indications: Quickens the blood, dispels stasis, and relieves pain. Treats pain in the abdomen and region of the heart caused by static blood, menstrual pain, non-descent of the lochia, and uterine bleeding. Dosage: 3–6 g 1–2 times a day (decoction: 9–12 g boiled in a bag).

241 *shi²-hu² san³* 石斛散 15
Dendrobium Powder
Source: 聖濟總錄 (*sheng⁴ ji⁴ zong³ lu⁴*)
Dendrobii Caulis *shi² hu²* 10 g
Epimedii Herba *yin² yang² huo⁴* 10 g
Atractylodis Rhizoma *cang¹ zhu²* (steeped in rice-water and stone-baked) 5 g
Actions and Indications: Treats night and twilight blindness.

242 *shi²-jue²-ming² san³* 石決明散 215
Abalone Shell Powder
Source: 聖濟總錄 (*sheng⁴ ji⁴ zong³ lu⁴*)
Haliotidis Concha *shi² jue² ming²* 4 g
Chrysanthemi Flos *ju² hua¹* 2 g
Lycii Fructus *gou³ qi³ zi³* 2 g
Mori Folium *sang¹ ye⁴* 1.5 g
Actions and Indications: Treats dizziness.

243 *shi² quan² da⁴ bu³ tang¹* 十全大補湯 2, 33, 76
Perfect Major Supplementation Decoction
Source: 和劑局方 (*he² ji⁴ ju² fang¹*)
Ginseng Radix *ren² shen¹* (or Codonopsitis Radix *dang³ shen¹*) 9–12 g

Atractylodis Ovatae Rhizoma *bai² zhu²* 6–9 g
Poria *fu² ling²* 9–12 g
Glycyrrhizae Radix *gan¹ cao³* (mix-fried) 2–3 g
Angelicae Sinensis Radix *dang¹ gui¹* 6–12 g
Rehmanniae Radix *di⁴ huang²* 9–12 g
Paeoniae Radix *shao² yao⁴* 6–9 g
Ligustici Rhizoma *chuan¹ xiong¹* 2–6 g
Astragali Radix *huang² qi²* 9–12 g
Cinnamomi Cortex *rou⁴ gui⁴* 1–3 g
Actions and Indications: Boosts qi and supplements the blood. Treats depletion of both qi and blood, dizziness, fatigue, withered yellow complexion, lack of strength in the feet and knees.

244 *shi² wei⁴ bai⁴ du² tang¹* 十味敗毒湯 ... 55, 194
Ten-Ingredient Toxin-Vanquishing Decoction
Source: 華岡青洲 (*hua² gang¹ qing¹ zhou¹*)
Bupleuri Radix *chai² hu²* 2–3 g
Trichosanthis Pericarpium *gua¹ lou² pi²* 2–3 g
Platycodonis Radix *jie² geng³* 2–3 g
Ligustici Rhizoma *chuan¹ xiong¹* 2–3 g
Poria *fu² ling²* 2–4 g
Ledebouriellae Radix *fang² feng¹* 1.5–3 g
Angelicae Duhuo Radix *du² huo²* 1.5–3 g
Glycyrrhizae Radix *gan¹ cao³* 1.4 g
Zingiberis Rhizoma Recens *sheng¹ jiang¹* 1–3 g
Schizonepetae Herba seu Flos *jing¹ jie⁴* 1–1.5 g
Forsythiae Fructus *lian² qiao²* 2–3 g (optional)
Actions and Indications: Treats yong, boils, clove sores, lymphadenitis, mastitis, dermatitis, urticaria, eczema, and otitis media.

245 *shi² zao³ tang¹* 十棗湯 37, 43, 111, 158
Ten Jujubes Decoction
Source: 傷寒論 (*shang¹ han² lun⁴*)
Euphorbiae Kansui Radix *gan¹ sui⁴* 1 g
Euphorbiae seu Knoxiae Radix *da⁴ ji³* 1 g
Daphnes Genkwa Flos *yuan² hua¹* 1 g
Zizyphi Fructus *da⁴ zao³* 4 g
Actions and Indications: Expels water-rheum. Treats: 1) Suspended rheum with water qi in the lateral costal region, with coughing causing local pain, hard glomus in below the heart, and pain in the chest and back making breathing difficult. 2) Repletion-type water swelling and abdominal distention. Dosage: 1–2 g once a day. Take in the morning on an empty stomach. Swallow powder with a decoction of jujubes.

246 *shi³-jun¹-zi³ wan²* 使君子丸 149
Quisqualis Pills
Source: 和劑局方 (*he² ji⁴ ju² fang¹*)
Quisqualis Fructus *shi³ jun¹ zi³* 10 g
Magnoliae Cortex *hou⁴ po⁴* 1 g
Citri Exocarpium *chen² pi²*   g

Ligustici Rhizoma *chuan¹ xiong¹* 1 g
Preparation method: Grind to a powder, mix with honey, and form into 500 mg pills. 1 pill for children over 3 years old, and half for children under 3 years old.
Actions and Indications: Treats the five gan in children with spleen-stomach disharmony, and bloating in the abdomen and region of the heart.

247 *shi⁴-di⁴ tang¹* 柿蒂湯 138
Persimmon Decoction
Source: 濟生方 (*ji⁴ sheng¹ fang¹*)
Caryophylli Flos *ding¹ xiang¹* 1–1.5 g
Kaki Calyx *shi⁴ di⁴* 5 g
Zingiberis Rhizoma Recens *sheng¹ jiang¹* 4 g
Actions and Indications: Warms the stomach and downbears counterflow. Treats gastric pain and thoracic fullness, and persistent hiccough.

248 *shu¹ jin¹ li⁴ an¹ san³* 舒筋立安散 32
Sinew-Soothing Peace-Bringing Powder
Source: 萬病回春 (*wan⁴ bing⁴ hui² chun¹*)
Ledebouriellae Radix *fang² feng¹* 1.2 g
Notopterygii Rhizoma *qiang¹ huo²* 1.2 g
Angelicae Duhuo Radix *du² huo²* 1.2 g
Poria *fu² ling²* 1.2 g
Ligustici Rhizoma *chuan¹ xiong¹* 1.2 g
Angelicae Dahuricae Radix *bai² zhi³* 1.2 g
Rehmanniae Radix Cruda *sheng¹ di⁴ huang²* 1.2 g
Atractylodis Ovatae Rhizoma *bai² zhu²* 1.2 g
Carthami Flos *hong² hua¹* 1.2 g
Persicae Semen *tao² ren²* 1.2 g
Arisaematis Rhizoma *tian¹ nan² xing¹* 1.2 g
Citri Exocarpium *chen² pi²* 1.2 g
Pinelliae Tuber *ban⁴ xia⁴* 1.2 g
Atractylodis Rhizoma *cang¹ zhu²* 1.2 g
Clematidis Radix *wei¹ ling² xian¹* 1.2 g
Achyranthis Radix *niu² xi¹* 1.2 g
Chaenomelis Fructus *mu⁴ gua¹* 1.2 g
Fangji Radix *fang² ji³* 1.2 g
Forsythiae Fructus *lian² qiao¹* 1.2 g
Scutellariae Radix *huang² qin²* 1.2 g
Mutong Caulis *mu⁴ tong¹* 1.2 g
Aconiti Tuber Laterale *fu⁴ zi³* 1 g
Bambusae Caulis in Taeniam *zhu² ru²* 1.2 g
Gentianae Scabrae Radix *long² dan³* 1,2 g
Actions and Indications: Treats acute and chronic rheumatism in the joints; numbness; hemiplegia.

249 *shu¹ jin¹ yao⁴ shui³* 舒筋藥水 19
Sinew-Soothing Medicinal Water
Source: 經驗方 (empirical formula)
Aconiti Tsao-wu-tou Tuber Crudum *sheng¹ cao³ wu¹* 400 g

Aconiti Tuber Crudum *sheng¹ chuan¹ wu¹* 400 g
Pinelliae Tuber Crudum *sheng¹ ban⁴ xia⁴* 400 g
Arisaematis Rhizoma Crudum *sheng¹ tian¹ nan² xing¹* 400 g
Camphorae Folium *zhang¹ nao³* 400 g
Gardeniae Fructus *shan¹ zhi¹ zi³* 400 g
Rhei Rhizoma *da⁴ huang²* 400 g
Chaenomelis Fructus *mu⁴ gua¹* 400 g
Notopterygii Rhizoma *qiang¹ huo²* 400 g
Angelicae Duhuo Radix *du² huo²* 400 g
Liquidambaris Fructus *lu⁴ lu⁴ tong¹* 400 g
Zanthoxyli Fructus *hua¹ jiao¹* 400 g
Sappan Lignum *su¹ mu⁴* 300 g
Typhae Pollen *pu² huang²* 300 g
Camphorae Lignum *zhang¹ mu⁴* 300 g
Paeoniae Radix Rubra *chi⁴ shao² yao⁴* 200 g
Carthami Flos *hong² hua¹* 200 g
Actions and Indications: Soothes the sinews and quickens the connecting vessels; dispels wind and relieves pain. Treats contusion and pain in the sinew and bone.

250 *shu¹ zao² yin³ zi³* 疏鑿飲子 161
Coursing and Piercing Beverage
Source: 濟生方 (*ji⁴ sheng¹ fang¹*)
Notopterygii Rhizoma *qiang¹ huo²* 5–12 g
Gentianae Macrophyllae Radix *qin² jiao¹* 5–12 g
Phytolaccae Radix *shang¹ lu⁴* 3–6 g
Arecae Semen *bin¹ lang²* 9–12 g
Alismatis Rhizoma *ze² xie⁴* 5–12 g
Mutong Caulis *mu⁴ tong¹* 2–5 g
Arecae Pericarpium *da⁴ fu² pi²* 6–9 g
Poria *fu² ling² pi²* 9–12 g
Phaseoli Calcarati Semen *chi⁴ xiao³ dou⁴* 15–30 g
Zanthoxyli Fructus *hua¹ jiao¹* 2–3 g
Zingiberis Rhizomatis Recentis Cortex *sheng¹ jiang¹ pi²* 2–3 g
Preparation method: Decoct with water.
Actions and Indications: Outthrusts pathogens and frees the interior; disinhibits water and disperses swelling. Treats generalized water swelling with dyspnea, thirst, and inhibited urination and defecation.

251 *si⁴ jun¹ zi³ tang¹* 四君子湯 ..33, 40, 42, 76, 236
Four Gentlemen Decoction
New name: 健脾益氣湯 *jian⁴ pi² yi⁴ qi⁴ tang¹* Spleen-Fortifying Qi-Boosting Decoction
Source: 和劑局方 (*he² ji⁴ ju² fang¹*)
Ginseng Radix *ren² shen¹* (or Codonopsitis Radix *dang³ shen¹*) 9–12 g
Atractylodis Ovatae Rhizoma *bai² zhu²* 6–9 g
Poria *fu² ling²* 9–12 g
Glycyrrhizae Radix *gan¹ cao³* (mix-fried) 2–3 g
Actions and Indications: Fortifies the spleen and

boosts qi. Treats spleen qi vacuity with withered white face, faint voice, lack of strength in the limbs, reduced appetite, thin stool, soft tongue with thin white tongue fur, and a soggy, forceless pulse.

252 *si⁴ ni⁴ san³* 四逆散 51
Counterflow Frigidity Powder
Source: 傷寒論 (*shang¹ han² lun⁴*)
Bupleuri Radix *chai² hu²* 6–9 g
Paeonia Radix Alba *bai² shao² yao⁴* 6–9 g
Aurantii Fructus Immaturus *zhi³ shi²* 4–9 g
Glycyrrhizae Radix *gan¹ cao³* 3–5 g
Actions and Indications: Harmonizes and resolves; discharges heat; courses the liver and resolves depression. Treats depressed yang qi failing to reach the outer body, characterized by counterflow frigidity of the limbs; liver-stomach disharmony with pain in the chest, lateral costal region, venter and abdomen; abdominal pain and diarrhea.

253 *si⁴ ni⁴ tang¹* 四逆湯 22, 42, 98
Counterflow Frigidity Decoction
Source: 傷寒論 (*shang¹ han² lun⁴*)
Aconiti Tuber Laterale *fu⁴ zi³* 6–15 g
Zingiberis Rhizoma *gan¹ jiang¹* 3–6 g
Glycyrrhizae Radix *gan¹ cao³* (mix-fried) 6–12 g
Preparation method: Decoct with water.
Actions and Indications: Returns yang and stems counterflow. Treats shao yin disease with debilitation of yang qi, characterized by inversion frigidity of the limbs, generalized cold sweat, clear-food diarrhea, frigid pain in the abdomen, and vomiting. Tongue: white and glossy. Pulse: deep and fine on the verge of expiry. Also treats yang collapse caused by profuse sweating or diarrhea.

254 *si⁴ shen² wan²* 四神丸 132, 151, 176, 181
Four Spirits Pills
Source: 證治準繩 (*zheng⁴ zhi⁴ zhun³ sheng²*)
Myristicae Semen *rou⁴ dou⁴ kou⁴* 100 g
Psoraleae Semen *bu³ gu³ zhi¹* 200 g
Schisandrae Fructus *wu³ wei⁴ zi³* 100 g
Evodiae Fructus *wu² zhu¹ yu²* 50 g
Zingiberis Rhizoma Recens *sheng¹ jiang¹* 200 g
Zizyphi Fructus *da⁴ zao³* 300 g
Preparation method: Grind to a fine powder, blend with a decoction of 80 g ginger and 60 g jujubes, and form into 300 mg pills.
Actions and Indications: Warms and supplements the spleen and kidney; astringes the intestines and stops diarrhea. Treats spleen-kidney vacuity cold with fifth watch diarrhea and no thought of food and drink, or enduring diarrhea with abdominal pain, aching lumbus and frigid limbs, fatigued spirit and lack of the

strength, a pale tongue with thin white fur, and a forceless deep, slow pulse.
Dosage: 10 pills on an empty stomach.

255 *si⁴ sheng¹ wan²* 四生丸 100
Four Raw Agents Pills
Source: 婦人良方 (*fu⁴ ren² liang² fang¹*)
Nelumbinis Folium Recens *xian¹ he² ye⁴*
Artemisiae Argyi Folium Recens *xian¹ ai⁴ ye⁴* 9–15 g
Biotae Folium et Ramulus *ce⁴ bo² ye⁴* 15–30 g
Rehmanniae Radix Recens *xian¹ sheng¹ di⁴* 30 g
Preparation method: Original source says prepare in pill form; now taken as free juice or boiled and taken as a decoction.
Actions and Indications: Cools the blood and staunches bleeding. Treats frenetic blood heat, coughing or vomiting of blood, or nosebleed with bright red blood, dry throat and mouth.

256 *si⁴ wu⁴ tang¹* 四物湯 25, 51, 59, 88
Four Agents Decoction
Source: 和劑局方 (*he² ji⁴ ju² fang¹*)
Angelicae Sinensis Radix *dang¹ gui¹* 6–12 g
Rehmanniae Radix *di⁴ huang²* 9–15 g
Paeoniae Radix *shao² yao⁴* 6–9 g
Ligustici Rhizoma *chuan¹ xiong²* 3–6 g
Actions and Indications: Supplements and quickens the blood; regulates the menses. Treats all types of vacuity and stagnation of construction-blood, menstrual irregularities, menstrual pain, and uterine bleeding etc.

257 *su¹-he²-xiang¹ wan²* 蘇合香丸 197, 203
Liquid Styrax Pills
Source: 和劑局方 (*he² ji⁴ ju² fang¹*)
Cinnabaris *zhu¹ sha¹* 60 g
Rhinocerotis Cornu *xi¹ jiao³* 60 g
Aristolochiae Debilis seu Contortae Radix *qing¹ mu⁴ xiang¹* 60 g
Piperis Longi Fructus *bi⁴ ba²* 60 g
Aquilariae Lignum *chen² xiang¹* 60 g
Santali Albi Lignum *tan² xiang¹* 60 g
Cyperi Rhizoma Crudum *sheng¹ xiang¹ fu⁴* 60 g
Caryophylli Flos *ding¹ xiang¹* 60 g
Chebulae Fructus *he¹ zi³* 60 g
Atractylodis Ovatae Rhizoma *bai² zhu²* 60 g
Benzoinum *an¹ xi² xiang¹* 60 g
Borneolum *bing¹ pian⁴* 30 g
Moschus *she⁴ xiang¹* 4.5 g
Olibanum *ru³ xiang¹* 30 g
Styrax Liquidus *su¹ he² xiang¹* 30 g
Actions and Indications: Opens the portals and exorcises foulness; rectifies qi and relieves pain. Treats sudden collapse, summerheat stroke, sha distention, sud-

den anger causing qi inversion, oppression in the chest and heart pain and other conditions involving exuberant internal phlegm-damp. Tongue fur: thick and slimy.

Dosage: Half to 1 pill 1–2 times a day. Swallow with water.

258 *su¹-zi³ jiang⁴ qi⁴ tang¹* 蘇子降氣湯...........146
Perilla Fruit Qi-Downbearing Decoction
Source: 和劑局方 (*he² ji⁴ ju² fang¹*)
Perillae Fructus *zi³ su¹ zi³*   9–12 g
Pinelliae Tuber *ban⁴ xia⁴*   6–9 g
Glycyrrhizae Radix *gan¹ cao³* (mix-fried)   3–4.5 g
Cinnamomi Cortex *rou⁴ gui⁴*   1.5–3 g
Angelicae Sinensis Radix *dang¹ gui¹*   6–9 g
Peucedani Radix *qian² hu²*   6–9 g
Magnoliae Cortex *hou⁴ po⁴*   3–6 g
Citri Exocarpium *chen² pi²*   6–9 g
Zingiberis Rhizoma Recens *sheng¹ jiang¹*   2 slices
Zizyphi Fructus *da⁴ zao³*   1 piece
Perillae Folium *zi³ su¹ ye⁴*   5 pieces
Preparation method: Decoct with water.
Actions and Indications: Downbears qi and calms dyspnea; transforms phlegm-rheum. Treats phlegm-rheum cough with shortness of breath and distressed, rapid, dyspneic breathing, oppression in the chest and copious phlegm. Tongue fur: white and moist.

259 *suan¹-zao³-ren² tang¹* 酸棗仁湯...............188
Spiny Jujube Decoction
Source: 金匱要略 (*jin¹ gui⁴ yao⁴ lue⁴*)
Zizyphi Spinosi Semen *suan¹ zao³ ren²*   7–15 g
Poria *fu² ling²*   5 g
Anemarrhenae Rhizoma *zhi¹ mu³*   3 g
Ligustici Rhizoma *chuan¹ xiong¹*   3 g
Glycyrrhizae Radix *gan¹ cao³*   1 g
Preparation method: Decoct with water.
Actions and Indications: Nourishes the blood and calms the spirit; clears heat and eliminates vexation. Treats vacuity vexation, insomnia or ungratifying sleep, excitability and irascibility, headache and feeling of distention in the head. Pulse: fine, wiry and rapid.

260 *tao²-he² cheng² qi⁴ tang¹* 桃核承氣湯...95, 177
Peach Kernel Qi-Infusing Decoction
Alternate name: 桃仁承氣湯 *tao²-ren² cheng²-qi⁴ tang¹* Peach Pit Purgative Decoction
Source: 傷寒論 (*shang¹ han² lun⁴*)
Persicae Semen *tao² ren²*   5 g
Rhei Rhizoma Crudum *sheng¹ da⁴ huang²*   4 g
Mirabilitum *mang² xiao¹*   1–2 g
Cinnamomi Ramulus *gui⁴ zhi¹*   4 g
Glycyrrhizae Radix *gan¹ cao³* (mix-fried)   1.5 g

Actions and Indications: Precipitates; expels stasis; frees the channels. Treats binding of heat and static blood with lower abdominal fullness and distention, black stool, fever, and in severe cases delirious or manic raving. Also used for blood stasis amenorrhea, and menstrual pain.

261 *tao² hua¹ tang¹* 桃花湯 228
Peach Blossom Decoction
Source: 傷寒論 (*shang¹ han² lun⁴*)
Halloysitum Rubrum *chi⁴ shi² zhi¹*   15–30 g
Zingiberis Rhizoma *gan¹ jiang¹*   3–6 g
Oryzae Semen *geng¹ mi³*   15–30 g
Actions and Indications: Warms the center and astringes the intestines. Treats persistent dysenteric efflux desertion with pus and pale colored blood in the stool and abdominal pain relieved by warmth, a pale tongue with white fur, and a weak, slow or fine, faint pulse.

262 *tian¹ wang² bu³ xin¹ dan¹* 天王補心丹56, 71, 188
Celestial Emperor Heart-Supplementing Elixir
Alternate name: 補心丹 *bu³ xin¹ dan¹* Heart-Supplementing Elixir
Source: 攝生秘剖方 (*she⁴ sheng¹ mi⁴ pou¹ fang¹*)
Rehmanniae Radix Cruda *sheng¹ di⁴ huang²*   20 g
Ginseng Radix *ren² shen¹* (or Codonopsitis Radix *dang³ shen¹*)   30 g
Asparagi Tuber *tian¹ men² dong¹*   30 g
Ophiopogonis Tuber *mai⁴ dong¹*   30 g
Scrophulariae Radix *xuan² shen¹*   15 g

Salviae Radix *dan¹ shen¹*   15 g
Poria *fu² ling²*   15 g
Polygalae Radix *yuan³ zhi⁴*   15 g
Angelicae Sinensis Radix *dang¹ gui¹*   30 g
Schisandrae Fructus *wu³ wei⁴ zi³*   30 g
Biotae Semen *bo² zi³ ren²*   30 g
Zizyphi Spinosi Semen *suan¹ zao³ ren²*   30 g
Platycodonis Radix *jie² geng³*   15 g
Cinnabaris *zhu¹ sha¹*   15 g
Acori Graminei Rhizoma *shi² chang¹ pu²*   15 g
Preparation method: Grind to a fine powder, blend with honey, and coat with cinnabar. Can also be prepared as a decoction.
Actions and Indications: Enriches yin and nourish the blood; supplements the heart and quiets the spirit. Treats insufficiency of yin-blood and disquieting of the heart spirit manifesting as vacuity vexation, palpitations, insomnia, poor memory, dry stool, and in some cases mouth and tongue sores or vacuity heat night sweats. Tongue: red with little fur. Pulse: fine and rapid.
Dosage: 6–9 g twice a day, or once before bed. Take with warm water.

263 *tiao² wei⁴ cheng² qi⁴ tang¹* 調胃承氣湯
.................................42, 95, 231
Stomach-Regulating Qi-Infusing Decoction
Source: 傷寒論 (*shang¹ han² lun⁴*)
Rhei Rhizoma *da⁴ huang²* 2–2.5 g
Mirabilitum *mang² xiao¹* 1 g
Glycyrrhizae Radix *gan¹ cao³* 1 g
Actions and Indications: Drains heat and abducts damp. Treats yang ming bowel repletion patterns with tidal fever, thirst, abdominal pain exacerbated by pressure, and constipation. Tongue fur: yellow. Pulse: slippery and rapid. Can also be used for food damage constipation in children, or for painful swelling of the gums and bad breath.

264 *tong¹ mai⁴ si⁴ ni⁴ tang¹* 通脈四逆湯 98
Vessel-Freeing Counterflow Frigidity Decoction
Source: 傷寒論 (*shang¹ han² lun⁴*)
Glycyrrhizae Radix *gan¹ cao³* 2 g
Zingiberis Rhizoma *gan¹ jiang¹* 3 g
Aconiti Tuber Laterale *fu⁴ zi³* 1 g
Actions and Indications: Frees yang and stems counterflow. Treats shao yin disease presenting as interior cold and exterior heat. Signs include inversion frigidity of the limbs, faint pulse verging on expiry, and red complexion. There may also be abdominal pain, vomiting, and sore throat.

265 *tuo¹ li³ xiao¹ du² yin³* 托裡消毒飲.......23, 114
Internal Expulsion Toxin-Dispersing Beverage
Source: 萬病回春 (*wan⁴ bing⁴ hui² chun¹*)
Angelicae Sinensis Radix *dang¹ gui¹* 5 g
Poria *fu² ling²* 5 g
Ginseng Radix *ren² shen¹* 3 g
Ligustici Rhizoma *chuan¹ xiong¹* 3 g
Platycodonis Radix *jie² geng³* 3 g
Atractylodis Ovatae Rhizoma *bai² zhu²* 3 g
Paeoniae Radix *shao² yao⁴* 3 g
Gleditsiae Spina *zao⁴ jiao³ ci⁴* 2 g
Astragali Radix *huang² qi²* 1.5 g
Lonicerae Flos *jin¹ yin² hua¹* 1.5 g
Angelicae Dahuricae Radix *bai² zhi³* 1 g
Glycyrrhizae Radix *gan¹ cao³* 1 g
Actions and Indications: Treats yong and ju.

266 *wai⁴ ke¹ chan² su¹ wan²* 外科蟾酥丸........211
External Medicine Toad Venom Pills
Source: 外科正宗 (*wai⁴ ke¹ zheng⁴ zong¹*)
Bufonis Venenum *chan² su¹* 6 g
Calomelas *qing¹ fen³* 1.5 g
Alumen Praeparatum *ku¹ fan²* 3 g
Calcitum *han² shui³ shi²* 3 g
Aeris Robigo *tong² lü⁴* (calcined) 3 g
Olibanum *ru³ xiang¹* 3 g

Myrrha *mo⁴ yao⁴* 3 g
Chalcanthitum *dan³ fan²* 3 g
Moschus *she⁴ xiang¹* 0·3 g
Realgar *xiong² huang²* 6 g
Eulota *wo¹ niu²* 21 pieces
Cinnabaris *zhu¹ sha¹* 9 g
Actions and Indications: Resolves toxin and disperses swelling; quickens the blood and relieves pain. Treats clove sores, brain ju, mammary yong, and bone ju.

267 *wei⁴ ling² tang¹* 胃苓湯 238
Stomach-Calming Poria Five Decoction
Source: 萬病回春 (*wan⁴ bing⁴ hui² chun¹*)
Combination of 五苓散 *wu³ ling² san³* Poria Five Powder and *ping² wei⁴ san³* Stomach-Calming Powder
Polyporus Sclerotium *zhu¹ ling²* 2.5–3 g
Alismatis Rhizoma *ze⁴ xie⁴* 2.5–3 g
Atractylodis Ovatae Rhizoma *bai² zhu²* 2.5–3 g
Atractylodis Rhizoma *cang¹ zhu²* 2.5–3 g
Magnoliae Cortex *hou⁴ po⁴* 2.5–3 g
Citri Exocarpium *chen² pi²* 2.5–3 g
Cinnamomi Ramulus *gui⁴ zhi¹* 2–2.5 g
Glycyrrhizae Radix *gan¹ cao³* 1–2 g
Zingiberis Rhizoma Recens *sheng¹ jiang¹* 1.5 g
Zizyphi Fructus *da⁴ zao³* 1.5–3 g
Amomi Semen *sha¹ ren²* 2 g
Coptidis Rhizoma *huang² lian²* 2 g
Actions and Indications: Dries damp and fortifies the spleen; disinhibits water and percolates damp. Treats watery diarrhea or vomiting with thirst and scant urine, such as due to summerheat.

268 *wen¹ dan³ tang¹* 溫膽湯 12
Gallbladder-Warming Decoction
Source: 三因方 (*san¹ yin¹ fang¹*)
Pinelliae Tuber *ban⁴ xia⁴* 6–9 g
Citri Exocarpium *chen² pi²* 6–9 g
Poria *fu² ling²* 9–12 g
Glycyrrhizae Radix *gan¹ cao³* 1.5–3 g
Bambusae Caulis in Taeniam *zhu² ru²* 6–9 g
Aurantii Fructus Immaturus *zhi³ shi²* 6–9 g
Zingiberis Rhizoma Recens *sheng¹ jiang¹* 3–6 g
Zizyphi Fructus *da⁴ zao³* 2–3 g
Actions and Indications: Clears the gallbladder and transforms phlegm; harmonizes the stomach and quiets the spirit. Treats phlegm-heat harassing the upper body with vacuity vexation, insomnia, dizziness, palpitation, copious phlegm, and vomiting. Tongue fur: slimy.

269 *wen¹ jing¹ tang¹* 溫經湯 9, 132
Channel-Warming Decoction
Source: 金匱要略 (*jin¹ gui⁴ yao⁴ lue⁴*)

Cinnamomi Ramulus *gui⁴ zhi¹*   3–9 g
Evodiae Fructus *wu² zhu¹ yu²*   3–6 g
Ligustici Rhizoma *chuan¹ xiong¹*   3–9 g
Angelicae Sinensis Radix *dang¹ gui¹*   6–12 g
Paeoniae Radix *shao² yao⁴*   6–12 g
Zingiberis Rhizoma Recens *sheng¹ jiang¹*   2–4 s
Moutan Radicis Cortex *mu³ dan¹ pi²*   6–9 g
Ophiopogonis Tuber *mai⁴ dong¹ zhi¹*   9–12 g
Pinelliae Tuber *ban⁴ xia⁴*   6–9 g
Ginseng Radix *ren² shen¹* (or Codonopsitis Radix
  dang³ shen¹)   9–12 g
Glycyrrhizae Radix *gan¹ cao³*   3–6 g
Asini Corii Gelatinum *e¹ jiao¹*   6–12 g
Preparation method: Decoct with water.
Actions and Indications: Warms the menses and
dissipates cold; nourishes the blood and dispels stasis.
Treats vacuity cold in the penetrating and conception
vessels, with static blood obstruction, menstrual ir-
regularities, frigid pain in the lower abdomen, and
infertility.

270 *wen¹-na⁴-qi² san³* 膃肭臍散 212
Seal Genitals Powder
Source: 聖濟總錄 (*sheng⁴ ji⁴ zong³ lu⁴*)
Callorhini Testis et Penis *hai³ gou³ shen⁴* (stone-
  baked and cut)   10 g
Evodiae Fructus *wu² zhu¹ yu²* (stone-baked)   10 g
Nardostachydis Rhizoma et Radix *gan¹ song¹* (stone-
  baked)   10 g
Citri Exocarpium *chen² pi²* (stone-baked)   10 g
Alpiniae Officinarum Rhizoma *gao¹ liang² jiang¹*
  10 g
Preparation method: Grind to a fine powder.
Actions and Indications: Vacuity taxation with ac-
cumulated frigidity.
Dosage: 2 g 3 times a day.

271 *wen¹ qing¹ yin³* 溫清飲 10
Warm Clearing Beverage
Source: 萬病回春 (*wan⁴ bing⁴ hui² chun¹*)
Angelicae Sinensis Radix *dang¹ gui¹*   3–4 g
Rehmanniae Radix *di⁴ huang²*   3–4 g
Paeoniae Radix *shao² yao⁴*   3–4 g
Ligustici Rhizoma *chuan¹ xiong¹*   3–4 g
Coptidis Rhizoma *huang² lian²*   1.5–2g
Scutellariae Radix   1.5–3 g
Gardeniae Fructus *huang² gin²shan¹ zhi¹ zi³* 1.5–2 g
Phellodendri Cortex *huang² bo²*   1.5–2 g
Actions and Indications: Treats difficult menstruation
and menopausal disorders.

272 *wu¹-mei² wan²* 烏梅丸 144, 157
Mume Pills
Source: 傷寒論 (*shang¹ han² lun⁴*)

Mume Fructus *wu¹ mei²*   300 g
Zanthoxyli Fructus *hua¹ jiao¹*   120 g
Coptidis Rhizoma *huang² lian²*   480 g
Phellodendri Cortex *huang² bo²*   180 g
Asiasari Radix *xi⁴ xin¹*   180 g
Zingiberis Rhizoma *gan¹ jiang¹*   300 g
Aconiti Tuber Laterale *fu⁴ zi³* (prepared)   180 g
Ginseng Radix *ren² shen¹*   180 g
Angelicae Sinensis Radix *dang¹ gui¹*   120 g
Cinnamomi Ramulus *gui⁴ zhi¹*   180 g
Preparation method: Form into 300 mg pills.
Actions and Indications: Quiets roundworm and
relieves pain. Treats roundworm inversion with
periodic abdominal pain, burning sensation below the
heart, vexation and oppression, nausea, vomiting that
sometimes brings up roundworm, cold limbs and a
hidden or tight, wiry pulse, and persistent diarrhea.

273 *wu¹-yao⁴ shun⁴ qi⁴ san³* 烏藥順氣散 47
Lindera Qi-Normalizing Powder
Source: 和劑局方 (*he² ji⁴ ju² fang¹*)
Linderae Radix *wu² yao⁴*   5 g
Ephedrae Herba *ma² huang²*   3 g
Platycodonis Radix *jie² geng³*   3 g
Glycyrrhizae Radix *gan¹ cao³*   1 g
Ligustici Rhizoma *chuan¹ xiong¹*   3 g
Aurantii Fructus *zhi³ ke²*   3 g
Angelicae Dahuricae Radix *bai² zhi³*   3 g
Zingiberis Rhizoma *gan¹ jiang¹*   1.5 g
Bombyx Batryticatus *bai² jiang¹ can²*   1.5 g
Zizyphi Fructus *da⁴ zao³*   3 g
Citri Exocarpium *chen² pi²*   5 g
Actions and Indications: Treats generalized pain; joint
pain; paralysis; difficulty in speaking; leg qi;
hemiplegia.

274 *wu²-zhu¹-yu² tang¹* 吳茱萸湯 132
Evodia Decoction
Source: 傷寒論 (*shang¹ han² lun⁴*)
Evodiae Fructus *wu² zhu¹ yu²*   3–6 g
Ginseng Radix *ren² shen¹* (or Codonopsitis Radix
  dang³ shen¹)   9–12 g
Zingiberis Rhizoma Recens *sheng¹ jiang¹*   3–5 slices
Zizyphi Fructus   *da⁴ zao³*   4–6 pieces
Preparation method: Decoct with water.
Actions and Indications: Warms the liver and stomach;
downbears counterflow and checks vomiting. Treats
liver-stomach vacuity cold with turbid yin rising
counterflow manifesting as pain in the venter and abdomen, desire to vomit after eating, acid regurgitation and clamoring stomach. Other possible signs include vertex headache, or dry retching with foamy
drool. Tongue: pale with glossy, white fur. Pulse: wiry
and slow.

275 wu³-bei⁴-zi³ san³ 五倍子散 62,199
Sumac Gallnut Powder
Source: 張潔古 (zhang¹ jie² gu³)
Galla Rhois wu³ bei⁴ zi³
Sanguisorbae Radix di⁴ yu²
Preparation method: Both agents in equal proportions.
Dosage: 1.5 g on a empty stomach.
Actions and Indications: Promotes contraction and resolves toxin. Treats prolapse of the rectum in children.

276 wu³ hu³ tang¹ 五虎湯 8
Five Tigers Decoction
Source: 萬病回春 (wan⁴ bing⁴ hui² chun¹)
Ephedrae Herba ma² huang² 4 g
Armeniacae Semen xing⁴ ren² 2 g
Glycyrrhizae Radix gan¹ cao³ 2 g
Gypsum shi¹ gao¹ 10 g
Mori Radicis Cortex sang¹ bai² pi² 2–3 g
Preparation method: Decoct with water.
Actions and Indications: Treats bronchial asthma.

277 wu³ ji¹ san³ 五積散 23
Five Accumulations Powder
Source: 和劑局方 (he² ji⁴ ju² fang¹)
Ephedrae Herba ma² huang² 1.2 g
Angelicae Dahuricae Radix bai² zhi³ 1.2 g
Zingiberis Rhizoma gan¹ jiang¹ 1.2 g
Cinnamomi Cortex rou⁴ gui⁴ 1.2 g
Aurantii Fructus zhi³ ke² 1.2 g
Platycodonis Radix jie² geng³ 1.2 g
Angelicae Sinensis Radix dang¹ gui¹ 1.2 g
Ligustici Rhizoma chuan¹ xiong¹ 1.2 g
Paeoniae Radix shao² yao⁴ 1.2 g
Atractylodis Rhizoma cang¹ zhu² 2 g
Magnoliae Cortex hou⁴ po⁴ 1.2 g
Glycyrrhizae Radix gan¹ cao³ 1.2 g
Citri Exocarpium chen² pi² 2 g
Pinelliae Tuber ban⁴ xia⁴ 2 g
Poria fu² ling² 2 g
Actions and Indications: Resolves the exterior and dissipates cold; warms the center and disperses accumulations. Treats contraction of external wind-cold engendering internal cold, with signs such as fever, aversion to cold, absence of sweating, headache and generalized pain, hypertonicity of neck and back, pain and distention in the chest and abdomen, no desire to eat, and in some cases nausea and vomiting. Tongue fur: slimy and white.

278 wu³-jia¹-pi² wan² 五加皮丸 1, 56
Acanthopanax Pills
Source: 瑞竹堂驗方 (rui⁴ zhu² tang² yan⁴ fang¹)

Acanthopanacis Radicis Cortex wu³ jia¹ pi² (steeped in wine) 4 g
Polygalae Radix yuan³ zhi⁴ 4 g
Preparation method: Make into pills with wine. Take with wine on an empty stomach.
Actions and Indications: Treats leg qi; pain and swelling of the joints.

279 wu³ lin² san³ 五淋散 236
Five Stranguries Powder
Source: 和劑局方 (he² ji⁴ ju² fang¹)
Poriae fu² ling² 6 g
Angelicae Sinensis Radix dang¹ gui¹ 3 g
Glycyrrhizae Radix gan¹ cao³ 3 g
Gardeniae Fructus shan¹ zhi¹ zi³ 2 g
Paeoniae Radix Rubra chi⁴ shao² yao⁴ 2 g
Actions and Indications: Treats the five stranguries (qi, blood, stone or sand, unctious, and toxin strangury, corresponding with Western medicine to urethritis, cystitis, bladder stones, and kidney stones).

280 wu³ ling² san³ 五苓散 2, 72, 76, 236, 238
Poria Five Powder
Source: 傷寒論 (shang¹ han² lun⁴)
Poria fu² ling² 9–15 g
Polyporus zhu¹ ling² 9–12 g
Alismatis Rhizoma ze² xie⁴ 9–15 g
Atractylodis Ovatae Rhizoma bai² zhu² 9–12 g
Cinnamomi Ramulus gui⁴ zhi¹ 3–6 g
Preparation method: Now usually prepared as a decoction.
Actions and Indications: Frees yang and promotes the transformative action of qi; fortifies the spleen and disinhibits water. Treats water-damp collecting internally with inhibited urination, and a moist, glossy tongue fur; sometimes there may be fever, vexation and thirst, and immediate vomiting of ingested fluid. Also treats swelling and fullness, and diarrhea due to water-damp.

281 wu³ pi² san³ 五皮散 8, 123, 236
Five Cortices Powder
Source: 麻科活人全書 (ma² ke¹ huo² ren² quan² shu¹)
Poria fu² ling² 12–30 g
Mori Radicis Cortex sang¹ bai² pi² 9–12 g
Citri Exocarpium chen² pi² 6–9 g
Zingiberis Rhizomatis Recentis Cortex sheng¹ jiang¹ pi² 3–6 g
Arecae Pericarpium da⁴ fu⁴ pi² 6–9 g
Preparation method: Decoct with water.
Actions and Indications: Disinhibits water; moves qi; dispels wind-damp. Treats: 1) Generalized water swelling with abdominothoracic distention and oppression, short scant urinary voidings. 2) Water swelling in

pregnancy. 3) Exuberant damp in summer giving rise to swelling of the instep.

282 wu³-wei⁴-zi³ wan² 五味子丸 151, 213
Schisandra Pills
Source: 衛生家寶 (wei¹ sheng¹ jia¹ bao³)
Schisandrae Fructus wu³ wei⁴ zi³ 4 g
Dipsaci Radix xu⁴ duan⁴ 4 g
Rehmanniae Radix di⁴ huang² 2 g
Cervi Cornu Parvum lu⁴ rong² 2 g
Aconiti Tuber Laterale fu⁴ zi³ 2 g
Actions and Indications: Treats vacuity taxation, shortness of breath, profuse dreaming, vexing pain in the flesh and bones, aching back and lumbus.

283 wu³ zi³ yan³ zong¹ wan² 五子衍宗丸 150
Five-Seed Procreation Pills
Alternate names: 五子丸 wu³ zi³ wan² Five Seeds Pills, 五子補腎丸 wu³ zi³ bu³ shen⁴ wan² Five Seeds Kidney-Supplementing Pills
Source: 證治準繩 (zheng⁴ zhi⁴ zhun³ sheng²)
Cuscutae Semen tu⁴ si¹ zi³ 240 g
Lycii Fructus gou³ qi³ zi³ 240 g
Rubi Fructus fu⁴ pen² zi³ 160 g
Schisandrae Fructus wu³ wei⁴ zi³ 30 g
Plantaginis Semen che¹ qian² zi³ 60 g
Actions and Indications: Supplements the kidney and secures essence. Treats kidney vacuity with signs such as seminal emission, impotence, premature ejaculation, female infertility, and male sterility.

284 xi¹-jiao³ di⁴-huang² tang¹ 犀角地黃湯 9, 59, 219
Rhinoceros Horn and Rehmannia Decoction
Source: 千金方 (qian¹ jin¹ fang¹)
Rhinocerotis Cornu xi¹ jiao³ 1–3 g
Rehmanniae Radix Cruda sheng¹ di⁴ huang² 15–30 g
Paeoniae Radix shao² yao⁴ 6–12 g
Moutan Radicis Cortex mu³ dan¹ pi² 6–12 g
Actions and Indications: Clears heat and resolves toxin; cools the blood and dissipates stasis. Treats: 1) Heat entering construction-blood in warm heat disease, with signs such as clouded spirit and delirious speech, red or crimson tongue, and fine rapid pulse; other possible signs include macules and papules, and vomiting of blood or hemafecia due to frenetic movement of hot blood. 2) Traveling clove sores.

285 xia⁴-ku¹-cao³ tang¹ 夏枯草湯 116
Prunella Decoction
Source: 攝生衆妙方 (she⁴ sheng¹ zhong⁴ miao⁴ fang¹)
Prunellae Spica xia⁴ ku¹ cao³ 30 g
Actions and Indications: Treats scrofulous lumps.
Dosage: Take after meals.

286 xiang¹ lian² wan² 香連丸 63, 80
Saussurea and Coptis Pills
Source: 和劑局方 (he² ji⁴ ju² fang¹)
Coptidis Rhizoma huang² lian² 20 g
Saussureae Radix mu⁴ xiang¹ (roasted) 5 g
Preparation method: Stir-fry the Coptidis Rhizoma with Evodiae Fructus (wu² zhu¹ yu²), which is discarded before both agents a ground to a powder, blended with honey and formed into pills.
Actions and Indications: Clears heat and checks dysentery; moves qi and relieves pain. Treats damp-heat dysentery with red and white stool, abdominal pain and tenesmus.

287 xiang¹ rong² wan² 香茸丸 213, 216
Musk and Velvet Deer Antler Pills
Source: 百一選方 (bai³ yi¹ xuan³ fang¹)
Moschus she⁴ xiang¹ 1.5 g
Cervi Cornu Parvum lu⁴ rong² 30 g
Preparation method: Mix-fry and grind the musk, and mix with Junci Medulla (deng¹ xin¹ cao³) boiled with jujubes, and form into 300 mg pills.
Actions and Indications: Treats severe diarrhea.
Dosage: Take 10 pills on an empty stomach.

288 xiang¹-ru² san³ 香薷散 173
Elsholtzia Powder
Source: 和劑局方 (he² ji⁴ ju² fang¹)
Elsholtziae Herba xiang¹ ru² 3–9 g
Lablab Semen bian³ dou⁴ 9–12 g
Magnoliae Cortex hou⁴ po⁴ 3–6 g
Actions and Indications: Dispels summerheat and resolves the exterior; transforms damp and harmonizes the center. Treats contraction of external cold with internal damp resulting from drinking of cold beverages in hot weather. Signs: aversion to cold, fever, headache, absence of sweating; oppression in the chest, nausea and upflow, or in severe cases vomiting and diarrhea. Tongue fur: slimy and white. Pulse: floating.

289 xiang¹ sha¹ er⁴ chen² tang¹ 香砂二陳湯 63, 160
Saussurea and Amomum Double Vintage Decoction
Source: 和劑局方 (he² ji⁴ ju² fang¹)
Pinelliae Tuber ban⁴ xia⁴ 2–3 g
Citri Exocarpium chen² pi² 2–3 g
Poria fu² ling² 3 g
Glycyrrhizae Radix gan¹ cao³ 1 g
Saussureae Radix mu⁴ xiang¹ 3 g
Amomi Semen sha¹ ren² 3 g
Actions and Indications: Supplements qi and fortifies the spleen; dries damp and dispels phlegm. Treats vomiting and retching due to stomach cold.

290 *xiang¹ sha¹ liu⁴ jun¹ zi³ tang¹* 香砂六君子湯
....160

Cyperus and Amomum Six Gentlemen Decoction
New name: 健脾和胃湯 *jian⁴ pi² he² wei⁴ tang¹*
Spleen-Fortifying Stomach-Harmonizing Decoction
Source: 內科摘要 (*nei⁴ ke¹ zhai¹ yao⁴*)
Ginseng Radix *ren² shen¹*   3–4 g
Poria *fu² ling²*   3–4 g
Atractylodis Ovatae Rhizoma *bai² zhu²*   3–4 g
Glycyrrhizae Radix *gan¹ cao³*   1 g
Pinelliae Tuber *ban⁴ xia⁴*   3–4 g
Citri Exocarpium *chen² pi²*   2 g
Agastaches sen Pogostemi Herba *huo⁴ xiang¹*   1–2 g
Cyperi Rhizoma *xiang¹ fu⁴ zi³*   1.5–2 g
Amomi Semen *sha¹ ren²*   1–2 g
Zingiberis Rhizoma Recens *sheng¹ jiang¹*   1.5–2 g
Zizyphi Fructus *da⁴ zao³*   1.5–2 g
Actions and Indications: Treats glomus below the heart, and indigestion.

291 *xiang¹ sha¹ ping² wei⁴ san³* 香砂平胃散 83,160
Saussurea and Amomum Stomach-Calming Powder
Source: 萬病回春 (*wan⁴ bing⁴ hui² chun¹*)
Cyperi Rhizoma *xiang¹ fu⁴ zi³*   3 g
Citri Exocarpium *chen² pi²*   3 g
Atractylodis Ovatae Rhizoma *bai² zhu²*   3 g
Aurantii Fructus Immaturus *zhi³ shi²*   2.5 g
Agastaches seu Pogostemi Herba *huo⁴ xiang¹*   2.5 g
Amomi Semen *sha¹ ren²*   1.5 g
Saussureae Radix *mu⁴ xiang¹*   1.5 g
Glycyrrhizae Radix *gan¹ cao³*   1.5 g
Zingiberis Rhizoma *gan¹ jiang¹*   1 g
Actions and Indications: Treats food damage; hyperchlorhydria.

292 *xiang¹ sha¹ yang³ wei⁴ tang¹* 香砂養胃湯 83,120
Saussurea and Amomum Stomach-Nourishing Decoction
Source: 萬病回春 (*wan⁴ bing⁴ hui² chun¹*)
Ginseng Radix *ren² shen¹*   1.5 g
Saussureae Radix *mu⁴ xiang¹*   1.5 g
Atractylodis Ovatae Rhizoma *bai² zhu²*   2.5 g
Citri Exocarpium *chen² pi²*   2.5 g
Poria *fu² ling²*   2.5 g
Magnoliae Cortex *hou⁴ po⁴*   2.5 g
Atractylodis Rhizoma *cang¹ zhu²*   2.5 g
Amomi Semen *sha¹ ren²*   2.5 g
Cyperi Rhizoma *xiang¹ fu⁴ zi³*   2.5 g
Glycyrrhizae Radix *gan¹ cao³*   1.5 g
Amomi Cardamomi Fructus *bai² dou⁴ kou⁴*   2 g
Zizyphi Fructus *da⁴ zao³*   2 g
Zingiberis Rhizoma *gan¹ jiang¹*   1 g
Actions and Indications: Treats gastrointestinal disorders with poor appetite, atony of the stomach, gastritis, and gastroptosis.

293 *xiang¹ sha¹ zhi³ zhu² wan²* 香砂枳朮丸
....63, 76, 125, 160
Saussurea, Amomum, Unripe Bitter Orange, and Atractylodes Ovata Pills
Source: 景岳全書 (*jing³ yue⁴ quan² shu¹*)
Aurantii Fructus Immaturus *zhi³ shi²*   10 g
Atractylodis Ovatae Rhizoma *bai² zhu²* (stir-fried with earth)   20 g
Saussureae Radix *mu⁴ xiang¹*   10 g
Amomi Semen *sha¹ ren²*   10 g
Actions and Indications: Rectifies qi and disperses glomus; opens the stomach and increases food intake. Treats spleen-stomach qi stagnation, with glomus and fullness in the venter and abdomen, no thought of food or drink, and in some cases distention.

294 *xiang¹ su¹ san³* 香蘇散 83, 104
Cyperus and Perilla Powder
Source: 和劑局方 (*he² ji⁴ ju² fang¹*)
Cyperi Rhizoma *xiang¹ fu⁴ zi³*   6–9 g
Perillae Folium *zi³ su¹*   6–9 g
Citri Exocarpium *chen² pi²*   3–6 g
Glycyrrhizae Radix *gan¹ cao³* (mix-fried)   3–6 g
Preparation method: Decoct with water.
Actions and Indications: Rectifies qi and resolves the exterior. Treats contraction of external wind-cold occurring with internal qi stagnation. Signs: Cold form and generalized fever, headache, glomus and fullness in the chest and venter, belching, no desire to eat or drink. Tongue fur: thin and white tongue fur.

295 *xiang¹ xiong¹ tang¹* 香芎湯 83, 88
Cyperus and Ligusticum (Cnidium) Decoction
Source: 儒門事親 (*ru² men² shi⁴ qin¹*)
Gypsum *shi² gao¹*   10 g
Cinnamomi Ramulus *gui⁴ zhi¹*   3 g
Ligustici Rhizoma *chuan¹ xiong¹*   3 g
Cyperi Rhizoma *xiang¹ fu⁴ zi³*   6 g
Menthae Herba *bo⁴ he²*   2 g
Glycyrrhizae Radix *gan¹ cao³*   2g
Actions and Indications: Treats fever and headache; hemilateral headache.

296 *xiao¹ yao² san³* 逍遙散 31
Free Wanderer Powder
Source: 和劑局方 (*he² ji⁴ ju² fang¹*)
Bupleuri Radix *chai¹ hu²*   6–9 g
Atractylodis Ovatae Rhizoma *bai² zhu²*   6–9 g
Angelicae Sinensis Radix *dang¹ gui¹*   9 g
Paeoniae Radix Alba *bai² shao² yao⁴*   9 g
Poria *fu² ling²*   9 g

Menthae Herba *bo⁴ he²* 3 g
Glycyrrhizae Radix *gan¹ cao³* 3 g
Zingiberis Rhizoma Recens *sheng¹ jiang¹* (roasted) 3 slices
Actions and Indications: Courses the liver and resolves depression; fortifies the spleen and nourishes the blood. Treats depressed liver blood vacuity with pain in both lateral costal regions, headache and visual dizziness, dry mouth and throat, fatigue and reduced food intake; in women, menstrual irregularities, menstrual pain, distended breasts; steaming bone taxation fever.

297 *xiao³ ban⁴-xia⁴ jia¹ fu²-ling² tang¹*
小半夏加茯苓湯..........................92, 98, 236
Minor Pinellia Decoction Plus Poria
Source: 金匱要略 (*jin¹ gui⁴ yao⁴ lue⁴*)
Pinelliae Tuber *ban⁴ xia⁴* 5–8 g
Zingiberis Rhizoma Recens *sheng¹ jiang¹* 5–8 g
Poria *fu² ling²* 3–5 g
Actions and Indications: Harmonizes the stomach and transforms rheum; downbears counterflow and stops vomiting. Treats counterflow ascent of phlegm-rheum with glomus and oppression in the chest and venter, vomiting, dizziness and palpitations.

298 *xiao³ chai²-hu² tang¹* 小柴胡湯............31, 65
Minor Bupleurum Decoction
Source: 傷寒論 (*shang¹ han² lun⁴*)
Bupleuri Radix *chai² hu²* 6–12 g
Scutellariae Radix *huang² qin²* 5–10 g
Pinelliae Tuber *ban⁴ xia⁴* 6–9 g
Ginseng Radix *ren² shen¹* (or Codonopsitis Radix *dang³ shen¹*) 9–12 g
Glycyrrhizae Radix *gan¹ cao³* (mix-fried) 3–6 g
Zingiberis Rhizoma Recens *sheng¹ jiang¹* 2–4 g
Zizyphi Fructus *da⁴ zao³* 4–6 g
Preparation method: Decoct with water.
Actions and Indications: Harmonizes and resolves the shao yang; supports the correct and eliminates pathogens. Treats shao yang disease with alternating fever and chills, bitter fullness in the chest and lateral costal region, no desire for food or drink, vexation, nausea and vomiting, bitter taste in the mouth, dry throat, and visual dizziness. Tongue fur: thin and white. Pulse: wiry. Also used for heat entering the blood chamber in women, malarial disease, and jaundice.

299 *xiao³ cheng² qi⁴ tang¹* 小承氣湯......7, 95, 125
Minor Qi-Infusing Decoction
Source: 傷寒論 (*shang¹ han² lun⁴*)
Rhei Rhizoma *da⁴ huang²* 2–4 g
Magnoliae Cortex *hou⁴ po⁴* 2–3 g

Aurantii Fructus Immaturus *zhi³ shi²* 2–4 g
Actions and Indications: Drains heat and abducts stagnation; disperses accumulation and eliminates fullness. Treats yang ming bowel repletion patterns with glomus and fullness, constipation, tidal fever. Tongue fur: yellow. Pulse: rapid and slippery. Also treats indigestion and food accumulation with diarrhea, as well as initial-stage dysentery with distention and fullness of the abdomen and tenesmus.

300 *xiao³ jian⁴ zhong¹ tang¹* 小建中湯..........158
Minor Center-Fortifying Decoction
Source: 傷寒論 (*shang¹ han² lun⁴*)
Cinnamomi Ramulus *gui⁴ zhi¹* 6–9 g
Paeoniae Radix Alba *bai² shao² yao⁴* 12–18 g
Glycyrrhizae Radix *gan¹ cao³* 3–6 g
Zingiberis Rhizoma Recens *sheng¹ jiang¹* 2–5 g
Zizyphi Fructus *da⁴ zao³* 5–7 g
Granorum Saccharon *yi² tang²* (infused) 30–60 g
Preparation method: Decoct with water, remove dregs, and add malt sugar (Saccharon Granorum), and allow it to melt, and then split the brew into two helpings. Actions and Indications: Warms the center and supplements vacuity; relaxes tension and relieves pain. Treats middle burner vacuity cold giving rise to crampy pain in the stomach that is relieved by warmth, pressure and food; vacuity taxation fever; palpitation and vacuity vexation due to insufficiency of heart qi.

301 *xiao³ jin¹ dan¹* 小金丹...................175, 203
Minor Golden Elixir
Source: 外科全生集 (*wai⁴ ke¹ quan² sheng¹ ji²*)
Momordicae Semen *mu⁴ bie¹ zi³* 150 g
Aconiti Tsao-wu-tou Tuber *cao³ wu¹ tou²* 150 g
Trogopteri seu Pteromi Excrementum *wu³ ling² zhi¹* 150 g
Liquidambaris Resina *bai² jiao¹ xiang¹* 150 g
Lumbricus *di⁴ long²* 150 g
Olibanum *ru³ xiang¹* 75 g
Myrrha *mo⁴ yao⁴* 75 g
Angelicae Sinensis Radix *dang¹ gui¹* 75 g
Moschus *she⁴ xiang¹* 3 g
Atramentum *xiang¹ mo⁴* 12 g
Oryzae Glutinosae *nuo⁴ mi³ fen³*
Actions and Indications: Disperses swelling and dissipates binds. Treats phlegm nodes, scrofulous lumps, breast nodes, and all early-stage yin ju.

302 *xiao³ qing¹ long² tang¹* 小青龍湯.......26, 151
Minor Green-Blue Dragon Decoction
New name: 溫肺化飲湯 *wen¹ fei⁴ hua⁴ yin³ tang¹*
Lung-Warming Rheum-Transforming Decoction
Source: 傷寒論 (*shang¹ han² lun⁴*)
Ephedrae Herba *ma² huang²* 6–9 g

Cinnamomi Ramulus *gui⁴ zhi¹* 6–9 g
Paeoniae Radix *shao² yao⁴* 6–9 g
Zingiberis Rhizoma *gan¹ jiang³* 3–6 g
Pinelliae Tuber *ban⁴ xia⁴* 6–9 g
Asiasari Radix *xi⁴ xin¹* 3–4.5 g
Schisandrae Fructus *wu³ wei² zi³* 3–6 g
Glycyrrhizae Radix *gan¹ cao³* (mix-fried) 3–6 g
Preparation method: Decoct with water.
Actions and Indications: Warms the lung and transforms rheum; suppresses cough and calms dyspnea. Treats external cold and internal rheum, with cough, dyspnea, and copious amounts of clear, thin phlegm. In severe cases, the dyspnea prevents the patient from lying down, there is a feeling of cold in the back, and there may be swelling of the limbs and face, and thirst. Tongue fur: thin, white, and moist.

303 *xie⁴ bai² san³* 瀉白散 6, 8
White-Draining Powder
Source:小兒藥證直訣(*xiao³ er² yao² zheng⁴ zhi² jue²*)
Mori Radicis Cortex *sang¹ bai² pi²* 6–12 g
Lycii Radicis Cortex *di⁴ gu³ pi²* 6–12 g
Glycyrrhizae Radix *gan¹ cao³* 3–6 g
Oryzae Semen *geng¹ mi³* 15–30 g
Preparation method: Now usually prepared as a decoction.
Actions and Indications: Clears lung heat; suppresses cough and dyspnea. Treats lung heat with cough and dyspnea, expectoration of blood, tidal fever, and dry mouth and lips. Tongue: red with thin fur. Pulse: fine and rapid.

304 *xie⁴ xin¹ tang¹* 瀉心湯 65, 80, 95
Heart-Draining Decoction
Alternate name:三黃瀉心湯*san¹ huang² xie⁴ xin¹ tang¹*
Three Yellows Heart-Draining Decoction
Source:金匱要略 (*jin¹ gui⁴ yao⁴ lue⁴*)
Rhei Rhizoma *da⁴ huang²* 3–9 g
Coptidis Rhizoma *huang² lian²* 3–9 g
Scutellariae Radix *huang² qin²* 6–12 g
Actions and Indications: Clear heat and dries damp. Treats exuberant internal pathogen fire or damp-heat, manifesting in general signs such as fever, vexation, red face and eyes, dark-colored urine, constipation, slimy yellow tongue fur, and in severe cases, clouded spirit and manic or delirious raving. Specific patterns include glomus and fullness below the heart, jaundice, diarrhea, dysentery, nosebleed or vomiting of blood due to frenetic movement of hot blood, swelling of the ears, sores of the mouth and tongue, swollen yong, and cinnabar toxin.

305 *xing² qi⁴ xiang¹ su¹ san³* 行氣香蘇散 ...83, 104
Qi-Moving Cyperus and Perilla Powder

Source:古今醫鑑 (*gu³ jin¹ yi¹ jian⁴*)
Cyperi Rhizoma *xiang¹ fu⁴ zi³* 2.5 g
Perillae Folium *zi³ su¹ ye⁴* 2.5 g
Citri Exocarpium *chen² pi²* 2.5 g
Linderae Radix *wu¹ yao⁴* 2.5 g
Notopterygii Rhizoma *qiang¹ huo²* 2.5 g
Ligustici Rhizoma *chuan¹ xiong¹* 2.5 g
Ephedrae Herba *ma² huang²* 2 g
Aurantii Fructus *zhi³ ke²* 2 g
Zingiberis Rhizoma *gan¹ jiang¹* 1 g
Glycyrrhizae Radix *gan¹ cao³* 1 g
Actions and Indications: Treats food damage, colds, arthritis, and abdominal pain.

306 *xing⁴ su¹ san³* 杏蘇散 104, 162
Apricot Kernel and Perilla Powder
Source:溫病條辨 (*wen¹ bing⁴ tiao² bian⁴*)
Armeniacae Semen *xing⁴ ren²* 6 g
Perillae Caulis et Calyx *zi³ su¹* 3 g
Pinelliae Tuber *ban⁴ xia⁴* 6 g
Citri Exocarpium *chen² pi²* 3 g
Poria *fu² ling²* 6 g
Glycyrrhizae Radix *gan¹ cao³* 1.5 g
Peucedani Radix *qian² hu²* 6 g
Platycodonis Radix *jie³ geng³* 3 g
Aurantii Fructus *zhi³ ke²* 3 g
Zingiberis Rhizoma Recens *sheng¹ jiang¹* 1 g
Zizyphi Fructus *da⁴ zao³* 1 g
Actions and Indications: Dissipates wind-cold with warm agents. Treats contraction of external wind-cold giving rise to cough with copious phlegm, headache and nasal congestion.

307 *xiong¹ gui¹ jiao¹ ai⁴ tang¹* 芎歸膠艾湯 99, 208
Ligusticum (Cnidium), Tangkuei, Ass Hide Glue, and Mugwort Decoction
Source:金匱要略 (*jin¹ gui⁴ yao⁴ lue⁴*)
Ligustici Rhizoma *chuan¹ xiong¹* 3 g
Asini Corii Gelatinum *e¹ jiao¹* 3 g
Glycyrrhizae Radix *gan¹ cao³* 3 g
Artemisiae Argyi Folium *ai⁴ ye⁴* 3 g
Angelicae Sinensis Radix *dang¹ gui¹* 4 g
Paeoniae Radix *shao² yao⁴* 4 g
Rehmanniae Exsiccatae Radix *gan¹ di⁴ huang²* 6 g
Actions and Indications: Treats bleeding hemorrhoids; uterine bleeding; hematuria; intestinal bleeding.

308 *xiong²-dan³ wan²* 熊膽丸 214
Bear's Gall Pills
Source:小兒衛生 (*xiao³ er² wei⁴ sheng¹*)
Fel Ursi *xiong² dan³*
Quisqualis Fructus *shi³ jun¹ zi³*
All agents in equal proportions.

Preparation method: Grind to a powder, steam, and form into 100 mg pills.

Actions and Indications: Treats child gan accumulation.

Dosage: 20 pills at a time.

309 xu⁴-duan⁴ wan² 續斷丸 36
Dipsacus Pills

Source: 萬病回春 (wan⁴ bing⁴ hui² chun¹)

Dipsaci Radix xu⁴ duan⁴ 10 g

Psoraleae Semen bu³ gu³ zhi¹ 5 g

Achyranthis Bidentatae Radix niu² xi¹ 5 g

Chaenomelis Fructus mu⁴ gua¹ 5 g

Eucommiae Cortex du⁴ zhong⁴ 5 g

Dioscoreae Hypoglaucae Rhizoma bei¹ xie⁴ 5 g

Actions and Indications: Treats lumbar pain.

310 xu⁴-sui²-zi³ wan² 續隨子丸 168
Caper Spurge Seed Pills

Source: 摘元方 (zhai¹ yuan² fang¹)

Euphorbiae Lathyridis Semen xu⁴ sui² zi³ 20 g

Rhei Rhizoma da⁴ huang² 10 g

Preparation method: Stir-fry the Euphorbiae Lathyridis Semen (caper spurge seed) and remove oil. Grind with the Rhei Rhizoma to a fine powder, blend with wine and water, and form into 150 mg pills.

Actions and Indications: Treats yang water swelling and distention.

Dosage: 20 pills at a time.

311 xuan²-fu⁴ dai⁴-zhe³ tang¹ 旋覆代赭湯 113, 227
Inula and Hematite Decoction

Source: 傷寒論 (shang¹ han² lun⁴)

Inulae Flos xuan² fu⁴ hua¹ 9–12 g

Haematitum dai⁴ zhe³ shi² 9–15 g

Pinelliae Tuber ban⁴ xia⁴ 6–12 g

Ginseng Radix ren² shen¹ (or Codonopsitis Radix dang³ shen¹) 9 g

Glycyrrhizae Radix gan¹ cao³ (mix-fried) 3–5 g

Zingiberis Rhizoma Recens sheng¹ jiang¹ 3–5 g

Zizyphi Fructus da⁴ zao³ 3 pieces

Preparation method: Decoct with water.

Actions and Indications: Harmonizes the stomach; downbears counterflow; transforms phlegm. Treats phlegm turbidity causing internal obstruction with counterflow ascent of stomach qi, characterized by oppression and distention in the venter, belching and hiccoughing, nausea and vomiting.

312 xuan²-shen¹ san³ 玄參散 64
Scrophularia Powder

Source: 聖惠方 (sheng⁴ hui² fang¹)

Scrophulariae Radix xuan² shen¹ 3 g

Belamcandae Rhizoma she⁴ gan¹ 3 g

Scutellariae Radix huang² qin² 3 g

Actions and Indications: Treats cold damage with upper burner vacuity and congesting toxin.

313 xuan²-shen¹ sheng¹-ma² tang¹ 玄參升麻湯 64,79
Scrophularia and Cimicifuga Decoction

Source: 活人書 (huo² ren² shu¹)

Scrophulariae Radix xuan² shen¹ 1.5 g

Cimicifugae Rhizoma sheng¹ ma² 1.5 g

Glycyrrhizae Radix gan¹ cao³ (mix-fried) 1.5 g

Actions and Indications: Resolves toxin and transforms macules. Treats macules and sore swollen throat due to heat toxin in warm disease.

314 yi¹ sao³ guang¹ 一掃光 129, 172, 175
Gone-In-One-Sweep

Source: 外科正宗 (wai⁴ ke¹ zheng⁴ zong¹)

Sophorae Radix ku³ shen¹ 500 g

Phellodendri Cortex huang² bo² 500 g

Coriarii Fuligo Oleacea yan¹ jiao¹ 1000 g

Alumen Praeparatum ku¹ fan² 30 g

Momordicae Semen mu⁴ bie¹ zi³ 30 g

Hydnocarpi Semen da⁴ feng¹ zi³ 30 g

Cnidii Monnieri Fructus she² chuang² zi³ 30 g

Zanthoxyli Fructus hua¹ jiao¹ 30 g

Camphora zhang¹ nao³ 30 g

Sulphur shi² liu² huang² 30 g

Alumen bai² fan² 30 g

Hydrargyrum shui³ yin² 30 g

Calomelas qing¹ fen³ 30 g

Arsenicum Trioxidum Album bai² pi¹ 15 g

Actions and Indications: Kills worms and relieves itching. Treats bald white scalp sores, jie, and white scaling wind.

315 yi⁴ gan¹ san³ 抑肝散 20
Liver-Repressing Powder

Source: 保嬰撮要 (bao³ ying¹ cuo¹ yao⁴)

Bupleuri Radix chai² hu² 2 g

Glycyrrhizae Radix gan¹ cao³ 1.5 g

Ligustici Rhizoma chuan¹ xiong¹ 3 g

Angelicae Sinensis Radix dang¹ gui¹ 3 g

Atractylodis Ovatae Rhizoma bai² zhu² 4 g

Poria fu² ling² 4 g

Uncariae Ramulus et Uncus gou¹ teng² 3 g

Actions and Indications: Resolves tetany; quickens the blood and transforms stasis; resolves heat. Treats liver channel vacuity heat with signs such as pain, fever, grinding of the teeth, fright palpitations, and fever and chills; wood overwhelming earth with vomiting of phlegm-drool, abdominal distention, reduced appetite, and troubled sleep.

316 *yi⁴-mu³ sheng⁴ jin¹ dan¹* 益母勝金丹 ...60, 139
Leonurus Metal-Overcoming Elixir
Source: 醫學心悟 (*yi¹ xue² xin¹ wu⁴*)
Leonuri Herba *yi⁴ mu³ cao³* 9–15 g
Leonuri Fructus *chong¹ wei⁴ zi³* 6–12 g
Angelicae Sinensis Radix *dang¹ gui¹* 6–12 g
Rehmanniae Radix Conquita *shou² di⁴ huang²*
    9–15 g
Paeoniae Radix *bai² shao² yao⁴* 6–12 g
Ligustici Rhizoma *chuan¹ xiong¹* 3–9 g
Salviae Radix *dan¹ shen¹* 9–15 g
Atractylodis Ovatae Rhizoma *bai² zhu²* 6–12 g
Cyperi Rhizoma *xiang¹ fu⁴ zi³* 6–12 g
Preparation method: Prepare as a decoction (original book says prepare in pill form).
Actions and Indications: Quickens the blood and regulates the menses. Treats menstruation at irregular intervals.

317 *yi⁴ qi⁴ cong¹ ming² tang¹* 益氣聰明湯 155
Qi-Boosting Sharp and Bright Decoction
Source: 證治準繩 (*zheng⁴ zhi⁴ zhun³ sheng²*)
Astragali Radix *huang² qi²* 4 g
Ginseng Radix *ren² shen¹* 4 g
Puerariae Radix *ge² gen¹* 3 g
Viticis Fructus *man⁴ jing¹ zi³* 1.5 g
Paeoniae Radix Alba *bai² shao² yao⁴* 3 g
Phellodendri Cortex *huang² bo²* 1 g
Cimicifugae Rhizoma *sheng¹ ma²* 3 g
Glycyrrhizae Radix *gan¹ cao³* (mix-fried) 3 g
Actions and Indications: Boosts qi and restores uplift; sharpens hearing and brightens the eyes. Treats blurred vision, eye screens, deafness, and tinnitus.

318 *yi⁴-yi³ fu⁴-zi³ bai⁴-jiang⁴ san³* 薏苡附子敗醬散
....166
Coix, Aconite, and Baijiangcao Powder
Source: 金匱要略 (*jin¹ gui⁴ yao⁴ lue⁴*)
Coicis Semen *yi⁴ yi³ ren²* 15–30 g
Aconiti Tuber Laterale *fu⁴ zi³* 9–12 g
Baijiangcao Radix *bai⁴ jiang⁴ cao³* 15–30 g
Actions and Indications: Expels pus and disperses yong; warms yang and eliminates binds. Treats suppurating intestinal yong with tense abdomen that is soft to the touch and not too tender, a somber white complexion and a fine, weak pulse.

319 *yi⁴-yi³-ren² tang¹* 薏苡仁湯 166
Coix Decoction
Source: 明醫指掌 (*ming² yi¹ zhi³ zhang³*)
Ephedrae Herba *ma² huang²* 4 g
Angelicae Sinensis Radix *dang¹ gui¹* 4 g
Atractylodis Ovatae Rhizoma *bai² zhu²* 4 g
Coicis Semen *yi⁴ yi³ ren²* 8–10 g

Cinnamomi Ramulus *gui⁴ zhi¹* 3 g
Paeoniae Radix *shao² yao⁴* 3 g
Glycyrrhizae Radix *gan¹ cao³* 2 g
Preparation method: Decoct with water.
Actions and Indications: Treats pain in the joints, the sinews, and the muscle.

320 *yi⁴-zhi⁴ san³* 益智散 119
Alpinia Fruit Powder
Source: 和劑局方 (*he² ji⁴ ju² fang¹*)
Aconiti Tuber *chuan¹ wu¹ tou²* 4 g
Alpiniae Oxyphyllae Fructus *yi⁴ zhi⁴ ren²* 2 g
Zingiberis Rhizoma *gan¹ jiang¹* 0.5 g
Citri Exocarpium Immaturum *qing¹ pi²* 3 g
Zingiberis Rhizoma Recens *sheng¹ jiang¹* 1 g
Zizyphi Fructus *da⁴ zao³* 1 g
Actions and Indications: Treats cold damage with exuberant yin, glomus and fullness in the abdomen and the region below the heart, vomiting, retching, and diarrhea, and inversion frigidity of the limbs.

321 *yin¹-chen²-hao¹ tang¹* 茵陳蒿湯 189
Capillaris Decoction
Source: 傷寒論 (*shang¹ han² lun⁴*)
Artemisiae Capillaris Herba *yin¹ chen² hao¹* 15–30 g
Gardeniae Fructus *zhi¹ zi³* 9–15 g
Rhei Rhizoma *da⁴ huang²* 6–12 g
Preparation method: Decoct with water.
Actions and Indications: Clears heat and disinhibits damp; abates jaundice. Treats damp-heat jaundice characterized by an orange yellow coloring of eyes, face and whole body, as well as thirst, mild abdominal fullness, dark yellow urine, inhibited stool or constipation. Tongue: red with yellow fur. Pulse: slippery and rapid or deep and replete.

322 *yin¹-chen² wu³ ling² san³* 茵陳五苓散 189
Capillaris and Poria Five Powder
Source: 金匱要略 (*jin¹ gui⁴ yao⁴ lue⁴*)
Poria *fu² ling²* 3–4.5 g
Polyporus *zhu¹ ling²* 3–4.5 g
Alismatis Rhizoma *ze² xie⁴* 4.5–6 g
Atractylodis Ovatae Rhizoma *bai² zhu²* 3–4.5 g
Cinnamomi Ramulus *gui⁴ zhi¹* 2–3 g
Artemisiae Capillaris Herba *yin¹ chen² hao¹* 3–4 g
Actions and Indications: Disinhibits damp-heat and abates jaundice. Treats any form of jaundice with scant voidings of yellow urine.

323 *yin² qiao² san³* 銀翹散 114, 122, 134
Lonicera and Forsythia Powder
Source: 溫病條辨 (*wen¹ bing⁴ tiao² bian⁴*)
Lonicerae Flos *jin¹ yin² hua¹* 9–15 g
Forsythiae Fructus *lian² qiao²* 9–15 g

Sojae Semen Fermentatum *dou⁴ chi³* 9–12 g
Arctii Fructus *niu² bang⁴ zi³*   9–12 g
Menthae Herba *bo⁴ he²* 3–5 g
Schizonepetae Herba seu Flos *jing¹ jie⁴* 6–9 g
Platycodonis Radix *jie² geng³* 3–5 g
Glycyrrhizae Radix Cruda *sheng¹ gan¹ cao³* 3–5 g
Lophatheri Folium *zhu² ye⁴* 9–12 g
Phragmititis Rhizoma Recens *xian¹ lu² gen¹* 15–30 g
Preparation method: Now usually prepared in decoction form, but should not be boiled too long.
Actions and Indications: Resolves the exterior with cool pungent agents; clears heat and resolves toxin. Treats initial-stage febrile disease. Signs: fever, aversion to cold, absence of sweating, or inhibited sweating, headache, and sore throat. Tongue: slightly red at the edges, with a white or yellow fur. Pulse: rapid and floating.

324 *yu³ gong¹ san³* 禹功散............................178
Hallowed Ancient Yu Powder
Source: 儒門事親 (*ru² men² shi⁴ qin¹*)
Pharbitidis Semen Atrum *hei¹ chou³* 40 g
Foeniculi Fructus *hui² xiang¹* (stir-fried) 10 g
Saussureae Radix *mu⁴ xiang¹* 10 g
Actions and Indications: Dissipates cold and moves water. Treats cold-damp water shan with swelling and distention of the scrotum, and inhibited urination and defecation.

325 *yu⁴-jin¹ san³* 鬱金散...............................34
Curcuma Powder
Source: 普濟方 (*pu³ ji⁴ fang¹*)
Curcumae Tuber *yu⁴ jin¹*
Rehmanniae Radix Exsiccata *gan¹ di⁴ huang²*
Typhae Pollen *pu² huang²*
In equal proportions.
Actions and Indications: Treats blood strangury, vexation, blood in the urine, and accumulated heat in the small intestine.

326 *yu⁴-jin¹ yin³ zi³* 鬱金飲子........................34
Curcuma Drink
Source: 聖惠方 (*sheng⁴ hui⁴ fang¹*)
Curcumae Tuber *yu⁴ jin¹* 1.5 g
Scutellariae Radix *huang² qin²* 3 g
Paeoniae Radix Rubra *chi⁴ shao² yao⁴* 3 g
Aurantii Fructus *zhi³ ke²* 3 g
Rehmanniae Radix *di⁴ huang²* 3 g
Arecae Pericarpium *da⁴ fu⁴ pi²* 3 g
Zingiberis Rhizoma Recens *sheng¹ jiang¹* 1 g
Actions and Indications: Treats vexation and fever in the five hearts; clouding of the spirit in febrile disease.

327 *yu⁴ ping² feng¹ san³* 玉屏風散........30, 45, 76
Jade Wind-Barrier Powder
Source: 丹溪心法 (*dan¹ xi¹ xin¹ fa³*)
Astragali Radix *huang² qi²* 9–18 g
Atractylodis Ovatae Rhizoma *bai² zhu²* 9–12 g
Ledebouriellae Radix *fang² feng¹* 6–9 g
Actions and Indications: Boosts qi and fortifies the spleen; secures the exterior and checks sweating. Treats exterior vacuity with spontaneous sweating, or constitutional vacuity with susceptibility to external pathogens.

328 *yu⁴ suo³ dan¹* 玉鎖丹...............199, 225, 235
Jade Lock Elixir
Source: 和劑局方 (*he² ji⁴ ju² fang¹*)
Galla Rhois *wu³ bei⁴ zi³* 40 g
Poria *fu² ling²* 10 g
Fossilia Ossis Mastodi (Draconis Os) *long² gu³* 5 g
Preparation method: Grind to a powder, mix with flour and water paste, and form into pills the size of firmiana seeds (*wu³ tong² zi³*).
Actions and Indications: Treats vacuity taxation with white turbidity (*bai² zhuo²*).

329 *yu⁴ zhen¹ san³* 玉眞散...........................75
True Jade Powder
Source: 外科正宗 (*wai⁴ ke¹ zheng⁴ zong¹*)
Aconiti Coreani seu Typhonii Gigantei Tuber
  bai² fu⁴ zi³
Arisaematis Rhizoma *tian¹ nan² xing¹*
Gastrodiae Rhizoma *tian¹ ma²*
Ledebouriellae Radix *fang² feng¹*
Angelicae Dahuricae Radix *bai² zhi³*
Notopterygii Rhizoma et Radix *qiang¹ huo²*
All agents in equal proportions.
Actions and Indications: Dispels wind-phlegm; settles tetany. Treats lockjaw with arched-back rigidity and clenched jaws. Pulse: wiry.
Dosage: Take 3 g 2–3 times a day with warm wine or water. For topical use, blend with yellow wine or rice vinegar.

330 *yu⁴-zhu² yin³* 玉竹飲............................94
Solomon's Seal Beverage
Source: 張氏醫通 (*zhang¹ shi⁴ yi¹ tong¹*)
Polygonati Officinalis Rhizoma *yu⁴ zhu²* 3 g
Poria *fu² ling²* 2 g
Glycyrrhizae Radix *gan¹ cao³* 1 g
Platycodonis Radix *jie² geng³* 1 g
Citri Exocarpium *ju² pi² you⁴* 1 g
Asteris Radix et Rhizoma *zi³ wan³* 2 g
Fritillariae Cirrhosae Bulbus *chuan¹ bei⁴ mu³* 3 g
Zingiberis Rhizoma Recens *sheng¹ jiang¹* 4 g
Actions and Indications: Treats phlegm-fire with cough, dyspnea and fullness.

331 _yun² nan² bai² yao⁴_ 雲南白藥...................61
Yunnan White
Source: 經驗方 (empirical formula)
Notoginseng Radix _san¹ qi¹_
Moschus _she⁴ xiang¹_
Rhinacanthi Ramulus et Folium _bai² he⁴ ling² zhi¹_
Actions and Indications: Quickens the blood, staunches bleeding, and relieves pain. Treats all forms of internal or external bleeding, pain due to impact trauma, stomach or menstrual pain. Each bottle additionally contains one "emergency pill," which is used only for more serious impact trauma. It is swallowed with yellow wine.
Dosage: 0.4–0.5 g twice a day (usually with water). For external injuries without bleeding, mix with yellow wine.

332 _zao⁴-jia² wan²_ 皂莢丸...........................136
Gleditsia Fruit Pills
Source: 金匱要略 (_jin¹ gui⁴ yao⁴ lue⁴_)
Gleditsiae Fructus _zao⁴ jia²_
Preparation method: Remove skin from the honey locust pod, smear with fat, and bake. Then grind to a powder, blend with honey, and form into pills.
Actions and Indications: Cold-type cough.
Dosage: 0.5 g. three times a day and once at night.

333 _ze²- xie⁴ tang¹_ 澤瀉湯........................72, 76
Alisma Decoction
Source: 金匱要略 (_jin¹ gui⁴ yao⁴ lue⁴_)
Alismatis Rhizoma _ze² xie⁴_   5 g
Atractylodis Ovatae Rhizoma _bai² zhu²_   2 g
Actions and Indications: Treats column rheum below the heart with severe dizziness.

334 _zeng¹ ye⁴ tang¹_ 增液湯.................50, 59, 64
Humor-Increasing Decoction
Source: 溫病條辨 (_wen¹ bing⁴ tiao² bian⁴_)
Scrophulariae Radix _xuan² shen¹_   9–30 g
Rehmanniae Radix Exsiccata _gan¹ di⁴ huang²_   9–24 g
Ophiopogonis Tuber _mai⁴ dong¹_   9–24 g
Actions and Indications: Nourishes yin, engenders liquid, and moistens the intestines. Treats a) damage to liquid due to exuberant heat in warm disease with signs such as thirst, sore throat, dry red or crimson tongue; b) yin vacuity with constipation due to intestinal dryness.

335 _zhen¹ wu³ tang¹_ 眞武湯........................ 22
True Warrior Decoction
New name:溫陽利水湯 _wen¹ yang² li⁴ shui³ tang¹_
Yang-Warming Water-Disinhibiting Decoction
Source: 傷寒論 (_shang¹ han² lun⁴_)
Aconiti Tuber Laterale _fu⁴ zi³_   6–9 g

Poria _fu² ling²_   9–12 g
Atractylodis Ovatae Rhizoma _bai² zhu²_   9–12 g
Paeoniae Radix Alba _bai² shao² yao⁴_   6–9 g
Zingiberis Rhizoma Recens _sheng¹ jiang¹_   3–5 slices
Preparation method: Decoct with water.
Actions and Indications: Warms yang and disinhibits water. Treats: 1) Debilitation of kidney yang with accumulation of water qi. Signs: inhibited urination, water swelling, pain and heaviness in the limbs, aversion to cold, abdominal pain, and diarrhea. Tongue fur: white and glossy. 2) Palpitations, dizziness, and general shaking due to damage to yang through profuse sweating and cold-water stirring internally.

336 _zhen⁴ gan¹ xi² feng¹ tang¹_ 鎮肝熄風湯.......27
Liver-Settling Wind-Extinguishing Decoction
Source:醫學衷中參西錄 (_yi¹ xue² ai¹ zhong¹ can¹ xi¹ lu⁴_)
Achyranthis Bidentatae Radix _niu² xi¹_   9–30 g
Haematitum _dai⁴ zhe³ shi²_   15–30 g
Ostreae Concha Cruda _sheng¹ mu³ li⁴_   15–30 g
Fossilia Ossis Mastodi(Draconis Os) Crudum _sheng¹ long² gu³_   9–15 g
Testudinis Plastrum Crudum _sheng¹ gui¹ ban³_   9–15 g
Paeoniae Radix Cruda _sheng¹ shao² yao⁴_   9–15 g
Scrophulariae Radix _xuan² shen¹_   9–15 g
Asparagi Tuber _tian¹ men² dong¹_   9–15 g
Meliae Toosendan Fructus _chuan¹ lian⁴ zi³_   5–9 g
Hordei Fructus Germinatus Crudus _sheng¹ mai⁴ ya²_   5–9 g
Artemisiae Capillaris Herba _yin¹ chen² hao¹_   5–9 g
Glycyrrhizae Radix _gan¹ cao³_   3–6 g
Preparation method: Decoct with water.
Actions and Indications: Settles the liver and extinguishes wind. Treats ascendant liver yang stirring liver wind. Signs: dizziness, headache with sensatin of heat in the brain, distended eyes, tinnitus, heat vexation in the heart, fright palpations, and insomnia, gradual inhibition of the limbs and deviation of the eyes and face, or sudden collapse leaving the limbs paralyzed after consciousness is regained. Pulse: long, wiry and forceful.

337 _zhi¹ bo² di⁴-huang² wan²_ 知柏地黃丸
....10, 59, 74, 84
Anemarrhena, Phellodendron, and Rehmannia Pills
Alternate name:知柏八味丸 _zhi¹ bo² ba¹ wei⁴ wan²_
Anemarrhena and Phellodendron Eight Pills
Source: 醫方考 (_yi¹ fang¹ kao³_)
Variant of 六味地黃丸 _liu⁴ wei⁴ di⁴-huang² wan²_
Rehmannia Six Pills
Rehmanniae Radix Conquita _shou² di⁴ huang²_   8 g
Corni Fructus _shan¹ zhu¹ yu²_   4 g

Dioscoreae Rhizoma *shan¹ yao⁴* 4 g
Alismatis *ze² xie⁴* 3 g
Moutan Radicis Cortex *mu³ dan¹ pi²* 3 g
Poria *fu² ling²* 3 g
Anemarrhenae Rhizoma *zhi¹ mu³* 2 g
Phellodendri Cortex *huang² bo²* 2 g
Actions and Indications: Enriches yin and drains fire. Treats effulgent yin vacuity fire with steaming bone tidal fever, seminal emission, night sweats, yellow or dark-colored urine.

338 *zhi¹-zi³ chi³ tang¹* 梔子豉湯............135, 185
Gardenia and Fermented Soybean Decoction
Alternate name:梔子豆豉湯 *zhi¹-zi³ dou⁴-chi³ tang¹*
Gardenia and Fermented Soybean Decoction
Source: 傷寒論 (*shang¹ han² lun⁴*)
Gardeniae Fructus *zhi¹ zi³* 6–9 g
Sojae Semen Praeparatum *dou⁴ chi³* 9–12 g
Preparation method: Decoct with water.
Actions and Indications: Clears heat and eliminates vexation. Treats: 1) Externally contracted pathogens in the qi aspect, characterized by fever, oppression in the chest, vexation, and slightly yellow tongue fur. 2) Vacuity vexation and insomnia after diaphoresis, ejection or precipitation in febrile diseases.

339 *zhi¹-zi³ da⁴-huang² tang¹* 梔子大黃湯 95, 135
Gardenia and Rhubarb Decoction
Source: 金匱要略 (*jin¹ gui⁴ yao⁴ lue⁴*)
Gardeniae Fructus *zhi¹ zi³* 2 g
Aurantii Fructus Immaturus *zhi³ shi²* 3 g
Sojae Semen Praeparatum *dou⁴ chi³* 6 g
Rhei Rhizoma *da⁴ huang²* 1 g
Actions and Indications: Clears heat and eliminates vexation; disperses accumulations, drains and precipitates. Treats jaundice with hot sensation in the rgion of the heart, sometimes with pain; relapse of disease due to dietary irregularity, with fever, and constipation.

340 *zhi¹-zi³ gan¹-cao³ chi³ tang¹* 梔子甘草豉湯
................................42, 135, 185
Gardenia, Licorice, and Fermented Soybean Decoction
Source: 傷寒論 (*shang¹ han² lun⁴*)
Gardeniae Fructus *zhi¹ zi³* 3 g
Sojae Semen Praeparatum *dou⁴ chi³* 5 g
Glycyrrhizae Radix *gan¹ cao³* 1 g
Actions and Indications: Clears heat and eliminates vexation; boosts qi. Treats Gardenia and Fermented Soybean Decoction (*zhi¹-zi³ chi³ tang¹*) patterns with shortness of breath.

341 *zhi³-shi² dao³ zhi⁴ wan²* 枳實導滯丸........125
Unripe Bitter Orange Stagnation-Abducting Pills

Source:內外傷辨惑論(*nei⁴ wai⁴ shan¹ bian⁴ huo⁴ lun⁴*)
Aurantii Fructus Immaturus *zhi³ shi²* (stir-fried with bran) 5 g
Massa Medicata Fermentata *shen² qu¹* (stir-fried) 5 g
Rhei Rhizoma *da⁴ huang²* 5 g
Scutellariae Radix *huang² qin²* 3 g
Coptidis Rhizoma *huang² lian²* 3 g
Atractylodis Ovatae Rhizoma *bai² zhu²* 3 g
Poria *fu² ling²* 3 g
Alismatis Rhizoma *ze² xie⁴* 2 g
Preparation method: Can also be prepared as a decoction.
Actions and Indications: Disperses accumulation and abducts stagnation; clears heat and disinhibits damp. Treats dietary irregularity giving rise to stagnation and accumulation with brewing damp-heat, manifesting as glomus, distention and oppression in the chest and venter, bitter taste in the mouth, constipation or inhibited diarrhea. Tongue fur: yellow and slimy. Pulse: deep and replete. May also be used for initial-stage dysenteric disease.
Dosage: 6–9 g twice daily.

342 *zhi³-shi² zhi¹-zi³ chi³ tang¹* 枳實梔子豉湯
................................125, 135, 185
Unripe Bitter Orange, Gardenia, and Fermented Soybean Decoction
Source: 傷寒論 (*shang¹ han² lun²*)
Aurantii Fructus Immaturus *zhi³ shi²* 2 g
Gardeniae Fructus *zhi¹ zi³* 4 g
Sojae Semen Praeparatum *dou⁴ chi³* 8 g
Actions and Indications: Clears heat and eliminates vexation; fortifies the stomach and disperses glomus. Treats relapse of disease due to taxation, with generalized fever and glomus and oppression beneath the heart.

343 *zhi³ sou⁴ san³* 止嗽散 28, 68
Cough Powder
Source: 醫學心悟 (*yi¹ xue² xin¹ wu⁴*)
Schizonepetae Herba seu Flos *jing¹ jie⁴* 6–9 g
Platycodonis Radix *jie² geng³* 3–6 g
Asteris Radix et Rhizoma *zi³ wan³* 6–9 g
Stemonae Radix *bai³ bu⁴* 6–9 g
Cynanchi Baiqian Radix et Rhizoma *bai² qian²* 6–9 g
Citri Exocarpium *chen² pi²* 6–9 g
Glycyrrhizae Radix *gan¹ cao³* 3–4.5 g
The original formula says Citri Exocarpium (tangerine peel) without the white part. Preparation method: Now normally prepared as a decoction.
Actions and Indications: Suppresses cough and transforms phlegm; courses wind and resolves the exterior. Treats persistent cough due to external contrac-

tion, with difficulty in expectorating phlegm, and in some cases slight aversion to cold, fever, and headache. Tongue fur: thin and white. Pulse: floating and moderate.

344 *zhi³ zhu² tang¹* 枳朮湯 125
Unripe Bitter Orange and Atractylodes Ovata Decoction
Source: 金匱要略 (*jin¹ gui⁴ yao⁴ lue⁴*)
Aurantii Fructus Immaturus *zhi³ shi²* 6 g
Atractylodis Ovatae Rhizoma *bai² zhu²* 2 g
Actions and Indications: Disperses glomus and eliminates rheum. Treats poor spleen-stomach movement and transformation with bloating after eating.

345 *zhi⁴-gan¹-cao³ tang¹* 炙甘草湯 42, 50, 164, 208
Honey-Fried Licorice Decoction
Alternate name: 復脈湯 *fu⁴ mai⁴ tang¹* Pulse-Restorative Decoction
Source: 傷寒論 (*shang¹ han² lun⁴*)
Glycyrrhizae Radix *gan¹ cao³* (mix-fried) 9–15 g
Ginseng Radix *ren² shen¹* (or Codonopsitis Radix *dang³ shen¹*) 6–9 g
Cinnamomi Ramulus *gui⁴ zhi¹* 6–9 g
Rehmanniae Radix Cruda *sheng¹ di⁴ huang²* 12–15 g
Ophiopogonis Tuber *mai⁴ dong¹ zhi¹* 6–9 g
Asini Corii Gelatinum *e¹ jiao¹* (dissolved in hot water) 6–9 g
Cannabis Semen *huo³ ma² ren²* 6–12 g
Zingiberis Rhizoma Recens *sheng¹ jiang¹* 3–5 slices
Zizyphi fructus *da⁴ zao³* 5–10 pieces
Granorum Vinum seu Spiritus *jiu³*
Actions and Indications: Nourishes the blood and restores the pulse. Treats qi and blood vacuity with palpitations and a bound or regularly interrupted pulse.

346 *zhu¹ ling²-tang¹* 豬苓湯 72, 208, 232, 236, 238
Polyporus Decoction
Source: 傷寒論 (*shang¹ han² lun⁴*)
Polyporus *zhu¹ ling²* 9–12 g
Poria *fu² ling²* 9–12 g
Alismatis Rhizoma *ze² xie⁴* 9–12 g
Asini Corii Gelatinum *e¹ jiao¹* 6–9 g
Talcum *hua² shi²* 9–12 g
Preparation method: Decoct with water.
Actions and Indications: Disinhibits water, enriches yin, and clears heat. Treats: 1) Water and heat binding together, with the heat causing damage to yin. Signs: inhibited urination, thirst with desire for fluid, vexation and insomnia. 2) Strangury with painful urination, blood in the urine, and pain, fullness and distention in the lower abdomen.

347 *zhu¹-sha¹ an¹ shen² wan²* 朱砂安神丸 224
Cinnabar Spirit-Quieting Pills
Source: 經驗方 (empirical formula)
Cinnabaris *zhu¹ sha¹* (water-ground) 100 g
Coptidis Rhizoma *huang² lian²* (stir-fried in wine) 150 g
Angelicae Sinensis Radix *dang¹ gui¹* 100 g
Glycyrrhizae Radix *gan¹ cao³* (mix-fried with honey) 50 g
Rehmanniae Radix *di⁴ huang²* 100 g
Preparation method: Grind to a fine powder, mix with water to form pills, and coat with cinnabar.
Actions and Indications: Settles the heart and quiets the spirit; drains fire and nourishes yin. Treats effulgent heart fire and damage to yin-blood. Signs: heat vexation in the chest, fright palpitations, and insomnia or profuse dreaming.
Dosage: 3–6 g taken with water before bed.

348 *zhu² han² dang⁴ jing¹ tang¹* 逐寒蕩驚湯 ...107
Cold-Dispelling Fright-Assuaging Decoction
Source: 福幼編 (*fu² you⁴ bian¹*)
Caryophylli Flos *ding¹ xiang¹* 1.5–3 g
Cinnamomi Cortex *rou⁴ gui⁴* 2–3 g
Piperis Nigri Fructus *hu² jiao¹* 1.5–3 g
Zingiberis Rhizoma *jiang¹* (blast-fried) 1.5–3 g
Terra Flava Usta *fu² long² gan¹* 60–90 g
Preparation method: Make a decoction of the Terra Flava Usta (fu² long² gan¹), and then use this to boil the other constituents. Split into a number of helpings and take warm.
Actions and Indications: Expels cold and eliminates fright. Treats enduring vomiting and diarrhea in children, with signs such as a white complexion with a green-blue tinge, cold breath from the nose and mouth, cold limbs, hypersomnia with incompletely closed eyes, long clear voidings of urine, thin stool, and signs of developing chronic fright.

349 *zhu²-ye⁴ shi²-gao¹ tang¹* 竹葉石膏湯 ..102, 226
Bamboo Leaf (Lophatherum) and Gypsum Decoction
Source: 傷寒論 (*shang¹ han² lun⁴*)
Lophatheri Folium *zhu² ye⁴* 2 g
Gypsum *shi² gao¹* 10 g
Ophiopogonis Tuber *mai⁴ dong¹ zhi¹* 6 g
Ginseng Radix *ren² shen¹* 3 g
Pinelliae Tuber *ban⁴ xia⁴* 4 g
Glycyrrhizae Radix *gan¹ cao³* 2 g
Oryzae Semen *geng¹ mi³* 6 g
Actions and Indications: Clears heat and engenders liquid; boosts qi and harmonizes the stomach. Treats: 1) Recovery stage of heat disease with residual heat and damage to both qi and liquid, manifesting in signs

such as vexation and thirst, desire to vomit, dry mouth and lips, smooth red tongue with little fur, and a rapid, fine pulse. 2) Stomach fire due to insufficiency of stomach yin giving rise to erosion of the mouth and tongue, a red or crimson dry tongue, thirst, nausea and retching. 3) Stomach fire wasting thirst. 4) Summerheat-heat with damage to qi and liquid.

350 zi^1 $shou^4$ jie^3 yu^3 $tang^1$ 資壽解語湯 207
Life-Prolonging Speech-Returning Decoction
Source: 沈氏尊生書 ($zhen^3$ shi^4 zun^1 $sheng^1$ shu^1)
Antelopis Cornu $ling^2$ $yang^2$ $jiao^3$ (grated and infused) 0.3–0.6 g
Gastrodiae Rhizoma $tian^1$ ma^2 3–9 g
Zizyphi Spinosi Semen $suan^1$ zao^3 ren^2 3–9 g
Ledebouriellae Radix $fang^2$ $feng^1$ 6–9 g
Notopterygii Rhizoma $qiang^1$ huo^2 6–9 g
Cinnamomi Ramulus gui^4 zhi^1 3–6 g
Aconiti Tuber Laterale fu^4 zi^3 3–6 g
Glycyrrhizae Radix gan^1 cao^3 3–6 g
Bambusae Succus Exsiccatus zhu^2 li^4 15–20 ml.
Zingiberis Succus $jiang^1$ zhi^1 aq.
Preparation method: Swallow mixed with fluid.
Actions and Indications: Calms the liver and extinguishes wind; dispels wind and frees the connecting vessels. Treats wind stroke with hemiplegia and stiffness of the tongue preventing speech.

351 zi^1 yin^1 $jiang^4$ huo^3 $tang^1$ 滋陰降火湯 27
Yin-Enriching Fire-Downbearing Decoction
Source: 萬病回春 (wan^4 $bing^4$ hui^2 $chun^1$)
Asparagi Tuber $tian^1$ men^2 $dong^1$ 2.5 g
Rehmanniae Radix di^4 $huang^2$ 2.5 g
Paeoniae Radix $shao^2$ yao^4 2.5 g
Angelicae Sinensis Radix $dang^1$ gui^1 2.5 g
Anemarrhenae Rhizoma zhi^1 mu^3 1.5 g
Phellodendri Cortex $huang^2$ bo^4 1.5 g
Ophiopogonis Tuber mai^4 $dong^1$ 2.5 g
Atractylodis Ovatae Rhizoma bai^2 zhu^2 3 g
Citri Exocarpium $chen^2$ pi^2 2.5 g.r
Zingiberis Rhizoma Recens $sheng^1$ $jiang^1$ 1 g
Zizyphi Fructus da^4 zao^3 1 g
Actions and Indications: Drains fire and enriches yin. Treats dry throat and spasmodic cough without phlegm.

352 zi^3-gen^1 mu^3-li^4 $tang^1$ 紫根牡蠣湯 48
Puccoon and Oyster Shell Decoction
Source: 黴疫新書 (mei^2 yi^4 xin^1 shu^1)
Angelicae Sinensis Radix $dang^1$ gui^1 5 g
Paeoniae Radix $shao^2$ yao^4 3 g
Ligustici Rhizoma $chuan^1$ $xiong^1$ 3 g
Lithospermi Radix zi^3 cao^3 3 g
Rhei Rhizoma da^4 $huang^2$ 1.5 g

Cimicifugae Rhizoma $sheng^1$ ma^2 2 g
Astragali Radix $huang^2$ qi^2 2 g
Ostreae Concha mu^3 li^4 4 g
Glycyrrhizae Radix gan^1 cao^3 1 g
Actions and Indications: Treats malignant tumors, gummae, and lymphomae.

353 zi^3-wan^3 san^3 紫菀散 28, 112
Aster Powder
Source: 聖濟總惠 ($sheng^4$ ji^4 $zong^3$ hui^4)
Asteris Radix et Rhizoma zi^3 wan^3 10 g
Armeniacae Semen $xing^4$ ren^2 1 g
Asiasari Radix xi^4 xin^1 1 g
Tussilaginis Flos $kuan^3$ $dong^1$ hua^1 1 g
Preparation method: Grind to a fine powder.
Actions and Indications: Treats cough counterflow qi ascent with rale in children.
Dosage: 1.5 g 3 times a day.

354 zi^3 xue^3 dan^1 紫雪丹 107
Purple Snow Elixir
Original name: 紫雪 zi^3 xue^3 Purple Snow
Source: 和劑局方 (he^2 ji^4 ju^2 $fang^1$)
Gypsum shi^2 gao^1 480 g
Calcitum han^2 $shui^3$ shi^2 480 g
Talcum hua^2 shi^2 480 g
Magnetitum ci^2 shi^2 480 g
Rhinocerotis Cornu xi^1 $jiao^3$ 50 g
Antelopis Cornu $ling^2$ $yang^2$ $jiao^3$ 50 g
Saussureae Radix $qing^1$ mu^4 $xiang^1$ 50 g
Aquilariae Lignum $chen^2$ $xiang^1$ 50 g
Caryophylli Flos $ding^1$ $xiang^1$ 10 g
Scrophulariae Radix $xuan^2$ $shen^1$ 160 g
Cimicifugae Rhizoma $sheng^1$ ma^2 160 g
Glycyrrhizae Radix gan^1 cao^3 (mix-fried) 80 g
Mirabilitum Poxiao po^4 $xiao^1$ 320 g
Nitrum $xiao^1$ shi^2 320 g
Cinnabaris zhu^1 sha^1 30 g
Moschus she^4 $xiang^1$ 12.5 g
Actions and Indications: Clears heat and resolves toxin; opens the portals and settles tetany. Treats: 1) Febrile disease with high fever, vexation and agitation, clouding of the spirit and delirious speech, dark-colored urine, constipation, convulsive spasm. 2) Child fright inversion with exuberant fever.

355 zi^3 yun^2 gao^1 紫雲膏 48
Purple Clouds Paste
Source: 華岡青洲 (hua^2 $gang^1$ $qing^1$ $zhou^1$)
Sesami Oleum Seminis ma^2 you^2 1,000 g
Cera mi^4 la^4 300–400 g
Suis Adeps zhu^1 zhi^1 gao^1 20–30 g
Angelicae Sinensis Radix $dang^1$ gui^1 60–100 g
Lithospermi Radix zi^3 cao^3 100–120 g

Lonicerae Ramus *ren³ dong¹ teng²* 1.5 g
Preparation method: Bring the sesame oil to the boil
and add bee's wax and lard to melt. Then add the and
allow it to turn amber (ca 140°C). Finally, add the
Lithospermum root, bring to the boil.
Actions and Indications: Treats wounds, chilblains,
and periproctitis.

356 *zuo³ jin¹ wan²* 左金丸 80, 132
Metal-Assisting Pills
Source: 丹溪心法 (*dan¹ xi¹ xin¹ fa³*)
Coptidis Rhizoma *huang² lian²* 18 g
Evodiae Fructus *wu² zhu¹ yu²* 3 g
Preparation method: Can also be prepared in decoc-
tion form.
Actions and Indications: Drains fire and downbears
counterflow. Treats liver fire and stomach heat
manifesting as bitter taste in the mouth and lateral
costal pain, vomiting of sour fluid, nausea, and
clamoring stomach. Tongue: red with yellow fur.
Pulse: rapid and wiry.
Dosage: 2–3 g 2–3 times a day.

Appendix IV Glossary of Chinese Medical Terms

abducting dispersion 消導 *xiao¹ dao³*: Disperse stagnant food, thereby enabling it to be carried down the digestive tract. Abducting dispersion agents include Crataegus Fructus *(shan¹ zha¹)*, Massa Medicata Fermentata *(shen² qu¹)*, and Raphani Semen *(lai² fu⁴ zi³)*, which are often combined with spleen-fortifying agents such as Atractylodis Ovatae Rhizoma *(bai² zhu²)*, Hoelen (fu² ling²), Dioscoreae Rhizoma *(shan¹ yao⁴)*, and Coicis Semen *(yi⁴ yi³ ren²)* to treat an underlying vacuity. A commonly used abducting dispersion formula is Harmony-Preserving Pills *(bao³ he² wan²)*.

arched-back rigidity 角弓反張 *jiao³ gong¹ fan³ zhang¹*: Spasm that causes arching of the back, as observed in fright wind. Synonym: opisthotonos.

articular wind 歷節風 *li⁴ jie² feng¹*: Disease name from *Essential Prescriptions of the Golden Coffer (jin¹ gui⁴ yao⁴ lue⁴)* denoting redness and swelling of the joints, with acute pain and difficulty bending and stretching. This disease is attributed to transformation of wind-cold-damp into heat in patients suffering from liver-kidney vacuity.

ascendant liver yang 肝陽上亢 *gan¹ yang² shang⁴ kang⁴*: Excessive upbearing and stirring of liver yang due to insufficiency of liver yin, characterized by headache, dizziness, flowery vision, tinnitus, vexation and agitation, irascibility, numbness of the limbs, tremor the hands, bitter taste in the mouth, and constipation.

astringe essence 澀精 *se⁴ jing¹*: To check seminal loss (semen being a form of essence). See *securing astriction.*

bi 痹 *bi⁴*: (1) Obstruction of the channels by a combination of externally contracted wind, cold, and dampness, giving rise to conditions of pain and numbness that correspond to biomedically defined diseases such as rheumatism, arthritis, sciatica. Three major forms are distinguished according to the predominant pathogen: *wind bi*, in which wind predominates, is characterized by migratory pain (swiftness and changeability being the attributes of wind); *cold bi*, in which the cold pathogen is dominant, is characterized by severe pain (pain being one of the pain attributes of cold); *damp bi*, in which dampness is the prevalent pathogen, is characterized by heavy cumbersome limbs (heaviness being an attribute of dampness). In addition to these forms, there is also *heat bi*, which is characterized by pain and heat in the joints, and which develops when wind, cold, and dampness transform into heat after having remained lodged in the body for a long time. (2) Other conditions of obstruction, e.g., throat bi (swelling of the throat that causes difficulty in swallowing).

blood amassment 蓄血 *xu⁴ xue⁴*: Binding depression of malign blood in the channels and organs, e.g., uterine blood amassment, which is marked by lower abdominal pain, alternating fever and chills, delirious speech, and disquietude of the spirit at night.

blood ejection 吐血 *tu⁴ xue⁴*: (1) Ejection of blood from the lung or stomach through mouth. (2) Specifically, vomiting of blood.

binding depression of liver qi 肝氣鬱結 *gan¹ qi⁴ yu⁴ jie²*: Stagnation of qi in the liver and liver channel resulting for impairment of the liver's normal free coursing action. It is mainly caused by insufficiency of yin-blood depriving the liver of nourishment, or by damp-heat. Its most general signs are wiry pulse and lateral costal pain. It may also manifest as plum-pit qi, scrofulous lumps, menstrual irregularities, and distension of the breasts. Depressed liver qi can invade the stomach, giving rise to nausea, vomiting etc., which can develop into a liver-spleen pattern with diarrhea.

bowstring and elusive masses 痃癖 *xian² pi⁴*: Bowstring masses are elongated masses located lateral to the navel; elusive masses are ones located in the lateral costal region that occur intermittently with pain and at other times are not detectable by palpation. The two conditions belong to the category of concretions, conglomerations, accumulations, and gatherings.

break blood 破血 *po⁴ xue⁴*: To dispel severe forms of blood stasis, with potent agents such as Rhei Rhizoma *(da⁴ huang²)*, Juglandis Semen *(hu² tao² ren²)*, Carthami Flos *(hong² hua¹)*, Manitis Squama *(chuan¹ shan¹ jia³)*, and Eupolyphaga seu Opisthoplatia *(zhe⁴ chong²)*.

break qi 破氣 *po⁴ qi⁴*: To dispel severe qi stagnation with potent qi-rectifiers such as Citri Exocarpium Immaturum *(qing¹ pi²)* and Aurantii Fructus Immaturus *(zhi³ shi²)*.

brighten the eyes 明目 *ming² mu⁴*: Enhance visual acuity.

calm the liver and extinguish wind 平肝熄風 *ping² gan¹ xi² feng¹*: To treat internal wind due to ascendant liver yang. Liver-calming wind-extinguishing agents include Uncariae Ramulus cum Uncus *(gou¹ teng²)*, Tribuli Fructus *(ci⁴ ji² li²)*, Chrysanthemi Flos *(ju² hua¹)*, Lumbricus *(di⁴ long²)*, Concha Margaritifera *(zhen¹ zhu¹ mu³)*, Ostreae Concha *(mu³ li⁴)*, and Haliotidis Concha *(shi² jue² ming²)*.

canthus outcrop 胬肉攀睛 *nu³ rou⁴ pan¹ jing¹*: A gray-white fleshy growth at the canthus that progressively grows over the eye, in severe cases affecting vision. It is attributed to heat congesting in the heart and lung channels. Corresponds to pterygium in Western medicine.

choleraic disease 霍亂 *huo⁴ luan⁴*: Disease marked by simultaneous fulminant vomiting and diarrhea, followed by severe cramps. It corresponds to cholera as defined by Western medicine, and to acute gastroenteritis characterized by similar signs. Also called *sudden turmoil.*

cinnabar toxin 丹毒 *dan¹ du²*: A disease characterized by clearly defined painful and palpably hot red pat-

346

ches on the skin that are slightly raised at the edges, in some cases with vesicles that exude yellow fluid, causing pain and itching when they burst. The condition develops rapidly after fever and aversion to cold, and is accompanied by general heat signs such as vexation and thirst, continuing generalized fever, constipation, dark-colored (reddish) urine. It is attributed to heat toxin in the blood aspect with accompanying wind if it affects the upper body (usually the head) or with accompanying dampness if it affects the lower body (usually the lower legs). Cinnabar toxin, so called because it gives the skin the appearance of having been smeared with cinnabar, corresponds to erysipelas in Western medicine, although the term is sometimes used as a general name for any similar red lesion, e.g., *snake fire cinnabar* (herpes zoster).

clamoring stomach 嘈雜 *cao² za²*: A sensation of discomfort in the venter or region of the heart described as being neither hunger nor pain. It may occur in food damage, stomach heat, stomach cold, or liver-stomach disharmony.

clear 清 *qing¹*: (1) Clean or pure, as in clear yang qi. (2) To eliminate heat, as in *clear the lung*, meaning eliminate lung heat.

concretion 癥 *zheng¹*: See *concretions, conglomerations, accumulations, and gatherings*.

concretions, conglomerations, accumulations, and gatherings 癥瘕積聚 *zheng¹ jia³ ji¹ ju⁴*: Abdominal masses associated with pain and distention. Concretions and accumulations are masses of definite form and fixed location, associated with pain of fixed location. They stem from disease in the five viscera and blood aspect. Conglomerations and gatherings are masses of indefinite form, which gather and dissipate at irregular intervals and are attended by pain of unfixed location. They are attributed to disease in the six bowels and qi aspect. Accumulations and gatherings chiefly occur in the middle burner. Concretions and conglomerations chiefly occur in the lower burner, and in many cases are gynecological disorders. In general, any of the four may arise when emotional depression or dietary irregularities cause damage to the liver and spleen. The resultant organ disorder leads to obstruction and stagnation of qi, which in turn causes the gradual collection of static blood.

constrain the lung 斂肺 *lian⁴ fei⁴*: To constrain sweating ascribed to lung vacuity that results from enduring cough.

constrain yin 斂陰 *lian⁴ yin¹*: To prevent loss of yin qi from the body, as in night sweating after abatement of fever in febrile disease. Yin-constraining agents include Corni Fructus (*shan¹ zhu¹ yu²*) and Schisandrae Fructus (*wu³ wei⁴ zi³*).

construction-defense disharmony 營衛不和 *ying² wei⁴ bu⁴ he²*: Exterior patterns characterized by spontaneous sweating and occurring in one of two forms: (1) strong defense and weak construction, where yang qi is depressed in the muscular exterior and forces yin-fluid (sweat) out of the pores, giving rise to perspira-tion whenever fever occurs; and (2) weak defense and strong construction, characterized by spontaneous sweating without fever, whereby sweat flows forth unconstrained by defense qi.

counterflow 逆 *ni⁴*: Flow counter to the normal direction. See inversion.

clear-eye blindness 青盲 *qing¹ mang²*: Gradual blindness that in severe cases can be total. Said in modern literature to correspond in Western medicine to optic atrophy (atrophy of the optic nerve), it is attributed to insufficiency of the liver and kidney and depletion of essence-blood, combined with spleen-stomach vacuity preventing essential qi from reaching to the eyes.

clove sore 疔瘡 *ding¹ chuang¹*: A small hard sore with a deep root like a clove or nail, appearing most commonly on the face and ends of the fingers. Clove sores arise when fire toxin enters the body through a wound, and then brews and binds in the skin and flesh.

course wind 疏風 *shu¹ feng¹*: To dissipate the wind pathogen. Wind-coursing agents are selected according to the accompanying pathogen. Ledebouriellae Radix (*fang² feng¹*) Angelicae Dahuricae Radix (*bai² zhi³*), and Ligustici Sinensis Rhizoma et Radix (*gao³ ben³*) are used for wind-cold, while Menthae Herba (*bo⁴ he²*) and Arctii Fructus (*niu² bang⁴ zi³*) are used for wind-heat. Notopterygii Rhizoma (*qiang¹ huo²*) and Cinnamomi Ramulus (*gui⁴ zhi¹*) are used for wind-damp joint pain (bi patterns). See also *course the exterior*.

course the exterior 疏表 *shu¹ biao³*: To free the exterior of pathogens without necessarily making the patient sweat. Agents used to course the exterior are mild exterior-resolving agents such as warm acrid Perillae Folium (*zi³ su¹ ye⁴*), Schizonepetae Herba seu Flos (*jing¹ jie⁴*), and Ledebouriella Radix (*fang² feng¹*), or the cool acrid Menthae Herba (*bo⁴ he²*), Mori Folium (*sang¹ ye⁴*), and Puerariae Radix (*ge² gens¹*).

course the liver and resolve depression 疏肝解鬱 *shu¹ gan¹ jie³ yu⁴*: To eliminate depression of liver qi and restore the liver's normal free coursing function. Bupleuri Radix (*chai² hu²*), Angelicae Sinensis Radix (*dang¹ gui¹*), Paeoniae Radix Alba (*bai² shao² yao⁴*), Cyperi Rhizoma (*xiang¹ fu⁴ zi³*), Toosendan Fructus (*chuan¹ lian⁴ zi³*), Corydalis Tuber (*yan² hu² suo³*), Magnoliae Cortex (*hou⁴ po⁴*). See *binding depression of liver qi*.

deep-source nasal congestion 鼻淵 *bi² yuan¹*: Nasal congestion with thick, turbid, fishy-smelling mucus, sometimes accompanied by pressure pain either side of the nose. It is caused by contraction of wind-cold, or deep-lying damp-heat in the gallbladder channel. Modern literature indicates correspondences to paranasal sinusitis and chronic rhinitis.

depression 鬱 *yu⁴*: Any form stagnation, i.e., absence of movement or activity. Traditional literature speaks of the six depressions: dampness, phlegm, food, blood, heat, and qi depression, the latter being the most important because it is invariably the underlying cause of the others. The term depression also describes inhibition of normal emotional activity, manifesting as feelings of oppression, frustration, and anger. In the case of depressed liver qi, these emotional signs accompany the physiologic manifestions.

desertion 脱 *tuo¹*: Life-threatening loss (of qi, blood, fluids).

diffuse the lung 宣肺 *xuan¹ fei⁴*: Restore the lung's function of diffusion (outward movement to the exterior of the body).

disinhibit 利 *li⁴*: To promote fluency, movement, or activity. E.g., *disinhibit the throat* means to relieve the throat of swelling that inhibits swallowing; *disinhibit the joints* means to restore their ability to bend and stretch freely. *Disinhibit water* means to drain excess fluid from the body, as in the treatment of water swelling (edema). See also *disinhibit* dampness.

disinhibit dampness 利濕 *li⁴ shi¹*: To eliminate dampness, especially from the lower burner, by allowing it to flow downward and pass out of the body through the urine. Dampness-disinhibiting agents include Talcum (*hua² shi²*), Alisma Rhizoma (*ze² xie⁴*), and Coicis Semen (*yi⁴ yi³ ren²*). Also called *percolate dampness*. See also *dispel dampness*.

dispel dampness 祛濕 *qu¹ shi¹*: To eliminate dampness. Distinction is made between transforming dampness, drying dampness, and disinhibiting dampness, which are methods of dealing with upper, middle, and lower burner dampness.

dispel phlegm 祛痰 *qu¹ tan²*: To eliminate phlegm. Dispelling phlegm includes transforming phlegm, dispersing phlegm and flushing phlegm, the first being the mildest and the latter being the strongest method.

disperse food 消食 *xiao¹ shi¹*: To eliminate food stagnation.

disperse phlegm 消痰 *xiao¹ tan²*: To eliminate stagnant turbid phlegm. See *dispel phlegm*.

dormant papules 癮疹 *yin³ zhen³*: Wheals that come and go, so named by their capacity to remain latent between eruptions. Dormant papules, which correspond to urticaria in Western medicine, are usually ascribed to wind or heat, but are also observed in cold patterns.

downbear 降 *jiang⁴* To descend, or cause to descend.

downbear qi 降氣 *jiang⁴ qi⁴*: To treat counterflow ascent of qi to treat cough or hiccough. Qi-downbearing agents include Perillae Fructus (*zi³ su¹ zi³*), Inulae Flos (*xuan² fu⁴ hua¹*), Pinelliae Tuber (*ban⁴ xia⁴*), Caryophylli Flos (*ding¹ xiang¹*), Haematitum (*dai⁴ zhe³ shi²*).

dream emission 夢遺 *meng⁴ yi²*: Spontaneous discharge of semen associated with dreaming. As a pathological phenomenon it occurs in effulgent heart fire and heart-spleen or heart-kidney vacuity. Dream emissions with occasional seminal efflux may occur in patterns of frenetic stirring of the ministerial fire or downpour of damp-heat. See *seminal loss*.

drinker's nose 酒齇 *jiu³ zha¹*: Reddening and thickening of the skin of the nose in those given to drinking. It is attributed to local blood stasis occurring when spleen damp-heat fumes up into the lung.

dry dampness 燥濕 *zao⁴ shi¹*: To eliminate dampness

with dry bitter agents. Drying dampness is the method used to treat dampness obstructing the middle burner, and takes one of two major forms: (1) drying dampness with warm bitter agents such as Magnoliae Cortex (*hou⁴ po⁴*), Pinelliae Tuber (*ban⁴ xia⁴*), Amomi Cardamomi Fructus (*bai⁴ dou⁴ kou⁴*), and Hoelen (*fu² ling²*), which is used to treat cold-damp obstructing the middle burner, characterized by oppression in the chest, nausea, abdominal distention, clear thin stool, and white tongue fur; and (2) drying dampness with cold bitter agents such as Coptidis Rhizoma (*huang² lian²*), Scutellariae Radix (*huang² qin²*), Aurantii Fructus (*zhi³ ke²*), and Polyporus (*zhu¹ ling²*), which is used to treat damp-heat obstructing the middle burner, characterized by abdominal pain and distention, thin stool that is hot and malodorous, and slimy yellow tongue fur. See also *eliminate dampness*.

dyspnea 喘 *chuan³*: Labored breathing with discontinuity between inhalation and exhalation and in serious cases with raising of the shoulders and flaring of the nostrils. It takes the form of repletion or vacuity. Wheezing dyspnea is dyspnea with a characteristic phlegm rale observed in what Western medicine calls asthma.

efflux 滑 *hua²*: Severe uncontrollable loss, especially of fluids (watery stool, semen).

efflux desertion 滑脱 *hua² tuo¹*: Critical weakening of the body with involuntary discharge of semen, urine, or watery stool.

effulgent 旺 *wang⁴*: Strong or exuberant (of heat or fire).

elusive masses 癖積 *pi⁴ ji¹*: See *bowstring and elusive masses*.

emolliate the liver 柔肝 *rou² gan¹*: To nourish the liver in order to address liver yin vacuity characterized by loss of visual acuity, dry eyes, night blindness, dizziness and tinnitus, pale nails, and a fine weak pulse. Liver-emolliating agents include Angelicae Sinensis Radix (*dang¹ gui¹*), Paeoniae Radix Alba (*bai² shao² yao⁴*), Rehmanniae Radix Exsiccata (*gan¹ di⁴ huang²*), Polygoni Multiflori Radix (*he² shou³ wu¹*), Lycii Fructus (*gou³ qi³ zi³*), Ligustri Fructus (*nu³ zhen¹ zi³*), Ecliptae Herba (*mo⁴ han⁴ lian⁴*), and Mori Fructus (*sang¹ shen⁴*).

engender liquid 生津 *sheng¹ jin¹*: To restore body fluids damaged by heat in febrile disease. Liquid-engendering agents include Scrophulariae Radix (*xuan² shen¹*), Ophiopogonis Tuber (*mai⁴ men² dong¹*), Rehmanniae Radix Exsicata (*gan¹ di⁴ huang²*), and Dendrobii Caulis (*shi² hu²*).

esophageal constriction 噎膈 *ye¹ ge²*: Constriction of the esophagus characterized by a sensation of blockage when swallowing, andor blockage at the diaphragm preventing the downflow of food. Upper esophageal constriction may occur along, although it usually portends the development of the dual condition. It is attributed to to stagnant qi, depressed heat, phlegm-rheum, and blood stasis, arising from damage to the spleen by excessive thought, excessive consumption of tobacco and alcohol, or consumption of hard abrasive foodstuffs.

externally contracted febrile disease 外感熱病 *wai⁴ gan³ re⁴ bing⁴*: Any disease caused by influences originating outside the body such as wind, cold, fire, summerheat, dampness, or dryness as in the system laid down in the *Treatise on Cold Damage (shang¹ han² lun⁴)* or wind warmth or damp warmth etc., discussed by the warm disease *(wen¹ bing⁴)* school.

external contraction 外感 *wai⁴ gan³*: See *externally contracted febrile disease.*

eyelid rim 弦 xian², 眼弦 *yan³ xian²* 目弦 *mu⁴ xian²*: The edge of the eyelid (palpebral margin) from which the eyelashes grow.

eye screen 目翳 *mu⁴ yi⁴*: Any visible visual impediment in the eyeball such as cataracts.

flush phlegm 滌痰 *di² tan²*: To eliminate stubborn phlegm with powerful agents such as Daphnes Genkwa Flos *(yuan² hua¹)* and Euphorbiae Kansui Radix *(gan¹ sui⁴)*. A phlegm-flushing formula is *shi² zao³ tang¹* (Ten Jujubes Decoction, 245). See *dispel phlegm.*

five stranguries 五淋 *wu³ lin²*: Stone, qi, unctuous, taxation, and blood strangury. The general features of strangury are urinary frequency and urgency, and difficult and painful voiding, as well as dribbling incontinence. Stone strangury, blood strangury, and unctuous strangury are attributed to lower burner damp-heat, and are characterized by additional signs of calculi in the urine, blood in the urine, or milky urine respectively. Qi strangury is usually attributable to bladder qi stagnation, and is characterized by inhibited urination with pain after voiding and lower abdominal fullness; less frequently it is attributed to spleen-kidney qi vacuity in which case there is lower abdominal fullness and dribble after urination. Taxation strangury is brought on by overexertion and is marked by dull pain in the urethra after voiding, and fatigued limbs. It often develops from other forms of strangury, and is the manifestation of spleen qi and/or kidney yang vacuity.

flowery vision 目花 *mu⁴ hua¹*: Blurred, dizzy, or mottled vision, including floaters.

food damage 傷食 *shang¹ shi²*: "Stomach upset" due to voracious eating. It is characterized by aversion to cold, nausea, vomiting and belching (with putrid-smelling vomitus and gas), diarrhea or constipation, painful bloating of the abdomen relieved by passing of stool or flatus. The tongue fur is slimy, or thick and yellow.

food accumulation 食積 *shi² ji¹*: Any form of accumulation or stagnation of food in the stomach and intestines. It includes food damage (see previous entry), as well as more severe gastrointestinal accumulations in which palpable lumps are to be felt in the abdomen. Patients suffering food accumulation patterns quite often display signs of spleen-stomach vacuity.

fortify the spleen 健脾 *jian⁴ pi²*: To supplement the spleen to treat impaired spleen movement and transformation. Spleen-fortifying agents include Codonopsitis Radix *(dang³ shen¹)*, Atractylodis Ovatae Rhizoma

(bai² zhu²), Hoelen *(fu² ling²)*, Dioscoreae Rhizoma *(shan¹ yao⁴)*, Coicis Semen *(yi⁴ yi³ ren²)*.

frenetic movement of hot blood 血熱妄行 *xie⁴ re⁴ wang⁴ xing²*: Abnormal movement or activity of the blood that manifests in bleeding or macules.

fright 驚 *jing¹*: (1) Sudden fear, shock, or alarm, often accompanied by a physical start. (2) The sudden spasms or convulsions associated with certain diseases (e.g., fright epilepsy), apparently so called by their resemblance to fright as a response to external stimulus. See following entries.

fright epilepsy 驚癇 *jing¹ xian²* (1) Epilepsy caused by fright. (2) Fright wind (in Tang and Song medical records).

fright inversion 驚厥 *jing¹ jue²*: (1) Syncope occurring when strong emotional stimulus disrupts the flow of qi and blood. (2) The signs associated with *fright wind.* See *inversion.*

fright palpitation 驚悸 *jing¹ ji⁴*: Heart palpitations brought on by strong emotional stimulus, attributable to heart qi vacuity or heart blood vacuity, often associated with kidney vacuity, and sometimes associated with blood stasis, water-rheum or phlegm-fire. Compare *racing of the heart.*

fright wind 驚風 *jing¹ feng¹*: Disease occurring in infants and and young children, marked by convulsive spasm, arched-back rigidity (opisthotonos), and loss of consciousness. Synonym: infantile convulsions.

fulminant 暴 *bao⁴*: Sudden and severe.

gan 疳 *gan:* (1) Gan accumulation. (2) Indented mucosal ulceration, often accompanied by putrefaction of the flesh and mild suppuration, e.g., gan of the teeth and gums.

gan accumulation 疳積 *gan¹ ji⁴*: A disease of infancy or childhood caused by spleen-stomach vacuity. Signs include yellow complexion, emaciation, dry hair, abdominal distention with visible superficial veins, and loss of vitality. It corresponds to child malnutrition as well as some parasitic and debilitating diseases in Western medicine.

glomus 痞 *pi³*: A localized subjective feeling of fullness and blockage in the chest or venter; sometimes called *focal distention.*

harmonize the stomach 和胃 *he² wei⁴*: To treat disharmony of stomach qi (oppression and distention in the venter, belching, acid regurgitation). Stomach-harmonizing agents include Citri Exocarpium *(chen² pi²)*, Pinelliae Tuber *(ban⁴ xia¹)*, Saussureae Radix *(mu⁴ xiang¹)*, Amomi Semen *(sha¹ ren²)*, Santali Albi Lignum *(tan² xiang¹)*.

heat bind 熱結 *re⁴ jie²*: Concentration of heat, usually in the stomach or intestines, giving rise to dry bound stool (constipation). The passage of looser stool passes around the blockage is called *heat bind with circumfluence.*

heat toxin 熱毒 *re⁴ du²*: Heat manifesting in the form of painful red swelling such as in severe sore throat or certain types of sores. Heat toxin is the cause to which

Chinese medicine attributes conditions that Western medicine describes as acute inflammation.

heat vexation 煩 *fan³*: Fever with vexation and related signs such as agitation and insomnia; occurs in exuberant interior heat with damage to both qi and yin. Heat vexation can be treated with formulas containing Gardeniae Fructus *(shan¹ zhi¹ zi³)* and Rehmanniae Radix Exsiccata *(gan¹ di⁴ huang²)*.

heavy settler 重鎮藥 *zhong⁴ zhen⁴ yao⁴*: Any mineral or shell product used, for example, to quiet the spirit in patterns characterized by palpitation and manic agitation.

hemilateral headache 偏頭痛 *pian¹ tou² tong⁴*: Pain on one side of the head, usually recurrent. Observed in ascendant liver yang, blood stasis, and cold rheum patterns.

hypertonicity 拘急 *ju¹ ji²*, 拘攣 *ju¹ luan²*: Stiffness and tension in the limbs inhibiting normal bending and stretching. It is usually attributable to wind, and occurs for example in bi disease.

innominate swollen toxin sore 無名腫毒 *wu² ming² zhong³ du²*: Any nondescript redness and swelling due to local accumulation of toxin.

internal wind 內風 *nei⁴ feng¹*: See *liver wind*.

intestinal wind 腸風 *chang² feng¹*: A condition in which fresh red blood is discharged from the anus prior to evacuation; there is no pain or swelling of the anus (such as in bleeding hemorrhoids or other disease of the anus); the tongue is red and the pulse is rapid. Note that in the term *intestinal wind*, the word wind describes the nature of the disease, not flatulence. In some older texts, intestinal wind can refer to other conditions such as bleeding hemorrhoids, or wind dysentery.

inversion 厥 *jue²*: The disruption of qi dynamic in which supplies of qi and blood suddenly fail to reach the head and extremities and which is marked by syncope (clouding inversion) and/or pronounced cold in the limbs (inversion frigidity of the limbs). Cold inversion refers to a pattern characterized by clouding inversion and inversion frigidity of the limbs, attributed to yang qi vacuity. Blood inversion refers to patterns caused by blood disease (vacuity or repletion) and characterized by the two signs of inversion. The notion of inversion is closely associated with that of counterflow. Inversion frigidity of the limbs and counterflow frigidity of the limbs are identical in meaning. However, counterflow otherwise describes disruption of the qi dynamic of organs such as the liver, stomach, and lung.

jie 疥 *jie⁴*: A sore that commonly occurs between the fingers of the hand, that is characterized by an insufferable penetrating, prickly itching sensation, and that can lead to suppuration when scratched. Attributed to ''worms'' (i.e., parasites) in the skin.

ju 疽 *ju¹*: A diffuse swelling of low elevation in which pus gathers. It is slow to develop and unassociated with pain or change in skin color. It may be due to stagnation of qi and blood that develops when externally contracted pathogens become depressed in the flesh, or to disturbance of qi and the blood attributable to internal

damage by the seven emotions, or to congealing phlegm and dampness that stems from eating rich fatty foods. Before pus has formed, it does not easily disperse, and after pus has formed it does not easily burst. Hence, it is hard to treat, especially in old age. Ju are classified as yin sores in contradistinction to yong, which are classified as yang.

lai 癩 *lai⁴*: (1) Leprosy. (2) Jie and xian etc., that lead to hair loss on the affected area.

leg qi 脚氣 *jiao³ qi⁴*: Disease attributed to dampness, cold-damp, or phlegm-damp, and characterized by numbness and swelling of the legs and fever, and in serious cases mental abstraction and deranged speech; equated by most modern Chinese texts with beriberi, and often simply translated as such.

lesser abdomen 少腹 *shao⁴ fu⁴*: (1) The lower abdomen. (2) The lateral areas of the lower abdomen.

liver wind 肝風內動 *gan¹ feng¹ nei⁴ dong⁴*: Clonic spasm, dizziness, and in severe cases loss of consciousness due to internal causes rather than contraction of external pathogens. Pathomechanisms include: liver yang transforming into wind, extreme heat engendering wind, blood vacuity engendering wind.

lower origin 下元 *xia⁴ yuan²*: The kidney, seen as the basis of physiologic activity.

lump glomus 痞塊 *pi³ kuai⁴*: Any lump in the abdomen that can be felt subjectively and palpated. C.f., *glomus*.

malarial disease 瘧疾 *nüe⁴ ji²* (or obsolete *yao⁴ ji²*): A recurrent disease marked by shivering, vigorous fever, and sweating, and classically attributed to contraction of summerheat during the hot season, contact with mountain forest miasma, or contraction of cold-damp. Malarial disease is explained as pathogenic qi latent at midstage (half exterior and half interior).

malign sore 惡瘡 *e⁴ chuang¹*: Any severe sore (lesion) that fails to heal and that is accompanied by generalized signs directly related to it (e.g., fever).

mania 狂 *kuang²*: See *mania and withdrawal*.

mania and withdrawal 癲狂 *dian¹ kuang²*: Mania and withdrawal are forms of mental derangement. Mania denotes states of excitement marked by noisy, unruly, and even aggressive behavior, offensive speech, constant singing and laughter, irascibility, springing walls and climbing roofs, and inability to remain tidily dressed. This is a yang pattern of the heart spirit straying outward owing to hyperactivity of yang qi. Withdrawal refers to emotional depression, indifference, deranged speech, taciturnity, and obliviousness of hunger or satiety. It is a yin pattern caused by binding of depressed qi and phlegm or heart-spleen vacuity.

menstrual block 經閉 *jing¹ bi⁴*: Pathological absence of periods. Synonym: amenorrhea.

mother of malaria 瘧母 *nüe⁴ mu³*: A lump glomus (abdominal mass) occurring in persistent malaria, equated with splenomegaly in Western medicine.

move qi 行氣 *xing² qi⁴*: Promote the movement of qi. See *rectify qi*.

muscular tetany 痙 *jing⁴*: Severe spasm taking the form of stiffness and tension in the neck, clenched jaw, convulsive spasm of the limbs, arched-back rigidity, and shaking of the head. Occurring in repletion patterns, it is explained as wind, cold, dampness and fire congesting the channels and connecting vessels. In vacuity patterns, it attributable to loss of supply of nourishment and moisture to the sinews and stirring of internal vacuity wind as a result of excessive sweating, loss of blood, constitutional vacuity, qi vacuity, and shortage of blood, and insufficiency of the fluids. Muscular tetany may occur as a symptom of a variety of different diseases including tetanus (lockjaw) and fright wind. Also called *tetany*.

open the portals 開竅 *kai¹ qiao⁴*: To restore normal operation of portals, e.g., by restoring normal urination or clearing the nose. Most commonly, opening the portals denotes opening the portals of the heart, i.e., full operation of the senses and normal consciousness. See *portal*. Exuberant heat in febrile disease, wind stroke, summerheat strike, and epilepsy can lead to patterns of heat entering the pericardium or phlegm turbidity clouding the portals of the heart, in which the patient's "portals are blocked" and his mind becomes clouded. Powerful portal-opening agents contain aromatic and pervasive substances such as Moschus (*she⁴ xiang¹*), Borneolum (*bing¹ pian⁴*), and Styrax Liquidus (*su¹ he² xiang¹*), that penetrate the block.

oral putrescence 口糜 *kou³ mi²*: A condition characterized by the appearance of white fur in the oral cavity with erosion spots and soreness that makes eating difficult. Attributed to accumulated heat in the spleen channel fuming up into the mouth.

oxhide xian 牛皮癬 *niu² pi² xian³*: Thickening and hardening of the skin, so called because the affected area resembles the skin of an ox's neck. It arises when wind and other pathogens gather, become depressed, and transform into heat, which in turn damages yin-blood, depriving the skin of nourishment. The condition is often emotionally related and worsens with emotional stimulus. It is sometimes accompanied by itching. It tends to be located on the neck, spreading to the head, arms, and shoulders.

outcrop 胬肉 *nu³ rou⁴*: See *canthus outcrop*.

outthrust the exterior 透表 *tou⁴ biao³*: To outthrust pathogens or outthrust papules.

outthrust papules 透疹 *tou⁴ zhen³*: To cause eruption of papules.

outthrust pathogens 透邪 *tou⁴ xie²*: To expel pathogens, especially wind-heat, from the exterior.

overcome dampness 勝濕 *sheng⁴ shi¹*: To dispel dampness, especially from the exterior, using agents such as Angelica Duhuo Radix (*du² huo²*), Lebedebouriellae Radix (*fang² feng¹*), and Ligustici Sinensis Rhizoma et Radix (*gao³ ben³*), as with Notopterygium Dampness-Overcoming Decoction (*qiang¹-huo² sheng⁴ shi¹ tang¹*).

pathomechanism 病機 *bing⁴ ji¹*: The process by which a disease or sign of disease arises and develops. Synonym: pathogenesis.

percolate dampness 滲濕 *shen⁴ shi¹*: Disinhibit dampness.

phlegm 痰 *tan²*: A pathological entity traditionally understood as a concentration of dampness arising when the lung, kidney, and especially the spleen fail to move and transform fluids properly, or when fluids are "boiled" by depressed fire. Since disease of the spleen is the most important single cause of phlegm patterns, this organ is said to be the "basis of phlegm formation." Phlegm commonly collects in the lung, giving rise to dyspnea or productive cough, but can also affect other parts of the body: it can lodge in the channels, binding to form scrofula and other types of subcutaneous phlegm nodes; it can lodge in the stomach, causing vomiting and nausea; it can rise upward to cause dizziness; and it can also "confound the portals of the heart," causing stupor and loss of consciousness. Phlegm is identified not only by increased expectorate, but also general signs like a slimy tongue and a slippery pulse. Phlegm in Chinese medicine is seen as the cause for a wide variety of diseases in which increased expectoration is often viewed by Western medicine as a secondary or incidental phenomenon. A thinner form of phlegm is called *rheum (yin)*.

phlegm-rheum 痰飲 *tan² yin³*: (1) Accumulation of fluid in the trunk or limbs, that occurs when the lung, spleen, and kidney fail to move fluids. (2) Specifically, such an accumulation in the chest and lateral costal region, the venter, and intestines.

portal 竅 *qiao⁴*: Any one of the openings (or locations) which, according to visceral manifestation theory (*zang⁴ xiang⁴ lun⁴*), connect with the environment. The nine portals include the upper or clear portals, i.e., the two eyes, two ears, two nostrils, and mouth, as well as the lower or turbid portals, i.e., anterior yin (urethra) and posterior yin (anus). According to another enumeration, the nine portals are the two eyes, two hearts, two nostrils, tongue, and throat. The term "portals of the heart" is commonly used, but is not clearly defined; since stupor and coma are traditionally described as a "confounding" or "clouding" of the portals of the heart, it may be assumed to denote the "senses" by which the heart spirit (the mind) is conscious of the environment, and hence partially synonymous with the clear portals. See *open the portals*.

precipitate 下 *xia⁴* To cause to descend, especially the stool (i.e., to purge). The term precipitation is used in preference to purge (which means to clean) in order to reflect the Oriental concept of causing downward movement to treat internal heat, fire, and stagnation. See also next two entries.

precipitation of blood 下血 *xia⁴ xue⁴*: Passage of blood after the stool (as opposed to being mixed with the stool).

precipitate qi 下氣 *xia⁴ qi⁴*: Downbear qi, i.e., reverse qi counterflow. See *rectify qi*.

pulmonary atony 肺痿 *fei⁴ wei³*: A condition characterized by cough with expectoration of foamy phlegm, accompanied by emaciation, dry lips and mouth, and vacuous rapid pulse.

qi pain 氣痛 *qi⁴ tong⁴*: Pain attributed to qi stagnation.

qi inversion 氣厥 *qi⁴ jue²*: Sudden loss of consciousness and inversion frigidity of the limbs due to qi vacuity or derangement of qi dynamic. Two pathomechanisms are known: (1) disruption of qi dynamic due to emotional stimulus, whereby congestion of qi in and the chest and heart gives rise to clouding of the clear portals; (2) insufficient food or excessive fatigue in patients regularly suffering from original qi vacuity, causing downward fall of qi and impaired upbearing of clear yang, manifesting as sudden loss of consciousness and inversion frigidity of the limbs, sweating, and a faint pulse. The first is a repletion pattern, while the latter is a vacuity pattern.

quicken the blood 活血 *huo² xue⁴*: To stimulate blood flow to eliminate blood stasis.

quiet the spirit 安神 *an¹ shen²*: To calm the heart spirit, thereby alleviating such disorders as insomnia, profuse dreaming, palpitations etc.

racing of the heart 怔忡 *zheng¹ chong¹*: Violent throbbing of the heart felt not only in the chest but even as far down as the umbilical region; attributable to heart blood or heart yin vacuity. Racing of the heart similar to, but more severe than palpitation. It generally forms part of a vacuity pattern, and is continuous in nature. Palpitation, by contrast, may be attributable either to vacuity or to repletion, and is paroxysmal (i.e., comes in bouts). Viewed from a biomedical perspective, palpitation is generally due to nervous or functional disorders, while racing of the heart is structural in nature. This distinction may not apply to the use of the terms in ancient texts.

repletion 實 *shi²*: The opposite of vacuity. See *vacuity and repletion* and *repletion pattern*.

rectify qi 理氣 *li³ qi⁴*: To restore normal qi dynamic. Rectifying qi takes two forms: (1) Moving qi, which is the method used to treat qi stagnation. Qi-moving agents include Cyperi Rhizoma (*xiang¹ fu⁴ zi³*), Curcumae Tuber (*yu⁴ jin¹*), Linderae Radix (*wu¹ yao⁴*), Meliae Toosendan Fructus (*chuan¹ lian⁴ zi³*). (2) Downbearing qi, i.e., restoring the normal downbearing of the qi especially of the lung or stomach. Agents that treat counterflow ascent of stomach qi, addressing nausea and vomiting, etc., include Pinelliae Tuber (*ban⁴ xia⁴*), Inulae Flos (*xuan² fu⁴ hua¹*), Haematitum (*dai⁴ zhe³ shi²*), and Aquilariae Lignum (*chen² xiang¹*), while those that treat counterflow ascent of lung qi characterized by dyspnea or cough, include Pinelliae Tuber (*ban⁴ xia⁴*), Perillae Fructus (*zi³ su¹ zi³*), and Arisaematis Rhizoma cum Felle Bovis (*dan³ xing¹*).

rectify the blood 理血 *li³ xue⁴*: To dispel stasis or staunch bleeding.

resolve the exterior 解表 *jie³ biao³*: To free the exterior of externally contracted pathogens using agents that promote sweating and dispel pathogens. Exterior resolution makes use of diaphoretic agents such as the powerful Ephedrae Herba (*ma² huang²*) and the slightly milder Cinnamomi Ramulus (*gui⁴ zhi¹*), and pathogen-dispelling agents such as Ledebouriellae Radix (*fang² feng¹*) for wind-cold and Menthae Herba (*bo⁴ he²*) for wind-heat. See also *course the exterior*.

return yang and stem counterflow 回陽救逆 *hui² yang² jiu⁴ ni⁴*: Restore yang qi and eliminate counterflow frigidity of the limbs in order to treat yang collapse patterns (persistent cold sweating, frigid extremities, faint breathing).

roundworm inversion 蚘厥 *hui² ju²*: Inversion pattern occurring in roundworm infestation, characterized by acute attacks of abdominal pain, nausea, and vomiting (sometimes vomiting of roundworm), with frigid limbs, and cold sweat. Usually observed in what Western medicine has determined as biliary ascariasis or intestinal obstruction due to ascariasis.

scrofulous lumps 瘰癧 *luo³ li⁴*: Lumps beneath the skin on the side of the neck and under the armpits that in severe cases can suppurate. They occur when phlegm produced by the scorching of fluids by lung and kidney vacuity fire.

securing astriction 固澀 *gu⁴ su⁴*: Method used to treat efflux desertion patterns (persistent spontaneous or night sweating; enduring diarrhea and prolapse of the rectum; seminal emission or premature ejaculation; uterine bleeding, or blood loss; vaginal discharge, etc.). Securing astriction includes: (1) constraining sweat and securing the exterior; (2) constraining the lung and suppressing cough; (3) astringing the intestines and checking diarrhea, (4) securing the kidney and astringing essence (used to treat increased urination and seminal loss); and (5) checking uterine bleeding and vaginal discharge. Ostreae Concha (*mu³ li⁴*) is commonly used to constrain sweat, Schisandrae Fructus (*wu³ wei⁴ zi³*) to constrain the lung, Chebulae Fructus (*he¹ zi³*) and Papaveris Pericarpium (*ying¹ su⁴ ke²*) to astringe the intestines, Nelumbinis Stamen (*lian² xu¹*) and Euryales Semen (*qian⁴ shi²*), to secure the kidney and astringe essence, Trachycarpi Stipulae Fibra Carbonisata (*zong¹ lu² tan⁴*), to stem uterine bleeding, and Cuscutae Semen (*tu⁴ si¹ zi³*), Mantidis Ootheca (*sang¹ piao¹ xiao¹*), Kaolin (*bai² shi² zhi¹*), and Ginkgo Semen (*bai² guo³*) to check vaginal discharge.

seminal efflux 滑精 *hua² jing¹*: Seminal loss occurring several times a day and night. It is a sign of insecure kidney qi (kidney qi failing to secure, i.e., retain, essence).

seminal emission 遺精 *yi² jing¹*: Seminal loss, especially during sleep, but unassociated with dreaming.

seminal loss 失精 *shi¹ jing¹*: (1) Loss of semen other than through sexual activity, and including: *seminal emission*, seminal loss during sleep; *dream emission*, seminal loss associated with dreaming; *seminal efflux*, severe emission several times a day; and *profuse spermatorrhea*, severe, continual loss. (2) Specifically, seminal emission.

shan 疝 *shan⁴*: Any of various diseases characterized by pain or swelling of the abdomen or scrotum, including but not limited to what Western medicine calls inguinal hernia and hydrocele. Also called *shan qi*.

spontaneous external bleeding 衄血 *nü⁴ xue⁴*: Spontaneous bleeding (i.e., bleeding not induced by lesions) from the eyes, nose, ears, or mouth, or from the skin; usually refers to nosebleed, the most common form.

staunch bleeding 止血 *zhi³ xue⁴*: To check any form of bleeding.

steaming bone tidal fever 骨蒸潮熱 *gu³ zheng¹ chao² re⁴*: Yin vacuity tidal fever, whereby heat qi thrusts out from the interior. This type of fever is invariably associated with night sweating.

stirring fetus 胎動不安 *tai¹ dong⁴ bu⁴ an¹*: A condition characterized by movement of the fetus, pain and downbearing sensation in the abdomen, and in severe cases the discharge of blood. It is attributed to impact injury (knocks and falls), yin vacuity blood heat, or vacuity of the penetrating and conception vessels, and is a sign of possible or impending miscarriage.

stomach reflux 反胃 *fan³ wei⁴*: A pattern of distention fullness after eating, athe vomiting in the evening of food ingested in the morning, or the vomiting in the morning of food ingested the previous evening, untransformed food in the vomitus, fatigued spirit, and lack of bodily strength. Its chief cause is spleen-stomach vacuity cold, but it may also occur when congealed damp-heat stagnation leads ot impaired harmonious downbearing of the stomach.

strangury 淋 *lin²*: Disease marked by signs such as urinary frequency and urgency, difficult voiding, and dribbling incontinence. See *five stranguries*.

subdue yang 潛陽 *qian² yang²*: To treat ascendant liver yang with heavy settling agents such as Ostreae Concha Cruda (*sheng¹ mu³ li⁴*), Draconis Os Crudum (*sheng¹ long³ gu³*), Haliotidis Concha Cruda (*sheng¹ shi² jue² ming²*), Concha Margaritifera (*zhen¹ zhu¹ mu³*), Magnetitium (*ci² shi²*), and Haematitum (*dai⁴ zhe³ shi²*).

suspended rheum 懸飲 *xuan² yin³*: Water in the chest and lateral costal region causing local pain and cough with copious phlegm.

taxation 勞 *lao²*: Overexertion or lack of exercise, and the wear and tear on the body that it causes; severe vacuity developing over a long period.

tetanic disease 痙病 *jing⁴ bing⁴*: See *muscular tetany*.

tetany 痙 *jing⁴*: See muscular tetany.

throat bi 喉痺 *hou² bi⁴*: Swelling, pain and a sensation of blockage in the throat that hinders swallowing and results from localized blockage of qi and blood. Causes include wind-heat, wind-cold, and yin vacuity.

throat moth 喉蛾 *hou² e²*: Sore, hot, red swellings in the throat with a white purulent exudate. It is attributable, amongst other things, to wind-heat or upflaming vacuity fire, and is equivalent to tonsilitis in Western medicine.

toxin swelling 腫毒 *zhong³ du²*: Swelling due to toxin, such as occurs in yong, sores, or sore throat. This term stands in contradistinction to water swelling, which is due to morbidity of the spleen, lung, and kidney. Corresponds roughly to inflammatory swelling in Western medicine.

transform 化 *hua⁴*: (1) To undergo (gradual) change. (2) To eliminate (dampness, phlegm, rehum, static blood, or accumulated food by mild action). In both senses, transform connotes gradual and gentle change.

transform dampness 化濕 *hua4 shi¹*: To eliminate dampness, especially from the upper burner. Transforming dampness includes: (1) Coursing the exterior and transforming dampness, the method used when the damp pathogen is in the upper burner or exterior giving rise to heavy-headedness, heavy aching limbs, slimy sersation in the mouth, absence of thirst, white slimy tongue fur and soggy pulse. Agents used include Ledebouriellae Radix (*fang² feng¹*), Gentianae Macrophyllae Radix (*qin² jiao¹*), Atractylodis Rhizoma (*cang¹ zhu²*), Agastaches seu Pogostemi Herba (*huo⁴ xiang¹*), Citri Exocarpium (*chen² pi²*), and raw Glycyrrhizae Radix (*gan¹ cao³*). (2) Clearing heat and transforming dampness, which is used in the early stages of damp warmth seasonal epidemic diseases when the pathogen is in the qi aspect giving rise to fever, aching limbs, absence of sweating with vexation or sweating that brings no abatement of fever, oppression in the chest and abdominal distention, dark-colored urine, constipation or diarrhea with hot malodorous stool, and a grimy slimy or dry yellow tongue fur. Agents used include Coptidis Rhizoma (*huang² lian²*), Scutellariae Radix (*huang² qin²*), and Polyporus (*zhu¹ ling²*).

transform phlegm 化痰 *hua⁴ tan²*: To eliminate phlegm. Warm phlegm-transforming agents include Pinelliae Tuber (*ban⁴ xia⁴*), Arisaematis Rhizoma (*tian¹ nan² xing¹*), Inulae Flos (*xuan² fu⁴ hua¹*), Asteris Radix et Rhizoma (*zi³ wan³*), Cynanchi Baiqian Radix et Rhizoma (*bai² qian²*), Platycodonis Radix (*jie² geng³*), and Polygalae Radix (*yuan³ zhi³*). Cool ones include Peucedani Radix (*qian² hu²*), Fritillariae Cirrhosae Bulbus (*chuan¹ bei⁴ mu³*), Trichosanthis Semen (*gua¹ lou² zi³*) and Bambusae Concretio Silicea (*tian¹ zhu² huang²*). See also *dispel phlegm*.

turbid strangury 淋濁 *turbid strangury*: Strangury characterized by turbid urine.

uterine bleeding 崩漏 *beng¹ lou⁴*: Pathological discharge of blood from the womb. Abnormally sudden and heavy bouts of bleeding (which may or may not be the product of menstruation) are termed *profuse uterine bleeding*. Scant bleeding after menstruation that continues after the abatement of menstruation or that starts between periods is called *scant uterine bleeding* or spotting. It the flow is deep red and clotted, it is usually a sign of heat. If pale red without clots, it indicates damage to the penetrating and conception vessels, or center qi fall (blood management failure).

vacuity and repletion 虛實 *xu¹ shi²*: Vacuity is weakness or emptiness; repletion is strength or fullness. Specifically (and most commonly), vacuity denotes weakness of correct qi (yin and yang components of the body in their active aspect of maintaining health), while repletion denotes strength of pathogenic qi. In this sense, vacuity is characterized by gradually developing physical weakness, loss of vitality, emaciation, and persistent or intermittent discomforts etc., while repletion is characterized by acute forms of pain, distention, fullness.

venter 脘 *guan³, wan³*: The physical stomach (and adjacent portions of the intestine and esophagus), as distinct from the stomach as a functional entity.

vertex headache 顛頂頭痛 *dian¹ ding³ tou² tong⁴*: Pain in the region of the vertex of the head.

vexation 煩 *fan²*, 心煩 *xin¹ fan²*: A feeling of restlessness and irritability that focuses in the area of the heart, is a very common symptom that occurs in either vacuity or repletion heat. In severe cases it is associated with agitation, i.e., increased physical movement.

visceral agitation 臟躁 *zang⁴ zao⁴*: A paroxysmal mental disorder most prevalent in women, and heralded by melancholy and depression, illusions, emotionalism, and increased or diminished sensitivity. Attacks are characterized by vexation and oppression, rashness and impatience, sighing for no apparent reason, and sadness with an urge to weep. In serious cases, there may be convulsive spasms, which, unlike those occurring in epilepsy, are accompanied by a white complexion or complete loss of consciousness. Heart-liver blood vacuity and emotional depression are the prime causes.

warm the center and dissipate cold 溫中散寒 *wen¹ zhong¹ san⁴ han²*: To treat interior cold patterns due to spleen-stomach yang vacuity. The center refers to the middle burner, i.e., the stomach and the spleen.

wasting thirst 消渴 *xiao¹ ke³*: Disease characterized by thirst, increased fluid intake, and increased urination. Biomedical correspondences include diabetes and hypoadrenocorticism. It is attributed to overexuberant heat in the lung, stomach, and kidney that arises from a combination of factors such as excessive consumption of sweet and rich foods and fatigue in patients with yin vacuity constitutions.

water swelling 水腫 *shui³ zhong³*: Diffuse swelling due to local accumulation of water that arises when the spleen, kidney, and/or lung fail to move and discharge fluids normally. It usually affects the feet and ankles or the eyes and face. Corresponds to edema in Western medicine.

white turbidity 白濁 *bai² zhuo²*: (1) Turbid white urine. (2) Turbid white discharge from the urethra, with pain on urination.

wind stroke 中風 *zhong⁴ feng¹*: (1) Disease marked by sudden loss of consciousness, hemaplegia, or deviated mouth, and impeded speech; occurs under the following circumstances. It is usually explained in terms of ascendant liver yang, liver wind, phlegm, and heat. (2) Contraction of external wind as in febrile disease.

wind water 風水 *feng¹ huo³*: External wind contraction with water swelling. Signs include rapid onset, floating pulse, pain in the joints, fever and aversion to cold, swelling, particularly in the head and face (the upper part of the body being affected by the wind pathogen). The disorder is the result of impairment of lung qi's depurative downbearing by the wind pathogen in patients suffering from spleen-kidney qi vacuity.

wind-fire eye 風火眼 *feng¹ huo³ yan³*: Reddening of the

eyes, sometimes associated with fever and headache. Corresponds to acute conjunctivitis in Western medicine. Synonym: fire eye.

wheezing dyspnea 哮喘 *xiao¹ chuan³*: See *dyspnea.*

white patch 白癜 *bai² dian⁴*: See *white patch wind.*

white patch wind 白癜風 *bai² dian⁴ feng¹*: White patches on the skin attributed to disharmony of the blood arising when the wind pathogen assails the exterior, causing the interstices (*cou⁴ li³*) to loose their tightness. It is most common in youth and the prime of life. It is marked by cream-colored white macules of varying size, clearly distinguishable for the normal skin coloring. Any hair growing in the patches also turns white. Some of the patches have a brown or pale red papule in the center. The condition is associated with neither pain nor itching. It is of gradual onset, and often persists for a long period. Corresponds to vitiligo in Western medicine.

xian 癬 *xian³*: Skin disease marked by elevation of the skin, serous discharge, scaling, and itching; often associated with dampness.

yellow perspiration 黃汗 *huang² han⁴*: Sweat that is thick and sticky, and the color of phellodendron juice and that can stain the clothes, accompanied by fever, thirst, swelling of the head, face, and limbs, fever, lumbar pain, frigid lower legs, heavy aching body, inhibited urination, and a deep slow pulse. Attributed to a combination of wind, water, dampness, and heat. If damp-heat causes damage to the blood aspect, it may also be accompanied by sores.

yellow swelling 黃胖 *huang² pang²*: Swelling of the face and ankles with a withered yellow complexion, together with fatigued spirit and lack of strength. In some cases it can be associated with nausea and vomiting of yellow water, and desire to eat uncooked rice, tea leaves, coal, and usually observed in what Western medicine calls hook worm infestation.

yellow wine 黃酒 *huang² jiu³*: Wine made from rice or millet that is "yelllow," i.e., the color or rum or whiskey.

yong 癰 *yong⁴*: (1) External yong: A painful swelling of the skin and flesh in which pus gathers. It arises when damp-heat or fire toxin stemming from excessive consumption of rich foods or toxin contracted through unclean wounds obstructs the channels, causing qi and blood congeal and stagnate. It starts with swelling and redness, and as pus gathers inside, the skin becomes redder, and forms a head that produces a rippling sensation under pressure. The healing process begins after the head bursts. Larger yong of the back are also referred to "effusions of the back" (*fa¹ bei⁴*). (2) Internal yong: A similar sore that develops within the body, including notably intestinal yong and pulmonary yong. External yong correspond largely to carbuncles in Western medicine, while intestinal and pulmonary yong correspond to appendicitis and pulmonary abscess respectively.

Index I Chinese

Index II English, Latin, Pinyin, and Japanese

CHINESE MEDICINE SERIES

(Nos. 1–6 include a preface by Professor Nathan Sivin especially for this series)

MW01 G.A. Stuart, *Chinese Materia Medica: Vegetable Kingdom.*
An important work in English on Chinese herb drugs. The drugs are listed under Latin names with Chinese characters and transcription given for each. A description of the drug along with its description and usage follows each entry. A romanized index of Chinese terms and Latin names is appended.
SMC repr. 1987; 21cm, cloth, 558pp.

MW02 Bernard E. Read, *Chinese Materia Medica: Insect Drugs, Dragon and Snake Drugs, and Fish Drugs.*
Insect Drugs (213pp.; trans. from chaps. 39–42 of *PKTM*)
Dragon and Snake Drugs (66pp.; trans. from chap. 43 of *PKTM*)
Fish Drugs (136pp.; trans. from chap. 44 of *PKTM*)
SMC repr. 1982; 21cm, cloth, 1 vol.

MW03 Bernard E. Read, *Chinese Materia Medica: Turtle and Shellfish Drugs, Avian Drugs, and a Compendium of Minerals and Stones.*
Turtle and Shellfish Drugs (95pp.; trans. from chaps. 45–46 of *PTKM*)
Avian Drugs (12pp.; trans. from chap. 47 of *PTKM*)
A Compendium of Minerals and Stones (viii+98pp.; trans. from vols. 8–12 of *PTKM*)
SMC repr. 1982; 21cm, cloth, 1 vol.

MW04 Bernard E. Read. *Chinese Materia Medica: Animal Drugs.*
Animal Drugs (ii+[146]+18pp.; trans. from chaps. 50–52 of *PTKM*)
SMC repr. 1982; 21cm, cloth, 1 vol.

MW05 Bernard E. Read. *Chinese Medicinal Plants from the Pen Ts'ao Kang Mu. A.D. 1597; 3rd of A Botanical, Chemical and Pharmacological Reference List.*
SMC repr. 1982; 21cm, cloth, 1 vol., xvi, 389pp.

MW06 Bernard E. Read. *Famine Foods, Ephedra, Food Fishes.*
Three other works by Read are brought together in: *Famine Foods Listed in the Chui Huang Pen Ts'ao* 救荒本草 *Giving their Identity, Nutritional Values and Notes on their Preparation.* *Ephedra* 麻黃 *Part 2. Common Food Fishes of Shanghai.*
SMC repr. 1982; 21cm, cloth, 1 vol.

MW07 K. Chimin Wong and Wu Lien-ten, *History of Chinese Medicine, Being a Chronicle of Medical Happenings in China from Ancient Times to the Present Period.*
SMC repr. 1985; 21cm, cloth, xxviii, 906pp.+53 half-tone plates.

MW08 Veith, Ilaz, trans., *Huang Ti Nei Ching Su Wen or The Yellow Emperor's Classic of Internal Medicine,* Chapters 1–34.
Translated from the Chinese with an introductory study.
SMC repr. 1982; 2nd ed., 21cm, cloth, 1 vol., xix, 253pp.

MW09 Giles, Herbert A., trans., *The Hsi Yuan Lu or Instructions to Coroners.*
SMC repr. 1982; 26cm, cloth, 49pp., illus.

*PTKM = *Pen Ts'ao Kang Mu* 本草綱目

SMC PUBLISHING INC.

P.O. Box 13-342, Taipei 10764
Taiwan, Republic of China
Tel: (886-2)362-0190 Fax:(886-2)362-3834